Fundamental Pharmacology for Pharmacy Technicians

Custom Edition

Jahangir Moini

W9-AHB-573

CENGAGE
Learning·

Australia • Brazil • Japan • Korea • Mexico • Singapore • Spain • United Kingdom • United States

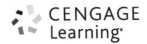

Fundamental Pharmacology for Pharmacy Technicians, Custom Edition

Fundamental Pharmacology for Pharmacy Technicians, 1st Edition
Jahangir Moini

Senior Project Development Manager:
  Linda deStefano

Market Development Manager:
  Heather Kramer

Senior Production/Manufacturing Manager:
  Donna M. Brown

Production Editorial Manager:
  Kim Fry

Sr. Rights Acquisition Account Manager:
  Todd Osborne

For product information and technology assistance, contact us at
Cengage Learning Customer & Sales Support, 1-800-354-9706

For permission to use material from this text or product,
submit all requests online at **cengage.com/permissions**
Further permissions questions can be emailed to
permissionrequest@cengage.com

This book contains select works from existing Cengage Learning resources and was produced by Cengage Learning Custom Solutions for collegiate use. As such, those adopting and/or contributing to this work are responsible for editorial content accuracy, continuity and completeness.

Compilation © 2013 Cengage Learning
ISBN-13: 978-1-285-56417-3

ISBN-10: 1-285-56417-0

Cengage Learning
5191 Natorp Boulevard
Mason, Ohio 45040
USA

Cengage Learning is a leading provider of customized learning solutions with office locations around the globe, including Singapore, the United Kingdom, Australia, Mexico, Brazil, and Japan. Locate your local office at:
international.cengage.com/region.
Cengage Learning products are represented in Canada by Nelson Education, Ltd.
For your lifelong learning solutions, visit **www.cengage.com/custom.**
Visit our corporate website at **www.cengage.com.**

Printed in the United States of America

Brief Contents

SECTION I

GENERAL ASPECTS OF PHARMACOLOGY

Introduction to Pharmacology, Drug Legislation, and Regulation

OBJECTIVES

After completing this chapter, the reader should be able to:

1. Define the key terms.
2. Explain the four stages of drug product development.
3. Explain the differences between the DEA and the FDA.
4. Name the first drug act passed in the United States for consumer safety, and give the year it was passed.
5. Distinguish between legend drugs, over-the-counter drugs, and controlled substances.
6. Summarize the provisions of the Controlled Substances Act of 1970, and define the C-I to C-V schedules.

GLOSSARY

Clinical pharmacology – an area of medicine devoted to the evaluation of drugs used for human benefit

Controlled substances – drugs recognized by the Drug Enforcement Agency (DEA) as having abuse potential

Drug Enforcement Agency (DEA) – the government agency concerned with controlled substances that enforces laws against drug activities, including illegal drug use, dealing, and manufacturing

Food and Drug Administration (FDA) – the branch of the U.S. Department of Health and Human Services that is responsible for the regulation of foods, drugs, cosmetics, and medical devices

Genetic engineering – techniques wherein genes from one organism are spliced into the chromosomes

of another organism; also known as recombinant DNA technology

Investigational new drug (IND) application – an application for human drug testing that is submitted to the FDA once enough data has been collected on a new drug

Legend drug – a prescription drug

Narcotics – drugs that produce a sedative or pain relieving affect

Over-the-counter (OTC) – nonprescription drugs

Pharmacology – the science concerned with drugs and their sources, appearance, chemistry, actions, and uses

Recombinant DNA technology – techniques wherein genes from one organism are spliced into the chromosomes of another organism; also known as genetic engineering

OVERVIEW

Pharmacology is defined as the study of the sources, appearance, chemistry, actions, uses, and manufacturing of drugs and medications. This chapter presents a basic overview of the history of pharmacology, drug development, and drug legislation affecting the dispensing and use of medications.

THE HISTORY OF PHARMACOLOGY

Historical records show that drug use has long been a part of human culture worldwide. A historical timeline showing major pharmacological developments provides a continuum that may be divided into three distinct periods: the age of natural substances, the age of synthetic substances, and the age of biotechnology.

Medical Terminology Review

pharmacology

pharmac/o = drugs, medicine
-logy = the study of
the study of drugs or medicine

The Age of Natural Substances

The age of natural substances is characterized by the use of plant derivatives (e.g., morphine, which is derived from opium). The use of natural substances evolved in China and Egypt. In 1875, George Ebers found one of the earliest written records of medicinal uses of plants in Egypt, the Ebers Papyrus. This document was written around 1500 B.C. It contained formulas for more than 800 remedies. About 2000 B.C., the Chinese began developing an interest in herbs as having value in the cure of diseases. Theophrastus, an early Greek philosopher and scientist (about 300 B.C.), wrote about observations on the classification of plants by their various parts.

The Age of Synthetic Substances

The age of synthetic substances is characterized by the mass production of synthetic medicines and drug screening techniques (e.g., antibiotics and insulin). The period from 1350 to 1650 A.D. (the later stages of the Middle Ages) is known as the Renaissance. During this period, Swiss-born physician Theoprastus Philippus Aureolus Bombastus von Hohenheim, also known as Paracelsus, began to emphasize a chemical rather than a botanical orientation to medicine. He believed that disease was a chemical manifestation and should be treated chemically.

The production of synthetic substances for medicinal uses continued into the twentieth century. It was at this time that synthetic drugs began to be mass-produced relatively cheaply in pharmaceutical laboratories. Once the molecular structure of a natural drug is identified, it may be more convenient to synthesize it wholly in the laboratory instead of extracting it in its natural form, or else modify it chemically for better absorption, greater effectiveness, or fewer side effects.

The Age of Biotechnology

Biotechnology is defined as the use of proteins from cells and tissues from humans, animals, and plants to produce medicines and therapeutic treatments. These proteins are highly complex compounds where the functional characteristics are determined by subtle chemical bonds and structural arrangements. Biotechnological techniques involve the manipulation of these bonds and structural arrangements from microbial and human genetic material. A human gene can be inserted into one bacterium or fungal cell, which in turn, divides to produce a colony in which each microbe contains the gene. This process is referred to as **recombinant DNA technology** or **genetic engineering** and was put into practice in the early 1970s. The best clinical example of this includes substances used in hormone replacement therapy (e.g., insulin and growth hormone).

DRUG PRODUCT DEVELOPMENT

In the United States, the development of new drugs and drug therapies can take anywhere from seven to fifteen years. The **Food and Drug Administration (FDA)**, a branch of the U.S. Department of Health and Human Services, is responsible for the regulation of foods, drugs, cosmetics, and medical devices. The FDA oversees the approval of new drugs, over-the-counter and prescription drug labeling, and standards related to the manufacture of drugs. The FDA considers a new chemical entity as an active pharmaceutical ingredient that has not been approved for marketing in the United States. Before a drug is approved for sale, it must go through several phases of drug product development.

- Pre-clinical Investigation (Stage 1)

    Animal pharmacology and toxicology data are obtained to determine the safety and effectiveness of the drug. It takes about one to three years, with the average being approximately eighteen months. An **investigational new drug (IND) application** for human testing is submitted to the FDA once enough data has been collected on the new drug.

- Clinical Investigation (Stage 2)

    Clinical testing on humans takes place in three different phases called clinical phase trials. This is the longest part of the drug approval process and involves **clinical pharmacology**, an area of medicine devoted to the evaluation of drugs used for human benefit. Clinical phase trials are essential because responses among patients vary. If a drug appears to be effective without causing serious side effects, approval for marketing may be accelerated, or the drug may be used for treatment immediately in special cases, with careful monitoring. In any case, an IND must be submitted before a drug is allowed to proceed to the next stage of the approval process. During the clinical phase trials, healthy volunteers are

used in large groups of selected patients to determine drug toxicity and tolerance. The trial phase takes about two to ten years with the average being five years.

- Investigational New Drug (IND) Review (Stage 3)
  A review of the IND is the third stage of drug approval. During this stage, the final phase of clinical trials and testing may continue, depending on the results obtained from preclinical testing. If the IND is approved, the process continues to the final stage. If the IND is rejected, the process stops until concerns are addressed. This stage takes about two months to seven years. The average is twenty-four months.

- Postmarketing Studies (Stage 4)
  Postmarketing surveillance is the fourth stage of the drug approval process. It takes place after clinical trials and the IND review process have been completed. Testing in humans is continued to check for any new side effects in larger and more diverse populations. Some adverse effects take longer to appear and are not identified until a drug is used by large numbers of patients.

REMOVAL OF A DRUG FROM THE MARKET

The FDA holds annual public meetings to hear comments from patients and professional and pharmaceutical organizations about the effectiveness and safety of new drug therapies. If the FDA discovers a serious problem, it will require that a drug be withdrawn from the market and its use discontinued.

PRESCRIPTION DRUGS

A prescription drug is a medication that can only be legally dispensed to a patient with a written order (prescription) from a physician or another individual licensed to prescribe medications. Most prescription drugs are so designated by the FDA; however, states can also designate specific drugs or devices as prescription items. Prescription drugs may only be dispensed by a pharmacist, pharmacy technician under direction of a pharmacist, or by the prescriber. Prescription drugs are also called **legend drugs**.

NONPRESCRIPTION DRUGS

When drugs are used over long periods of time and demonstrate "wide" margins of safety, prescription drugs may become nonprescription or **over-the-counter (OTC)** drugs. Unlike prescription drugs, OTC drugs do not require a physician's order. Patients may treat themselves safely if they carefully follow the instructions included with these OTC drugs. If patients do not follow these guidelines, OTC drugs can have serious side effects.

CONTROLLED SUBSTANCES

A **controlled substance** is a medicinal product that has a high potential for abuse and is regulated by the **Drug Enforcement Agency (DEA)**, a part of the U.S. Department of Justice. The DEA is tasked with the enforcement of laws regulating drug activities, illegal drug use, illegal drug dealing and sale, and illegal manufacture of drugs. A controlled substance can only legally be obtained with a physician's prescription. Many **narcotics**, drugs producing sedative or pain relieving affects, are classified as controlled substances.

FEDERAL DRUG LEGISLATION

Many laws and regulations have been enacted during the past century regulating pharmacy practice. These laws include: the Pure Food and Drug Act; the Harrison Narcotic Act; the Pure Food, Drug, and Cosmetic Act; and the Comprehensive Drug Abuse Prevention and Control Act. These laws have been passed to control the use of prescription drugs, nonprescription drugs, and controlled substances.

The Pure Food and Drug Act of 1906

The Pure Food and Drug Act was the government's first attempt to control and regulate the manufacture, distribution, and sale of drugs. Before this law, the purity and potency of many drugs were questionable, and some of these agents were even dangerous for human consumption.

The Harrison Narcotic Act of 1914

The Harrison Narcotic Act regulated the importation, manufacture, sale, and use of opium, codeine, and their derivations and compounds. Before this law, any narcotic could be purchased without a prescription. In 1970, the Harrison Narcotic Act was replaced by the Comprehensive Drug Abuse Prevention and Control Act.

The Pure Food, Drug, and Cosmetic Act of 1938

In 1938, further amendments were made to the Pure Food and Drug Act of 1906, resulting in the Pure Food, Drug, and Cosmetic Act, which created the FDA. The FDA provided additional control over the manufacture and sale of cosmetics. Under this act, manufacturers must be concerned with the purity, strength, effectiveness, safety, and packaging of drugs. Foods and cosmetics are also regulated. By this act, the FDA has the power to approve or deny new drug applications and even to conduct inspections to ensure compliance. The FDA approves the investigational use of drugs on humans and ensures that all approved drugs are safe and effective.

The Comprehensive Drug Abuse Prevention and Control Act of 1970

The Comprehensive Drug Abuse Prevention and Control Act, also called the Controlled Substances Act (CSA), regulates the manufacture, distribution, and dispensation of drugs with a potential for abuse. This law deals with control and enforcement of pharmaceuticals and places this control and enforcement under the jurisdiction of the DEA.

The CSA classifies drugs with the potential for abuse into five schedules designated with a C and a Roman numeral (I–V) to indicate their level of control (Table 1-1). Drugs in Schedule I have the highest potential for abuse and addiction. Those in Schedule V have the least potential for abuse. Records must be kept on the transactions of all pharmaceuticals that are classified as controlled substances. This is also regulated by the DEA.

TABLE 1-1 Schedules of Controlled Substances

Schedule	Manufacturer's Label	Abuse Potential	Prescription Requirement	Examples
I	C-I	high; no accepted medical use	no prescription permitted	heroin, LSD (lysergic acid diethylamide), marijuana, mescaline, and peyote
II	C-II	high; accepted medical use	prescription required; no refills permitted without a new written prescription	codeine, fentanyl, methadone hydrochloride, methamphetamine, methylphenidate, morphine, and opium (deodorized)
III	C-III	moderate; accepted medical use	prescription required; 5 refills permitted in 6 months	certain drugs compounded with small quantities of narcotics; also other drugs with strong potential for abuse (Tylenol® with codeine), and certain barbiturates
IV	C-IV	low; accepted medical use	prescription required; 5 refills permitted in 6 months	barbital, chloral hydrate, chlordiazepoxide, diazepam, and pentazocine hydrochloride
V	C-V	low; accepted medical use	no prescription required for individuals 18 or older unless quantities are greater than 4 fluid ounces.	cough syrups with codeine, diphenoxylate hydrochloride with atropine sulfate, and kaolin/pectin/opium

SUMMARY

Pharmacology deals with the discovery, chemistry, effects, uses, and manufacturing of drugs. History shows that drug use has long been a part of human culture worldwide. Three distinct periods in the development of pharmacology have included: the age of natural substances, the age of synthetic substances, and the age of biotechnology.

The development of a new drug is controlled by the FDA, and consists of several phases. Drug product development is a long and difficult process, taking anywhere from seven to fifteen years.

In the past century, Congress has passed many laws to control and regulate the importation, manufacture, sale, and use of drugs. Any new drug that is developed must be safe and effective for the human body.

EXPLORING THE WEB

Visit *www.drugs.com*

- Look for information on drugs going through drug trials for FDA approval. Choose one drug and review the study and approval process from start to finish.

Visit *www.fda.gov*

- Search using the term drug development. Review documents and articles that provide details about the process of developing new drugs.

- Search using the term pulled drugs/Review articles on why drugs may be pulled off the market and how this is determined.

Visit *www.napra.org*

- Click on "Federal Drug Legislation." Review the information on the Controlled Drugs and Substances Acts as well as the Food and Drugs Acts.

REVIEW QUESTIONS

Short Answer

1. What types of drugs are listed in the C-II and C-V schedules?

   _____

   _____

2. Define the role of the DEA.

   _____

   _____

3. List three responsibilities of the FDA.

_____

_____

_____

4. In what year was the first major U.S. drug act passed and what was it called?

_____

_____

5. Define the following:
   a. The Controlled Substances Act (CSA)

   _____

   b. The Pure Food and Drug Act of 1906

   _____

   c. The Harrison Narcotic Act of 1904

   _____

   d. Legend drugs

   _____

Multiple Choice

1. The drugs with the highest potential for abuse and addiction, which are not accepted for medical use, are classified as which of the following schedules?
   A. I
   B. II
   C. IV
   D. V

2. Which of the following agencies oversees controlled substances and prosecutes individuals who illegally distribute them?
   A. FDA
   B. CDC
   C. DHHS
   D. DEA

3. Which of the following was the first period of historical drug development?
   A. synthetic substances
   B. natural substances
   C. biotechnical substances
   D. genetic engineering

4. The FDA is a branch of which department that controls all drugs for legal use?

   A. U.S. Department of Health
   B. U.S. Department of Health and Human Services
   C. U.S. Department of Agriculture
   D. U.S. Department of Labor

5. The best clinical example of a "genetic engineering" substance is which of the following?

   A. insulin
   B. penicillin
   C. aspirin
   D. vitamin A

6. Which type of schedule drugs has a high potential for abuse but is currently accepted for medical treatment in the United States?

   A. Schedule I
   B. Schedule II
   C. Schedule III
   D. Schedule IV

7. Which of the following drug schedules do heroine, LSD, and marijuana fall into?

   A. Schedule IV
   B. Schedule III
   C. Schedule II
   D. Schedule I

8. Stage 1 of drug product development may take:

   A. 2-7 months
   B. 18-24 months
   C. 1-3 years
   D. 2-10 years

9. Which of the following phases of drug product development may be improved as a result of equipment, regulatory, supply, or market demands?

   A. Stage 1
   B. Stage 2
   C. Stage 3
   D. Stage 4

10. Which of the following laws was the first to regulate the importation, manufacture, sale, and use of narcotic drugs?

    A. Harrison Narcotic Act
    B. Pure Food, Drug, and Cosmetic Act
    C. Controlled Substances Act
    D. Pure Food and Drug Act

11. An investigational new drug application for human testing is submitted to which of the following?

    A. DEA
    B. DHHS
    C. FDA
    D. JCAHO

12. Which of the following federal laws may control the use of prescription drugs, nonprescription drugs, and controlled substances?

    A. The Harrison Narcotic Act
    B. The Comprehensive Drug Abuse Prevention and Control Act
    C. The Pure Food and Drug Act
    D. All of the above

Matching

_____ 1. Schedule C-I   A. low abuse potential; accepted medical use

_____ 2. Schedule C-II   B. moderate abuse potential; accepted medical use

_____ 3. Schedule C-III   C. high abuse potential; accepted medical use

_____ 4. Schedule C-V   D. high abuse potential; no accepted medical use

Critical Thinking

Tom is a student in the pharmacy technician program who is taking the final exam for law and ethics. Many of his questions are related to federal drug acts.

1. What would be the correct name of the act that regulates the importation, manufacturing, sale, and use of opium, codeine, and their derivations and compounds?

2. Which agency has the power to approve or deny new drug applications?

3. What was the first federal drug act Congress passed in 1906?

Drug Sources and Dosage Forms

OBJECTIVES

After completing this chapter, the reader should be able to:

1. Differentiate between the chemical name, generic name, and trade name of drugs.
2. Explain the classification of drug sources.
3. Name three animal sources of drugs.
4. Distinguish between engineered and synthetic drug sources.
5. Describe the various dosage forms of drugs.
6. Distinguish between syrups and elixirs.

GLOSSARY

Aromatic water – a mixture of distilled water with an aromatic volatile oil

Buffered tablet – a type of tablet manufactured to prevent irritation of the stomach

Caplet – a tablet shaped like a capsule

Capsule – a solid dosage form in which the drug is enclosed in either a hard or soft shell of soluble material

Chemical name – a drug's full name, that refers to its complete chemical makeup

Cream – a semisolid emulsion of either the oil-in-water or the water-in-oil type, ordinarily intended for topical use

Elixir – a clear, sweetened, flavored, hydroalcoholic liquid medication intended for oral use

Emulsion – a system containing two liquids that cannot be mixed together in which one is dispersed in the form of very small globules throughout the other

Enteric-coated tablet – a tablet covered in a special coating to protect it from stomach acid, allowing the drug to dissolve in the intestines

Fluidextract – a pharmacopoeial liquid preparation of vegetable drugs, made by filtration, containing alcohol as a solvent or as a preservative, or both

Gel – a jelly or the solid or semisolid phase of a colloidal solution

Gelcap – an oil-based medication that is enclosed in a soft gelatin capsule

Generic name – a drug not protected by a trademark, but regulated by the FDA. Also called the *official name*

Granule – a very small pill, usually gelatin- or sugar-coated, containing a drug to be given in a small dose

Liniment – a liquid preparation for external use, usually applied by friction to the skin

Lozenge – a small, disk-shaped tablet composed of solidifying paste containing an astringent, an antiseptic, or an oil-based drug used for local treatment of the mouth or throat and is held in the mouth until dissolved; also known as a troche

Mixture – a mutual incorporation of two or more substances, without chemical union, in which the physical characteristics of each of the components are retained

Ointment – a semisolid preparation usually containing medicinal substances and is intended for external application

Pill – a small, globular mass of soluble material containing a medicinal substance to be swallowed

Plaster – a solid preparation that can be spread when heated and then becomes adhesive at the temperature of the body

Powder – a dry mass of minute separate particles of any substance

Solution – a liquid dosage form in which active ingredients are dissolved in a liquid vehicle

Spirits – alcoholic or hydroalcoholic solutions of volatile substances

Suppository – a small, solid body shaped for ready introduction into one of the orifices of the body other than the oral cavity (e.g., rectum, urethra, or vagina), made of a substance, usually medicated, that is solid at ordinary temperature but melts at body temperature

Suspension – a liquid dosage form that contains solid drug particles floating in a liquid medium

Sustained release (SR) capsule – a capsule with a controlled release of the dosage over a special period of time

Syrup – a liquid preparation in a concentrated aqueous solution of a sugar used for medicinal purposes or to add flavor to a substance

Tablet – a solid dosage form containing medicinal substances with or without suitable diluents

Tincture – an alcoholic solution prepared from vegetable materials or from chemical substances, used as a skin disinfectant

Trade name – brand name given to a drug by its manufacturer (such drugs are marked with the symbol®). Trade names are also called *proprietary* or *brand* names

Troche – a small, disk-shaped tablet composed of solidifying paste containing an astringent, antiseptic, or oil-based drug used for local treatment of the mouth or throat and is held in the mouth until dissolved; also known as a lozenge

OVERVIEW

The pharmacy technician must be familiar with many different forms of medication. There are varieties of sources from which drugs are derived and forms in which drugs are prepared. A working knowledge of these sources and forms will aid the pharmacy technician in understanding how drugs are used and administered.

DRUG NAMES

It is not unusual for each drug entity to be known by several designations. Usually, a single drug may have up to three names: chemical, generic, and trade. The first type of name, usually applied to compounds of known composition, is the **chemical name**. For substances of plant or animal

origin that cannot be classified as pure chemical compounds, scientific identification is given in terms of precise biochemical or zoological names. Chemical names are generally not useful to the physician, pharmacist, or other users of the drug.

When a new drug is proven to be useful through successive research stages to the point at which it appears that it may become a marketable product, a **trade name** is developed by the manufacturer. Properly registered trade names become the legal property of their owners, are protected by copyright laws, and cannot be used freely in the public domain. These two types of names do not fulfill the need for a single, simple, informative designation available for unrestricted public use. The nonproprietary name is the only name intended to function in this capacity.

The nonproprietary name often is referred to as the **generic name**. A generic name is the official name of the drug. This name is much simpler than the chemical name, and it is not protected by copyright. The use of generic names is encouraged over trade names to avoid confusion. Generic drugs are cheaper than brand name drugs. They are usually easier to remember and less complicated. However, because generic drug formularies may be different, the inert ingredients may be somewhat different and consequently may affect the ability of the drug to reach the target cells and produce an effect.

DRUG SOURCES

There are basically five sources of drugs: plants, animals (including humans), minerals or mineral products, synthetic (chemical substances), and engineered drugs (investigational drugs). Today, chemicals and even human tissues such as those used in stem-cell therapy can be manipulated to create new drug sources.

Plant Sources

Plant sources are grouped by their physical and chemical properties. Alkaloids are organic compounds combined with acids to make a salt. Nicotine, morphine sulfate, and atropine sulfate are examples of these chemical compounds. An important cardiac glycoside is digoxin. Digoxin is made from digitalis, a derivative of the foxglove plant.

Animal Sources

Animal sources, such as the body fluids and glands of animals, can act as drugs. The drugs obtained from animal sources include enzymes such as pancreatin and pepsin. Hormones such as thyroid and insulin are also from animal sources.

Medical Terminology Review

biochemical
bio = life; living systems
chemical = drug; agent
drug created from a living system

Key Concept

Chemical names and generic names are unique to each drug — there is only one chemical name and one generic name for any specific drug. However, any drug may have dozens of trade (or brand) names, with similar ingredients.

Medical Terminology Review

alkaloid
alkal = alkaline
oid = compound
an alkaline based compound

Mineral Sources

Minerals from the earth and soil are used to provide inorganic materials unavailable from plants and animals. They are used as they occur in nature. Examples include iron, potassium, silver, and gold, which are used to prepare medications. Sodium chloride (table salt) is one of the best-known examples in this category. Gold is used to prevent severe rheumatoid arthritis, and coal tar is used to treat seborrheic dermatitis and psoriasis.

Synthetic Sources

New drugs may come from living organisms (organic substances) or nonliving materials (inorganic substances). These drugs are called synthetic or manufactured drugs. They are created through the application of chemistry and biology. Because they are not found in nature, these medications come from artificial substances. Common examples of synthetic drugs include meperidine (Demerol®), sulfonamides, and oral contraceptives. Certain organic drugs such as penicillin are semisynthetic and are made by altering their natural compounds or elements. Some drugs are both organic and inorganic, such as propylthiouracil, which is an antithyroid hormone.

Medical Terminology Review

inorganic
  in = not
  organic = relating to living organisms
not related to live organisms

Engineered Sources

The newest area of drug origin is gene splicing or genetic engineering. The newer forms of insulin for use in humans have been produced with this technique. Other engineered drugs include: tissue plasminogen activator, growth hormones, cancer drugs, and drugs that combat HIV. The replacement of missing or nonfunctional genes is an emerging area of genetic engineering.

DOSAGE FORMS OF DRUGS

Pharmaceutical principles are the underlying physiochemical principles that allow a drug to be incorporated in a pharmaceutical dosage form such as tablets and solutions. These principles apply whether the drug is extemporaneously compounded by the pharmacist or manufactured for commercial distribution as a drug product. Drug dosage forms are classified according to their physical state and chemical composition. They may include gases, liquids, solids, and semisolids. Some substances can undergo a change of state or phase, from solid to liquid states (melting) or from liquid to gaseous states (vaporization). Certain drugs are soluble in water, some are soluble in alcohol, and others are soluble in a mixture of liquids.

Medical Terminology Review

physiological
  physio = relating to nature or physiology
  chemical = drug; agent
drug related to nature

Solid Drugs

Intermolecular forces of attraction are stronger in solids than in liquids or gases. Solid drugs include tablets, pills, plaster, capsules, caplets, gelcaps, powder, granules, troches, or lozenges (Figure 2-1).

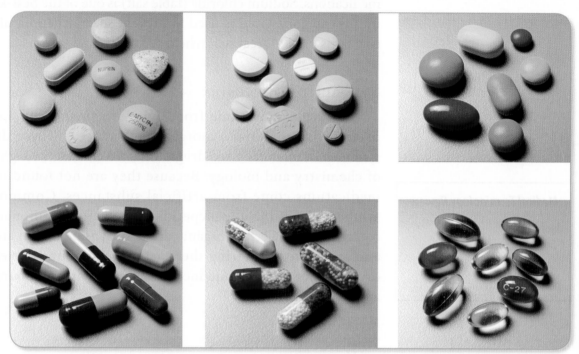

Figure 2-1 Solid dosage forms.

Tablet

A **tablet** is a pharmaceutical preparation made by compressing the powdered form of a drug and bulk filling material under high pressure (Figure 2-1). Most tablets are intended to be swallowed whole for dissolution and absorption from the gastrointestinal tract. Some are intended to be dissolved in the mouth or dissolved in water. Many times tablets are mistakenly called pills. Tablets come in various sizes, shapes, colors, and composition. The various forms of tablets include chewable, sublingual, buccal, enteric-coated, and buffered tablets.

Chewable tablets *must* be chewed. They contain a flavored or sugar base. Chewable tablets are commonly used for antacids and antiflatulents, and for children who cannot swallow medication. Sublingual tablets must be dissolved under the tongue for rapid absorption. An example is nitroglycerin for angina pectoris. Buccal tablets are placed between the cheek and the gum until they are dissolved and absorbed. An **enteric-coated tablet** has a special coating to protect against stomach acid, allowing the drug to dissolve in the alkaline environment of the intestines. A **buffered tablet** can prevent ulceration or severe irritation of the stomach wall. Antacids have been added to reduce irritation to the stomach by the active ingredients. Some tablets are coated with a volatile liquid that is meant to dissolve in the mouth, such as antacid tablets.

Key Concept

Enteric-coated tablets are often given to patients who cannot take certain medications, such as aspirin, which are irritating to the stomach. For example, many elderly people who have stomach ulcers cannot tolerate aspirin unless it has an enteric-coating.

Medical Terminology Review

nitroglycerin

nitro = nitrate; nitrogen
glycerin = preparation obtained from fats and oils
drug preparation containing nitrogen

Pill

A single-dose unit of medicine made by mixing the powdered drug with a liquid, such as syrup and rolling it into a round or oval shape is called a **pill**.

Plaster

Any composition of a liquid and a powder that hardens when it dries is called a **plaster**. Plasters may be solid or semisolid. An example is the salicylic acid plaster used to remove corns.

Capsule

A **capsule** is a medication dosage form in which the drug is contained in an external shell (Figure 2-1). Capsule shells are usually made of hard cylindrical gelatin and enclose or encapsulate powder, granules, liquids, or some combinations of these. Liquids may be placed in soft gelatin capsules, such as vitamin E capsules and cod liver oil capsules. They are used when medications have an unpleasant odor or taste. Capsules can be pulled apart, and the entire contents can be added as powder to food for individuals who have difficulty swallowing. Some forms of capsules come with a controlled-release dosage and are used over a defined period of time. These are called **sustained-release (SR)** or timed-release capsules. These drugs should never be crushed or dissolved, because this would negate their timed-release action.

Caplet

A **caplet** is shaped like a capsule but has the form of a tablet. The shape and film-coated covering make swallowing easier.

Gelcap

A **gelcap** is an oil-based medication that is enclosed in a soft gelatin capsule (Figure 2-1).

Powder

A drug that is dried and ground into fine particles is called a **powder**. An example is potassium chloride powder (Kato Powder).

Granule

A small pill, usually accompanied by many others most commonly encased within a gelatin capsule is called a **granule**. In most cases, granules within capsules are specially coated to gradually release medication over a period of up to 12 hours (Figure 2-1).

Troche or Lozenge

A hard or semisolid dosage form containing a medication intended for local application in the mouth or throat is called a **troche** or **lozenge**. These

---

Medical Terminology Review

chloride
 chlor = chlorine
 ide = compound
substance containing chlorine

are flattened disks. Typically, a troche is placed on the tongue or between the cheek and gum and left in place until it dissolves. The medications most commonly administered by means of troches include cough suppressants and treatments for sore throat.

Semisolid Drugs

Semisolid drugs are often used as topical applications. These drugs are soft and pliable. Semisolid drugs include suppositories, ointments, and gels.

Suppository

A bullet-shaped dosage form intended to be inserted into a body orifice is called a **suppository**. Suppositories contain medication usually intended for a local effect at the site of insertion. Suppositories maintain their shape at room temperature but melt or dissolve when inserted. The most common sites of administration for suppositories are the rectum, vagina, and urethra.

Ointment

An **ointment** is a semisolid, greasy medication intended for external application, usually by rubbing (Figure 2-2). Medications that may be administered in ointment form include anti-inflammatory drugs, topical anesthetics, and antibiotics. Examples are zinc oxide ointment and Ben-Gay® ointment.

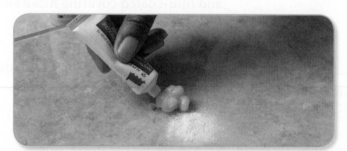

Figure 2-2 Semisolid dosage forms.

Cream

A **cream** is a semisolid preparation that is usually white and nongreasy; it has a water base. It is applied externally to the skin or administered via an applicator intravaginally.

Gel

A **gel** is a jelly-like substance that may be used for topical medication. Some gels have a high alcohol content and can cause stinging if applied to broken skin.

Liquid Drugs

Liquid preparations include drugs that have been dissolved or suspended. Examples of liquid drugs are syrups, spirits, elixirs, tinctures, fluid extract, liniments, emulsions, solutions, mixtures, suspension, aromatic waters, sprays, and aerosols (Figure 2-3). They are also classified by site or route of

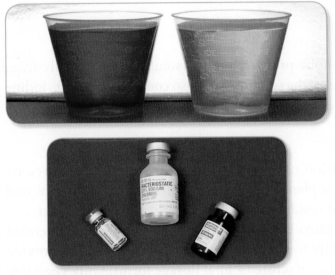

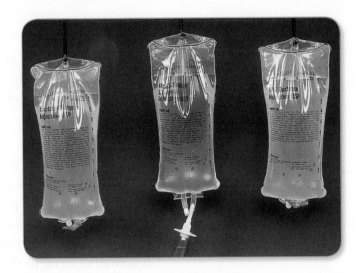

Figure 2-3 Liquid dosage forms.

Key Concept

Liquid drugs are very popular for use in children because other oral forms, such as tablets and capsules, are harder to swallow. Children have far less difficulty in taking liquid drugs.

administration such as local (topical) on or through the skin, through the mouth, through the eye (ophthalmic), through the ear (otic), or through the rectum, urethra, or vagina. Liquid drugs may also be administered systemically by mouth or by injection throughout the body.

Syrup

A drug dosage form that consists of a high concentration of a sugar in water is called a **syrup**. It may or may not have medicinal substances added (e.g., simple syrup, ipecac syrup).

Solution

A **solution** is a drug or drugs dissolved in an appropriate solvent. An example of a solution is normal saline, which is salt dissolved in water.

Spirit

An alcohol-containing liquid that may be used pharmaceutically as a solvent is called a **spirit**. It is also known as essence (e.g., essence of peppermint, camphor spirit).

Elixir

A drug vehicle that consists of water, alcohol, and sugar is known as an **elixir**. It may or may not be aromatic and may or may not have active

medicinal properties. The alcohol content makes elixirs convenient liquid dosage forms for many drugs that are only slightly soluble in water. In these cases, the drug is first dissolved in alcohol and the other elixir components are added. All elixirs contain alcohol (e.g., terpin hydrate elixir, phenobarbital elixir). Elixirs differ from tinctures in that they are sweetened. They should be used with caution in patients with diabetes or a history of alcohol abuse.

Tincture

A **tincture** is an alcoholic preparation of a soluble drug, usually from plant sources. In some cases, the solution may also contain water (e.g., iodine tincture, digitalis tincture).

Fluidextract

A concentrated solution of a drug removed from a plant source by mixing ground parts of the plant with a suitable solvent, usually alcohol, and then separating the plant residue from the solvent is called a **fluidextract**. Typically, 1 mL (1 cc) contains 1 g of the drug. Fluidextracts are not intended to be administered directly to a patient. Instead, they are used to provide a source of drug in the manufacture of final dosage forms. Only vegetable drugs are used (e.g., glycyrrhiza fluidextract).

Liniment

A **liniment** is a mixture of drugs with oil, soap, water, or alcohol, intended for external application with rubbing. Most liniments are counterirritants intended to treat muscle or joint pain (e.g., camphor liniment, chloroform liniment).

Emulsion

A pharmaceutical preparation in which two agents that cannot ordinarily be combined are mixed is called an **emulsion**. In the typical emulsion, oil is dispersed inside water, however they can also be water dispersed inside oil. Most creams and lotions are emulsions (e.g., Petrogalar Plain).

Mixtures and Suspensions

In a **mixture** or a **suspension**, an agent is mixed with a liquid but not dissolved. These preparations must be shaken before the patient takes them. An example is Milk of Magnesia®.

Aromatic Water

In pharmacy, a mixture of distilled water with an aromatic volatile oil is called an **aromatic water**. Aromatic waters may be used for medicinal purposes (e.g., peppermint water, camphor water).

Gaseous Drugs

Pharmaceutical gases include the anesthetic gases such as nitrous oxide and halothane. Compressed gases include oxygen for therapy (Figure 2-4) or carbon dioxide.

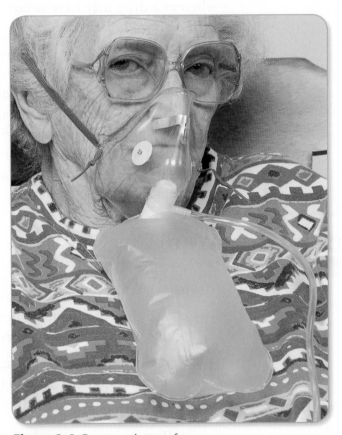

Figure 2-4 Gaseous dosage forms.

SUMMARY

A single drug may have up to three names: chemical, generic, and trade. There is only one chemical name and one generic name for each drug, whereas a drug may have several trade names, with similar ingredients in each marketed drug product.

Drug sources may include: plants, animals (including humans), minerals, synthetics (chemical substances), and engineered drugs (investigational drugs). Drug dosage forms are classified according to their physical state and chemical composition. They may include solids, semisolids, liquids, and gases. Some substances may change from solid to liquid states (melting) or from liquid to gaseous states (vaporization). Certain drugs are water soluble, some are soluble in alcohol, and others are soluble in a mixture of liquids.

EXPLORING THE WEB

Visit *www.fda.gov*

- Search using the term dosage forms defined. Review information that outlines the characteristics of the dosage forms.

- Search for the various drug sources and review information related to the drugs derived from those sources.

Visit *www.ismp.org*

- Review information listed under the link "Medication Safety Tools and Resources." Discover the common types of errors that can occur with drugs and what strategies can be used to avoid them.

Visit *www.mapharm.com*

- Click on "medical drug sources." What additional information can you find here on the various forms of medications available?

REVIEW QUESTIONS

Multiple Choice

1. Which of the following is an important cardiac glycoside?
   - A. nicotine
   - B. digoxin
   - C. morphine sulfate
   - D. atropine sulfate

2. Tablets are mistakenly called:

    A. pills

    B. powders

    C. buffered

    D. gelcaps

3. Which of the following is an example of semisolid drugs?

    A. caplets

    B. gelcaps

    C. gels

    D. granules

4. Which of the following is an example of plant drug sources?

    A. insulin

    B. pepsin

    C. meperidine

    D. morphine

5. Any composition of a liquid and a powder that hardens when it dries is called a:

    A. capsule

    B. plaster

    C. gelcap

    D. granule

6. Which of the following is an example of spirits?

    A. phenobarbital liquids

    B. peppermint and camphor liquids

    C. iodine and digitalis liquids

    D. Milk of Magnesia®

7. A preparation that can be used rectally is called a:

    A. powder

    B. gel

    C. pill

    D. suppository

8. A solution containing alcohol is called a(n);

    A. emulsion

    B. solution

    C. syrup

    D. elixir

9. A small, disk-shaped medication, which is composed of a solidifying paste and used for local treatment is called a(n):

    A. lozenge

    B. liniment

    C. ointment

    D. gelcap

10. Nicotine, morphine sulfate, and atropine sulfate are examples of which of the following compounds?

    A. engineered (investigational drugs)
    B. animals or humans
    C. plants
    D. synthetics

11. Which of the following is an advantage of generic drugs over equivalent trade-name drugs?

    A. less toxic
    B. absorbed slower
    C. taste better
    D. cheaper

12. A dry mass of minute separate particles of any substance is called a:

    A. powder
    B. plaster
    C. pill
    D. granule

Matching

_____ 1. Not intended to be administered directly to a patient

_____ 2. A bullet-shaped dosage form intended to be inserted into a body orifice

_____ 3. A drug or drugs dissolved in an appropriate solvent

_____ 4. Can prevent ulceration or severe irritation of the stomach wall

_____ 5. An alcoholic preparation of a soluble drug, usually from plant sources

_____ 6. A semisolid, greasy medication intended for external application, usually by rubbing

_____ 7. Placed between the cheek and the gum until dissolved

_____ 8. A mixture of distilled water with a volatile oil

_____ 9. Shells usually made of hard cylindrical gelatin

_____ 10. Most creams and lotions

A. emulsion

B. aromatic water

C. ointment

D. buccal tablet

E. buffered tablet

F. tincture

G. capsule

H. solution

I. suppository

J. fluidextract

Critical Thinking

A pharmacist decides to switch from a trade-name drug that was ordered by a physician to a generic-equivalent drug instead.

1. What advantages does this substitution have for the patient?

2. What disadvantages might the switch cause?

3. What must the pharmacist do before switching from a trade-name drug to a generic-equivalent drug?

Biopharmaceutics

OBJECTIVES

After completing this chapter, the reader should be able to:

1. Describe the mechanisms of drug action and define pharmacokinetic and pharmacodynamic.
2. Explain the importance of the first-pass effect.
3. Explain the significance of the blood-brain barrier to drug therapy.
4. Identify the major processes by which drugs are eliminated from the body.
5. Describe the process of filtration, secretion, and reabsorption for renal excretion of drugs.
6. Describe factors affecting drug action.
7. Explain how rate of elimination and plasma half-life (t ½) are related to the duration of drug action.
8. Define idiosyncratic and anaphylactic reactions.

GLOSSARY

Absorption – the movement of a drug from its site of administration into the bloodstream

Active transport – a process that moves particles in fluid through membranes from a region of lower concentration to a region of high concentration

Agonist – the drug that produces a functional change in a cell

Anaphylactic reaction – a severe, life-threatening allergic reaction to a drug

Antagonist – the drug blocks a functional change in the cell

Antimetabolite – a substance that is produced to alter the actions of liver enzymes

Bioavailability – measurement of the rate of absorption and total amount of drug that reaches the systemic circulation

Biotransformation – the conversion of a drug within the body; also known as metabolism

Diffusion – the process of particles in a fluid moving from an area of higher concentration to an area of lower concentration, resulting in an even distribution of the particles in the fluid

Dose-effect relationship – the relationship between drug dose and blood, or other biological fluid concentrations

Drug clearance – elimination rate over time divided by the drug's concentration

Excretion – the process whereby the undigested residue of food and waste products of metabolism are eliminated, material is removed to regulate composition of body fluids and tissues, or substances are expelled to perform functions on an exterior surface

Filtration – the movement of water and dissolved substances from the glomerulus to the Bowman's capsule

First-pass effect – drugs reaching the liver where they are partially metabolized before being sent to the body

Glomerular filtration rate (GFR) – the rate of filtration in the kidneys

Half-life – the time it takes for the plasma concentration (e.g., of a drug) to be reduced by 50 percent

Hepatic portal circulation – the circulation of blood through the liver

Idiosyncratic reaction – experience of a unique, strange, or unpredicted reaction to a drug

Lipid solubility – the ability to dissolve in a fatty medium

Metabolism – the conversion of a drug within the body; also known as biotransformation

Passive transport – the most common and important mode of traversal of drugs through membranes; diffusion

Pharmacodynamics – the study of the biochemical and physiological effects of drugs

Pharmacokinetics – the study of the absorption, distribution, metabolism, and excretion of drugs

Placebo – sugar pill

Reabsorption – the movement of water and selected substances from the tubules to the peritubular capillaries

Target sites – the areas where a drug's greatest action takes place at the cellular level

Tolerance – reduced responsiveness of a drug because of adaptation to it

Tubular secretion – the active secretion of substances such as potassium from the peritubular capillaries into the tubules

OVERVIEW

Drugs differ widely in their biochemical and physiological properties, as well as their mechanisms of action. In clinical applications, a drug must be absorbed, transported to the target tissue or organ, and then it must penetrate into the cell membranes, their organelles, and alter the ongoing processes. The drug may be distributed to a number of tissues, bound or stored, then metabolized to inactive or active products. Then it must be excreted. The usual route of drug administration, distribution, and elimination are factors in the effectiveness of a drug's ability to produce a desired outcome. The principles explaining the manner in which drugs act within the body are explained in this chapter.

PHARMACOKINETICS

Pharmacokinetics is the study of the action and movement of drugs within the body, including the mechanisms of absorption, distribution, metabolism, and excretion of drugs. It defines the processes by which the body ingests a drug, breaks down the drug, distributes it throughout the body, uses it, and then excretes the waste products of the drug.

Drug Absorption

The movement of a drug from its site of administration into the bloodstream is **absorption**. In most cases, this is the first step the body takes to begin processing a drug. For absorption to occur, a drug must be transported across one or more biological membranes to reach the blood circulation. This process can take place via passive (diffusion) or active transport.

Passive Transport

The most common and important mode of traversal of drugs through membranes is **passive transport** or **diffusion**. Diffusion is the process in which particles in a fluid move from an area of higher concentration to an area of lower concentration, resulting in an even distribution of the particles in the fluid (Figure 3-1). This mechanism requires little or no energy. In the body, diffusion depends upon **lipid solubility** (ability to be dissolved in a fatty substance) of the drug. Cell membranes consist of a fatty bi-layer through which drugs must pass for diffusion to occur. Agents that are relatively lipid-soluble diffuse more rapidly than less lipid-soluble drugs.

> ### *Medical Terminology Review*
>
> **pharmacokinetics**
>
> *pharmac/o* = drugs, medicine
> *-kinet-* = movement
> *-ic* = pertaining to
> the movement of drugs through the body

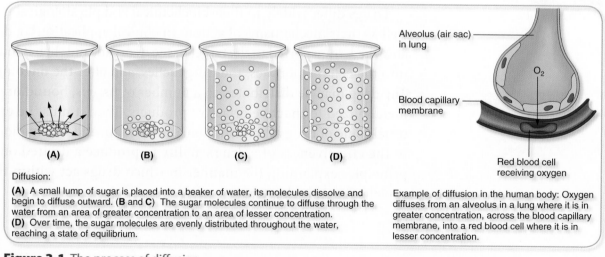

Diffusion:

(A) A small lump of sugar is placed into a beaker of water, its molecules dissolve and begin to diffuse outward. **(B and C)** The sugar molecules continue to diffuse through the water from an area of greater concentration to an area of lesser concentration. **(D)** Over time, the sugar molecules are evenly distributed throughout the water, reaching a state of equilibrium.

Example of diffusion in the human body: Oxygen diffuses from an alveolus in a lung where it is in greater concentration, across the blood capillary membrane, into a red blood cell where it is in lesser concentration.

Figure 3-1 The process of diffusion.

Active Transport

Active transport is a process that moves particles in fluid through membranes from a region of lower concentration to a region of high concentration. It uses specific carrier molecules (proteins) in the cell membranes and requires energy (Figure 3-2).

Absorption of Medications Through the Digestive System

Oral administration of drugs is the most convenient, economical, and common route of administration. Absorption of most drugs administered orally takes place through the digestive system. Drugs given orally are usually absorbed across the stomach or upper intestinal wall and enter blood vessels

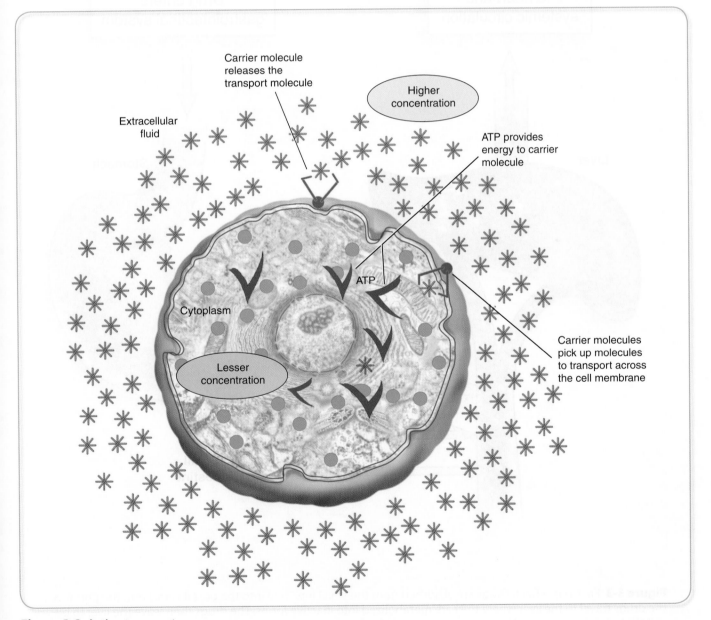

Figure 3-2 Active transport.

Medical Terminology Review

hepatic
  hepat/o = liver
  -ic = pertaining to
related to the liver

of **hepatic portal circulation** (Figure 3-3). Hepatic portal circulation carries blood directly to the liver where it is immediately exposed to metabolism by the liver enzymes before reaching the systemic circulation. This exposure is called the **first-pass effect**; the drug reaches the liver, where it is partly metabolized before being sent to the body for systemic effects. Drugs that are administered parenterally or sublingually do not undergo a first-pass effect. Therefore, parenteral medications are often given in lower doses than those given orally.

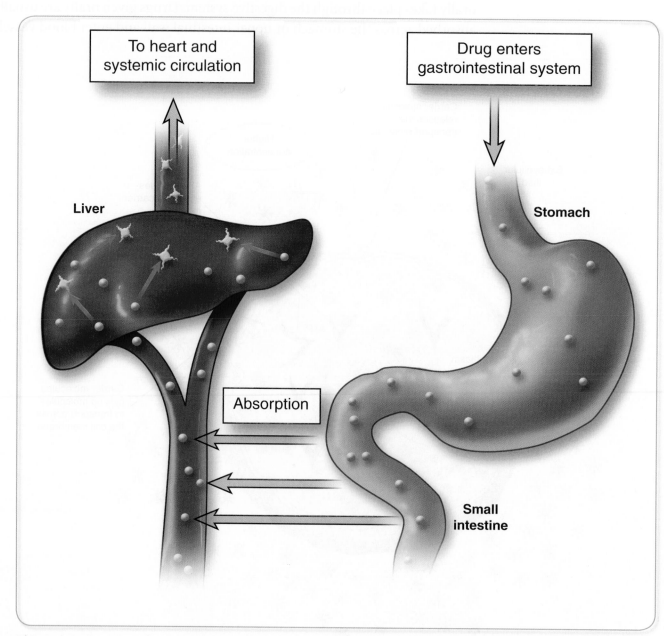

Figure 3-3 First-pass effect. Drugs are absorbed from the small intestine into the portal vein. From the portal vein, the drugs travel to the liver where they are metabolized into inactive forms. The drugs then leave the liver to be distributed through general circulation.

Factors Influencing Absorption

There are many factors that may alter the rate of absorption of drugs into the body. Such factors to consider are the acidity of the stomach, presence of food in the stomach, dosage of drugs, bioavailability, and the routes of administration.

- Acidity of the Stomach

  Drugs with an acidic pH, such as aspirin, are easily absorbed in the acid environment of the stomach, whereas alkaline medications are more readily absorbed in the alkaline environment of the small intestine. Milk products and antacids tend to change the pH of the stomach. Therefore, some drugs are not absorbed properly. The infant who is taking formula or milk may need to take medications on an empty stomach because the regular feedings will change the stomach acid level.

- Presence of Food in the Stomach

  The presence of food in the stomach or intestine can have a profound influence on the rate and extent of drug absorption. Food in the stomach decreases the absorption rate of medications, while an empty stomach increases the rate. Sometimes the drug must be put into effect quickly, requiring the stomach to be empty. If the medication causes irritation of the stomach, food should be eaten to serve as a buffer and decrease irritation.

- Dosage of Drugs

  Drugs administered in high concentrations tend to be more rapidly absorbed than those administered in low concentrations. The relationship between drug dose and blood, or other biological fluid concentrations, is called the **dose-effect relationship**.

- Drug Bioavailability

  Bioavailability is a term that indicates measurement of both the rate of drug absorption and total amount of drug that reaches the systemic blood circulation from an administered dosage form. The route of drug administration in this matter is essential. If a drug is administered by intravenous injection, all of the dose enters the blood circulation. This is not true for drugs administered by other routes, especially for drugs given orally. Solid drugs such as tablets and capsules must dissolve. This is a major source of difference in drug bioavailability. Poor solubility of a drug or incomplete absorption of a drug in the gastrointestinal tract, and rapid metabolism of a drug during its first pass through the liver are other factors that influence bioavailability.

• Routes of Administration

 Absorption will vary based upon the route of administration. Some oral drugs are administered sublingually (under the tongue) or buccally (inner lining of cheek); these drugs are absorbed through the mucous membranes directly into the bloodstream to protect the drug from decomposition and deterioration in the stomach or liver. Topical drugs may be absorbed through several layers of skin for local absorption. For example, nitroglycerin commonly is applied to the skin in the form of an ointment or transdermal patches; it is absorbed rapidly, and provides sustained blood levels. When the drug is injected directly into the bloodstream (vein or artery) and distributes throughout the body, it acts rapidly; the process of absorption is bypassed. The drug may be injected deeply into a skeletal muscle. The rate of absorption depends on the vascularity of the muscle site, and the lipid solubility of the drug. If it is injected beneath the skin, drug absorption is less rapid, because the subcutaneous region is less vascular than the muscle tissues.

Drug Distribution

 The process by which drug molecules leave the bloodstream and enter the tissues of the body is called distribution. When a drug reaches the bloodstream, it is ready to travel through blood, lymphatics, and other fluids to its site of action. Drugs interact with specific receptors. Some drugs are frequently bound to plasma proteins (albumin) in the blood. If these drugs are bound to albumin, they are known as inactive drugs, while those that are unbound are called pharmacologically-active drugs. If binding is extensive and firm, it will have a considerable impact upon the distribution and excretion of the drug in the body. Only when the protein molecules release the drug can it diffuse into the tissues, interact with receptors, and produce a therapeutic effect. The brain and placenta possess special anatomical barriers that prevent many chemicals and drugs from entering. These barriers are referred to as the blood-brain barrier and fetal-placental barrier.

Drug Metabolism

 Drug **metabolism** is a chemical reaction wherein a drug is converted into compounds, and then easily removed from the body. It occurs once the drug reaches the liver, before the drug reaches its intended site within the body. Most drugs are acted upon by enzymes in the body, and are converted to metabolic derivatives during metabolism. The process of conversion is called **biotransformation**. The liver is the major site of biotransformation. Many biotransformations in the liver occur in the smooth endoplasmic reticulum of the hepatocytes. Liver enzymes react with the drugs creating metabolites. The majority of these metabolites are inactive and toxic. Drug metabolism

influences drug action, such as duration of drug action, drug interactions, drug activation, and toxicity or side effects. In most cases, biotransformation can terminate the pharmacological action of the drug and increase removal of the drug from the body.

Drug Excretion

The final step of pharmacokinetics is **excretion**, which is the removal of drugs from the body. Drugs may be excreted from the body by many routes, including urine, feces (unabsorbed drugs, and those secreted in the bile), saliva, sweat, milk, lungs (alcohols and anesthetics), and tears. Any route may be important for a given drug, but the kidney is the major site of excretion for most drugs. Unchanged drugs or drug metabolites can be eliminated by the kidneys. The main role of the kidney is to remove all non-natural and harmful agents in the bloodstream while keeping a balance of other natural substances. Kidney impairment can significantly prolong drug action and causes drug toxicity. Renal excretion of drugs and their metabolites may undergo three processes: (1) filtration, (2) secretion, and (3) reabsorption.

Drug Filtration

Urine formation begins in the glomerulus and Bowman's capsule in the kidneys. **Filtration** causes water and dissolved substances to move from the glomerulus into Bowman's capsule. Filtration occurs when the pressure on one side of a membrane is greater than the pressure on the opposite side. Small substances such as water, sodium, potassium, chloride, glucose, uric acid, and creatinine move through the wall of the glomerulus very easily. These substances are filtered in proportion to their plasma concentration. In other words, if the concentration of a particular substance or drug in the plasma is high, many of these substances are filtered (Figure 3-4). Approximately one-fifth of the plasma reaching the kidney is filtered. The rate of filtration is referred to as the **glomerular filtration rate (GFR)** and is normally 125–130 milliliters per minute (mL/min).

Drug Secretion

Although most of the water and dissolved substances enter the tubules of the kidneys as a result of filtration across the glomerulus, a second process moves very small amounts of substances from the blood into the tubules. This is called **tubular secretion**. It involves the active secretion of substances such as potassium ions (K^+), hydrogen ions (H^+), uric acid, the ammonium ion, and drugs from the peritubular capillaries into the tubules. Secretion occurs primarily in the proximal convoluted tubule (Figure 3-4). This is an active process mediated by two carrier systems, one specific for organic acids and one specific for organic bases. Therefore, the pH of the urine may affect the rate of drug excretion by changing the chemical form of a drug to one that can be more readily excreted or to one that can be reabsorbed. Penicillins

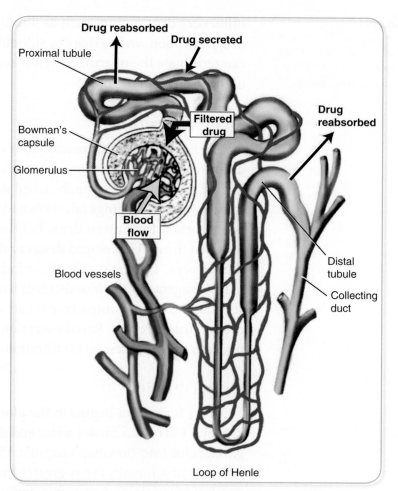

Figure 3-4 Renal excretion of drugs. Note sites where drugs are secreted and reabsorbed.

or barbiturates are weak acids, and available as sodium or potassium salts. These agents can be better excreted if the urine pH is less acid.

On the other hand, any drug which is available as sulfate, hydrochloride, or nitrate salts, such as atropine or morphine, can be excreted better if the urine is more acidic. By altering the pH of urine, increased elimination of certain drugs can be facilitated, thus preventing prolonged action or overdosage of a toxic compound. Another technique to alter the rate of excretion of a drug is to produce a competitively blocking effect. For example, probenecid may be used to block the renal excretion of penicillin. This prolongs the effect of the antibiotic by maintaining a higher therapeutic plasma level. Secretions of drugs are active transport systems. They require energy and may become saturated.

Drug Reabsorption

Reabsorption may occur throughout the tubules of the nephrons (Figure 3-4). It causes water and selected substances to move from the tubules into the peritubular capillaries. The mechanism is passive diffusion, therefore, only the unionized form of a drug is reabsorbed.

It is dependent upon its lipid solubility. For example, the kidneys selectively reabsorb substances such as glucose, proteins, and sodium, which they have already secreted into the renal tubules. These reabsorbed substances return to the blood.

Drug Clearance

Drug clearance describes drug elimination (excretion plus metabolism). It is defined as elimination rate over time divided by the drug's concentration. Drug clearance can also be described as being equal to the volume of fluid completely cleared of a drug per a unit of time. It is usually expressed in mL/minute or L/hour. Plasma clearance divided by blood clearance equals blood concentration divided by plasma concentration. Total clearance equals the sum of clearances of individual body processes. The eliminated drug amount is proportional to the clearance of the respective elimination process.

Pharmacodynamics

Pharmacodynamics is the study of the biochemical and physiological effects of drugs. It is also defined as the study of a drug's mechanism of action. After administration, most drugs enter the blood circulation, and expose almost all body tissues to their possible effects. All drugs produce more than one effect in the body. The primary effect of a drug is the desired or therapeutic effect. Secondary effects are all other effects, whether desirable or undesirable (causing harmful effects), produced by the drug. Most drugs have an affinity for certain organs or tissues, and exert their greatest action at the cellular level in those specific areas, which are called **target sites**.

Most often, there are links between pharmacokinetics and pharmacodynamics that demonstrate the relationship between drug dose and blood, or other biological fluid concentration. The pharmacologic response by itself does not provide information about some very important determinants of that response; for example, dose, drug concentration in plasma or at the site of action. Pharmacokinetic and pharmacodynamics can determine the dose-effect relationship (see Figure 3-5).

Drug Action

Drugs produce their effects by altering the normal function of the cells and tissues of the body. They do not create new cellular functions. Instead, they change existing cellular functions. Drug action is generally described relative to a physiological state that was in existence when a drug was administered. Some drugs accumulate in specific tissues because they have an affinity for a tissue component. The most common way that drugs exert their

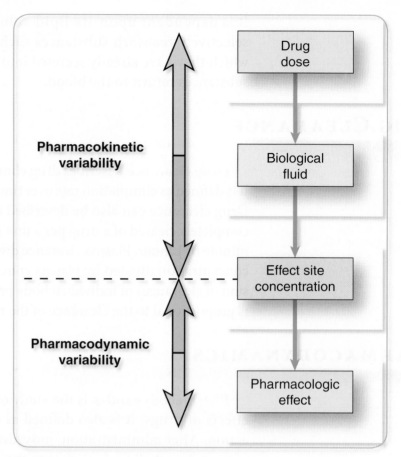

Figure 3-5 The dose-effect relationship.

action is by forming chemical bonds with certain receptors in the body. This usually occurs only if the drug and its receptor have a compatible chemical shape. Drugs with molecules that fit precisely into a given receptor elicit a comparable drug response and are known as **agonists**. Those that do not fit perfectly produce only a weak response or no response at all (Figure 3-6).

Not all drugs that bind to specific cells cause a functional change in the cell. These drugs act as **antagonists** to the natural process and work by blocking a sequence of biochemical events.

Some drugs may act by affecting the enzyme functions of the body. When drugs are metabolized in the liver, they produce **antimetabolites**. These antimetabolites interrupt or inhibit the actions of particular enzymes, thus producing a desired therapeutic effect.

Factors Affecting Drug Action

There are various factors that are important in determining the correct drugs for a patient, such as drug half-life, age, sex, body weight, time of day administered (diurnal), presence of illnesses, psychological factors, tolerance, toxicity of drugs, idiosyncrasy, and drug interactions.

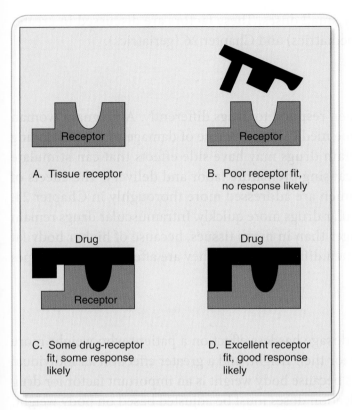

Figure 3-6 Drug-receptor interaction. Binding with specific receptors occurs only when the drug and its receptors have a compatible chemical shape.

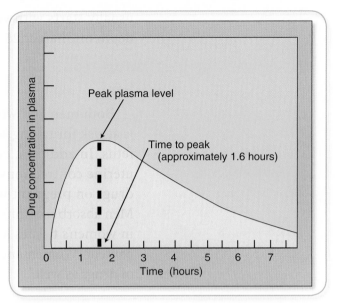

Figure 3-7 Plot of drug concentration in plasma versus time after single oral administration of a drug.

Drug Half-Life

The **half-life** of a drug is a related measurement used to ensure that maximum therapeutic dosages are given. The half-life of a drug is the time it takes for the concentration of the drug in plasma to be reduced by one-half (50 percent). It is an indication of how long a medication will produce its effect in the body. The larger the half-life value, the longer it takes for a drug to be eliminated. This is one of the most common methods used to explain drug actions. The half-life of each drug may be different: for example, a drug with a short half-life, such as two or three hours, will need to be administered more often than one with a long half-life, such as eight hours. Another method of describing drug action is by the use of graphic depiction of the plasma concentration of the drug versus time (see Figure 3-7).

Age

Newborns and elderly individuals show the greatest effects of a drug's actions. Because of their ages and either immature or impaired body systems, they are more sensitive to medications that affect the central nervous system, and are at risk for developing toxic drug levels. Calculations of drug dosages for these two groups must be carefully measured, and treatment

usually starts with very small doses. These factors are discussed in greater depth in Chapter 25 (pediatrics) and Chapter 26 (geriatrics).

Sex

Both men and women respond to drugs differently. A pregnant woman is at risk for taking some medications because of damage to the developing fetus. In addition, certain drugs may have side effects that can stimulate uterine contractions, causing premature labor and delivery. The effects of drugs on pregnant women are addressed more thoroughly in Chapter 24. Men absorb intramuscular drugs more quickly. Intramuscular drugs remain in women's tissues longer than in men's tissues, because of higher body fat content. Women and men differ in the way they are affected by other types of drugs as well.

Body Weight

Basically, the same dosage has less effect on a patient who weighs more than the normal range for their height, and a greater effect on an individual who weighs less. This is because body weight is an important factor for drug action, and some medication doses must be adjusted based on body weight. Pediatric medications are designed for the body weight or body surface of children. If adult medications are used for children, the correct dosage must be calculated and adjusted for the child's body weight.

Diurnal Body Rhythms

Diurnal (during the day) body rhythms play an important part in the effects of some drugs, because they can affect the intensity of a person's response to a drug. For example, sedatives given in the morning will not be as effective as when administered before bedtime. On the other hand, corticosteroid administration is preferred in the morning, because this best mimics the body's natural pattern of corticosteroid production and elimination.

Presence of Illnesses

Patients with liver or kidney disease may respond to drugs differently, because the body is not able to detoxify and excrete chemicals properly. The liver and kidneys are the major sites of elimination of chemical substances. Other illnesses that affect the physical health of the liver and kidneys must also be considered.

Psychological Factors

Psychological factors involve how patients feel about the drug(s) they are prescribed, and the different ways they respond to them. If an individual believes in the therapy, even a **placebo** (sugar pill, or sterile water thought to be a drug) may help to bring about relief. Some patients cooperate in

Key Concept

Acute or chronic illnesses of the liver in elderly patients may cause severe toxicity. For example, diazepam may cause coma in severely liver-damaged patients when given in average doses.

following the directions for a specific drug, and a patient's mental attitude can reduce or increase an expected response to a drug.

Tolerance

Tolerance is the phenomenon of reduced responsiveness to a drug. The body becomes so adapted to the presence of the drug that it cannot function properly without it. The only way to prevent drug tolerance from occurring is to avoid the repeated use of a drug. The signs of drug tolerance consist of an increased amount required by the body to achieve the desired effects. Certain drugs that stimulate or depress the central nervous system are prone to causing drug tolerance.

Drug Toxicity

Almost all drugs are capable of producing toxic effects. There is a range between the therapeutic dose of a drug and its toxic dose. This range is measurable by the therapeutic index, which is used to explain the safety of a drug. The therapeutic index is expressed in the form of a ratio:

$$\text{Therapeutic Index (TI)} = \frac{\text{median lethal dose:} \quad LD_{50}}{\text{median effective dose:} \quad ED_{50}}$$

The larger the difference between the two doses, the greater the therapeutic index. For example, if the therapeutic index is 3 (such as 30 mg ÷ 10 mg), it means that three times the dose of a drug will be lethal to a patient.

Idiosyncratic Reactions

When a patient has experienced a unique, strange, or unpredicted reaction to a drug, this is termed an **idiosyncratic reaction**. Idiosyncratic reactions may be caused by underlying enzyme deficiencies from genetic or hormonal variation.

Drug Interactions

Drug interactions are defined as effects of medications taken together. When two or more drugs are prescribed together, this generally results in one of the following:

1. The drugs have no effects on each other's action.
2. The drugs increase each other's effect.
3. The drugs decrease each other's effect.

Any of these results may also be affected by the ingestion of food. Most drugs do not interact with other drugs or food, but when such interactions do occur, some may be life-threatening. Plasma protein binding can be a source of drug interaction if several drugs compete for binding sites on

protein molecules. Drug interactions may result in elevated concentrations of drugs by displacement of protein-bound drugs or by reduced rates of drug disposition, therefore, resulting in toxic drug concentrations.

Some drug interactions are wanted, and the medications are prescribed together to produce the desired effect. For example, probenecid is given with penicillin to increase the absorption of penicillin. Other interactions are unintended and unwanted, producing possible dangers for the patient. Drug interactions may also cause a more rapid drug disappearance, with plasma concentrations decreasing to below minimum effective values. For example, some antibiotics make birth control pills less effective.

Side Effects and Adverse Effects of Drugs

Side effects are usually referred to as mild but annoying responses to the medication. Adverse reactions or adverse effects usually imply more severe symptoms or problems that develop because of a drug. Adverse effects may require the patient to be hospitalized, or may even threaten the patient's life. Certain side effects such as nausea may disappear if the dosage is reduced. Some side effects such as drowsiness may go away after the patient takes the medication for a while. Occasionally, side effects are very problematic, thus the dispensing of the drug to the patient is stopped or changed to a different drug. An example of this can be hyperactivity or inability to sleep, bleeding, nephrotoxicity, or hepatoxic development.

Hypersensitivity or Allergy

Allergies or hypersensitivity reactions are another unpredictable reaction that some drugs such as aspirin, penicillin, or sulfa products may cause in some patients. Hypersensitivity reactions generally occur when a patient has received a drug and the body has developed antibodies against it. After this process of antibody production, if the patient is re-exposed to the drug, the antigen-antibody reaction produces, itching, hives, rash, or swelling of the skin. This is a common type of allergic reaction.

Anaphylactic Reaction

An **anaphylactic reaction** to a drug is a severe form of allergic reaction that is life threatening. The patient develops severe shortness of breath, and may even have cardiac collapse. An anaphylactic reaction is a medical emergency because the patient may suffer paralysis of the diaphragm, swelling of the oropharynx, and an inability to breathe.

SUMMARY

A biologic response is induced within a living organism when a drug is administered to that organism. This chapter reviews the study of the absorption, distribution, metabolism, and excretion of drugs. It also reviews the study of the biochemical and physiological effects of drugs. The mechanisms of drug action depend on several factors that affect pharmaceutical, pharmcokinetic, and pharmacodynamic phases. Drug interaction is another major consideration. Multiple-drug therapy should never be employed without a convincing indication that each drug is beneficial and less harmful. In addition, drugs may induce side effects or adverse reactions. An adverse drug effect is more serious and its effect is unintended, undesirable, and often unpredictable.

EXPLORING THE WEB

Visit *www.aafp.org*

- Search using the term drug interactions. What common foods may interfere with the actions of some drugs? What drugs when taken together may cause adverse effects?

- Search using the term adverse drug reactions. What information can you find related to identifying and reducing these reactions?

Visit *www.fda.gov*

- Search using the following terms: drug absorption, drug distribution, drug metabolism, drug excretion. What additional information can you find to help reinforce your understanding of these concepts?

Visit *www.medscape.com*

- Click on the link "pharmacists." Review the resources available on this page.

Visit *www.nlm.nih.gov/medlineplus*

- Become familiar with the resources and information available at this site.

REVIEW QUESTIONS

Multiple Choice

1. For action to occur, a drug must be _____, transported to tissues or organs, and penetrate cell membranes.

   A. filtered
   B. secreted
   C. absorbed
   D. therapeutic

2. The study of the action of drugs within the body is known as:

    A. metabolism
    B. pharmacokinetics
    C. pharmacology
    D. pharmacodynamics

3. The most common and important mode of traversal of drugs through membranes is:

    A. filtration
    B. transportation
    C. diffusion
    D. transaction

4. Idiosyncratic reactions may be caused by which of the following factors?

    A. genetics
    B. obesity
    C. gender
    D. age

5. The process by which drug molecules leave the bloodstream and enter the tissues of the body is called:

    A. solubility
    B. distribution
    C. suitability
    D. concentration

6. The process of converting drugs to metabolic derivatives during metabolism is known as:

    A. ionization
    B. binding
    C. excretion
    D. biotransformation

7. The major site of excretion for most drugs is the:

    A. spleen
    B. sweat glands
    C. gall bladder
    D. kidney(s)

8. A second process that moves very small amounts of substances such as potassium and hydrogen from the blood into the renal tubules is known as:

    A. tubular secretion
    B. pH alteration
    C. increased elimination
    D. blocking effect

9. Which of the following is the study of the biochemical and physiological effects of drugs?

   A. pathophysiology
   B. pharmacology
   C. pharmacodynamics
   D. pharmacokinetics

10. A drug that has a specific affinity for a particular cell receptor is known as the:

    A. antagonist
    B. agonist
    C. blocker
    D. biochemical event

11. Which of the following pharmacokinetic phases may cause a major problem in patients with liver impairment?

    A. excretion
    A. distribution
    C. absorption
    D. metabolism

12. All of the following factors may influence the effectiveness of drug therapy, except:

    A. time of administration
    B. route of administration
    C. food-drug interaction
    D. temperature

13. Sedatives given in the morning will not be as effective as when they are administered before bedtime. This is due to the effect of:

    A. diurnal (during the day) body rhythms
    B. nocturnal (during the night) body rhythms
    C. corticosteroids
    D. placebos

14. The phenomenon of reduced responsiveness to a drug is known as:

    A. adaptation
    B. toxicity
    C. tolerance
    D. therapeutic index

15. When a patient has experienced a unique, strange, or unpredicted reaction to a drug, this reaction is called:

    A. hormonal
    B. idiosyncratic
    C. hypersensitive
    D. biologic

Fill in the Blank

1. A mechanism whereby drugs are absorbed across the intestinal wall and enter into blood vessels known as the hepatic portal circulation is called _____.

2. The effectiveness of a drug in producing a more intense response as its concentration is increased is known as _____.

3. The study of how the body responds to drugs and natural substances is called _____.

4. The rate of filtration is referred to as the _____.

5. Lipid-soluble drugs enter the central nervous system _____.

6. _____ and elderly individuals show the greatest effects of a drug.

7. Sugar pills or sterile water are thought to be a drug referred to as a _____.

Critical Thinking

A 75-year-old man was diagnosed with a urinary tract infection and a high fever. After the results of a urine culture, his physician ordered IV gentamicin 2 mg/kg loading dose, followed by 3–5 mg/kg/day in divided doses. Consider the nephrotoxicity of this agent to elderly patients, and answer the following questions.

1. What formula should be used to calculate drug toxicity?

2. Since the patient is 75 years old, what precautions must the physician take in calculating the correct dosage?

3. Besides nephrotoxicity, name the other potential adverse effects of this drug for elderly patients.

PHARMACOLOGY RELATED TO SPECIFIC BODY SYSTEMS AND DISORDERS

CHAPTER 4

Drug Therapy for the Nervous System: Antipsychotic and Antidepressant Drugs

OBJECTIVES

After completing this chapter, the reader should be able to:

1. List the main parts of the brain.
2. Describe the principal functions of the cerebrum and hypothalamus.
3. List the major chemical transmitters of the CNS.
4. Describe the major role of acetylcholine in the CNS.
5. Explain the role of dopamine in the brain.
6. Define schizophrenia, bipolar disorder, and depression.
7. List major groups of drugs that are used for schizophrenia.
8. Identify the drugs used for bipolar disorder.
9. List three major groups of drugs used to treat depression.
10. Describe the major adverse effects of MAOIs.

GLOSSARY

Acetylcholine – a neurotransmitter that plays a major role in cognitive function and memory formation as well as motor control

Anorexia nervosa – an eating disorder characterized by a psychological fear of being overweight; view of body image is distorted

Antidepressants – drugs used to treat depression

Antipsychotic drugs – the major therapeutic modality for psychotic disorders; also known as neuroleptic drugs

Bipolar disorder – a type of mental illness characterized by periods of extreme excitation, or mania, and deep depression.

Bulimia nervosa – an eating disorder characterized by recurrent (at least

twice a week) episodes of binge eating, during which the patient consumes large amounts of food and feels unable to stop eating

Dementia – a chronic deterioration of intellectual function and other cognitive skills severe enough to interfere with the ability to perform activities of daily living

Depression – a mood disorder

Dopamine – a neurotransmitter that is naturally produced in the brain, affecting motor control, memory, attention span, the ability to problem solve, motivation, pleasure, and creative thought

Extrapyramidal – nerves in the brain that control movement

Gamma-aminobutyric acid (GABA) – a neurotransmitter distributed throughout the brain and spinal cord; now considered to be the major inhibitory neurotransmitter in the CNS, acting to modulate the activity of excitatory pathways

Glutamate – an amino acid that acts as a neurotransmitter and is a key molecule in cellular metabolism, playing an important role in the body's disposal of excess or waste nitrogen

Hallucinations – false or distorted sensory experiences that appear to be real perceptions

Mania – a severe medical condition characterized by extremely elevated mood, energy, and unusual thought patterns; a characteristic of bipolar disorder

Monoamine oxidase inhibitor (MAOI) – a class of drug effective for the treatment of depression

Neuroleptic drugs – the major therapeutic modality for psychotic disorders; also known as antipsychotic drugs

Neurotransmitter – a biochemical that is formed in and released from a neuron in order to stimulate or inhibit the actions of another cell

Nocturnal enuresis – nighttime bedwetting

Norepinephrine – a neurotransmitter that regulates appetite, sleep, arousal, mood, temperature, and hormone release

Schizophrenia – a mental illness characterized by distortion of reality, disorganized thought patterns, social withdrawal, hallucinations, and poor judgment

Selective serotonin reuptake inhibitor (SSRI) – a class of drugs used as antidepressants; they block resorption of serotonin in nerve cells in the brain

Serotonin – a neurotransmitter that regulates appetite, sleep, arousal, mood, temperature, and hormone release

Serotonin syndrome – a rare condition resulting from intentional self-poisoning with serotonin, use of the drug therapeutically, or from inadvertent drug interactions characterized by progressively worsening symptoms such as: mental confusion, shivering or muscle twitching, sweating or fever, hallucinations, hypertension, tachycardia, headache, tremor, nausea, diarrhea, coma, and death; also known as serotonin toxicity

Serotonin toxicity – a rare condition resulting from intentional self-poisoning with serotonin, use of the drug therapeutically, or from inadvertent drug interactions characterized by progressively worsening symptoms such as: mental confusion, shivering or muscle twitching, sweating or fever, hallucinations, hypertension, tachycardia, headache, tremor, nausea, diarrhea, coma, and death; also known as serotonin syndrome

Tricyclic antidepressant (TCA) – a class of antidepressants; they inhibit reabsorption of serotonin, norepinephrine, and dopamine in the brain

OVERVIEW

The human brain is an extremely complex organ. It is responsible for all affective (emotional) and cognitive (thinking) processes, and is as capable of coordinating bodily functions (eating, sleeping, walking, talking) as it is of pursuing abstract thought. Sometimes imbalances in mental functioning occur that can result in one of a number of brain disturbances, producing disorders such as schizophrenia, depression, anxiety, or parkinsonism. The onset of such conditions can make normal functioning within society difficult, if not impossible. The use of psychopharmacology in the treatment of these conditions may be a necessary part of the reintegration of affected individuals in the community.

Mental health problems involve significant dysfunction in the areas of behavior or personality that interfere with a person's ability to function. Biochemical and structural abnormalities in the brain appear to contribute to the pathologies. Many disorders have a genetic component. Stressors may play a role in the development of mental illness. Psychotic illnesses include the more serious disorders such as schizophrenia, delusional disorders, and some affective or mood disorders. Many patients with psychotic disorders receive large doses of drugs with significant adverse effects. Other common mental disorders include anxiety, insomnia, and panic disorders, which are less severe but nevertheless disruptive.

ANATOMY REVIEW

The nervous system is composed of the brain, spinal cord, and nerves (Figures 4-1 and 4-2).

- The nervous system has two divisions: the central nervous system (CNS) and the peripheral nervous system (PNS).

- The brain and spinal cord make up the CNS. The nerves make up the peripheral nervous system.

- The brain is divided into specific regions; each region is responsible for the performance of specific functions within the body (Figures 4-3A and 4-3B).

- The brain consists of four parts: the cerebrum, diencephalon (thalamus and hypothalamus), cerebellum, and brain stem.

- The main functions of the cerebrum include the controlling of consciousness, memory, emotions, sensations, and voluntary movements.

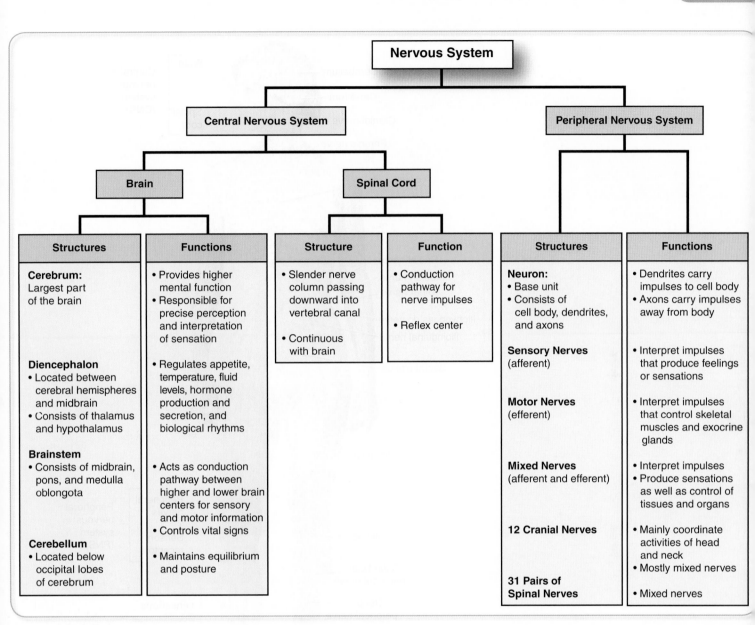

Figure 4-1 Overview of the structure and function of the nervous system.

- The thalamus receives sensory stimuli (except the sense of smell), relaying them to the cerebral cortex.

- The hypothalamus (located just below the thalamus) activates, controls, and integrates the peripheral autonomic nervous system. It also controls endocrine system processes, body temperature, appetite, sleep, and other sensory functions.

- The cerebellum, attached to the brain stem, maintains muscle tone, and coordinates balance and movement.

- The brain stem controls blood pressure, respiration, pulse, and other body functions; it connects the hypothalamus with the spinal cord.

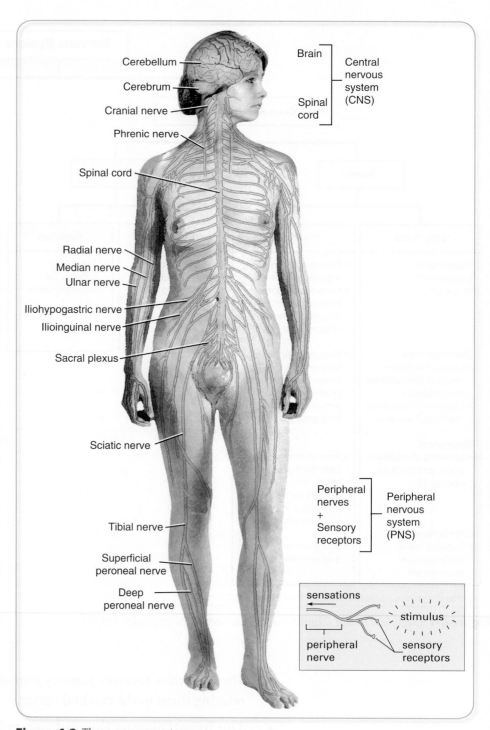

Figure 4-2 The nervous system.

- The basic functional unit of the nervous system is the neuron (Figure 4-4).
- There are three types of nerves: sensory nerves transmit information that produces sensation and feelings, motor nerves transmit

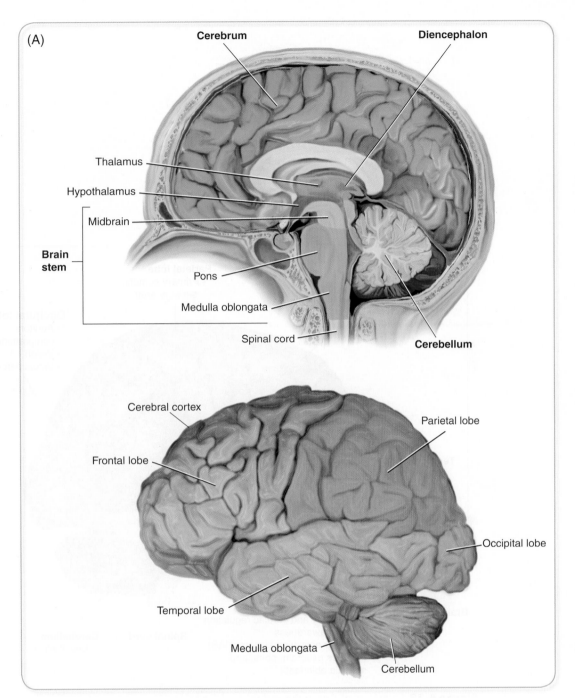

Figure 4-3A Divisions of the brain and related functions.

information that produces movement and function, mixed nerves transmit information that produces both sensation and movement.

- The spinal cord provides a two-way communication system between the brain and body parts outside of the nervous system (Figure 4-5).

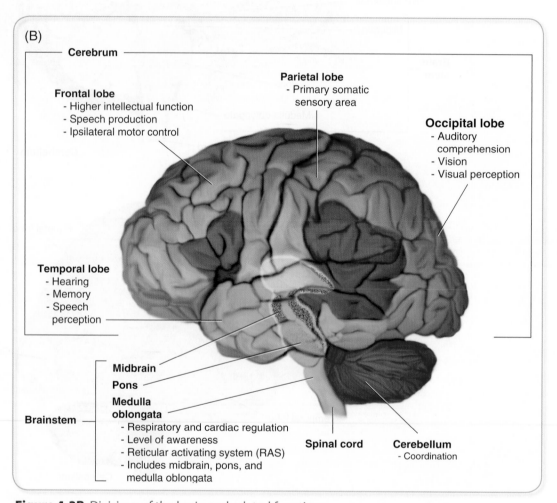

(B)

Cerebrum

Frontal lobe
- Higher intellectual function
- Speech production
- Ipsilateral motor control

Parietal lobe
- Primary somatic sensory area

Occipital lobe
- Auditory comprehension
- Vision
- Visual perception

Temporal lobe
- Hearing
- Memory
- Speech perception

Midbrain
Pons
Medulla oblongata

Brainstem
- Respiratory and cardiac regulation
- Level of awareness
- Reticular activating system (RAS)
- Includes midbrain, pons, and medulla oblongata

Spinal cord

Cerebellum
- Coordination

Figure 4-3B Divisions of the brain and related functions.

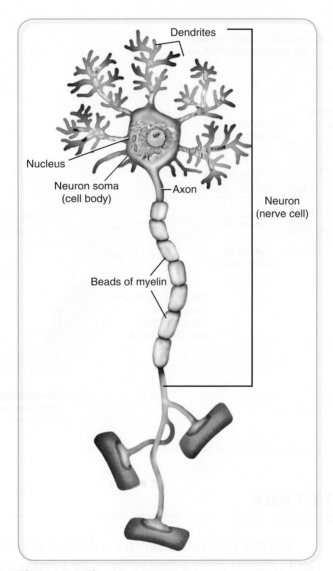

Figure 4-4 The neuron.

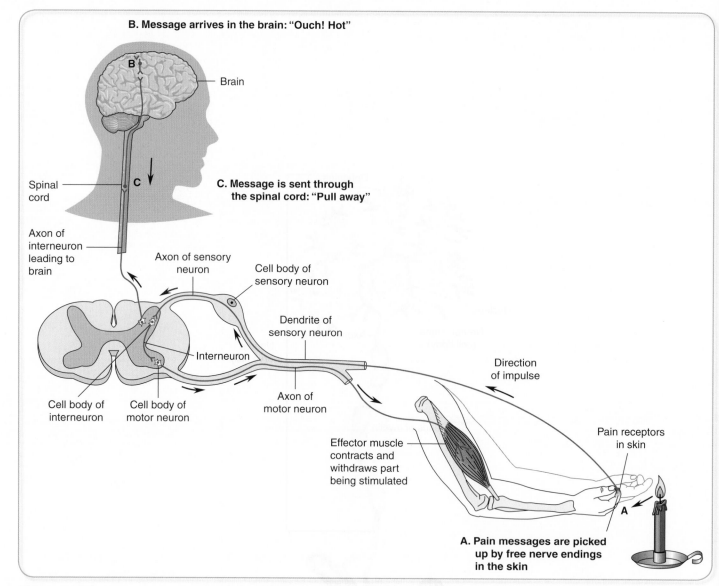

B. Message arrives in the brain: "Ouch! Hot"

B

Brain

Spinal cord

C. Message is sent through the spinal cord: "Pull away"

C

Axon of interneuron leading to brain

Axon of sensory neuron

Cell body of sensory neuron

Dendrite of sensory neuron

Interneuron

Direction of impulse

Cell body of interneuron

Cell body of motor neuron

Axon of motor neuron

Pain receptors in skin

Effector muscle contracts and withdraws part being stimulated

A

A. Pain messages are picked up by free nerve endings in the skin

Figure 4-5 The two-way communication system of the brain and nerve function.

NEUROTRANSMITTERS

The term **neurotransmitter** is defined as a biochemical that is formed in and released from a neuron in order to stimulate or inhibit the actions of another cell. Examples of neurotransmitters include acetylcholine, dopamine, noradrenaline, serotonin, glutamate, and GABA. Disorders in the production and function of neurotransmitters may contribute to psychiatric illnesses.

Acetylcholine

Acetylcholine plays a major role in cognitive function and memory formation as well as motor control. It was the first neurotransmitter to be identified. Acetylcholine allows neurons to communicate with each other. This neurotransmitter is released by the axon terminals in response to a nerve impulse. In relation to motor function, the release of acetylcholine

will cause a change in the muscle cell and elicit a contraction of the muscle, producing movement.

Dopamine

Dopamine is a naturally produced agent that, in the brain, functions as a neurotransmitter. Dopamine release and dopamine levels within the brain affect motor control, memory, attention span, the ability to problem solve, motivation, pleasure, and creative thought. Alterations in dopamine production and secretion play a role in disorders such as Parkinson's disease (see Chapter 7), attention deficit disorder, and schizophrenia. It is also believed to play a role in addiction to drugs.

Norepinephrine and Serotonin

Both **norepinephrine** and **serotonin** seem to be involved in similar functions within the brain: regulation of appetite, sleep, arousal, mood, temperature, and hormone release.

Norepinephrine is also known as noradrenaline. As a stress hormone, it affects parts of the human brain where attention and responding actions are controlled. It is released from the medulla of the adrenal glands as a hormone into the blood, but is also a central and sympathetic nervous system neurotransmitter.

Serotonin is a neurotransmitter synthesized in the CNS as well as the gastrointestinal tract. It is believed to play an important role in regulating anger, aggression, body temperature, mood, sleep, vomiting, sexuality, and appetite. It was initially identified as a vasoconstrictor present in blood serum, and it was from here that its name was derived. Serotonin (also known as 5-hydroxytryptamine or 5-HT) may also have a role in pain perception and behavior. It acts as an inhibitory neurotransmitter.

A rare condition known as **serotonin syndrome**, also known as **serotonin toxicity**, can result from intentional self-poisoning with serotonin, use of the drug therapeutically, or from inadvertent drug interactions. This condition includes progressively worsening symptoms such as: mental confusion, shivering or muscle twitching, sweating or fever, hallucinations, hypertension, tachycardia, headache, tremor, nausea, diarrhea, coma, and death.

Glutamate

Glutamate is an amino acid, however, not one of the essential amino acids. It is a key molecule in cellular metabolism. Glutamate plays an important role in the body's disposal of excess or waste nitrogen. It is important for the ability to perceive taste sensations.

Glutamate is distributed throughout the CNS. It is considered the major excitatory CNS neurotransmitter. It can stimulate a number of receptor types in the brain and spinal cord. Glutamate is involved in the facilitation of learning and memory. The brain is very vulnerable to glutamate-mediated

---

Medical Terminology Review

glutamate

glutam = glutamic acid
ate = salt or ester
a salt containing glutamic acid

over-excitation. This results in excitotoxicity, which causes cell integrity to be disrupted and nerve cells to die. Excitotoxicity has been demonstrated in strokes and some neuro-degenerative diseases. Glutamate has also been implicated in the development of epilepsy (see Chapter 9).

Gamma-Aminobutyric Acid

Gamma-aminobutyric acid (GABA) is distributed throughout the brain and spinal cord. It is now considered to be the major inhibitory neurotransmitter in the CNS and it acts to modulate the activity of excitatory pathways. It is formed from the excitatory neurotransmitter glutamate. Motor control, consciousness, levels of arousal, and memory formation are all inhibited by GABA.

GABA has mostly excitatory effects during early development. It has been purported to increase the amounts of human growth hormone. It is unknown if GABA can cross the blood-brain barrier.

MENTAL DISORDERS

Mental illness is defined as any disturbance of emotional equilibrium, as manifested in maladaptive behavior and impaired functioning of behavior or personality. Biochemical and structural abnormalities in the brain appear to contribute to these disorders. Some of these disorders have a genetic component. Stressors may play a role in the development of these types of illnesses. Psychotic illnesses include the more serious disorders such as schizophrenia, bipolar disorder, and depression. Other common mental disorders including dementia and eating disorders (discussed here) as well as anxiety and sleep disorders (discussed in Chapter 5), are less severe but nevertheless disruptive.

Schizophrenia

Schizophrenia is a mental illness characterized by distortion of reality, disorganized thought patterns, social withdrawal, **hallucinations**, and poor judgment. Schizophrenia is one of the most devastating forms of mental illnesses. It occurs in approximately 1 percent of the population.

Schizophrenia includes a variety of syndromes, presented differently in each individual. Although the cause of this disorder has not been fully determined, some common changes do occur in the brains of patients suffering from schizophrenia, including reduction of the cortex (outer portion) of the temporal lobes, enlargement of the third and lateral ventricles, excessive dopamine secretion, and decrease blood flow to the front of the brain.

The cause of schizophrenia may be genetic, along with brain damage in the fetus caused by perinatal complications or viral infections in the mother during pregnancy. The onset of schizophrenia usually occurs between ages 15 and 25 in men, and between 25 and 35 in women. Stressful events appear to initiate the onset and recurrence of the disorder.

Medical Terminology Review

schizophrenia

schizo = split
phrenia = mind condition
condition in which the mind is divided

perinatal

peri = around
nat = birth
-al = pertaining to
around the time of birth

Bipolar Disorder

Bipolar disorder is a mental illness characterized by periods of extreme excitation or **mania**, and deep depression. It is not commonly understood why it takes months to move from one of these extremes to the other. Some patients have predominantly manic episodes or predominantly depressive episodes. Few patients experience the classic swing from mania to depression and back. Bipolar disorder is also called manic-depressive illness.

Depression

Depression is classified as a mood disorder, of which there are several subgroups. Major depression, or unipolar disorder, is a chemical deficit within the brain, and a precise diagnosis is based on biologic factors or personal characteristics. The causes of depression include genetic and psychosocial stressors. Depression may also occur as a reactive episode, a response to a life event, or secondarily to many systemic disorders (including cancer, diabetes, heart failure, and AIDS). This condition is a common problem, and many patients with milder forms may be misdiagnosed and not receive treatment.

Eating Disorders

Anorexia nervosa is a complex psychological state characterized by the fear of being overweight. Often, patients' perceptions are distorted to the extent that they believe they are overweight despite appearing emaciated to others. Without proper treatment, anorexia nervosa may be fatal.

Bulimia nervosa is another eating disorder that is characterized by recurrent (at least twice a week) episodes of binge eating, during which the patient consumes large amounts of food and feels unable to stop eating. This is followed by inappropriate compensatory effects to avoid weight gain, such as self-induced vomiting, laxative or diuretic abuse, vigorous exercise, or fasting.

Dementia

Dementia is a chronic deterioration of intellectual function and other cognitive skills severe enough to interfere with the ability to perform activities of daily living. Dementia may occur at any age and can affect young people as the result of injury or hypoxia. However, it is mostly a disease of the elderly.

ANTIPSYCHOTIC DRUGS

Antipsychotic drugs, also called **neuroleptic drugs**, are a major therapeutic modality for psychotic disorders, often in conjunction with psychotherapy and psychosocial rehabilitation. The antipsychotic drugs (conventional and atypical agents) are listed in Table 4-1.

TABLE 4-1   Antipsychotic Drugs

Generic Name	Trade Name	Route of Administration	Average Adult Dosage
Conventional Agents			
chlorpromazine hydrochloride	Thorazine®	PO, IM, IV, PR (suppository)	50–400 mg/day
fluphenazine	Prolixin®	PO, IM	1–30 mg/day
haloperidol	Haldol®	PO, IM	1–50 mg/day
loxapine succinate	Loxitane®	PO	10–160 mg/day
molindone (no longer available)	Moban®	PO	15–225 mg/day
perphenazine	Trilafon®, Etrafon®	PO	12–24 mg/day
pimozide	Orap®	PO	1–10 mg/day
prochlorperazine	Compazine®	PO, IM, PR	2.5–25 mg/day
thioridazine hydrochloride	Mellaril®	PO	50–800 mg/day
thiothixene hydrochloride	Navane®	PO	6–60 mg/day
trifluoperazine	Stelazine®	PO, IM	4–60 mg/day
Atypical Agents			
aripiprazole	Abilify®	PO	10–15 mg/day
clozapine	Clozaril®, Fazaclo®	PO	300–900 mg/day
olanzapine	Zyprexa®	PO, IM	5–20 mg/day
quetiapine fumarate	Seroquel®	PO	50–400 mg/day
risperidone	Risperdal®	PO, IM	2–6 mg/day
ziprasidone hydrochloride	Geodon®	PO, IM	40–120 mg/day

Medical Terminology Review

antipsychotic

anti = against
psych/o = mind
tic = pertaining to
against the mind

neuroleptic

neuro = nerve
lep = seizure, attack
tic = pertaining to
attack of the nerves

Key Concept

Antipsychotic drugs do not alter the underlying pathology of schizophrenia. Therefore, treatment is not curative.

Mechanism of Action

Antipsychotic drugs act by blocking receptors for dopamine, acetylcholine, histamine, and norepinephrine. The current suggestions are that conventional antipsychotic drugs suppress symptoms of psychosis by blocking dopamine receptors in the brain.

Indications

Schizophrenia is the primary indication for antipsychotic drugs. These agents effectively suppress symptoms during acute psychotic episodes and, when taken chronically, can greatly decrease the risk of relapse. Selection among these drugs is based primarily on their adverse effect profiles, rather than on therapeutic effects.

In addition to their antipsychotic properties, some of these drugs, such as prochlorperazine, are also used as antiemetics. Chlorpromazine is

used for treating hiccups and lithium for managing bipolar disorders. Small doses of neuroleptics can be effective to control acute agitation in the elderly.

Adverse Effects

Antipsychotic drugs frequently cause a wide variety of adverse effects, which include dry mouth, blurred vision, urinary retention, orthostatic hypotension, tachycardia, sedation, headache, and behavior changes. These drugs may also produce agitation, confusion, lethargy, and paranoid reactions. Antipsychotic agents commonly cause adverse effects related to excessive **extrapyramidal** (nerves in the brain controlling movement) activity (or parkinsonian signs). Involuntary muscle spasms in the face, neck, arms, or legs (dystonia) may be present. Tardive dyskinesia may be present, such as chewing or grimacing, repetitive jerky or writhing movements of the limbs, tremors, or a shuffling gait. Extrapyramidal effects usually diminish with a decreased dosage of the antipsychotic medication.

Contraindications and Precautions

Antipsychotic drugs are contraindicated in patients with a known hypersensitivity, severe depression, blood dyscrasias, liver dysfunction, severe hypotension or hypertension, and Parkinson's disease.

Safe use of antipsychotic drugs during pregnancy and lactation has not been established. These agents in pregnancy are category C (except for clozapine, which is category B).

Antipsychotic agents should be used with caution in patients with glaucoma, asthma, epilepsy, prostatic hypertrophy, peptic ulcer, renal dysfunction, and in those who have been exposed to extreme heat.

Drug Interactions

Antipsychotic medications may have drug interactions with antihistamines, alcohol, tranquilizers, narcotics, and barbiturates. They may result in additive CNS depression.

MOOD ALTERING DRUGS

Bipolar disorder was formerly known as manic-depressive illness. According to the National Institutes of Health, more than 5.7 million Americans are suffering from this disease. Bipolar disorder is a chronic condition that requires treatment for life.

Bipolar disorder is treated with three major groups of drugs: mood stabilizers, antipsychotics, and antidepressants. The mainstays of therapy are lithium and valproic acid, drugs with the ability to stabilize mood. In addition, benzodiazepines are commonly used for sedation. Antipsychotic drugs were discussed before, and antidepressants will be discussed later in this chapter. The following is a discussion of mood stabilizers.

The principal mood stabilizers are lithium and two drugs originally developed for epilepsy: valproic acid and carbamazepine (see Chapter 8). Lithium has a low therapeutic index. As a result, toxicity can occur at blood levels only slightly greater than therapeutic levels. Accordingly, monitoring of lithium levels is mandatory.

Mechanism of Action

The precise mechanism of action of lithium is unknown. The lithium ion behaves in the body much like the sodium ion, but its exact mechanism of action is unclear. Lithium competes with various physiologically important cations: Na^+, K^+, Ca^{++}, and Mg^{++}. At the synapse, it accelerates catecholamine destruction, inhibits the release of neurotransmitters, and decreases sensitivity of postsynaptic receptors.

Indications

Lithium is a drug of choice for controlling acute manic episodes in patients with bipolar disorder, and for long-term prophylaxis against recurrence of mania or depression. In manic patients, lithium reduces euphoria, hyperactivity, and other symptoms, but does not cause sedation. Anti-manic effects begin five to seven days after the onset of treatment, but full benefits may not develop for two to three weeks.

Adverse Effects

Adverse effects of lithium, such as nausea, diarrhea, abdominal bloating, and anorexia are common but transient. The other adverse effects include fatigue, muscle weakness, headache, confusion, memory impairment, polyuria, and thirst. Lithium-induced tremors can be augmented by stress and fatigue.

Contraindications and Precautions

Lithium is contraindicated in patients with known hypersensitivity, in those with significant cardiovascular or kidney disease, brain damage, dehydration, or sodium debilitation. Lithium is also contraindicated in pregnancy, especially during the first trimester (category D), lactation, and in children younger than 12 years of age.

Lithium should be used with caution in older adults and in patients suffering from thyroid disease, epilepsy, cardiac disease, dehydration, diarrhea, renal impairment, and seizure disorders.

Drug Interactions

Diuretics promote sodium loss and can thereby increase the risk of lithium toxicity. Nonsteroidal anti-inflammatory drugs can increase lithium levels and increase renal reabsorption of lithium. Anticholinergics can cause urinary hesitancy coupled with lithium-induced polyuria.

Key Concept

Lithium is not a true antipsychotic drug, but it is used in regulating the severe fluctuations of the manic phase of bipolar disorder.

ANTIDEPRESSANTS

As previously mentioned in this chapter, depression is classified as a mood disorder with several subgroups. Severe depression, or unipolar disorder, is endogenous (originating from within), and a precise diagnosis is based on biologic factors or personal characteristics. Etiologic factors include genetic, developmental, and psychosocial stressors. Bipolar disorder involves alternating periods of depression and mania. Depression may also occur as an exogenous or reactive episode, a response to a life event, or secondarily to many systemic disorders, including cancer, diabetes, heart failure, and systemic lupus erythematosus.

The scene is now set to discuss the action of **antidepressant** drugs in the context of nerve physiology within the brain. Four major drug classifications are used to treat depression, which include: tricyclic antidepressants, selective serotonin reuptake inhibitors (SSRIs), monoamine oxidase inhibitors (MAOIs), and atypical antidepressant drugs (see Table 4-2).

TABLE 4-2 Drugs Used to Treat Depression

Generic Name	Trade Name	Route of Administration	Average Adult Dose
Tricyclic Antidepressants (TCAs)			
amitriptyline hydrochloride	Elavil®, Enovil®	PO	75–100 mg/day (max: 150–300 mg/day)
amoxapine	Asendin®	PO	200–400 mg/day
desipramine hydrochloride	Norpramin®	PO	75–100 mg/day (max: 300 mg/day)
doxepin hydrochloride	Sinequan®	PO	30–150 mg/day h.s. (max: 300 mg/day)
imipramine hydrochloride	Tofranil®	PO	75–100 mg/day (max: 300 mg/day)
maprotiline	Ludiomil®	PO	25–150 mg/day
nortriptyline hydrochloride	Aventyl®	PO	25 mg t.i.d.-q.i.d. (max: 150 mg /day)
protriptyline	Vivactil®	PO	15–40 mg/day in 3-4 div. doses (max: 60 mg/day)
trimipramine	Surmontil®	PO	75–100 mg/day (max: 300 mg/day)
Selective Serotonin Reuptake Inhibitors (SSRIs)			
citalopram hydrobromide	Celexa®	PO	Start at 20 mg/day (max: 40 mg/day)
escitalopram oxalate	Lexapro®	PO	10 mg/day (max: 20 mg/day after 1 wk)

(continues)

TABLE 4-2 Drugs Used to Treat Depression—*continued*

Generic Name	Trade Name	Route of Administration	Average Adult Dose
fluoxetine hydrochloride	Prozac®	PO	20 mg/day in a.m. (max: 80 mg/day)
fluvoxamine	Luvox®	PO	Start at 50 mg/day (max: 300 mg/day)
paroxetine	Paxil®	PO	10–50 mg/day (max: 60 mg/day)
sertraline hydrochloride	Zoloft®	PO	Start at 50 mg /day (max: 200 mg/day)
Monoamine Oxidase Inhibitors (MAOIs)			
isocarboxazid	Marplan®	PO	10–30 mg/day (max: 30 mg/day)
phenelzine	Nardil®	PO	15 mg t.i.d. (max: 90 mg/day)
tranylcypromine	Parnate®	PO	30 mg/day (20 mg in a.m. and 10 mg in p.m.) (max: 60 mg/day)
Atypical Antidepressants			
bupropion hydrochloride	Wellbutrin®	PO	75–100 mg t.i.d. (max: 450 mg/day)
mirtazapine	Remeron®	PO	15 mg/day h.s. (max: 45 mg/day)
nefazodone hydrochloride	Serzone®	PO	50–100 mg b.i.d. (max: 600 mg/day)
trazodone hydrochloride	Desyrel®, Trialodine®	PO	150 mg/day (max: 600 mg/day)
venlafaxine	Effexor®	PO	25–125 mg t.i.d.

Tricyclic Antidepressants

Historically, **tricyclic antidepressants** (TCAs) were the first choice in the treatment of depression, until SSRI's entered the market. The term tricyclic derives from the common three-ringed structure of the drug molecule itself.

Mechanism of Action

Tricyclic antidepressants inhibit the reuptake of serotonin and noradrenaline into nerve terminals (Figure 4-6).

Indications

Tricyclic antidepressants are mainly used for major depression, and imipramine may be used for the treatment of **nocturnal enuresis** (nighttime bedwetting) in children.

Medical Terminology Review

tricyclic
tri = three
cyclic = related to cycles, circles, rings
three cycles

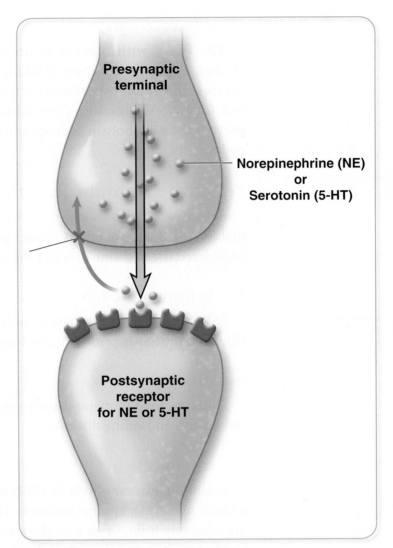

Figure 4-6 Mechanism of action for tricyclic antidepressants.

Adverse Effects

Common adverse effects of tricyclic antidepressants include dry mouth, blurred vision, postural hypotension, constipation, and urinary retention. Other adverse effects may be sedation, drowsiness, cardiovascular symptoms (such as dysrhythmias), and extreme hypertension.

Contraindications and Precautions

The TCAs are contraindicated in patients with known hypersensitivity to these drugs. They are also contraindicated in patients with glaucoma, hypertrophy of prostate gland, and during pregnancy or lactation.

Like other antidepressants, the tricyclics should be used with caution in patients who have heart disease (angina or paroxysmal tachycardia), hepatic or renal dysfunction, or a history of seizures.

Drug Interactions

The TCAs, with concurrent use of other CNS depressants, including alcohol, may cause sedation. If taking clonidine, patients may experience a decrease in the antihypertensive effects of the drug and are at an increased risk for CNS depression. Cimetidine (a histamine blocking agent) may prevent the metabolism of imipramine, leading to increased serum levels and toxicity.

Selective Serotonin-Reuptake Inhibitors

Selective serotonin-reuptake inhibitors (SSRIs) are antidepressants that have had a tremendous impact on prescribing patterns. They are now considered the first-line drugs in the treatment of major depression.

Mechanism of Action

SSRIs block the presynaptic amine reuptake pump, as do the TCAs. However, the SSRIs primarily affect serotonin reuptake (see Figure 4-7).

Indications

SSRIs are used in major depression and may be prescribed for obsessive-compulsive and eating disorders.

Adverse Effects

Common adverse effects of SSRIs include headache, vomiting, diarrhea, nausea, insomnia, and nervousness. Generally, the adverse effects of SSRIs are relatively mild, of shorter duration, and cease as treatment continues. Cardiac toxicity and the risk of death after overdose are less likely than with the TCAs.

Contraindications and Precautions

SSRIs are contraindicated in patients with known hypersensitivity to these agents and during pregnancy. SSRIs should be used with caution in patients with hepatic or renal dysfunction, diabetes mellitus, and during lactation.

Drug Interactions

Concurrent use of SSRIs with benzodiazepines may cause increased adverse CNS effects. Beta blockers may cause decreased elimination of SSRIs, resulting in hypotension or bradycardia. Clozapine, phenytoin, and theophylline may interact with SSRIs and decrease their elimination and their toxicity.

Monoamine Oxidase Inhibitors

Monoamine oxidase inhibitors (MAOIs) were the first drugs approved for the treatment of depression.

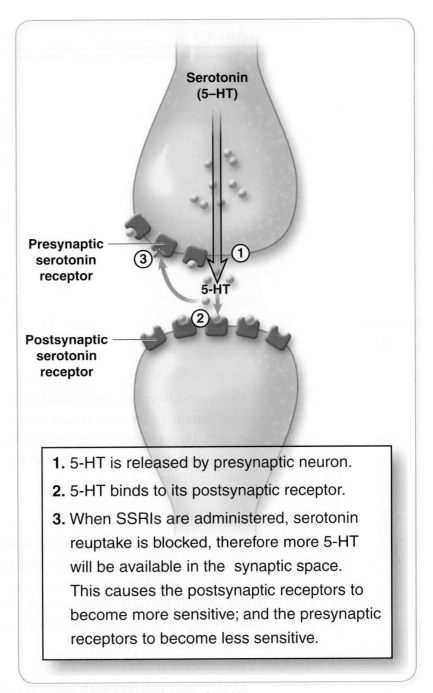

Serotonin
(5–HT)

Presynaptic
serotonin
receptor

③   ①

5-HT

②

Postsynaptic
serotonin
receptor

1. 5-HT is released by presynaptic neuron.

2. 5-HT binds to its postsynaptic receptor.

3. When SSRIs are administered, serotonin
   reuptake is blocked, therefore more 5-HT
   will be available in the synaptic space.
   This causes the postsynaptic receptors to
   become more sensitive; and the presynaptic
   receptors to become less sensitive.

Figure 4-7 Mechanism of action for SSRIs.

Mechanism of Action

MAOIs inhibit monoamine oxidase (an enzyme) that stops the actions of dopamine, norepinephrine, epinephrine, and serotonin. Therefore, these drugs intensify the effects of norepinephrine in adrenergic synapses.

Indications

MAOIs are used to manage symptoms of depression not responsive to other types of pharmacotherapy. The effect of these drugs may continue for two to three weeks after therapy is discontinued.

TABLE 4-3 Foods that Contain Tyramine

Type of Food	Tyramine-Containing Foods
alcohol	beer, wines (especially red wines and Chianti)
dairy products	cheese (except for cottage cheese), sour cream, yogurt
fruits	avocados, bananas, canned figs, papaya products (including meat tenderizers), raisins
meats	beef or chicken liver, bologna/hot dogs, meat extracts, pate, pepperoni, pickled or kippered herring, salami, sausage
other	chocolate
sauces	soy sauce
vegetables	pods of broad beans (fava beans)
yeast	all yeast or yeast extracts

Adverse Effects

Common adverse effects of the MAOIs include dizziness, vertigo, dry mouth, nausea, diarrhea or constipation, loss of appetite, orthostatic hypotension, and insomnia. Hypertensive crisis (severe hypertension) may occur if ingesting foods containing tyramine while taking MAOIs. Table 4-3 lists foods that contain tyramine.

Contraindications and Precautions

MAOI agents are contraindicated in patients with known hypersensitivity to these drugs; in patients with hepatic or renal disease, hypertension, congestive heart failure, cerebrovascular disease, and in the elderly. MAOI drugs should be used with caution in patients with liver dysfunction, diabetes, hyperthyroidism, and history of seizures.

Drug Interactions

MAOIs may interact with other antidepressant drugs such as SSRIs and TCAs, resulting in elevation of body temperature and seizures. Meperidine should be avoided with MAOIs due to increased risk of respiratory failure or hypertensive crisis.

Atypical Antidepressants

Atypical antidepressants are also called miscellaneous agents. They are frequently prescribed to alleviate symptoms of depression for patients with bipolar disorder. Atypical antidepressants are chemically unrelated to other antidepressants. They include trazodone, mirtazapine, and bupropion.

Mechanism of Action

Atypical antidepressants inhibit the reabsorption of serotonin and norepinephrine. They elevate mood by increasing the levels of dopamine, serotonin, and norepinephrine in the central nervous system.

Indications

Atypical antidepressants are indicated for mental depression. Since bupropion has been associated with increased risk of seizures, it is not the agent of first choice. It is also used as an adjunct for smoking cessation. Venlafaxine is also used for generalized anxiety disorder and social anxiety disorder.

Adverse Effects

Common adverse effects of atypical antidepressants include dry mouth, blurred vision, dizziness, headache, nausea, vomiting, orthostatic hypotension, increased appetite, and insomnia.

Contraindications and Precautions

Atypical antidepressants are contraindicated in patients with known hypersensitivity to these agents. These drugs should be avoided in patients with hepatic diseases, pregnancy (category C), lactation, suicidal thoughts, and in children less than 8 years of age.

Atypical antidepressants must be used cautiously in patients with renal failure, hepatic impairment, history of mania, acute closed-angle glaucoma, cardiac disorders, hypertension, hyperthyroidism, and history of seizures or seizure disorders.

Drug Interactions

Atypical antidepressants may increase metabolism of carbamazepine, cimetidine, phenytoin, and phenobarbital. They may increase incidence of adverse effects of levodopa and MAOIs. They may cause additive cognitive and motor impairment with alcohol or benzodiazepines, and increase risk of hypertensive crisis with MAOIs. Antihypertensive agents may potentiate hypotensive effects of atypical antidepressants. Levels of digoxin or phenytoin may be increased if used concurrently. Levels and toxicity of ketoconazole, indinavir, and ritonavir may be increased with concurrent use.

SUMMARY

The nervous system is composed of two divisions: the CNS (brain and spinal cord) and the peripheral nervous system (nerves). The major parts of the human brain are the cerebrum, diencephalon, brainstem, and cerebellum. The cerebrum is involved in motor and sensory function, and is the seat of intellect. The diencephalon comprises the thalamus, which acts as an information sorting area, and hypothalamus, which is an integration area for visceral functioning. The brainstem contains control centers for heart rate, respiratory rate, and blood pressure. The cerebellum controls muscle tone and posture, and facilitates smooth and coordinated muscle movements. Acetylcholine, dopamine, noradrenaline, serotonin, and GABA are key neurotransmitters in the brain.

Antipsychotics are used in the treatment of psychoses such as schizophrenia, dementia, and restlessness. All antipsychotics exert their effect on dopamine receptors and antagonize dopaminergic activity in the CNS. Antipsychotics have a diverse and potentially debilitating adverse effect profile.

Depression is a state of profound sadness. It can be reactive, in response to a life event, or endogenous, without an apparent trigger. Antidepressant drugs act by raising the levels of one or both of these neurotransmitters. This is achieved by blocking a subtype of postsynaptic serotonin receptors (selective serotonin receptor blockers) or MAOIs.

EXPLORING THE WEB

Visit *www.fda.gov*

- Search using the term antipsychotics. Look for drug information sheets for patients. You can also search for information on specific drug names for additional information on specific drugs.

Visit *www.mentalhealth.com*

- Click on the link "disorders." Choose one of the disorders discussed in the text and research what is known about the disorder and the treatments that are used to address it.

Visit *www.nimh.nih.gov*

- Choose one of the disorders discussed in the text and research what is known about the disorder and the treatments that are used to address it.

Visit *www.nlm.nih.gov/medlineplus*

- Choose one of the types of drugs discussed in the chapter and research the uses, mechanisms of action, adverse effects, contraindications and

precautions, and drug interactions to further your understanding of the drug. Make index cards with the pertinent information to help you review and study.

Visit *www.rxlist.com*

- Bookmark this site to be used as a reference. It is one of several drug information sites available on the Web. What additional websites are available for drug information? Make sure the sites are reputable.

REVIEW QUESTIONS

Multiple Choice

1. Which of the following parts of the brain is responsible for the precise perception and interpretation of sensation?

   A. cerebellum
   B. cerebrum
   C. diencephalon
   D. brainstem

2. Which of the following disorders is the *primary* indication for antipsychotic drugs?

   A. insomnia
   B. anxiety
   C. manic-depressive
   D. schizophrenia

3. Lithium is a *drug of choice* for controlling which of the following mental disorders?

   A. schizophrenia
   B. restlessness
   C. acute manic episodes
   D. brain injury

4. Which of the following antidepressants have relatively mild adverse effects, and are the *newest* of these drugs?

   A. monoamine oxidase inhibitors
   B. tricyclic antidepressants
   C. atypical antidepressants
   D. selective serotonin reuptake inhibitors

5. Which of the following neurotransmitters is distributed *throughout* the central nervous system?

   A. GABA
   B. dopamine
   C. acetylcholine
   D. serotonin

6. Which of the following is the largest part of the brain?
   A. hypothalamus
   B. cerebellum
   C. brainstem
   D. cerebrum

7. Which of the following neurotransmitters is involved in hormone release, motor control, behavior, and emesis?
   A. serotonin
   B. dopamine
   C. acetylcholine
   D. GABA

8. Which of the following neurotransmitters' functions within the brain is *similar* to noradrenaline?
   A. dopamine
   B. GABA
   C. serotonin
   D. acetylcholine

9. Bipolar disorder involves alternating periods of which of the following?
   A. depression and insomnia
   B. depression and mania
   C. depression and anxiety attacks
   D. insomnia and anxiety

10. Which of the following is the *cure* for schizophrenia?
    A. lithium
    B. chlorpromazine
    C. benzodiazepine
    D. no cure

Matching

_____ 1. Involved in the facilitation of learning and memory

_____ 2. Plays a major role in cognitive function and memory function

_____ 3. Involved in behavior and emesis

_____ 4. Formed from the excitatory neurotransmitter glutamate

_____ 5. Principally involved in the regulation of sleep

A. dopamine

B. serotonin

C. GABA

D. acetylcholine

E. glutamate

Fill in the Blank

1. Serotonin is also known as 5-hydroxytryptamine or _____.

2. Antipsychotic drugs are also called _____ drugs.

3. Schizophrenia is one of the most devastating forms of _____.

4. Lithium is used for managing _____ disorders.

5. Bipolar disorder was formerly known as _____ illness.

6. The principal mood stabilizer is _____.

7. SSRIs are now considered the first-line drugs in the treatment of _____.

Critical Thinking

A 45-year-old female has been diagnosed with major depression based on biologic factors and personal characteristics. Her physician has several options for prescribing the best drugs to treat her. These are TCAs, SSRIs, MAOIs, and atypical antidepressants.

1. Which of these classes of antidepressants is the drug of choice?

2. Which of these classes of drugs are the newest types of antidepressants?

3. If the patient is taking MAOIs, which type of foods would be contraindicated?

Drug Therapy for the Nervous System: Antianxiety and Hypnotic Drugs

OBJECTIVES

After completing this chapter, the reader should be able to:

1. Identify the major classifications of anxiety disorders.
2. Describe the difference between a sedative or anxiolytic and a hypnotic.
3. Identify the various types of anxiolytics and hypnotics.
4. Explain the problems associated with anxiolytics and hypnotics.
5. List four benzodiazepine-like drugs and their mechanisms of action.
6. Discuss the therapeutic effects and adverse effects of the major barbiturates.
7. Explain miscellaneous drugs that are used for insomnia.

GLOSSARY

Antianxiety agents – drugs that relieve anxiety; also known as anxiolytics

Anxiety – state of apprehension and autonomic nervous system activation resulting from exposure to a nonspecific or unknown cause

Anxiolytics – drugs that relieve anxiety; also known as antianxiety agents

Compulsion – a ritualized behavior or mental act that a patient is driven to perform in response to his or her obsessions

Barbiturates – drugs that depress multiple aspects of central nervous system function and can be used for sleep, seizures, and general anesthesia

Benzodiazepines – drugs of first choice for treating anxiety and insomnia

Buspirone – an anxiolytic drug that differs significantly from the benzodiazepines

Generalized anxiety disorder – difficult-to-control, excessive anxiety that lasts six months or more

Hypnotics – drugs given to promote sleep

Insomnia – the inability to fall asleep or stay asleep

Melatonin – an important hormone secreted from the pineal gland that is believed to induce sleep

Obsession – a recurrent, persistent thought, impulse, or mental image that is unwanted and distressing, and comes involuntarily to mind despite attempts to ignore or suppress it

Obsessive-compulsive disorder – anxiety characterized by recurrent, repetitive behaviors that interfere with normal activities or relationships

Panic attacks – of sudden onset, reaching peak intensity within ten

minutes; symptoms may include trembling, shortness of breath, heart palpitations, chest pain (or chest tightness), sweating, nausea, dizziness (or slight vertigo), light-headedness, hyperventilation, paresthesias (tingling sensations), and sensations of choking or smothering

Panic disorder – anxiety characterized by intense feelings of immediate apprehension, fearfulness, and terror

Post-traumatic stress disorder – anxiety characterized by a sense of helplessness and the re-experiencing of a traumatic event

Sedative-hypnotics – drugs that when given in lower doses, produce a calming effect, and when given in higher doses, produce sleep

Social anxiety disorder – characterized by an intense, irrational fear of situations in which one might be scrutinized by others, or might do something that is embarrassing or humiliating; also known as social phobia

Social phobia – characterized by an intense, irrational fear of situations in which one might be scrutinized by others, or might do something that is embarrassing or humiliating; also known as social anxiety disorder

OVERVIEW

Medical Terminology Review

preanesthetic
pre = before
an- = without, not
-esthesi/o = feeling, sensation
-tic = pertaining to
a drug administered before an anesthetic

Anxiety disorders are common occurrences in society today. These disorders can prove stressful and disruptive to those suffering from them. There are a variety of anxiety disorders for which drug therapy may be therapeutic. Antianxiety drugs or hypnotics are the most common classifications of medications that may be used to treat these disorders.

Sleep disturbances are also extremely common. If continuous, they have the potential to seriously disrupt normal day-to-day living. Many people suffering from a sleep disorder want to turn to drugs to solve their problem. The use of drugs in many of these situations is usually undesirable.

Many of the medications discussed in this chapter are also administered as muscle relaxants, preanesthetic medications, anticonvulsants, and therapeutic aids in psychiatry.

ANXIETY

Medical Terminology Review

tachycardia
tachy- = fast, rapid
cardia = the heart
rapid heart beat

According to the Anxiety Disorders Association of America, anxiety disorders are the most common psychiatric illnesses in the United States, affecting 40 million people, with a higher incidence of anxiety seen in women than in men. **Anxiety** is an uncomfortable state that has both psychological and physical components. The psychological component can be characterized with terms such as fear, apprehension, dread, and uneasiness. The physical component may exhibit as tachycardia, palpitations, trembling, dry mouth, sweating, weakness, fatigue, and shortness of breath. Fortunately, anxiety disorders respond well to treatment either with behavior therapy, psychotherapy, or drug therapy.

Anxiety disorders may be classified as generalized anxiety disorder, panic disorder, obsessive-compulsive disorder, social anxiety disorder, or post-traumatic stress disorder. Brief explanations of the different types of anxiety follow.

Generalized Anxiety Disorder

Generalized anxiety disorder is a chronic condition characterized by uncontrollable worrying. Most patients with generalized anxiety disorder also have another psychiatric disorder, usually depression. The hallmark of this disorder is unrealistic or excessive anxiety about several events or activities (e.g., work or school performance). Generalized anxiety disorder may last for six months or longer.

Panic Disorder

Panic disorder is characterized by recurrent, intensely uncomfortable episodes known as **panic attacks**. Panic attacks have a sudden onset, reaching peak intensity within ten minutes. Symptoms may include trembling, shortness of breath, heart palpitations, chest pain (or chest tightness), sweating, nausea, dizziness (or slight vertigo), light-headedness, hyperventilation, paresthesias (tingling sensations), and sensations of choking or smothering. These symptoms typically disappear within 30 minutes. Many patients go to an emergency department because they think they are having a heart attack. Some patients experience panic attacks daily; others have only one or two per month. According to the *American Journal of Psychiatry*, the incidence of panic disorders in women is two to three times that seen in men. Onset of panic disorder usually occurs in the late teens or early twenties.

Obsessive-Compulsive Disorder

Obsessive-compulsive disorder is a potentially disabling condition characterized by persistent obsessions and compulsions that cause marked distress, consume at least one hour per day, and significantly interfere with daily living. An **obsession** is defined as a recurrent, persistent thought, impulse, or mental image that is unwanted and distressing, and comes involuntarily to mind despite attempts to ignore or suppress it. A **compulsion** is a ritualized behavior or mental act that a person is driven to perform in response to his or her obsessions.

Social Anxiety Disorder

Social anxiety disorder, formerly known as **social phobia**, is characterized by an intense, irrational fear of situations in which one might be scrutinized by others, or might do something that is embarrassing or humiliating. Exposure to the feared situation almost always elicits anxiety. As a result, the person avoids the situation, or, if it cannot be avoided, endures

it with intense anxiety. Manifestations include blushing, stuttering, sweating, palpitations, dry throat, and muscle tension.

Social anxiety disorder is one of the most common psychiatric disorders and the most common anxiety disorder. This disorder typically begins during the teenage years, and if left untreated, is likely to continue lifelong.

Post-Traumatic Stress Disorder

Post-traumatic stress disorder develops following a traumatic event that elicited an immediate reaction of fear, helplessness, or horror. It is more common in women than in men, and is the fourth most common psychiatric disorder. Traumatic events that involve interpersonal violence (e.g., assault, rape, or torture) are more likely to cause post-traumatic stress disorder than are traumatic events that do not (e.g., car accidents or natural disasters).

SLEEP DISORDERS

Insomnia is the inability to fall asleep or stay asleep. Difficulty in falling asleep or disturbed sleep patterns both result in insufficient sleep. Sleep disorders are common and may be short in duration or may be longstanding. They may have little or no apparent relationship to other immediate disorders. Sleep disorders can be secondary to emotional problems, pain, physical disorders, and the use or withdrawal of drugs. Excess alcohol consumed in the evening can shorten sleep and lead to withdrawal effects in the early morning.

Medical Terminology Review

insomnia
in = lack of
somnia = ability to sleep
lacking the ability to sleep

SEDATIVES AND HYPNOTICS

The **sedative-hypnotics** are agents that depress central nervous system (CNS) function. These drugs are widely used primarily to treat anxiety and insomnia. Agents given to relieve anxiety are known as **antianxiety agents** or **anxiolytics**. They were previously known as tranquilizers. Drugs given to promote sleep are known as **hypnotics**. The distinction between antianxiety and hypnotic effects is often a matter of dosage. Sedative-hypnotics relieve anxiety in low doses and induce sleep in higher doses. Therefore, a single drug may be considered both an antianxiety agent and a hypnotic agent, depending upon the reason for its use and the dosage employed.

Sedative-hypnotic drugs include barbiturates, benzodiazepines, and benzodiazepine-like drugs. Anxiety and insomnia are treated primarily with the benzodiazepines. Benzodiazepines are used primarily for one condition (generalized anxiety disorder). In contrast, the selective serotonin reuptake inhibitors (SSRIs) are now used for all anxiety disorders. It should be noted that, although SSRIs were developed as antidepressants, they are highly effective against anxiety (with or without depression). SSRIs are discussed in Chapter 4.

TABLE 5-1 First-Line Drugs for Anxiety Disorders

Type of Anxiety Disorder	Benzodiazepines	SSRIs	Others
Generalized Anxiety Disorder	alprazolam	escitalopram oxalate	buspirone hydrochloride
	chlordiazepoxide	paroxetine hydrochloride	venlafaxine hydrochloride
	clorazepate dipotassium	paroxetine mesylate	
	diazepam		
	lorazepam		
	oxazepam		
Panic Disorder	alprazolam	paroxetine	
	clonazepam	sertraline hydrochloride	
	lorazepam		
Obsessive-Compulsive Disorder		citalopram hydrobromide	
		escitalopram oxalate	
		fluoxetine hydrochloride	
		fluvoxamine maleate	
		paroxetine	
		sertraline hydrochloride	
Post-Traumatic Stress Disorder		paroxetine	
		sertraline hydrochloride	

Table 5-1 shows the first-line drugs that are used for specific anxiety disorders. Table 5-2 shows sedative-hypnotics, including barbiturates, benzodiazepines, and miscellaneous agents used to treat anxiety and insomnia.

Benzodiazepines

Benzodiazepines are the drugs of first choice for treating anxiety and insomnia. The popularity of the benzodiazepines as sedatives and hypnotics stems from their clear superiority over the alternatives, such as barbiturates and other general CNS depressants. The benzodiazepines are safer than the general CNS depressants and have a lower potential for abuse.

Mechanism of Action

The mechanism of action of benzodiazepines on the CNS appears to be closely related to their ability to potentiate GABA (gamma-aminobutyric acid)-mediated neural inhibition. Recent research has identified specific

TABLE 5-2 Drugs for Anxiety and Insomnia

Generic Name	Trade Name	Route of Administration	Average Adult Dosage
Barbiturates (Short-Acting)			
pentobarbital	Nembutal®	PO	Sedative: 20–30 mg b.i.d.-t.i.d. Hypnotic: 120–200 mg/day
secobarbital	Seconal®	PO	Sedative: 100–300 mg/day in 3 div. doses Hypnotic: 100–200 mg/day
(Intermediate-Acting)			
amobarbital	Amytal®	PO	Sedative: 30–50 mg b.i.d.-t.i.d. Hypnotic: 65–200 mg (max: 500 mg/day)
aprobarbital	Alurate®	PO	Sedative: 40 mg t.i.d. Hypnotic: 40–160 mg/day
butabarbital	Butisol®	PO	Sedative: 15–30 mg t.i.d.-q.i.d. Hypnotic: 50–100 mg h.s.
(Long-Acting)			
mephobarbital	Mebaral®	PO	Sedative: 32–100 mg t.i.d.
phenobarbital	Luminal®	PO	Sedative: 30–120 mg/day
Benzodiazepines			
alprazolam	Xanax®	PO	0.25–2 mg t.i.d.
chlordiazepoxide	Librium®	PO	5–25 mg t.i.d.-q.i.d.
clonazepam	Klonopin®	PO	1–2 mg/day in div. doses (max: 4 mg/day)
clorazepate dipotassium	Tranxene®	PO	15 mg/day h.s. (max: 4 mg/day)
diazepam	Valium®	PO	2–10 mg b.i.d.-q.i.d.
estazolam	ProSom®	PO	1 mg h.s. (max: 2 mg prn)
flurazepam	Dalmane®	PO	15–30 mg h.s.
halazepam (no longer available)	Paxipam®	PO	20–40 mg t.i.d.-q.i.d.
lorazepam	Ativan®	PO	1–3 mg b.i.d.-t.i.d.
oxazepam	Serax®	PO	10–30 mg t.i.d.-q.i.d.
quazepam	Doral®	PO	7.5–15 mg h.s.
temazepam	Restoril®	PO	15 mg h.s.
triazolam	Halcion®	PO	0.125–0.25 mg h.s. (max: 0.5 mg/day)

(continues)

TABLE 5-2   Drugs for Anxiety and Insomnia—*continued*

Generic Name	Trade Name	Route of Administration	Average Adult Dosage
Benzodiazepine-like Drugs			
eszopiclone	Lunesta®	PO	2–3 mg h.s.
ramelteon	Rozerem®	PO	8 mg within 30 min of h.s.
zaleplon	Sonata®	PO	5–10 mg h.s.
zolpidem tartrate	Ambien®	PO	10 mg h.s.
Miscellaneous Drugs: Antiseizure Medication			
valproic acid, (divalproex sodium, sodium valproate)	Depakote®, Depakene®, Depacon®	PO PO PO	250 mg t.i.d. (max: 60 mg/kg/day)
Special Anxiolytic			
buspirone hydrochloride	BuSpar®	PO	7.5–15 mg in div.doses (max: 60 mg/day)
Beta Blockers (rarely indicated for treatment of anxiety)			
atenolol	Tenormin®	PO	25–100 mg 1x/day
propranolol hydrochloride	Inderal®	PO	40 mg b.i.d. (max: 320 mg/day)

binding sites for benzodiazepines in the CNS, and has established the close relationship between the sites of action of the benzodiazepines and GABA.

Indications

Benzodiazepines are useful for the short-term treatment panic disorder, generalized anxiety, phobias, and insomnia. Chlordiazepoxide (Librium) and diazepam (Valium) are the most widely prescribed in medicine. The benzodiazepines are categorized as Schedule IV drugs. Benzodiazepines are also used in absence seizures and myoclonic seizures. Parenteral diazepam is used to terminate status epilepticus.

Adverse Effects

Adverse effects of benzodiazepines are drowsiness, ataxia, impaired judgment, dry mouth, fatigue, visual disturbances, rebound insomnia, and development of tolerance. Overdosage may result in CNS and respiratory depression as well as hypotension and coma. Gradual withdrawal of these drugs is recommended. Although the use of any of the benzodiazepines during pregnancy is likely to cause fetal abnormalities, flurazepam is entirely contraindicated during pregnancy. Benzodiazepines produce

---

Medical Terminology Review

ataxia
a- = without, not
tax/o = order
-ia = condition
without muscular coordination

considerably less physical dependence and result in less tolerance than barbiturates.

Contraindications and Precautions

Benzodiazepines are contraindicated in patients with known hypersensitivity to the drugs. Benzodiazepines are also contraindicated in patients with acute narrow-angle glaucoma, psychosis, liver or kidney disease, and neurological disorders.

Benzodiazepines should be used cautiously during pregnancy (category D), and in elderly or debilitated patients.

Drug Interactions

Benzodiazepines increase CNS depression with alcohol and omeprazole. They also increase pharmacological effects if combined with cimetidine, disulfiram, or hormonal contraceptives. The effects of benzodiazepines decrease with theophyllines and ranitidine.

Benzodiazepine-like Drugs

Nonbenzodiazepines have become quite popular as sleep aids. They are not indicated for anxiety (see Table 5-2).

Mechanism of Action

Benzodiazepine-like drugs are structurally different from the benzodiazepines, but nonetheless share the same mechanism of action. They all act as agonists at the benzodiazepine receptor site on the GABA receptor-chloride channel complex. These drugs are highly effective hypnotics, and have a low potential for tolerance, dependence, or abuse. Ramelteon has a unique mechanism of action that activates the receptors of **melatonin**.

Indications

Benzodiazepine-like drugs, especially zolpidem (Ambien) and buspirone (BuSpar) are widely used for sleep disorders and anxiety. Buspirone is discussed in detail later in this chapter. Benzodiazepine-like drugs are approved only for short-term management of insomnia, except eszopiclone, which was approved by the FDA in 2005 with no limitation on how long it can be used. Ramelteon is approved for treating chronic insomnia, and long-term use is permitted.

Adverse Effects

Zolpidem has adverse effects similar to those of benzodiazepines. Daytime drowsiness and dizziness are the most common, and these occur

in only 1 to 2 percent of patients. At therapeutic doses, benzodiazepine-like drugs cause little or no respiratory depression. Safety during pregnancy has not been established.

Zaleplon and eszopiclone are well tolerated. The most common side effects are headache, nausea, drowsiness, dizziness, myalgia, and abdominal pain.

Ramelteon can increase levels of prolactin and reduce levels of testosterone. As a result, the drug has the potential to cause galactorrhea, amenorrhea, reduced libido, and fertility problems.

Contraindications and Precautions

Benzodiazepine-like drugs are contraindicated in patients with a known hypersensitivity, acute narrow-angle glaucoma, shock, and psychoses. These drugs are also contraindicated in patients with acute alcoholic intoxication, depressed vital signs, and in comatose patients.

Benzodiazepine-like agents are contraindicated in patients during pregnancy (category B) and the drug metabolite freely crosses the placenta. These drugs are used with caution in patients who have impaired liver or kidney function, and in the elderly.

Drug Interactions

Benzodiazepine-like drugs cause less additive CNS depression than other antianxiety drugs, but should still be avoided with concurrent use of a CNS depressant. Buspirone may increase serum digoxin levels, increasing the risk of digitalis toxicity.

Barbiturates

The **barbiturates** depress multiple aspects of CNS function and can be used for sleep, seizures, and general anesthesia. Barbiturates cause tolerance and dependence, have high abuse potential, and are subject to multiple drug interactions. Moreover, barbiturates are powerful respiratory depressants that can be fatal in overdose. Because of these undesirable properties, barbiturates are used much less than in the past, having been replaced by newer and safer drugs—primarily the benzodiazepines and benzodiazepine-like drugs. However, although their use has declined greatly, barbiturates still have important applications in seizure control and anesthesia.

Mechanism of Action

All barbiturates exert a depressant effect on the CNS. These drugs act by changing the action of GABA, the primary inhibitory neurotransmitter in the brain. Barbiturates mimic the effects of GABA by stimulating an influx of chloride ions that interact with the GABA receptor through chloride channel

---

Medical Terminology Review

myalgia
  My/o = muscle
  -algia = pain
  muscle pain

Medical Terminology Review

metabolite
  metabol = metabolism
  ite = produced substance
  substance produced through metabolism

Medical Terminology Review

anesthesia
  an- = without
  -esthesia = sensation, feeling
  without sensation

molecules. When the receptors of barbiturate are stimulated, chloride ions move into the cells, therefore suppressing the ability of neurons to fire.

Indications

Barbiturates are used as sedatives and as hypnotics (short term, up to two weeks) for insomnia. Long-term treatment with certain barbiturates is prescribed for generalized tonic-clonic and cortical focal seizures. They are also indicated for emergency control of some acute convulsive episodes such as status epilepticus, eclampsia, meningitis, tetanus, and toxic reactions to local anesthetics. Thiopental and other highly lipid-soluble barbiturates are given to induce general anesthesia. Unconsciousness develops within seconds of IV injections. After prolonged use of barbiturates, withdrawal symptoms may occur.

Phenobarbital and mephobarbital are used for seizure disorders, congenital hyperbilirubinemia, and neonatal jaundice. Indications for intermediate-acting barbiturates are regional anesthesia, sedation, and hypnosis. Ultra-short-acting barbiturates are used for intravenous general anesthesia.

> ### *Medical Terminology Review*
>
> **neonatal**
> *neo = new*
> *natal = pertaining to birth*
> **new birth, newborn**

Adverse Effects

Barbiturates may cause numerous adverse effects on several different body systems. The manifestation of adverse effects includes ataxia, drowsiness, dizziness, and hangover effect. Some patients may have nausea and vomiting, insomnia, constipation, headache, night terrors, and faintness. Long-term use of barbiturates may cause bone pain, anorexia, muscle pain, and weight loss.

Contraindications and Precautions

Barbiturates are contraindicated in patients with known hypersensitivity to these agents, pregnancy (category D), or lactation. Barbiturates are also contraindicated in parturition, fetal immaturity, and uncontrolled pain.

Barbiturates should be used cautiously in patients with liver or kidney impairments and those with neurological disorders. These drugs are used with caution in patients with pulmonary disorders and in hyperactive children.

Drug Interactions

Barbiturates increase serum levels and therapeutic and toxic effects with valproic acid. They also increase CNS depression with alcohol, narcotic analgesics, and antidepressants. Barbiturates decrease effects of the following drugs: theophyllines, oral anticoagulants, β-blockers, doxycycline, griseofulvin, corticosteroids, hormonal contraceptives, and metronidazole.

Miscellaneous Drugs

There are several CNS drugs used for anxiety and insomnia that are categorized as miscellaneous drugs. These agents are chemically unrelated to either benzodiazepines, benzodiazepine-like drugs, or barbiturates.

The antiseizure drug valproate (Chapter 8), the beta blockers atenolol and propranolol (Chapter 11), and the CNS depressant buspirone are also used for anxiety or sleep disorders (see Table 5-2). Buspirone is unique and is commonly prescribed for antianxiety.

Buspirone

Buspirone (BuSpar) is an anxiolytic drug that differs significantly from the benzodiazepines. Buspirone is as effective as the benzodiazepines and has three distinct advantages:

- It does not cause sedation
- It has no abuse potential
- It does not intensify the effects of CNS depressants

Mechanism of Action.   The anxiolytic effect of buspirone is mainly on the brain's D_2-dopamine receptors. It has agonist effects on presynaptic dopamine receptors. It also has a high affinity for serotonin receptors.

Indications.   Buspirone is prescribed for management of anxiety disorders and for short-term treatment of generalized anxiety.

Adverse Effects.   Buspirone is generally well tolerated. The most common reactions are dizziness, nausea, headache, nervousness, lightheadedness, and excitement. The drug is nonsedating and does not interfere with daytime activities.

Contraindications and Precautions.   Buspirone is contraindicated in patients with known hypersensitivity to this medication. It is also contraindicated with concomitant use of alcohol and buspirone. Safety during pregnancy (category B), labor, delivery, lactation, and in children younger than 18 years is not established. Buspirone should be used with caution in patients with moderate to severe renal or hepatic impairment.

Drug Interactions.   Blood levels of buspirone can be greatly increased by erythromycin and ketoconazole. Levels of buspirone can also be increased by grapefruit juice. Buspirone does not enhance the depressant effects of alcohol, barbiturates, and other general CNS depressants.

SUMMARY

Sedatives affect the CNS, which can relieve anxiety, hence they are often called anxiolytics. Hypnotic is the term used to describe a substance that induces sleep. Both anxiety and insomnia are extremely common in the United States.

There are three major groups of anxiolytics and hypnotics: barbiturates, benzodiazepines, and benzodiazepine-like drugs. Benzodiazepines act on the GABA receptor complex. These drugs are relatively nontoxic, but can have several undesirable adverse effects. With most anxiolytics, the antianxiety effect is related to their sedative effect. The use of barbiturates as hypnotics is no longer advised, and they are gradually being phased out from use. Their availability today is mainly because some are still used in the treatment of epilepsy, and as anesthetics. Hypnotic drugs should be used for short-term therapy only.

Nonbenzodiazepine drugs have become very popular as sleep aids. They are not indicated for anxiety use. Benzodiazepine-like drugs are structurally different from the benzodiazepines, but their mechanism of action is the same. Nonbenzodiazepine drugs, especially zolpidem and buspirone, are widely used for anxiety and sleep disorders.

Miscellaneous drugs that are used for anxiety and insomnia are chemically unrelated to either benzodiazepines or barbiturates. These agents include antiseizure drugs (valproate) and beta blockers (atenolol and propranolol).

EXPLORING THE WEB

Visit *www.medicinenet.com*

- Search using the term post-traumatic stress disorder. Review relevant articles related to the treatment of this disorder.

Visit *www.nlm.nih.gov*

- Choose one of the disorders discussed in this chapter and research the treatments used to address the disorder.

Visit *www.usdoj.gov*

- Search using the term benzodiazepines. Look for information published by the DEA on this drug. What are the concerns with use of this drug? What is the potential for abuse?

REVIEW QUESTIONS

Multiple Choice

1. Which of the following are the first-line drugs used in the treatment of anxiety and insomnia?

   A. benzodiazepines and barbiturates
   B. benzodiazepines and SSRIs
   C. benzodiazepines and MAOIs
   D. benzodiazepines and chloral hydrate

2. Which of the following is the main concern for a patient that stopped taking barbiturates suddenly?

   A. shock
   B. hypotension
   C. severe withdrawal
   D. respiratory depression

3. Which of the following may increase the effects of sedatives?

   A. chocolate
   B. cheese
   C. nicotine
   D. alcohol

4. Benzodiazepines act by binding to the GABA receptor of which of the following channel molecules?

   A. chloride
   B. sodium
   C. potassium
   D. calcium

5. Generalized anxiety disorder may last for:

   A. 3 weeks
   B. 6 weeks
   C. 3 months
   D. 6 months

6. Symptoms of panic disorder typically disappear within:

   A. 30 seconds
   B. 30 minutes
   C. 30 days
   D. 90 days

7. Benzodiazepine-like drugs are the preferred agents for treating:

   A. insomnia
   B. depression
   C. panic disorder
   D. obsessive-compulsive disorder

8. Which of the following benzodiazepine-like drugs may increase levels of prolactin and reduce levels of testosterone?

    A. ramelteon
    B. zolpidem
    C. zaleplon
    D. all of the above

9. The newest drugs used for anxiety and sleep disorders include which of the following?

    A. Nembutal and Depakote
    B. Seconal and Inderal
    C. Tofranil and Librium
    D. BuSpar and Ambien

10. Adverse effects of zolpidem (Ambien) are similar to which of the following?

    A. antihypertensives
    B. barbiturates
    C. benzodiazepines
    D. beta blockers

11. The indications for barbiturates have declined greatly, but they still have important applications in which of the following disorders or conditions?

    A. insomnia
    B. major depression
    C. anxiety
    D. anesthesia

12. Which of the following hormones is believed to induce sleep?

    A. prolactin
    B. thyroxin
    C. melanin
    D. melatonin

13. The trade name of diazepam is:

    A. Librium
    B. Valium
    C. Xanax
    D. Serax

14. The generic name of Luminal is:

    A. butabarbital
    B. pentobarbital
    C. phenobarbital
    D. secobarbital

15. Long-term treatment with certain barbiturates is prescribed for which of the following disorders?

    A. insomnia
    B. anxiety attacks
    C. general anesthesia
    D. generalized tonic-clonic seizures

Fill in the Blank

1. Benzodiazepines are the drugs of first choice for treating _____ and _____.

2. Barbiturates cause tolerance and _____.

3. All barbiturates act by changing the action of _____.

4. Panic disorder is known as _____.

5. The sedative-hypnotics are used primarily to treat _____ and _____.

6. Antianxiety agents were previously known as _____.

7. Barbiturates are contraindicated in pregnancy because they are in category _____.

Critical Thinking

Kaleen is a nurse who was injured in a car accident on her way home from the hospital where she works. She was hospitalized for three weeks and developed post-traumatic stress disorder after approximately six months.

1. What would be the first-line drug for this condition?

2. If she also developed a panic disorder, does her physician have to change her medication or add other drugs to her regimen?

3. If her physician is prescribing the correct first-line drug, what would be the most severe adverse effect?

Drug Therapy for the Autonomic Nervous System

OUTLINE

OBJECTIVES

After completing this chapter, the reader should be able to:

1. Describe the subdivisions of the ANS.
2. Explain the various types of receptors.
3. Differentiate sympathomimetics from sympatholytic agents and give two examples for each.
4. Outline five beta$_2$-adrenergic drugs.
5. Explain the action of adrenergic blockers.
6. Describe the use of cholinergic agonist drugs.
7. Differentiate between cholinergics and cholinergic blockers.
8. Explain the major adverse effects of anticholinergic drugs.
9. Explain the contraindications of cholinergic blockers.
10. List three neurotransmitters that employ the ANS.

GLOSSARY

Adrenergic blocker agents – drugs that antagonize the secretion of epinephrine and norepinephrine from sympathetic terminal neurons; also known as sympatholytics

Adrenergic receptor – receptors that mediate responses to epinephrine (adrenaline) and norepinephrine

Alpha-receptors – an adrenergic receptor; there are two types: alpha$_1$ and alpha$_2$

Beta-receptors – an adrenergic receptor; there are two types: beta$_1$ and beta$_2$

Catecholamines – a group of chemically related compounds having a sympathomimetic action

Cholinergic receptor – receptors that mediate responses to acetylcholine

Congenital megacolon – congenital dilation and hypertrophy of the colon due to reduction in motor neurons of the parasympathetic nervous system, resulting in extreme constipation, and if untreated, growth retardation; also known as Hirschsprung's disease

Cycloplegia – paralysis of the ciliary muscles of the eye, resulting in loss of visual accommodation

Dopamine receptors – an adrenergic receptor

Epinephrine – a major transmitter released by the adrenal medulla

Iritis – inflammation of the iris

Miosis – contraction of the pupil of the eye

Mydriasis – dilation of the pupil

Necrosis – death of a group of cells or tissues

Norepinephrine – the chemical transmitter released by all postganglionic neurons of the sympathetic nervous system

Parasympathomimetic – producing effects similar to those produced when a parasympathetic nerve is stimulated

Pheochromocytoma – a usually benign tumor of the adrenal medulla or the sympathetic nervous system in which the affected cells secrete increased amounts of epinephrine or norepinephrine

Somnolence – prolonged drowsiness that may last hours to days

Sympatholytic – inhibiting or opposing adrenergic nerve function; sympatholytic agents are also known as *adrenergic blocker agents*

Sympathomimetic – adrenergic, or producing an effect similar to that obtained by stimulation of the sympathetic nervous system

Uveitis – inflammation of the uvea (the vascular middle layer of the eye, including the iris, ciliary body, and choroid)

OVERVIEW

The peripheral nervous system regulates both voluntary and involuntary functions in the human body. This chapter focuses on those drugs that are used to regulate and control disorders in the involuntary functions. The therapeutic agents discussed here are used to treat many disorders and conditions such as hypertension, hypotension, asthma, dysrhythmia, glaucoma, and even runny nose.

ANATOMY REVIEW

- The peripheral nervous system has two divisions the somatic nervous system (SNS) and the autonomic nervous system (ANS) (Figure 6-1).

- The SNS regulates voluntary or conscious functions such as motor movement.

- The autonomic nervous system regulates all involuntary functions such as secretion of hormones; contraction of the heart muscle, blood vessels and bronchioles; and the ability to move substances through the digestive tract.

- The ANS can be further divided into the sympathetic and parasympathetic nervous systems (PNS) (Figures 6-2 and 6-3).

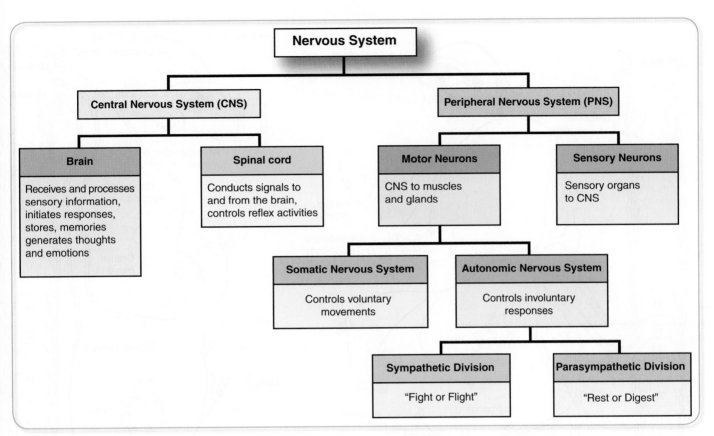

Figure 6-1 Divisions of the nervous system.

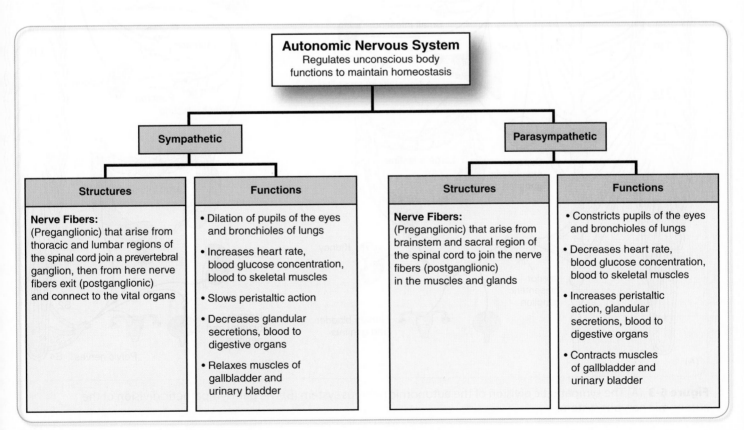

Figure 6-2 The autonomic nervous system.

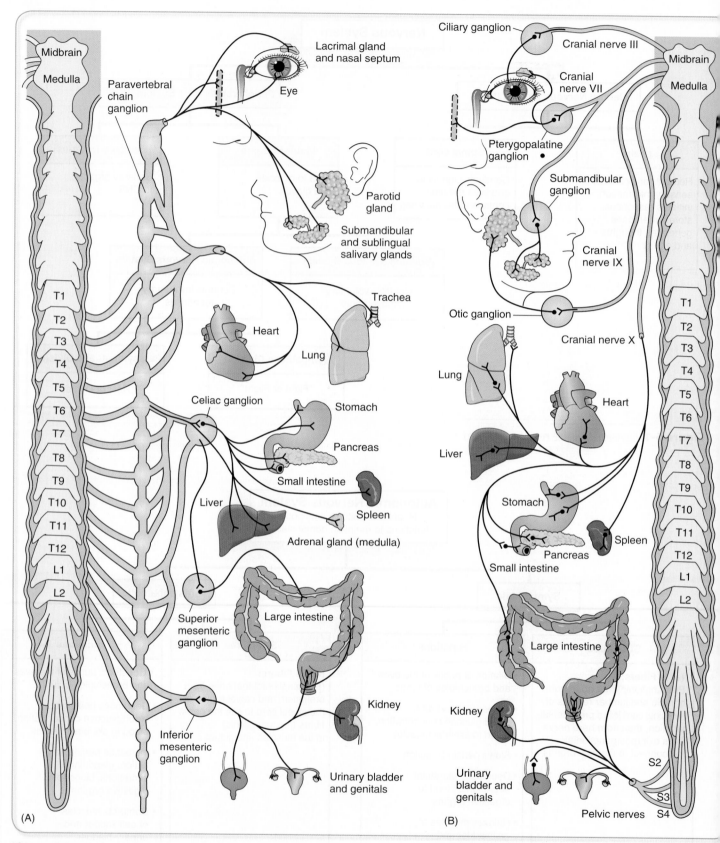

Figure 6-3 (A) The sympathetic division of the autonomic nervous system (B) The parasympathetic division of the autonomic nervous system.

- These divisions work antagonistically, for example, activation of the sympathetic division will increase heart rate while activation of the parasympathetic division will decrease heart rate.

- The sympathetic division responds in emergencies or during stressful situations and is called the fight-or-flight response.

- The parasympathetic division responds as a restorative function and is called the rest-and-digest response.

NEUROTRANSMITTERS ASSOCIATED WITH THE AUTONOMIC NERVOUS SYSTEM

In previous chapters, neurotransmitters are discussed related to the role alterations that these neurotransmitters play in psychiatric illnesses and the treatments of these illnesses. This chapter focuses on the role of neurotransmitters in the involuntary functions of the body regulated by the autonomic nervous system. The three main neurotransmitters discussed are acetylcholine, norepinephrine, and epinephrine. Any given junction in the autonomic nervous system uses only one of these transmitter substances. A fourth compound, dopamine, may also serve as a transmitter, but this role has not been demonstrated conclusively.

In order to understand the mechanism of action of drugs that act upon these neurotransmitters, it is necessary to know the identity of the transmitter employed at each of the junctions of the autonomic nervous system (Figure 6-4).

Acetylcholine is the chemical transmitter employed at most junctions of the ANS as well as at the skeletal muscles. Acetylcholine is the transmitter released by:

1. All preganglionic neurons of the PNS
2. All preganglionic neurons of the SNS
3. All postganglionic neurons of the PNS
4. Most postganglionic neurons of the SNS that go to sweat glands
5. All motor neurons to skeletal muscles

Norepinephrine is the chemical transmitter released by all postganglionic neurons of the SNS. The only exceptions are the postganglionic sympathetic neurons that go to sweat glands, which employ acetylcholine as their transmitter. **Epinephrine** is a major transmitter released by the adrenal medulla.

Medical Terminology Review

preganglionic

pre = before
ganglionic = nerve tissue masses
nerves that lead to nerve tissue masses

postganglionic

post = after
ganglionic = nerve tissue masses
nerves that lead to the specific organs

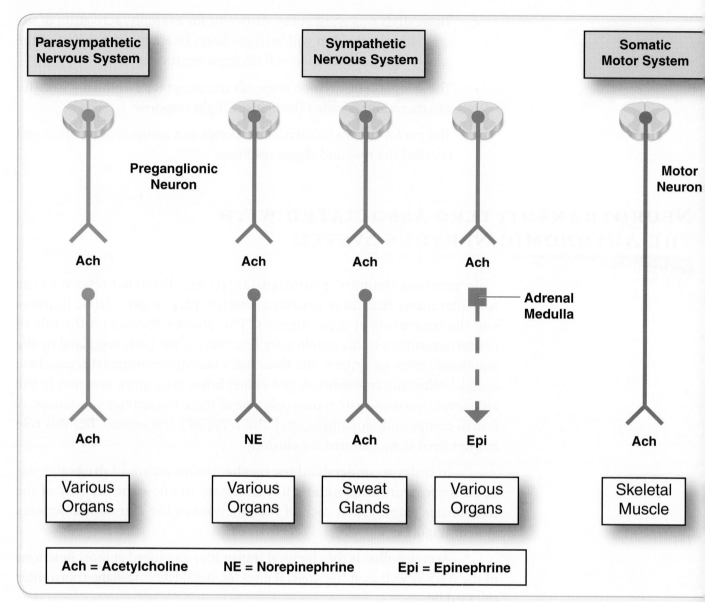

Figure 6-4 Chemical transmitters employed at specific junctions of the peripheral nervous system.

RECEPTORS

The peripheral and autonomic nervous systems work through various types of receptors. Understanding these receptors is essential to understanding nervous system pharmacology.

There are two basic types of receptors associated with the PNS: adrenergic and cholinergic receptors. Each of these receptors is divided into different subtypes. Activation of each subtype of these receptors causes a characteristic set of physiological responses. Some drugs affect all receptor subtypes while others only affect one type of receptor. Different doses of a drug may activate one type of receptor, while increased doses may activate other receptor subtypes. It is important to memorize the various receptor types and their responses.

Cholinergic Receptors

Cholinergic receptors are defined as receptors that mediate responses to acetylcholine. These receptors mediate responses at all junctions where acetylcholine is the transmitter. There are three major subtypes of cholinergic receptors, which are referred to as nicotinic$_N$, nicotinic$_M$, and muscarinic.

Adrenergic Receptors

Adrenergic receptors are defined as receptors that mediate responses to epinephrine (adrenaline) and norepinephrine. These receptors mediate responses at all junctions where norepinephrine or epinephrine is the transmitter. Adrenergic receptors are divided into two types: **alpha-receptors** (α-receptors) and **beta-receptors** (β-receptors). Alpha-receptors are divided into alpha$_1$ and alpha$_2$ receptors, and beta-receptors are divided into beta$_1$ and beta$_2$ receptors.

In addition to the four major subtypes of adrenergic receptors, there is another adrenergic receptor type, referred to as the **dopamine receptor**. Dopamine receptors respond only to dopamine, a neurotransmitter found primarily in the CNS. Tables 6-1 and 6-2 summarize functions of cholinergic and adrenergic receptor subtypes.

TABLE 6-1 Cholinergic Receptor Subtype Functions

Receptor Subtype	Location	Response to Receptor Stimulation
nicotinic$_N$	all autonomic nervous system ganglia and the adrenal medulla	stimulation of both parasympathetic and sympathetic postganglionic nerves and release of epinephrine from the adrenal medulla
nicotinic$_M$	neuromuscular junction	contraction of skeletal muscle
muscarinic	all parasympathetic target organs:	
	eyes	contraction of the ciliary muscle focuses the lens for near vision, and contraction of the iris sphincter muscle causes **miosis** (contraction of the pupil)
	heart	decreased rate
	lungs	constriction of bronchi and increased secretions
	GI tract	salivation, increased gastric secretions, increased intestinal tone and motility, defecation
	sweat glands	generalized sweating
	urinary bladder	increased bladder pressure, relaxation of smooth muscles and sphincter, allowing urine to leave the bladder
	sex organs	erection
	blood vessels	vasodilation

TABLE 6-2   Adrenergic Receptor Subtype Functions

Receptor Subtype	Location	Response to Receptor Stimulation
alpha₁	eyes	contraction of the radial muscle of the iris causes **mydriasis** (pupil dilation)
	arteries	constriction
	veins	constriction
	male sex organs	ejaculation
	prostate capsule	contraction
	bladder	contraction of bladder and sphincter
alpha₂	presynaptic nerve terminals	inhibition of transmitter release
beta₁	heart	increased rate and force of contraction
	kidneys	renin release
beta₂	arterioles of the:	
	heart	dilation
	lungs	dilation
	skeletal	dilation
	muscles of:	
	bronchi	dilation
	uterus	relaxation
	skeletal	increased contraction
	muscle	glycogenolysis (the breakdown of glycogen into glucose, releasing it back into the circulating blood in response to a very low blood sugar level)
	liver	
dopamine	kidneys	dilation of kidney vasculature

DRUGS AFFECTING THE AUTONOMIC NERVOUS SYSTEM

Drugs that affect the ANS may be classified into four categories:

- Sympathomimetics (Adrenergics)

- Sympatholytics (Adrenergic blockers)

- Parasympathomimetics (Cholinergics)

- Parasympatholytics (Anticholinergics)

Sympathomimetics (Adrenergic Drugs)

Sympathomimetic agents are also called adrenergic agonists. These agents produce their effects by activating adrenergic receptors. Since the SNS acts through these same receptors, responses to adrenergic agonists and responses to stimulation of the SNS are very similar.

Adrenergic agonist drugs may affect both alpha- and beta-receptors. The classification seems confusing, therefore, adrenergic drugs on each receptor will be discussed separately. Selected adrenergic agonist drugs are listed in Table 6-3.

Key Concept

Although dopamine receptors are classified as adrenergic, these receptors do not respond to epinephrine or norepinephrine.

Medical Terminology Review

Sympathomimetic

sympatho = related to the sympathetic nervous system
mimetic = an agent that mimics
a drug agent that mimics the actions of the sympathetic nervous system

TABLE 6-3   Sympathomimetics (Adrenergic Drugs)

Generic Name	Trade Name	Route of Administration	Average Adult Dosage
albuterol	Proventil® Ventolin®	PO, Inhalation	PO: 2.4 mg 3-4 times/day; Inhalation: 1-2 q4-6h
dobutamine	Dobutrex®	IV	2.5-10 mcg/kg/min
dopamine hydrochloride	Intropin® Dopamine®	IV	2-5 mcg/kg/min
epinephrine	EpiEZPen®, Primatene Mist Suspension®	SC, Inhalation	SC: 0.1-0.5 mL of 1:1000 q10-15 min prn; Inhalation: 1 inhalation q4h prn
isoproterenol hydrochloride	Isuprel® Dispos-a-Med®	IV, MDI	IV: 0.01-0.02 mg prn; MDI: 1-2 inhalations 4-6 times/day
metaproterenol sulfate	Alupent® Metaprel®	PO, MDI, Nebulizer	PO: 20 mg q6-8h; MDI: 2-3 inhalations q3-4h; Nebulizer: 5-10 inhalations
methyldopa	Aldomet®	PO, IV	PO/IV: 250-500 mg bid or tid
norepinephrine bitartrate	Levarterenol® Levophed®	IV	Start with 8-12 mcg/min; maintenance dose 2-4 mcg/min
oxymetazoline	Afrin®	Intranasal	2-3 drops or 2-3 sprays of 0.05% solution bid
phenylephrine hydrochloride	Neo-Synephrine® Alconefrin®	IM, IV, SC	IM/SC: 1-10 mg q10-15 min prn; IV: 0.1-0.18 mg/min
pseudoephedrine hydrochloride	Sudafed® Cenafed®	PO	60 mg q4-6h
ritodrine	Yutopar®	PO, IV	PO: 10 mg q2h; IV: 50-350 mcg/min
salmeterol xinafoate	Serevent®	Inhalation	2 inhalations of aerosol (42 mcg) bid
terbutaline sulfate	Brethine® Brethaire®	PO, Inhalation, SC	PO: 2.5-5 mg tid; Inhalation: 2 inhalations q4-6h; SC: 0.25 mg q15-30 min up to 0.5 mg in 4h

Mechanism of Action

Adrenergic drugs stimulate both alpha$_1$ and beta$_2$ receptor sites. The alpha-adrenergic receptor sites are located in the smooth muscle of blood vessels, the gastrointestinal tract, and the genitourinary tract. They produce vasoconstriction when stimulated by adrenergic drugs. The beta$_1$-adrenergic receptors are located in the heart muscle. When stimulated by adrenergic drugs, they produce increased contractility (resulting in increased heart rate).

Beta$_2$-adrenergic receptors in the respiratory system, located in the bronchial muscle, produce bronchodilation when stimulated by adrenergic agents.

Indications

Adrenergic agonist drugs that affect alpha-adrenergic receptors are used in patients with hypotension, hemostasis, to relieve nasal congestion, as adjuncts to local anesthesia (to reduce bleeding), and for dilation of the pupils (which facilitates eye examinations and ocular surgery). The beta-adrenergic drugs are used in the treatment of asthma and bronchitis.

Adverse Effects

All of the adverse effects caused by alpha$_1$ activation result directly or indirectly from vasoconstriction. The most common adverse effects include hypertension, **necrosis** (death of a group of cells or tissues) if an IV line is employed to administer an alpha$_1$ agonist, and slowness of the heart rate.

Common adverse effects of beta-adrenergic drugs include headache, tremors, mild leg cramps, nervousness, fatigue, hypertension, palpitation, nausea, vomiting, and shortness of breath.

Contraindications and Precautions

Adrenergic drugs are contraindicated in patients with known hypersensitivity to these agents. These drugs are also contraindicated in the elderly, who are more sensitive to the effects of adrenergic drugs. These drugs should not be given to patients with symptoms such as blurred vision, seizures, chest pain, and palpitations.

Alpha-adrenergic drugs are contraindicated in children younger than 2 years of age. Safe use during pregnancy (category C) or lactation is not established.

Beta adrenergic drugs are contraindicated in cardiac arrhythmias associated with tachycardia, hyperthyroidism, pregnancy (category C), and lactation.

Adrenergic drugs should be used with caution in older adults, hypertension, cardiovascular disorders (including coronary artery disease), hyperthyroidism, and diabetes.

Drug Interactions

No clinically significant drug interactions have been established for alpha-adrenergic agents. Beta-adrenergic drugs may interact with general anesthetics (especially cyclopropane and halothane).

Sympatholytics (Adrenergic Blockers)

Sympatholytic agents (or **adrenergic blocker agents**) produce many of the same responses as the parasympathomimetics. These drugs are the most commonly prescribed class of autonomic drugs. Adrenergic blocker agents are also effective on all adrenergic alpha- and beta-receptors. Selected adrenergic antagonists or adrenergic blockers are listed in Table 6-4.

TABLE 6-4 Sympatholytics (Adrenergic Blockers)

Generic Name	Trade Name	Route of Administration	Average Adult Dosage
acebutolol	Sectral®	PO	400-800 mg/day
atenolol	Tenormin®	PO	25-50 mg/day
carteolol	Cartrol®	PO	2.5 mg once/day
carvedilol	Coreg®	PO	3.125 mg b.i.d.
doxazosin mesylate	Cardura®	PO	1-16 mg h.s.
esmolol hydrochloride	Brevibloc®	IV	500 mcg/kg loading dose followed by 50 mcg/kg/min
metoprolol tartrate	Lopressor®	PO	50-100 mg/day
nadolol	Corgard®	PO	40 mg once/day
phentolamine	Regitine®	IM, IV	IM/IV: 5 mg 1-2h before surgery
prazosin hydrochloride	Minipress®	PO	Start with 1 mg h.s., then 1 mg b.i.d. or tid
propranolol hydrochloride	Inderal®	PO, IV	PO: 10-40 mg b.i.d.; IV: 0.5-3 mg q4h prn
sotalol hydrochloride	Betapace®	PO	40-160 mg b.i.d.
tamsulosin hydrochloride	Flomax®	PO	0.4 mg q.d. 30 min. after a meal
terazosin	Hytrin®	PO	1-5 mg/day
timolol maleate	Blocadren®, Timoptic®	PO	10-60 mg b.i.d.

Medical Terminology Review

sympatholytic

sympatho = related to the sympathetic nervous system
lytic = opposing effects
a drug that acts to oppose the actions of the sympathetic nervous system

---

Mechanism of Action

Adrenergic blockers reduce delivery of **catecholamines** to the adrenergic receptors by disrupting catecholamine synthesis, storage, or release.

Indications

Adrenergic blockers are used in treatment of hypertension, dysrhythmias, angina, heart failure, glaucoma, and migraines.

Adverse Effects

Adverse effects of adrenergic blockers include orthostatic hypotension, edema, headache, dizziness, vertigo, **somnolence** (prolonged drowsiness), fatigue, nervousness, and anxiety. These agents may also cause abdominal pain, nausea, vomiting, diarrhea, and exacerbation of peptic ulcer.

Adverse effects of beta-adrenergic blockers include respiratory disturbances, bradycardia, peripheral vascular insufficiency, palpitations, postural hypotension, behavioral changes, blurred vision, and dry eyes.

Contraindications and Precautions

Alpha adrenergic blockers are contraindicated in patients with known hypersensitivity to these agents, and those patients with hypotension or syncope. Safe use during pregnancy (category D) or in children is not established.

Beta adrenergic blockers are contraindicated in patients with sinus bradycardia, heart failure, peripheral vascular disease, hypotension, or pulmonary edema. Safety during pregnancy (category D) or lactation is not established.

Alpha adrenergic blockers must be used cautiously in patients with hepatic impairment, renal disease, or lactation.

Beta adrenergics are used with caution in hypertensive patients with congestive heart failure controlled by digitalis, and with diuretics, in vasospastic angina, asthma, bronchitis, emphysema, major depression, diabetes mellitus, impaired renal function, myasthenia gravis, hyperthyroidism, pheochromocytoma, and in older adults.

> **Medical Terminology Review**
>
> **pheochromocytoma**
> *pheo = dusky or gray*
> *chromo = related to chromaffin cells*
> *cytoma = cell tumor*
> a pigmented tumor of the chromaffin cells (adrenal gland)

Drug Interactions

Atropine and other anticholinergics may increase absorption of adrenergic blockers from the gastrointestinal (GI) tract.

Parasympathomimetics (Cholinergic Drugs)

Parasympathomimetic or cholinergic agonist drugs are able to mimic action of the PNS. Table 6-5 shows selected parasympathomimetic drugs.

Mechanism of Action

Some cholinergic drugs increase concentration of acetylcholine at cholinergic transmission sites, which prolongs and exaggerates their action. Others produce reversible cholinesterase inhibition and have direct stimulant action on voluntary muscle fibers.

Indications

Cholinergic agonist drugs are used most commonly in glaucoma by inducing miosis. Specific muscarinic agonist drugs may be used in the treatment of atonic constipation, **congenital megacolon**, and in postoperative or postpartum adynamic intestinal ileus. Bethanechol has been used to increase the tone of the lower esophageal sphincter in the diagnosis or treatment of reflux esophagitis. Muscarinic agonists are useful in the treatment of nonobstructive urinary retention and neurogenic atony of the urinary bladder with retention. Cholinergic agonist drugs are also used for dysrhythmias and for Alzheimer's disease.

TABLE 6-5 Parasympathomimetics (Cholinergic Drugs)

Generic Name	Trade Name	Route of Administration	Average Adult Dosage
bethanechol chloride	Urecholine®	PO	10-50 mg b.i.d. to q.i.d.
cevimeline hydrochloride	Evoxac®	PO	30 mg t.i.d.
neostigmine	Prostigmin®	PO, IM, IV	PO: 15-375 mg/day; IM: 0.022 mg/kg; IV: 0.5-2.5 mg slowly
physostigmine salicylate	Antilirium®	IM, IV	IM/IV: 0.5-3 mg
pilocarpine hydrochloride	Isopto Carpine®, Salagen®	PO, Ophthalmic	PO: 5-10 mg t.i.d.; Ophthalmic: 1 drop of 1-2% solution in affected eye q5-10 min for 3-6 doses
pyridostigmine	Mestinon®	PO	60 mg-1.5 g/day
rivastigmine tartrate	Exelon®	PO	1.5-6 mg b.i.d.
tacrine	Cognex®	PO	10 mg q.i.d.

Adverse Effects

Undesirable effects of cholinergic agonist drugs include flushing, sweating, abdominal cramps, difficulty in visual accommodation, headache, and convulsions (at high doses). Specific GI adverse effects include epigastric distress, diarrhea, involuntary defecation, nausea and vomiting, and colic. Other adverse effects are asthma and excessive salivary, nasopharyngeal, and bronchial secretions.

Contraindications and Precautions

Cholinergic agonist drugs are contraindicated in patients with known hypersensitivity to these agents: hypertension, coronary insufficiency, **pheochromocytoma** (benign tumor of adrenal medulla that increases production of epinephrine and norepinephrine), hyperthyroidism, asthma, and peptic ulcer.

Muscarinic drugs should be used cautiously in patients with hypertension, coronary disease, asthma, and hyperthyroidism.

Drug Interactions

Procainamide, quinidine, atropine, and epinephrine antagonize the effects of bethanechol. Beta-adrenergic agonists may cause conduction disturbances that may have additive effects with cholinergic drugs.

Neostigmine antagonizes effects of tubocurarine, atracurium, procainamide, quinidine, and atropine. Physostigmine may antagonize effects of echothiophate and isoflurophate.

Parasympatholytics (Anticholinergics or Cholinergic Blockers)

All parasympathetic effectors, some sympathetic effectors, all autonomic ganglia, and voluntary muscles bear cholinergic receptors. As a consequence, cholinergic drugs may affect the function of both divisions of the autonomic nervous system. Anticholinergic drugs are shown in Table 6-6.

Mechanism of Action

Cholinergic blockers act by selectively blocking all muscarine responses to acetylcholine, whether excitatory or inhibitory. Cholinergic blockers depress the CNS and relieve rigidity and tremor of Parkinson's syndrome.

TABLE 6-6 Parasympatholytics (Anticholinergics or Cholinergic Blockers)

Generic Name	Trade Name	Route of Administration	Average Adult Dosage
atropine sulfate	Atropisol®, Isopto Atropine®	IV, IM, SC, Ophthalmic	IV/IM/SC: 0.4–0.6 mg 30-60 min before surgery; Ophthalmic: 1-2 drops t.i.d.
benztropine mesylate	Cogentin®	PO	0.5-6 mg/day
cyclopentolate	Cyclogyl®	Topical	1 drop of 1% solution in eye 40-50 min. before procedure, followed by 1 drop in 5 min.
dicyclomine hydrochloride	Bentyl®	PO, IM	PO: 20-40 mg q.i.d.; IM: 20 mg q.i.d.
glycopyrrolate	Robinul®	PO, IM, IV	PO: 1-2 mg t.i.d.; IM/IV: 0.1-0.2 mg as single dose t.i.d. or q.i.d.
ipratropium bromide	Atrovent®	Inhalation	2 inhalations of MDI q.i.d. at no less than 4h intervals
oxybutynin	Ditropan®	PO	5 mg b.i.d. or t.i.d.
propantheline	Pro-Banthine®	PO	15 mg 30 min. a.c. and 30 mg h.s.
scopolamine	Hyoscine®, Transderm-Scop®	PO, IM, IV, SC	PO: 0.5-1 mg; IM/IV/SC: 0.3-0.6 mg
tiotropium bromide	Spiriva®	Inhalation	Inhale the contents of one capsule daily using hand inhaler device provided

Antisecretory action of cholinergic blockers includes suppression of sweating, lacrimation, salivation, and secretions from the nose, mouth, and bronchi.

Indications

Cholinergic blockers are used as adjuncts in the symptomatic treatment of GI disorders (i.e., peptic ulcer, pylorospasm, GI hypermotility, irritable bowel syndrome, and spastic disorders of the biliary tract). Cholinergic blockers are prescribed to produce mydriasis, **cycloplegia** (paralysis of the ciliary muscles of the eye) before refraction, and for the treatment of anterior **uveitis** (inflammation of the middle layer of the eye) and **iritis** (inflammation of the iris). These agents are also used in general anesthesia, bradycardia, or asystole during CPR.

Adverse Effects

The main adverse effects of cholinergic blockers include headache, ataxia, dizziness, excitement, irritability, convulsions, drowsiness, fatigue, weakness, mental depression, confusion, disorientation, hallucinations, hypertension or hypotension, ventricular fibrillation, inability to swallow, difficulty passing urine, skin eruption, and loss of power in the ciliary muscles of the eye.

Contraindications and Precautions

Cholinergic blockers are contraindicated in patients with hypersensitivity to belladonna alkaloids, synechiae, angle-closure glaucoma, parotitis, obstructive uropathy, intestinal atony, paralytic ileus, obstructive GI tract diseases, severe ulcerative colitis, toxic megacolon, tachycardia, acute hemorrhage, or myasthenia gravis. Safety during pregnancy (category C) or lactation is not established.

Cholinergic blockers are used with caution in patients with myocardial infarction, hypertension or hypotension, coronary artery disease, congestive heart failure (CHF), and irregular heart rhythms. Other conditions wherein cholinergic blockers should be used cautiously include: gastric ulcer, GI infections, hiatal hernia with reflux esophagitis, hyperthyroidism, chronic lung disease, and hepatic or renal disease. These blockers should be used cautiously in the following types of patients: older adults, debilitated patients, children under the age of 6 years, Down syndrome patients, those with autonomic neuropathy or spastic paralysis, children with brain damage, those exposed to high environmental temperatures, and in patients with fever.

Drug Interactions

Key Concept

Because the thermal regulatory system in elderly patients declines, hyperthermia is possible with anticholinergics. This happens because these drugs decrease sweating.

Cholinergic blockers may interact with amantadine, antihistamines, tricyclic antidepressants, quinidine, and procainamide, which may add to the anticholinergic effects. The effects of levodopa are decreased with cholinergic blockers. Methotrimeprazine may precipitate extrapyramidal effects. The antipsychotic effects of phenothiazines are decreased due to decreased absorption.

SUMMARY

The portion of the PNS serving involuntary effectors is called the autonomic nervous system or ANS. The sympathetic and parasympathetic nervous systems are subdivisions of the ANS.

Three neurotransmitters play a role in the functions regulated by the autonomic nervous system: acetylcholine, norepinephrine, and epinephrine. Dopamine may also serve as a nervous system transmitter.

There are two basic types of receptors associated with the ANS: cholinergic receptors and adrenergic receptors. There are three major subtypes of cholinergic receptors, which are referred to as nicotinic$_N$, nicotinic$_M$, and muscarinic. There are four major subtypes of adrenergic receptors, which include alpha$_1$, alpha$_2$, beta$_1$, and beta$_2$.

Drugs that affect the ANS may be classified into four categories: sympathomimetics (adrenergic agonists), sympatholytics (adrenergic blockers), parasympathomimetics (cholinergic agonists), and parasympatholytics (anticholinergics).

EXPLORING THE WEB

Visit *http://cvpharmacology.com*

- Click on the link "vasodilators." Research additional information on this drug class and the variations of drugs within this class. Record your findings to help further your understanding of the topics discussed in this chapter.

Visit *www.anaesthetist.com*

- Click on the link "autonomic physiology." Read additional information about the autonomic nervous system to enhance your understanding of its functions.

Visit *www.pharmacology2000.com*

- Click on the link "Chapter 4: Autonomic Introduction." Explore the discussions related to the autonomic nervous system and the drug classes that affect this system.

REVIEW QUESTIONS

Multiple Choice

1. Dopamine, epinephrine, and isoproterenol are classified as which of the following types of drug?

   A. sympatholytics
   B. anticholinergics

    C. adrenergics
    D. cholinergic-blockers

2. Which of the following agents are used to treat patients with myasthenia gravis?

    A. sympathomimetics (adrenergics)
    B. sympatholytics (adrenergic blockers)
    C. parasympatholytics (anticholinergics)
    D. parasympathomimetics (cholinergics)

3. Propranolol, metoprolol, and atenolol are:

    A. parasympathomimetics
    B. adrenergic drugs
    C. anticholinergic drugs
    D. beta-adrenergic blocking drugs

4. Elderly patients receiving anticholinergic drugs should be monitored closely for which of the following adverse effects?

    A. hyperthermia
    B. diuresis
    C. bradycardia
    D. hypothermia

5. The ANS employs all of the following neurotransmitters, *except*:

    A. epinephrine
    B. serotonin
    C. norepinephrine
    D. acetylcholine

6. Sympathomimetic drugs are also known as:

    A. cholinergics
    B. anticholinergics
    C. adrenergics
    D. adrenergic blockers

7. Which of the following adrenergic receptor subtypes may cause mydriasis?

    A. $alpha_1$
    B. $alpha_2$
    C. $beta_1$
    D. $beta_2$

8. Dobutamine is used to treat cardiac decompensation because of its action as a(n):

    A. beta adrenergic
    B. adrenergic blocking agent
    C. anticholinergic
    D. cholinergic

9. Atenolol may best be described as a(n):

    A. $beta_2$-adrenergic blocker
    B. $alpha_1$-adrenergic blocker

C. beta$_1$-and beta$_2$-adrenergic blocker

D. beta$_1$-adrenergic blocker

10. Which of the following agents is indicated for the treatment of anterior uveitis and iritis?

    A. timolol

    B. atropine

    C. nadolol

    D. bethanechol

11. Which of the following drugs are contraindicated in patients with hypertension, asthma, hyperthyroidism, and peptic ulcer?

    A. cholinergic agonists

    B. anticholinergics

    C. adrenergic blockers

    D. adrenergic agonists

12. Which of the following describes pilocarpine?

    A. direct-acting mydriatic agent

    B. direct-acting miotic agent

    C. reduces the delivery of catecholamine

    D. stimulates alpha receptor sites

13. Which of the following agents is classified as a sympatholytic?

    A. neostigmine (Prostigmin)

    B. cevimeline (Evoxac)

    C. pilocarpine (Isopto Carpine)

    D. prazosin (Minipress)

14. Which of the following statements is true of scopolamine?

    A. it is an anticholinergic

    B. it is an anticoagulant

    C. it is a thrombolytic agent

    D. it is an adrenergic blocker

15. Which of the following agents is used prior to anesthesia?

    A. scopolamine

    B. cyclopentolate

    C. atropine

    D. oxybutynin

True or False

_____ T _____ 1. All of the adverse effects caused by alpha$_1$ activation result in vasoconstriction.

_____ F _____ 2. Sympathomimetics are also called adrenergic blockers.

_____ F _____ 3. Adrenergic blockers are used in the treatment of hypotension.

_____ F _____ 4. The sympathetic nervous system's responses are also called rest-and-digest responses.

_____ 5. Norepinephrine is released by all postganglionic neurons of the sympathetic nervous system.

_____ 6. Muscarinic cholinergics may cause miosis.

_____ 7. Adrenergic agonist drugs may affect both alpha- and beta-receptors.

_____ 8. Prostigmin is the trade name of neostigmine.

_____ 9. All preganglionic neurons of the parasympathetic nervous system release acetylcholine.

_____ 10. Acetylcholine is a major transmitter released by the adrenal medulla.

Critical Thinking

A 61-year-old man has been diagnosed with glaucoma. He has recently had abdominal surgery. He has developed postoperative adynamic intestinal ileus.

1. Which class of autonomic nervous system drugs is the best for glaucoma and postoperative adynamic intestinal ileus?

2. If the patient is taking the drug of choice for these two conditions, what would be the most common adverse effects?

3. If the patient has asthma and hyperthyroidism, can the drug of choice still be used?

Drug Therapy for Parkinson's and Alzheimer's Diseases

OBJECTIVES

After completing this chapter, the reader should be able to:

1. Identify the most common degenerative diseases of the CNS.
2. Explain the cause of Parkinson's disease.
3. Classify the drugs that are used for the treatment of Parkinson's disease.
4. Describe the roles of dopamine and acetylcholine in Parkinson's disease.
5. Identify the characteristics of dopamine and levodopa.
6. Discuss the actions and adverse effects of dopaminergic drugs when used in the treatment of Parkinson's disease.
7. Discuss the actions and contraindications of cholinergic blocker drugs when used in the treatment of Parkinson's disease.
8. Identify the characteristics of Alzheimer's disease.
9. Explain the role of acetylcholinesterase inhibitors in the treatment of Alzheimer's disease.

GLOSSARY

Alzheimer's disease – a disorder causing severe cognitive dysfunction in older persons in which the brain experiences atrophy (shrinkage) and exhibits senile plaques

Atrophy – wasting away or "without development"

Basal nuclei – clusters of nerve cells at the base of the brain; responsible for body movement and coordination

Bradykinesia – a decrease in spontaneity and movement, as seen in Parkinson's disease

Corpus striatum – a layer of nervous tissue within the brain

Encephalitis – inflammation of the brain's connective tissue framework

Parkinson's disease – a neurological syndrome usually resulting from deficiency of dopamine because of degenerative, vascular, or inflammatory changes in the basal ganglia

Substantia nigra – pigmented cells in the midbrain responsible for the production of dopamine

Tremor – repetitive, often regular, oscillatory movements caused by alternate, or synchronous, but irregular contraction of opposing muscle groups

OVERVIEW

Degenerative diseases of the central nervous system (CNS) include Alzheimer's disease, multiple sclerosis, Huntington's chorea, and Parkinson's disease. In this chapter, focus will be on Parkinson's and Alzheimer's diseases, which are more common than other related diseases and affect millions of people (mostly elderly patients) in the United States.

PARKINSON'S DISEASE

Parkinson's disease is a progressive degenerative disorder affecting motor function through the loss of extrapyramidal activity. This disease is characterized by muscle **tremor**, muscle rigidity, and **bradykinesia**, and disturbances of posture and equilibrium are often present (see Figure 7-1).

> **Medical Terminology Review**
>
> **bradykinesia**
> *brady = slow*
> *kinesia = ability of movement*
> slowing in the ability to move

According to the National Parkinson's Alliance, it is estimated that as many as 1.5 million Americans have Parkinson's disease. This disorder causes dysfunction and changes in the **basal nuclei** (clusters of nerve cells at the base of the brain), principally in the **substantia nigra** (pigmented cells in the midbrain responsible for the production of dopamine). In this condition, a decreased number of neurons in the brain secrete dopamine, an inhibitory neurotransmitter, leading to an imbalance between excitation and inhibition in the basal nuclei. The cause of the disease is not fully understood, but it is believed to be associated with an imbalance of the neurotransmitters acetylcholine and dopamine in the brain (see Figure 7-2).

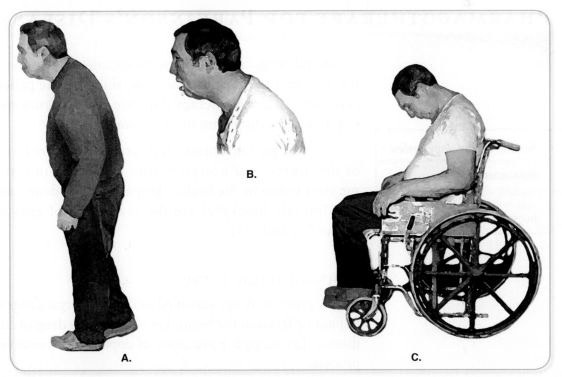

A.   B.   C.

Figure 7-1 Parkinson's disease is characterized by a shuffling gait and early postural changes.

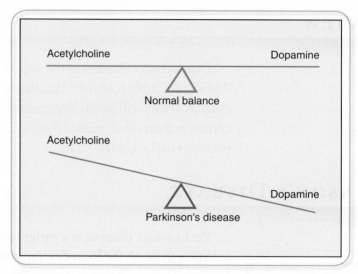

Figure 7-2 Dopamine imbalance exhibited in Parkinson's disease.

The excess stimulation affects movement and posture by increasing muscle tone and activity, leading to resting tremors, muscular rigidity, difficulty in initiating movement, and postural instability. Parkinson's disease usually develops after age 60 and occurs in both men and women. It may occur following **encephalitis**, trauma, or vascular disease. Drug-induced Parkinson's disease is particularly linked to use of phenothiazines (e.g., chlorpromazine). Pharmacotherapy is often successful in reducing some of the distressing symptoms of this disease.

Medical Terminology Review
encephalitis
encephal = brain
itis = inflammation
inflammation of the brain

PHARMACOTHERAPY FOR PARKINSON'S DISEASE

Several drugs can be used for Parkinson's disease; the goal of drug therapy for this condition is to increase the ability of the patient to perform daily activities. Pharmacotherapy does not cure Parkinson's disease, but it can dramatically reduce symptoms in some patients.

Anti-parkinsonism drugs are administered to restore the balance of dopamine and acetylcholine in the **corpus striatum** (layers of nervous tissue in the brain). Dopaminergic drugs and anticholinergics (cholinergic blockers) are the mainstays of anti-parkinsonism (see Tables 7-1 and 7-2).

Medical Terminology Review
dopaminergic
dopamin = dopamine
ergic = related to
drugs affecting dopamine

Dopaminergic Drugs

The group of drugs classified as dopaminergic drugs are used to increase dopamine levels in the brain. Levodopa is the drug of choice for Parkinson's disease. Levodopa is a precursor of dopamine formation and stimulates this process.

TABLE 7-1 Dopaminergic Drugs for Parkinsonism

Generic Name	Trade Name	Route of Administration	Average Adult Dosage
amantadine hydrochloride	Symmetrel®	PO	200 mg/day or 100 b.i.d.
bromocriptine mesylate	Parlodel®	PO	1.25–2.5 mg/day (max: 7.5 mg/day in div. doses)
carbidopa-levodopa	Sinemet®	PO	1 tablet of 10 mg carbidopa/ 100 mg levodopa, or 25 mg carbidopa/100 mg levodopa t.i.d. (max: 6 tablets/day)
levodopa	Larodopa®	PO	500 mg–1 g/day, may be increased by 750 mg q3–7 days
pergolide mesylate	Permax®	PO	Start with 0.05 mg/day for 2 days, increase by 0.1–0.15 mg/day q3 days for 12 days, then increase by 0.25 mg every third day (max: 5 mg/day)
pramipexole	Mirapex®	PO	Start with 0.125 mg t.i.d. for 1 week; double dose for the next week, increasing by 0.25 mg/dose t.i.d. q week to a max dose of 1.5 mg t.i.d.
ropinirole hydrochloride	Requip®	PO	Start with 0.25 mg t.i.d., increasing by 0.25 mg/dose t.i.d. q week to a max dose of 1 mg t.i.d.
selegiline hydrochloride	Carbex®, Eldepryl®	PO	5 mg/dose b.i.d. – Note: doses greater than 10 mg/day are potentially toxic
tolcapone	Tasmar®	PO	100 mg t.i.d. (max: 600 mg/day)

TABLE 7-2 Anticholinergic Drugs for Parkinsonism

Generic Name	Trade Name	Route of Administration	Average Adult Dosage
benztropine mesylate	Cogentin®	PO	0.5–1 mg/day, increasing p.r.n. (max: 6 mg/day)
biperiden hydrochloride	Akineton®	PO	2 mg/day to q.i.d.
diphenhydramine hydrochloride	Benadryl®	PO	25–50 mg t.i.d.-q.i.d. (max: 300/day)
procyclidine hydrochloride	Kemadrin®	PO	2.5 mg t.i.d. pc; may increase to 5 mg t.i.d. if tolerated, with an additional 5 mg at bedtime (max: 45–60 mg/day)
trihexyphenidyl	Artane®, Trihexy®	PO	1 mg for day 1; doubled for day 2; increased by 2 mg q3–5 days up to 6–10 mg/day (max: 15 mg/day)

Mechanism of Action

Dopaminergic agents restore the neurotransmitter dopamine in the extrapyramidal region of the brain. Levodopa can cross the blood-brain barrier, but dopamine cannot. Therefore, dopamine by itself is not used for the treatment of Parkinson's disease. The mechanism of action of amantadine and selegiline in the treatment of Parkinsonism is not fully understood.

Indications

Levodopa is considered the drug of choice for Parkinson's disease. Either carbidopa is combined with levodopa, or they are prescribed as two separate drugs. Amantadine is less effective than levodopa as a drug therapy for Parkinson's disease, but more effective than the cholinergic blockers. Amantadine is given alone or in combination with another anti-parkinsonism drug with cholinergic activity. Amantadine is also indicated for drug therapy for viral disorders.

Adverse Effects

Adverse effects of levodopa include increased, uncontrollable rhythmic hand shaking or trembling, grinding of teeth (bruxism), muscle incoordination, numbness, fatigue, and headache. Levodopa may also cause upright position hypotension, tachycardia, hypertension, nausea, vomiting, dry mouth, bitter taste, and hepatotoxicity.

Adverse effects of bromocriptine include headache, dizziness, vertigo, fainting, sedation, nightmares, and insomnia. It may also produce blurred vision, hypertension, palpitation, arrhythmias, nausea, vomiting, and diarrhea. The most serious adverse effects of amantadine are orthostatic hypotension, congestive heart failure, depression, psychosis, convulsions, leukopenia, and urinary retention.

Contraindications and Precautions

The dopaminergic drugs are contraindicated in patients with known hypersensitivity to these agents. Levodopa should be avoided in patients with narrow-angle glaucoma, those receiving an MAO inhibitor (MAOI) and during lactation.

Dopaminergic drugs are used with caution in patients with renal or hepatic disease, bronchial asthma, cardiovascular disease, and peptic ulcer. These agents should be used cautiously during pregnancy (category C) and lactation.

Drug Interactions

Levodopa increases therapeutic effects and possibility of a hypertensive crisis with MAOIs. Withdrawal of MAOIs is necessary at least 14 days before levodopa therapy is started. Levodopa exhibits decreased efficacy with pyridoxine (vitamin B_6) and phenytoin.

Medical Terminology Review

hepatotoxicity
  hepato = liver
  toxicity = state of being toxic or poisonous
liver poisoning

leukopenia
  leuk/o = white
  -penia = decrease in
decrease in white blood cells

Key Concept

Hallucinations occur commonly in older adults when taking dopamine receptor agonists.

Key Concept

Patients taking levodopa should be monitored for orthostatic hypotension and cardiac arrhythmias, and also watched for psychiatric disturbances.

Key Concept

Patients taking levodopa should avoid foods and medications containing substantial amounts of pyridoxine (vitamin B_6).

Cholinergic Blockers

Cholinergic blockers, or anticholinergic drugs, are able to change the balance between dopamine and acetylcholine in the brain.

Mechanism of Action

Cholinergic blockers act by inhibiting excess cholinergic stimulation of neurons in the brain. Anticholinergic drugs inhibit acetylcholine in the central nervous system.

Indications

Cholinergic blockers are used as adjunctive therapy to relieve Parkinsonism symptoms and in the control of drug-induced disorders such as postural tremor and chorea.

Adverse Effects

Cholinergic blockers produce dry mouth, blurred vision, sedation, dizziness, tachycardia, and constipation. Other adverse effects include urinary retention, dysuria, muscle weakness, confusion, disorientation, and skin rash.

Contraindications and Precautions

Anticholinergic drugs are contraindicated in patients with known hypersensitivity to these agents. These drugs are also contraindicated in those with peptic ulcers, duodenal obstruction, glaucoma (angle-closure), prostatic hypertrophy, myasthenia gravis, and an extreme dilation of the large intestine.

Anticholinergic drugs should be used cautiously in patients with cardiac arrhythmias, hypertension, hypotension, and liver or kidney dysfunction.

Drug Interactions

Cholinergic blockers interact with many drugs. These agents should not be taken with alcohol, MAO inhibitors (MAOIs) tricycline, procainamide, phenothiazines, or quinidine because of combined sedative effects.

> **Medical Terminology Review**
>
> **dysuria**
>
> *dys- = difficult*
> *-uria = characteristic of urine*
> difficult urination

> **Key Concept**
>
> *Elderly people are very sensitive to anticholinergics, and these drugs must be used only when the patient can be carefully observed, because confusion and disorientation are often reported.*

ALZHEIMER'S DISEASE

Alzheimer's disease (senile disease complex) has been demonstrated to be one of the most common causes of severe cognitive dysfunction in older persons. Pathologically, the brain experiences **atrophy** (shrinkage) and exhibits senile plaques. The exact cause of Alzheimer's disease is unknown, but current theories include loss of neurotransmitter stimulation by choline acetyltransferase.

Alzheimer's disease is a devastating illness characterized by progressive memory failure, impaired thinking, confusion, disorientation, personality

changes, restlessness, speech disturbances, and the inability to perform routine tasks. Unfortunately, the disease is incurable and, according to the American Health Assistance Foundation, affects about 350,000 new individuals per year in the United States. The current pharmacotherapy is focused on improving cognitive functioning or limiting the disease progression and controlling symptoms. In Alzheimer's disease, acetylcholine is decreased (this chemical substance is necessary for neurotransmission and for forming memories). There is no specific test for this disease; therefore, a definitive diagnosis is possible only upon autopsy.

PHARMACOTHERAPY FOR ALZHEIMER'S DISEASE

The FDA has approved only a few medications for Alzheimer's disease. Table 7-3 lists drugs used for the treatment of this disease. These agents are classified as acetylcholinesterase inhibitors.

Mechanism of Action

Acetylcholinesterase inhibitors are centrally acting agents, leading to elevated acetylcholine levels in the brain. Therefore, their action slows the neuronal degradation that occurs in Alzheimer's disease, and improves memory in cases of mild to moderate Alzheimer's dementia. Patients should receive pharmacotherapy for at least six months prior to assessing the maximum benefits of drug therapy.

Indications

Acetylcholinesterase inhibitors are used in the treatment of mild to moderate dementia of the Alzheimer's type.

TABLE 7-3   Drugs Used to Treat Alzheimer's Disease

Generic Name	Trade Name	Route of Administration	Average Adult Dosage
donepezil hydrochloride	Aricept®	PO	5–10 mg h.s.
galantamine hydrobromide	Razadyne®	PO	Start with 4 mg b.i.d. (at least 4 weeks); increase by 4 mg b.i.d. q4wk to 12 mg b.i.d. (max: 8–16 mg b.i.d.)
rivastigmine tartrate	Exelon®	PO	Start with 1.5 mg b.i.d. with food; increase by 1.5 mg b.i.d. q2wk if tolerated to 3–6 mg b.i.d. (max: 12 mg b.i.d.)
tacrine	Cognex®	PO	10 mg q.i.d.; increase in 40 mg/day increments q6wk (max: 160 mg/day)

Adverse Effects

There is a significant risk of liver damage from using tacrine, but increases in liver enzymes (which indicate damage) can be monitored with regular blood tests. Adverse effects of acetylcholinesterase inhibitors generally include nausea and vomiting, diarrhea, heartburn, muscle pain, and headache. Donepezil may cause darkened urine. Other adverse effects of acetylcholinesterase inhibitors include an inability to sleep, a sudden drop in blood pressure, depression, irritability, and headache.

Contraindications and Precautions

Acetylcholinesterase inhibitors are contraindicated in patients with known hypersensitivity to these agents. Acetylcholinesterase inhibitors are also contraindicated in patients with liver or kidney impairment, in pregnancy (category B), and lactation.

Acetylcholinesterase inhibitors should be used cautiously in patients with cardiac disorders, asthma, enlargement of the prostate, a history of seizures or GI bleeding, and renal or hepatic disease.

Drug Interactions

Donepezil and tacrine increase effects and risk of toxicity with theophylline and cholinesterase inhibitors. They decrease effects of anticholinergics and increase risk of GI bleeding with NSAIDs. Phenobarbital, phenytoin, dexamethasone, and rifampin may speed elimination of donepezil. Tacrine may prolong the action of succinylcholine.

Key Concept

Ginkgo is a natural remedy, and one of the oldest known herbs in the world. Gingko extract is most commonly used in treating dementia. Adverse effects include gastrointestinal upset, muscle cramps, bleeding, and headache.

SUMMARY

Parkinson's and Alzheimer's diseases are among the most common degenerative diseases of the CNS. Multiple sclerosis and Huntington's chorea are other degenerative diseases. **Parkinson's** disease is a degenerative disorder of the CNS resulting in the death of neurons that produce dopamine. It affects over 1.5 million Americans. Parkinson's disease is primarily seen in patients over the age of 60, and occurs in both men and women.

The goal of drug therapy for Parkinson's disease is to increase the ability of the patient to perform daily activities. Anti-parkinsonism agents are given to restore the balance of dopamine and acetylcholine in the brain. Dopaminergic drugs and anticholinergics are the mainstays of anti-parkinsonism.

Alzheimer's disease is another degenerative disorder of the CNS, and is characterized by progressive memory failure, impaired thinking, confusion, disorientation, and speech disturbances. It is very common, and affects about 350,000 new individuals per year in the United States. In Alzheimer's disease, acetylcholine (which is necessary for forming memories) is decreased. Unfortunately, the disease is incurable. The FDA has approved only a few medications for Alzheimer's disease to reduce its symptoms. These drugs are known as acetylcholinesterase inhibitors.

EXPLORING THE WEB

Visit *http://jaapa.com*

- Find the August 2006 issue, and read the article "Pharmacotherapy for Parkinson's Disease: Current Options, Promising Future Therapies."

Visit *www.alz.org*

- Learn more about Alzheimer's disease and review information on treatments and research related to pharmacological therapies.

Visit *www.nlm.nih.gov*

- Click on the link "Medline Plus". Search for additional information on Parkinson's disease and Alzheimer's disease.

REVIEW QUESTIONS

Multiple Choice

1. Which of the following drugs may induce Parkinson's disease?
   - A. pyridoxine (vitamin B_6)
   - B. chlorpromazine
   - C. dopamine
   - D. levodopa

2. The mechanism of action of amantadine in the treatment of Parkinsonism is
   A. to inhibit the effect of GABA
   B. to prevent the production of dopamine
   C. to inhibit the effect of acetylcholine
   D. unknown

3. Which of the following agents is the drug of choice for Parkinson's disease?
   A. levodopa
   B. aspirin
   C. amantadine
   D. pyridoxine

4. Anticholinergic drugs are contraindicated in patients who have which of the following conditions?
   A. Parkinsonism
   B. glaucoma
   C. hypocalcemia
   D. cataracts

5. Dopaminergic drugs should be used cautiously during pregnancy because they are included in which of the following pregnancy categories?
   A. D
   B. C
   C. B
   D. A

6. Which of the following brain chemicals, necessary for forming memories, is decreased in Alzheimer's disease?
   A. dopamine
   B. epinephrine
   C. melatonin
   D. acetylcholine

7. Which of the following agents is used in Alzheimer's disease?
   A. bromocriptine (Parlodel)
   B. amantadine (Symmetrel)
   C. tacrine (Cognex)
   D. ropinirole (Requip)

8. The Alzheimer's patient is given tacrine. Which of the following adverse effects is a major consideration?
   A. weight loss
   B. liver toxicity
   C. extrapyramidal side effects
   D. myalgia

9. Cholinesterase inhibitors are used to treat which of the following conditions associated with Alzheimer's disease?
   A. depression
   B. dementia
   C. urinary incontinence
   D. peripheral paralysis

10. Which of the following is an adverse effect of gingko (an herbal substance used for Alzheimer's disease)?

    A. insomnia and dizziness
    B. tremors
    C. gastrointestinal upset and headache
    D. an inability to speak normally

Fill in the Blank

1. Parkinson's disease causes dysfunction and changes in the _____ of the brain.

2. Parkinson's disease usually develops after age _____.

3. Anti-parkinsonism drugs are given to restore the balance of dopamine and _____.

4. Acetylcholinesterase inhibitors are used in the treatment of mild dementia for _____.

5. Agents used for Alzheimer's disease are classified as _____ inhibitors.

6. There is a significant risk of liver damage from using _____, one of the acetylcholinesterase inhibitors.

7. Levodopa should be avoided in patients with _____, those receiving an MAO inhibitor (MAOI), and during lactation.

8. Cholinergic blockers are used as adjunctive therapy to relieve _____ symptoms.

9. Dopamine is a precursor of norepinephrine and _____.

10. Patients taking levodopa should avoid foods and medications containing substantial amounts of vitamin _____.

11. There is no specific test for _____, and a definitive diagnosis is possible only upon autopsy.

12. Levodopa is considered the drug of choice for _____.

Critical Thinking

A 72-year-old female is diagnosed with Parkinson's disease. In her past medical history, she has had chronic hepatitis C and hypertension.

1. Which drug is considered the drug of choice for Parkinson's disease?

2. With the history of hepatitis C, what precautions should be taken if the physician ordered this drug of choice?

3. If the patient is suffering from narrow-angle glaucoma, can this drug of choice still be used for this patient?

Drug Therapy for Seizures

OBJECTIVES

After completing this chapter, the reader should be able to:

1. Distinguish between partial and generalized seizures.
2. Classify generalized seizures.
3. Explain tonic-clonic (grand mal) seizure.
4. Discuss the most commonly used anti-seizure drugs.
5. Discuss indications and major adverse effects of phenytoin.
6. Explain the mechanism of action of succinimides and their indications.
7. Recognize major phenytoin-like drugs.
8. Discuss treatment of status epilepticus.
9. Explain the type of seizures which are common in children.
10. List the drugs that may increase the toxicity of valproic acid.

GLOSSARY

Absence seizure – generalized seizure that does not involve motor convulsions; also referred to as "petit mal"

Anticonvulsant – a drug that prevents or stops a convulsive seizure

Convulsions – abnormal motor movements

Electrical threshold – an individual's balance between excitatory and inhibitory forces in the brain; also known as "seizure threshold"

Epilepsy – condition characterized by periodic or recurrent seizures or convulsions

Generalized seizure – seizure originating and involving both cerebral hemispheres

Grand mal – generalized seizure characterized by full-body tonic and clonic motor convulsions

Partial seizure – seizure originating in one area of the brain that may spread to other areas

Seizure – abnormal discharge of brain neurons that causes alteration of behavior and/or motor activity

Status epilepticus – an emergency situation characterized by continual seizure activity with no interruptions (another term for seizure)

Tonic-clonic seizure – an alternate contraction (tonic phase) and relaxation (clonic phase) of muscles, a loss of consciousness, and abnormal behavior

OVERVIEW

Today, nearly 2.3 million people in the United States have been diagnosed with **epilepsy** (a disorder characterized by **seizures**) in one of its many forms, according to the National Institute of Neurological Disorders and Stroke (NINDS). Epilepsy is the old term for recurrent seizures, rarely used today because of the stigma once attached to patients suffering from this disorder. *Seizure* is a term for all epileptic events, while **convulsion** relates to abnormal motor movements. NINDS statistics report that 75% to 90% of seizure patients have their first seizure before age 20. Fortunately, scientific discoveries about how the brain works have enabled about 80% of those diagnosed with epilepsy to benefit from modern medicines, and implantable devices regulated by the FDA can help many patients to live productive lives. Anti-seizure drugs prevent or stop a convulsive seizure.

CLASSIFICATIONS OF SEIZURES

Seizures are a group of disorders that are characterized by hyperexcitability of neurons in the brain. The abnormal stimuli can produce many symptoms, from short periods of unconsciousness to violent convulsions. Seizures are usually brief, with a beginning and an end. The activity may be localized or generalized. Seizures may result acutely from any of a number of neurological disorders, as well as from metabolic disturbances, trauma, and exposure to certain toxins. Each seizure lasts for a few seconds or minutes, and the excessive activity of the neurons then ceases spontaneously. The altered pattern of electrical activity, or brain waves, during a seizure can be demonstrated on the electroencephalogram (EEG), indicating the type of seizure. Patients may experience post-seizure impairment.

Seizure disorders are classified by their location in the brain and their clinical features, including characteristic EEG patterns during and between seizures. The international classification of seizures is summarized in Table 8-1.

TABLE 8-1   Classifications of Seizures

Partial Seizures (focal)	Generalized Seizures
A. Simple	A. Tonic-clonic (grand mal)
1. Motor (includes Jacksonian)	B. Absence (petit mal)
2. Sensory (e.g., visual, auditory)	C. Myoclonic
3. Autonomic	D. Infantile spasms
4. Psychic	E. Atonic (akinetic)
B. Complex (impaired consciousness)	
1. Psychomotor	

Medical Terminology Review

encephalogram
electro = electronic
encephalo = brain
gram = x-ray
electronic x-ray of the brain

Key Concept

Absence seizures (generalized seizures that do not involve motor convulsions; also referred to as "petit mal"), which are common in children, may decrease or be replaced by tonic-clonic or psychomotor seizures.

This is a commonly accepted classification that incorporates current terminology and divides seizures into two basic categories: generalized and partial.

Generalized seizures have multiple foci that may cause loss of consciousness, whereas **partial seizures** have a single or focal origin, often in the cerebral cortex (Figure 8-1). Partial seizures may or may not involve altered consciousness. However, partial seizures may progress to generalized seizures. The terms *epilepsy*, *convulsions*, and *seizures* are commonly used interchangeably, although they each have a slightly different medical meaning.

Complications may arise from generalized **tonic-clonic (grand mal)** seizures that are severe and frequent. Injuries may occur during a seizure. Recurrent or continuous seizures without recovery of consciousness are termed **status epilepticus**. This condition may lead to serious consequences if not treated promptly, and it is always an emergency condition.

ANTI-SEIZURE DRUGS

Several major groups of medications are used to treat seizure disorders. The choice of medication varies according to individual patient conditions and physician preference. In treatment of epilepsy, it takes weeks to establish drug plasma levels and to determine the adequacy of therapeutic improvement. Usually the most effective drug with the least adverse effects is used initially. Drug treatment is not always necessary for the lifetime of the patient. Medications for seizures include barbiturates and benzodiazepines, which are the most useful **anticonvulsants** (drugs that stop a seizure). Other medications include hydantoins, phenytoin-like agents, and succinimides, which are detailed below.

Barbiturates

Barbiturates are chemical derivatives of barbituric acid. They are classified into four groups: ultra-short-acting, short-acting, intermediate-acting, and long-acting. They are also classified as either Schedule II or III medications. More than 2,500 barbiturates have been synthesized, but only about 50 have been approved for clinical use in the United States, and fewer than a dozen are commonly used. Barbiturates were discussed in detail in Chapter 5. Specific barbiturates used solely in the treatment of seizures are summarized in Table 8-2.

TABLE 8-2 Summary of Barbiturates Used in Seizure Disorders

Generic Name	Trade Name	Route of Administration	Average Adult Dosage
phenobarbital	Barbital®, Solfoton®	PO	50–100 mg b.i.d.-t.i.d.
phenobarbital sodium	Luminal®	IM, IV	30–320 mg; may repeat in 6 h

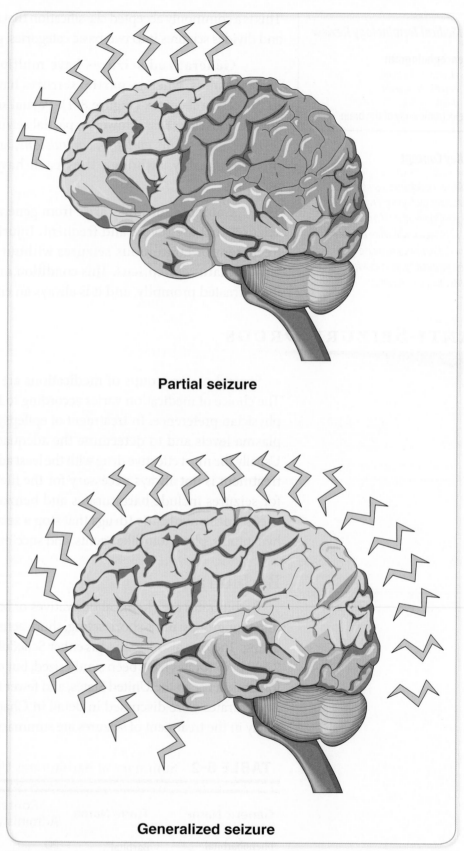

Partial seizure

Generalized seizure

Figure 8-1 A partial seizure is characterized by chaotic firing occurring in one portion of the brain, while a generalized seizure is characterized by chaotic firing all over the brain.

TABLE 8-3   Benzodiazepines Used in Seizure Disorders

Generic Name	Trade Name	Indications	Average Adult Dosage
clonazepam	Klonopin®	Seizure disorders	0.5–1.5 mg/day in divided doses
clorazepate dipotassium	Tranxene®	Partial seizures	15–60 mg/day in divided doses
diazepam	Valium®	Status epilepticus	2–10 mg b.i.d. – q.i.d.

Benzodiazepines

Benzodiazepines are one of the most widely prescribed classes of drugs. They are used not only to control seizures but also for the treatment of anxiety, skeletal muscle spasms, and alcohol withdrawal symptoms. Benzodiazepines are drugs of choice to treat anxiety and are used for hypnosis because of their great margin of safety. Benzodiazepines were discussed in detail in Chapter 5. Specific benzodiazepines used in the treatment of seizures are listed in Table 8-3.

Hydantoins

The most recognizable and used drug in the hydantoin class is phenytoin, and fosphenytoin is the newest. Phenytoin is a potent broad-spectrum anti-seizure medication. Fosphenytoin is used parenterally when substitution for oral anti-seizure medications is necessary, such as after surgery (see Table 8-4).

Mechanism of Action

Hydantoins act by desensitizing sodium channels in the CNS responsible for neuronal responsiveness. This desensitization prevents the spread of disruptive electrical charges in the brain that cause seizures.

Indications

Phenytoin is used for tonic-clonic seizures, psychomotor seizures, and seizures after head trauma. Fosphenytoin is converted to phenytoin in the body and is parenterally used for control of status epilepticus; it is a short-term substitute for oral phenytoin.

Adverse Effects

Adverse effects of phenytoin are related to plasma concentrations and include inability to coordinate muscle activity, mental confusion, dizziness, inability to sleep, headache, uncontrollable rhythmic movement of the eyes, gingival hyperplasia, toxic hepatitis, and reduction of the blood cells. Phenytoin may also cause dysrhythmias such as slow heart rate or ventricular fibrillation, abnormally low blood pressure, and hyperglycemia (excess blood glucose).

Medical Terminology Review

hypnosis

hypno = sleep
sis = condition
a sleep-like state

Key Concept

Phenytoin is administered orally and fosphenytoin is administered intravenously.

Medical Terminology Review

hyperplasia

hyper = over; above; beyond
plasia = growth; development
overgrowth

hyperglycemia

hyper = over; above; beyond
glyc/o = sugar, sweet
emia = blood condition
overproduction of sugar in the blood

Key Concept

Gingival hyperplasia is one of the major adverse effects of long-term use of phenytoin (Dilantin). Patients who use this agent should be periodically examined for an excessive growth of gum tissue.

TABLE 8-4 Hydantoins, Phenytoin-Like Drugs, and Succinimides

Generic Name	Trade Name	Route of Administration	Average Adult Dosage
Hydantoins			
fosphenytoin sodium	Cerebyx®	IV	Initial dose: 15–20 mg/kg at 100–150 mg/min, then 4–6 mg/kg/day
phenytoin sodium	Dilantin®	PO	15–18 mg/kg or 1 g initial dose, then 300 mg/day in 1–3 div. doses; may be gradually increased 100 mg/week
Phenytoin-Like Drugs			
carbamazepine	Tegretol®	PO	200 mg b.i.d., gradually increased to 800–1200 mg/day in 3–4 div. doses
felbamate	Felbatol®	PO	Initial: 1200 mg/day in 3–4 div. doses; may increase by 600 mg/day q2 weeks (max: 3600 mg/day)
lamotrigine	Lamictal®	PO	50 mg/day for 2 weeks, then 50 mg b.i.d. for 2 weeks; may increase gradually to 300–500 mg/day in 2 div. doses (max: 700 mg/day)
pregabalin	Lyrica®	PO	100 mg/day in 3 divided doses
primidone	Mysoline®	PO	Up to 500 mg q.i.d.
tiagabine hydrochloride	Gabitril®	PO	4–56 mg/day
topiramate	Topamax®	PO	200–400 mg/day in divided doses
valproic acid	Depakene® Depakote®	PO, IV	15 mg/kg/day in div. doses when total is >250 mg/day; increase 5–10 mg q week (max: 60 mg/kg/day)
zonisamide	Zonegran®	PO	100–600 mg/day
Succinimides			
ethosuximide	Zarontin®	PO	250 mg b.i.d., increased q4–7 days (max: 1.5 g/day)
methsuximide	Celontin®	PO	300 mg/day, may increase q4–7 days (max: 1.2 g/day in div. doses)

Contraindications and Precautions

Hydantoin products are contraindicated in patients with known hypersensitivity to these drugs. Hydantoin products are also contraindicated in patients with rash, seizures due to low blood glucose, pregnancy (category D), and lactation.

Hydantoin products should be used cautiously in older adults and in patients with impaired liver or kidney function, alcoholism, blood dyscrasias, hypotension, bradycardia, severe myocardial insufficiency, pancreatic adenoma, and diabetes mellitus.

Drug Interactions

Phenytoin has increased pharmacologic effects with chloramphenicol, cimetidine, isoniazid, and sulfonamides. Complex drug interactions and effects occur when phenytoin and valproic acid are given together. Severe hypotension may occur when phenytoin is given intravenously with dopamine. Alcohol decreases fosphenytoin effects. This drug may decrease absorption and increase metabolism of oral anticoagulants.

Phenytoin-Like Agents

Several commonly used drugs are classified as phenytoin-like drugs, including carbamazepine and valproic acid. Newer anti-seizure drugs, which have more limited uses, include zonisamide, felbamate, and lamotrigine, which are categorized as phenytoin-like drugs (see Table 8-4).

Mechanism of Action

In general, the mechanisms of action of phenytoin-like agents are not known, but resemble the mechanism of action of phenytoin.

Indications

Phenytoin-like drugs are useful for a wide range of seizure types, including absence seizures and mixed types of seizures. Valproic acid is used for prevention of migraine headaches and treatment of bipolar disorder.

Adverse Effects

Phenytoin-like drugs may result in adverse effects such as drowsiness, sedation, GI upsets, and prolonged bleeding time. Other adverse effects are visual disturbances, muscle weakness, bone marrow suppression, rash, fatal liver toxicity, weight gain, loss of hair, and abdominal pain.

Contraindications and Precautions

Phenytoin-like drugs are contraindicated in patients with known hypersensitivity to these agents, and in cardiac, hepatic, or renal disease. These drugs are also contraindicated in pregnancy (category D) and lactation. Carbamazepine should be used with caution in older adults and those with a history of cardiac disease. Valproic acid is used cautiously in patients with a history of kidney disease or renal impairment. This drug should be used with caution in patients with severe epilepsy and hypoalbuminemia.

Medical Terminology Review

hypoalbuminemia
hypo = low; under; beneath
albumin = plasma protein
emia = blood condition
low albumin in the blood plasma

Drug Interactions

Valproic acid interacts with many drugs. For example, chlorpromazine, felbamate, erythomycin, cimetidine, and aspirin may increase valproic acid toxicity. Lamotrigine, phenytoin, and rifampin lower valproic acid levels.

Succinimides

Succinimide drugs are another class of anti-convulsant drugs. Ethosuximide is generally considered to be the safest of the succinimide drugs, and is the most commonly prescribed drug in this class. The succinimide drugs are also listed in Table 8-4.

Mechanism of Action

Succinimides delay the entry of calcium into neurons by blocking calcium channels. Simply, anti-seizure drugs of this group increase the **electrical threshold**. Succinimides suppress the EEG pattern associated with lapses of consciousness in absence (petit mal) seizures. Its mechanism of action is not understood, but it may act to inhibit neuronal systems.

Indications

Succinimide drugs are used to control absence seizures and myoclonic seizures. They may be given in combination with other anticonvulsants.

Adverse Effects

Adverse effects of succinimides include ataxia, dizziness, nervousness, headache, and blurred vision. Behavioral changes are more prominent in patients with a history of psychiatric illness. Ethosuximide can also cause abnormal reduction of all circulating blood cells, vaginal bleeding, gingival hyperplasia, muscle weakness, and abnormal liver and kidney function tests.

Contraindications and Precautions

Succinimide drugs are contraindicated in patients with known hypersensitivity to these agents. Succinimides are also contraindicated in patients with bone marrow depression, or with hepatic or renal dysfunction. Ethosuximide should be used cautiously in pregnancy (category C) and lactation.

Drug Interactions

Drug interactions include ethosuximide, which increases phenytoin serum levels. Valproic acid causes ethosuximide serum levels to fluctuate (decrease or increase).

Medical Terminology Review

myocolonic

myo = muscle
clonic = contraction and relaxation
contraction and relaxation
of the muscles

Key Concept

The FDA approved a deep brain stimulator in 1997. This implanted device delivers electrical stimulations to the brain to reduce seizures in people who do not respond well to medication.

Serious injury or death can occur in patients with implanted neurologic stimulators who undergo magnetic resonance imaging (MRI) procedures.

SUMMARY

Seizures are a group of disorders that are characterized by hyperexcitability of neurons in the brain. Nearly 2.3 million people in the United States have seizure disorders. *Seizure* is a term for all epileptic events, while *convulsion* relates to abnormal motor movements.

Seizure disorders are classified into two basic categories: generalized and partial. Generalized seizures include tonic-clonic (grand mal), absence (petit mal), myoclonic, infantile spasms, and atonic (akinetic). Partial seizures (focal) may be divided into two categories: simple or complex (psychomotor).

Anti-seizure drugs are classified into five groups, which include: barbiturates, benzodiazepines, hydantoins, phenytoin-like agents, and succinimides. Phenytoin is the most recognizable and most used drug in the class of hydantoins. The newest drug in this class is fosphenytoin. Phenytoin is used for tonic-clonic and psychomotor seizures. Fosphenytoin is used for control of status epilepticus. Phenytoin-like drugs are useful for a wide range of seizure types, including absence seizures and mixed types of seizures.

EXPLORING THE WEB

Visit *http://professionals.epilepsy.com*

- Under the heading diagnosis and treatment, look for additional information on drug therapies used to treat epilepsy.

Visit *www.brainexplorer.org*

- Click on the link to "focus on brain disorders," then click on the link to epilepsy. Read more about this disorder and how the brain is affected.

Visit *www.coolnurse.com*

- Search for "benzodiazepines" or "seizures" review for additional information on these topics.

Visit *www.emedicine.com*

- Click on the specialty of neurology, then click on the link "seizures and epilepsy." Choose articles related to this topic to read for a greater understanding of the disorder and methods used to treat it.

Visit *www.mayoclinic.com*

- Under Diseases and Condition center click on "nervous system" and then "seizures." Review the additional information available on this topic.

Visit *www.nlm.nih.gov*

- Click on Medline Plus and search for information related to seizures and epilepsy.

REVIEW QUESTIONS

Multiple Choice

1. Which of the following adverse effects can be caused by ethosuximide (Zarontin)?

   A. tremors
   B. depression
   C. gingival hyperplasia
   D. hyperplasia of the prostate

2. Which of the following seizures is characterized by alternating contractions and relaxation of the muscles?

   A. febrile
   B. absence
   C. psychomotor
   D. tonic-clonic

3. Which of the following anti-seizure drugs increases phenytoin serum levels?

   A. carbamazepine (Tegretol)
   B. valproic acid (Depakene)
   C. ethosuximide (Zarontin)
   D. felbamate (Felbatol)

4. Which of the following seizures is classified as a simple seizure?

   A. infantile spasms
   B. absence (petit mal)
   C. psychic
   D. tonic-clonic (grand mal)

5. Which of the following seizures is the most dangerous, and requires prompt treatment?

   A. status epilepticus
   B. Jacksonian
   C. psychomotor
   D. absence

6. The newest drugs in the group of hydantoins is:

   A. phenytoin (Dilantin)
   B. fosphenytoin (Cerebyx)
   C. felbamate (Felbatol)
   D. valproic acid (Depakene)

7. Most anti-seizure drugs should be used cautiously in pregnancy because they are in which of the following categories?

   A. A
   B. B
   C. C
   D. D

8. Which of the following is the trade name for ethosuximide?

   A. Milontin
   B. Celontin
   C. Zarontin
   D. Zonegran

9. A specific barbiturate used solely in the treatment of seizures is known as:

   A. clonazepam
   B. clorazepate
   C. phenobarbital
   D. diazepam

10. Which of the following hydantoins is used for tonic-clonic, psychomotor, and head trauma–related seizures?

    A. carbamazepine
    B. phenytoin
    C. valproic acid
    D. fosphenytoin

11. Diazepam (Valium) is indicated for which type of seizure disorder?

    A. partial
    B. tonic-clonic
    C. absence
    D. status epilepticus

12. The most recognizable and most used drug in the category of hydantoins is:

    A. ethosuximide
    B. valproic acid
    C. phenytoin
    D. carbamazepine

13. Ethosuximide delays the entry of which of the following minerals into neurons by blocking its channels?

    A. calcium
    B. sodium
    C. potassium
    D. chloride

14. Which of the following agents is the drug of choice for absence seizures?

    A. valproic acid (Depakene)
    B. ethosuximide (Zarontin)
    C. felbamate (Felbatol)
    D. phenytoin (Dilantin)

15. Which of the following agents is the trade name of primidone?
   A. Gabitril
   B. Mysoline
   C. Lyrica
   D. Topamax

Fill in the Blank

1. The trade name of valproic acid is _____.

2. The choice of drugs to treat seizure disorders depends on patient conditions and _____ preference.

3. Tonic-clonic seizures are classified as _____ seizures.

4. An example of a complex seizure which impairs consciousness is a _____ seizure.

5. Fosphenytoin is the newest drug of the hydantoin group and is converted to _____ in the body.

6. Absence seizures are also known as _____.

7. Examples of phenytoin-like drugs include: carbamazepine, felbamate, lamotrigine, _____, and _____.

Critical Thinking

A 36-year-old female has been suffering from migraine headaches for almost two years. Her physician orders an anti-seizure, phenytoin-like medication for prevention of migraines.

1. Can you name which of the phenytoin-like drugs is used for the prevention of migraines?

2. If this patient were suffering from absence seizures, what phenytoin-like drugs may be prescribed?

3. If this patient is taking phenytoin-like drugs, name the most dangerous adverse effects.

Anesthetic Drugs

OBJECTIVES

After completing this chapter, the reader should be able to:

1. List the stages of anesthesia.
2. Define the importance of preanesthesia.
3. Outline the effects of general anesthetics.
4. Explain the mechanism of action of local anesthetics.
5. List the problems associated with the use of local anesthetics.
6. Describe the common local anesthetics and their uses.
7. Compare and contrast the five major routes for administering local anesthetics.
8. Define malignant hyperthermia.
9. Explain a malignant hyperthermia kit.
10. Define balanced anesthesia.

GLOSSARY

Anesthesia – a loss of feeling or sensation

Anesthetic – an agent that partially or completely numbs or eliminates sensitivity with or without loss of consciousness

Epidural anesthesia – injection of an anesthetic into the space immediately outside of the dura mater that contains a supporting cushion of fat and other connective tissues

General anesthesia – provision of a pain-free state for the entire body

Hypermetabolic – burning energy and nutrients at a higher rate than normal

Local anesthesia – provision of a pain-free state in a specific area of the body

Infiltration anesthesia – anesthesia produced by injecting a local anesthetic drug into tissues

Lipophilic – able to dissolve much more easily in lipids than in water

Malignant hyperthermia – a rare, genetic hypermetabolic condition that is characterized by severe overproduction

of body heat with rigidity of skeletal muscles

Nystagmus – rhythmical oscillation of the eyeballs

Preanesthetic medications – drugs given before the administration of anesthesia

Spinal anesthesia – a type of regional anesthesia produced by injecting a local anesthetic drug into the subarachnoid space of the spinal cord

Volatile liquids – liquids that evaporate upon exposure to the air

OVERVIEW

For several centuries, opiates and alcohol were the mainstays of **anesthetics** (substances used to reduce sensation of pain) in the control of pain. These substances had limited success, but were probably better than nothing. It was not until the 1840s that surgical **anesthesia** (reduction or elimination of pain) became possible, with the introduction of three agents: chloroform, ether, and nitrous oxide. These three substances, upon inhalation, quickly lead to a state of unconsciousness in which pain is not felt. Nitrous oxide is still one of the most widely used gaseous anesthetics, and diethyl ether is still occasionally used. Chloroform is rarely used today because of its toxicity, but other, newer halogenated hydrocarbons, such as halothane, are extremely common.

Gaseous anesthetics are the principal agents used in the maintenance of anesthesia, but agents given by other routes are still used in the induction of anesthesia. Anesthesia is basically characterized by four reversible actions: unconsciousness, analgesia, immobility, and amnesia. The critical factor is that there should be no significant impairment of cardiovascular or respiratory functions, especially those supplying the brain and other vital organs with adequate blood, nutrients, and gases.

General anesthetics are used to produce loss of consciousness before and during surgery. **Local anesthetics** numb small areas of the body tissue where a minor procedure is to be done, and are commonly used in dentistry for minor surgery. Regional anesthesia affects a larger (but still limited) part of the body, but does not make the person unconscious. Spinal and epidural anesthesia are examples of regional anesthesia.

> **Medical Terminology Review**
>
> **epidural**
>
> *epi* = on; upon; at; near; among
> *dural* = dura mater; the outermost layer of the meninges
> near the outermost layer of the meninges

PREANESTHETIC MEDICATIONS

Preanesthetic medications are used prior to the administration of an anesthetic to facilitate induction of anesthesia and to relieve anxiety and pain. They may also be used to minimize some of the undesirable effects of anesthetics, such as excessive salivation, bradycardia, and vomiting.

To accomplish these objectives, several drugs are often used at the same time. The following medications are commonly used as preoperative drugs:

- Sedative-hypnotics such as hydroxyzine, promethazine (Chapter 5)
- Antianxiety agents such as diazepam, droperidol (Chapter 5)
- Opioid analgesics such as morphine, meperidine, fentanyl (Chapter 21)
- Anticholinergics such as atropine, scopolamine (Chapter 6)

STAGES AND PLANES OF ANESTHESIA

Before patients reach surgical anesthesia, they go through several stages. The use of these stages and planes of anesthesia helps to describe the levels and progression of anesthesia produced by anesthetics. There are four stages of general anesthesia:

Stage I: This stage begins when the agent is administered and lasts until loss of consciousness. Stage I is characterized by:

- Analgesia
- Euphoria
- Perceptual distortions
- Amnesia

Stage II: Delirium begins with loss of consciousness and extends to the beginning of surgical anesthesia. There may be excitement and involuntary muscular activity. The skeletal muscle tone increases and breathing is irregular. At this stage, hypertension and tachycardia may occur. It is important that the passage from Stage I to Stage III be attained as quickly as possible. Sudden death can occur during Stage II.

Stage III: Surgical anesthesia lasts until spontaneous respiration ceases. It is further divided into four planes based on:

- Respiration
- The size of the pupils
- Reflex characteristics
- Eyeball movements

This stage is characterized by progressive muscular relaxation. Muscle relaxation is important during many surgical procedures as reflex movements can occur when a scalpel slices through the tissues.

Stage IV: Medullary paralysis begins with respiratory failure and can lead to circulatory collapse. Through careful monitoring, this stage is avoided.

GENERAL ANESTHETICS

General anesthetics are drugs that immediately produce unconsciousness and complete analgesia. These agents are generally administered by intravenous or inhalation routes. Preanesthetic and adjunct drugs are given before, during, and after surgery.

Inhalation Anesthetics

Certain drugs that are gases or **volatile liquids** at room temperature are administered by inhalation in combination with air or oxygen. The only gas used routinely for anesthesia is nitrous oxide, commonly called laughing gas. It is usually administered in combination with oxygen. Nitrous oxide provides analgesia equivalent to 10 mg of morphine sulfate but may cause occasional episodes of nausea and vomiting. Volatile liquids are converted into a vapor and inhaled to produce their anesthetic effects. Commonly administered volatile agents are halothane, enflurane, and isoflurane. The most potent of these is halothane (see Table 9-1).

Mechanism of Action

Inhaled general anesthetics are all very **lipophilic** (able to dissolve much more easily in lipids than in water). When the lipophilic anesthetic enters the lipid membrane, the whole membrane is slightly distorted and closes

> ### *Medical Terminology Review*
>
> **lipophilic**
> *lipo* = lipids (fats)
> *philic* = having an affinity for
> having an affinity for fats

TABLE 9-1   Inhaled General Anesthetics

Generic Name	Trade Name	Uses
Gas		
nitrous oxide	(generic only)	Used alone in dentistry, obstetrics, and short medical procedures Used in combination with more potent inhaled anesthetics
Volatile Liquids		
desflurane	Suprane®	Induction and maintenance of general anesthesia
enflurane	Ethrane®	Induction and maintenance of general anesthesia
halothane	Fluothane®	Induction and maintenance of general anesthesia; since safer agents have become available, its use has declined
isoflurane	Forane®	Induction and maintenance of general anesthesia; it is the most widely used inhalation anesthetic
methoxyflurane	Penthrane®	Used during labor; it does not suppress uterine contractions as greatly as other agents
sevoflurane	Ultane®	Induction and maintenance of general anesthesia

the sodium channels, causing a marginal blockage, which prevents neural conduction.

Indications

Volatile anesthetics are rarely used as the sole agents for both induction and maintenance of anesthesia. Most commonly, they are combined with intravenous agents in regimens of so-called balanced anesthesia. Of the inhaled anesthetics, nitrous oxide, desflurane, and sevoflurane are the most commonly used in the United States.

Adverse Effects

Nitrous oxide at higher doses causes anxiety, excitement, and aggressiveness. It also produces nausea, vomiting, and difficulty in breathing. Volatile anesthetics may cause headache, shivering, muscle pain, mental or mood changes, sore throat, and nightmares.

Contraindications and Precautions

Inhaled general anesthetics are contraindicated in patients with known hypersensitivity to these agents. They are also contraindicated in patients who have received monoamine oxidase inhibitors (MAOIs) within the previous 14 days (refer to Chapter 4). They should not be used by those who are intolerant to benzodiazepines, or have myasthenia gravis, acute narrow-angle glaucoma, acute alcohol intoxication, status asthmaticus, and acute intermittent porphyria.

Inhaled general anesthetics should be used cautiously during pregnancy, and in children younger than 12.

Drug Interactions

Inhaled general anesthetic drugs may interact with levodopa and increase the level of dopamine in the CNS. Skeletal muscle weakness, respiratory depression, or apnea may occur if halothane is administered with polymyxins, lincomycin, or aminoglycosides.

Injectable General Anesthetics

Intravenous anesthetics are often administered with inhaled general anesthetics. Administration of intravenous and inhaled anesthetics together allows the dose of the inhaled drug to be reduced, resulting in a decreased probability of serious side effects. They also provide more analgesia and muscle relaxation than is provided by an inhaled anesthetic alone. Drugs used as intravenous anesthetics include opioids, barbiturates, and benzodiazepines (see Table 9-2).

TABLE 9-2 Intravenous Anesthetics

Generic Name	Trade Name	Comments
Barbiturates and Barbiturate-Like Agents		
etomidate	Amidate®	For induction of anesthesia and for short medical procedures
methohexital sodium	Brevital®	Ultra–short-acting; for induction of anesthesia and as a supplement to other anesthetics
propofol	Diprivan®	For induction and maintenance of general anesthesia, and for short medical procedures
thiopental sodium	Pentothal®	Ultra–short-acting; for induction of anesthesia and as a supplement to other anesthetics
Benzodiazepines		
diazepam	Valium®	For induction of anesthesia; the prototype benzodiazepine
lorazepam	Ativan®	For induction of anesthesia, to produce conscious sedation, and for short medical procedures or surgery
midazolam hydrochloride	Versed®	For induction of anesthesia; to produce conscious sedation, and for short diagnostic procedures
Opioids		
alfentanil hydrochloride	Alfenta®	Rapid onset and short onset of action; for induction of anesthesia; used as a supplement to other anesthetics
fentanyl citrate	Sublimaze®, others	Short-acting; used during operative and perioperative periods; to supplement both general and regional anesthesia
remifentanil hydrochloride	Ultiva®	Short-acting; for induction and maintenance of general anesthesia
sufentanil citrate	Sufenta®	For induction and maintenance of anesthesia; approximately 7 times as potent as fentanyl with more rapid onset and duration of action
Others		
ketamine hydrochloride	Ketalar®	For sedation, amnesia, analgesia in short diagnostic, therapeutic, or surgical procedures; most often used in children

LOCAL ANESTHETICS

Local anesthetics are drugs that block the transmission of nerve impulses between the peripheral nervous system and the central nervous system. Their main purpose is to prevent pain impulses from pain receptors reaching the higher centers. They are mainly used in minor surgical procedures and are especially common in dentistry. Many minor surgical procedures such as suturing, excision of superficial growths, and removal of cataracts

are commonly performed using a local anesthetic injected intradermally or subcutaneously. Even deeper-excision operations such as hernias are performed occasionally using local anesthetics. Local anesthesia is more accurately called surface anesthesia or regional anesthesia.

Classification of Local Anesthetics

The two major groups of local anesthetics are esters and amides (see Table 9-3). The ester-type anesthetics, represented by procaine, contain an

TABLE 9-3 Common Local Anesthetics

Generic Name	Trade Name	Use	Comments
Esters			
benzocaine	Americaine®, Solarcaine®	Topical	For earache, hemorrhoids, sore throat, sunburn, and minor skin conditions
chloroprocaine	Nesacaine®	Epidural, infiltration, and nerve block	Short duration
cocaine	(generic only)	Topical	For ear, nose, and throat procedures
procaine hydrochloride	Novocain®	Epidural, infiltration, nerve block, and spinal	Short duration
tetracaine	Pontocaine®	Spinal and topical	Long duration
Amides			
bupivacaine hydrochloride	Marcaine®	Epidural and infiltration	Long duration
dibucaine	Nupercainal®	Spinal and topical	Long duration
etidocaine hydrochloride	Duranest®	Epidural, infiltration, and nerve block	Long duration
lidocaine hydrochloride	Xylocaine®	Epidural, infiltration, nerve block, spinal, and topical	May be combined with prilocaine (EMLA cream) for topical application
mepivacaine	Carbocaine®	Epidural, infiltration, and nerve block	Intermediate duration
prilocaine	Citanest®	Epidural, infiltration, and nerve block	Intermediate duration
ropivacaine	Naropin®	Epidural, infiltration, and nerve block	Long duration
Miscellaneous Agents			
dyclonine	Dyclone®	Topical	For ear, nose, and throat procedures
pramoxine	Tronolane®	Topical	For minor medical procedures

ester linkage in their chemical structure. In contrast, the amide-type drugs, represented by lidocaine, contain an amide linkage.

The amides have several advantages over the esters. Hypersensitivity to amide local anesthetics is rare. Most of the local anesthetics in common use today belong to the amide class.

Ester-type local anesthetics have been in use longer than amides. They tend to have a rapid onset and short duration of activity (except tetracaine). Esters are associated with a higher incidence of allergic reactions due to one of their metabolites, para-amino benzoic acid (PABA). PABA is structurally similar to methylparaben.

Mechanism of Action

Local anesthetics stop nerve conduction by inhibiting movement of sodium through channels in the membrane of a neuron. Therefore, neurons cannot fire because these agents block sodium channels.

Indications

> **Medical Terminology Review**
>
> **endoscopy**
> endo = inside
> scopy = looking
> procedure for looking
> inside the body

Local anesthetics are used for minor surgery, dental procedures, suturing small wounds, or making an incision into a small area for removing a superficial tissue sample for biopsy. Local anesthetics may also be used for obstetrics during labor and delivery, for diagnostic procedures such as gastrointestinal endoscopy, wart treatment, vasectomy, and neonatal circumcision.

Adverse Effects

True allergic reactions to local anesthetics are rare, and usually involve ester agents. Toxic effects are usually dose-related. Adverse effects include restlessness, dizziness, disorientation, light-headedness, **nystagmus** (rhythmical oscillation of the eyeballs), and psychosis. Slurred speech and tremors often precede seizures. Slower-than-normal heart rate, an abnormally low blood pressure, and cardiac arrest may occur.

Contraindications and Precautions

Local anesthetics are contraindicated in patients with known hypersensitivity, in the elderly, severe hemorrhage, hypotension, and shock. These agents are also contraindicated in patients with cerebrospinal deformities, blood dyscrasias, and hypertension.

Drug Interactions

Barbiturates may decrease activity of lidocaine. Increased effects of lidocaine may occur if taken with beta blockers, cimetidine, and quinidine. If lidocaine is used on a regular basis, its effectiveness may diminish when used with other medications.

Routes of Administration of Local Anesthetics

There are five major routes for applying local anesthetics (see Figure 9-1). These routes are summarized as follows:

1. Topical
2. Nerve block
3. Infiltration
4. Spinal
5. Epidural

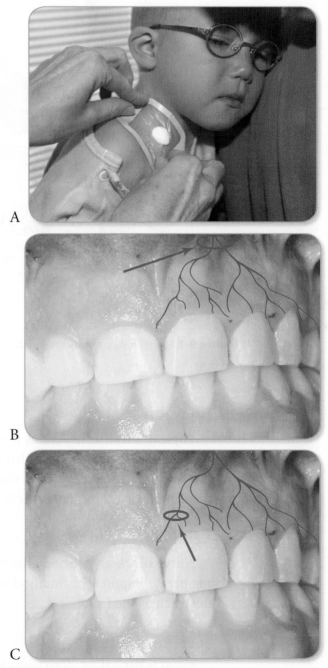

Figure 9-1 (A) Tegaderm topical anesthetic (B) nerve block anesthesia (C) local infiltration anesthesia.

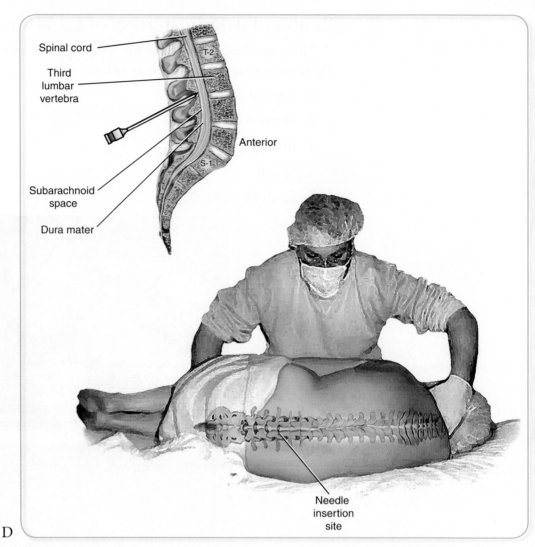

Spinal cord

Third lumbar vertebra

T-2

Anterior

S-1

Subarachnoid space

Dura mater

Needle insertion site

D

Figure 9-1 (D) spinal or epidural anesthesia (B and C courtesy of Dr. Gary Shellerud).

Topical Anesthesia

Topical anesthesia acts as a nerve conduction—blocking agent on the skin or mucus membranes. This procedure can provide anesthesia on skin and the mucus membranes of the rectum, urethra, and vagina. Lidocaine is an example of a topical anesthetic agent.

Nerve Block Anesthesia

Nerve block anesthesia affects the bundle of nerves serving the area to be operated upon. This method is used to block sensation in a limb or large area such as the face.

Local Infiltration Anesthesia

Local **infiltration anesthesia** blocks a specific group of nerves in a small area very close to the area to be operated on. Local infiltration is probably the

most common route used to administer local anesthetics, and is the simplest form of regional anesthesia. Lidocaine is a popular choice for infiltration anesthesia, but bupivacaine is used for longer procedures.

Spinal Anesthesia

During **spinal anesthesia**, an anesthetic agent is injected into the subarachnoid space (beneath the arachnoid membrane or between the arachnoid and pia mater, and filled with cerebrospinal fluid) through a spinal needle. Drugs injected in this manner affect large regional areas such as the lower abdomen and legs.

Epidural Anesthesia

Epidural anesthesia involves injection of the local anesthetic into the epidural (lumbar or caudal) space via a catheter that allows repeated infusions. After injection, the anesthetic agent is very slowly absorbed into the cerebrospinal fluid. This method is most commonly used in obstetrics during labor and delivery.

Medical Terminology Review

arachnoid

arach = spider
noid = like
spider-like

MALIGNANT HYPERTHERMIA

Malignant hyperthermia is a rare, genetic **hypermetabolic** condition that is characterized by severe overproduction of body heat with rigidity of skeletal muscles. It is a serious adverse effect of anesthesia (relating to inhalation anesthetics) that must be treated immediately. Treatment includes administration of large doses of dantrolene sodium and 100% oxygen, followed by immediate cooling, cessation of surgery, and correction of hyperkalemia. Dantrolene has a very short shelf life and must be restocked regularly so that, when needed, its action will be potent. Malignant hyperthermia may cause the death of the patient due to brain damage, cardiac arrest, internal bleeding, or damage to other body systems. A malignant hyperthermia kit must include:

- Dantrolene
- Furosemide
- Glucose
- Procainamide
- Sodium bicarbonate (7.5%)
- Sterile water

Medical Terminology Review

hyperkalemia

hyper = over; above; beyond
kalemia = condition of potassium ions in the blood
increased number of potassium ions in the blood

Key Concept

Patients susceptible to malignant hyperthermia must be informed of the condition and potentially susceptible relatives of the patient should also be screened.

SUMMARY

Preanesthetic drugs are used to facilitate induction of anesthesia and to relieve anxiety and pain. There are four stages of anesthesia. Stage I is characterized by analgesia, euphoria, and amnesia. Stage II increases the skeletal muscle tone and breathing is irregular. It is important that the passage from Stage I to Stage III be attained as quickly as possible. Stage III is called surgical anesthesia, which produces muscular relaxation. Stage IV causes medullary paralysis, and this stage should be avoided.

General anesthesia is a reversible stage of unconsciousness as a result of medication. It can be induced by inhalation or by injection of drugs. The combination of injectable anesthetics with inhaled general anesthetics together allows a decreased probability of serious side effects.

The two major groups of local anesthetics are esters and amides. The amides have several advantages over the esters. Local anesthetics are used for minor surgery, dental procedures, suturing small wounds, or removing a superficial tissue sample for biopsy.

EXPLORING THE WEB

Visit **www.emedicine.com**

- Click on the specialty "Emergency Medicine," then click on toxicology and look for information related to the drugs covered in this chapter.

Visit **www.healthline.com**

- Search by "anesthesia," and review information that related to this topic.

Visit **www.mayoclinic.com**

- Search by "anesthesia," and review information that related to this topic.

REVIEW QUESTIONS

Multiple Choice

1. The main purpose of local anesthetics is to prevent which of the following?

   A. falling asleep and muscle contraction
   B. allergic reaction and anaphylactic shock
   C. pain impulses from pain receptors reaching the lower limbs
   D. pain impulses from pain receptors reaching the higher centers

2. The ester-type anesthetics are represented by which of the following substances?

    A. procaine
    B. prolactin
    C. pro-hormone
    D. pro-vitamin

3. Which of the following is the most common route used to administer local anesthetics?

    A. epidural
    B. topical
    C. local infiltration
    D. nerve block

4. Which of the following stages of anesthesia must be avoided?

    A. Stage I
    B. Stage II
    C. Stage III
    D. Stage IV

5. Which of the following preanesthetic medications relieve anxiety?

    A. scopolamine
    B. promethazine
    C. diazepam
    D. atropine

6. Which of the following stages of anesthesia is characterized by euphoria and perceptual distortions?

    A. Stage I
    B. Stage II
    C. Stage III
    D. Stage IV

7. Which of the following is the only gas that is routinely used for anesthesia?

    A. chloroform
    B. ether
    C. nitrous oxide
    D. halothane

8. Which of the following volatile agents is the most potent?

    A. isoflurane
    B. halothane
    C. sevoflurane
    D. enflurane

9. All of the following agents are used as inhaled anesthetics, except:

    A. desflurane
    B. nitrous oxide
    C. halothane
    D. sevoflurane

10. Local anesthesia is more accurately called:

    A. surface anesthesia
    B. preanesthetic medication
    C. maintenance of anesthesia
    D. surgical anesthesia

11. Which of the following agents is in the local anesthetic amide group?

    A. procaine (Novocain)
    B. lidocaine (Xylocaine)
    C. tetracaine (Pontocaine)
    D. benzocaine (Americaine)

12. Which of the following is the stage of surgical anesthesia?

    A. Stage I
    B. Stage IV
    C. Stage II
    D. Stage III

Matching

Generic Names	Trade Names
_____ 1. sevoflurane	**A.** Penthrane
_____ 2. isoflurane	**B.** Suprane
_____ 3. halothane	**C.** Fluothane
_____ 4. enflurane	**D.** Ethrane
_____ 5. desflurane	**E.** Forane
_____ 6. methoxyflurane	**F.** Ultane

Fill in the Blank

1. A woman in labor will most likely receive _____.

2. Anticholinergics used to minimize some of the undesirable after effects of anesthetics, such as excessive salvation, vomiting, and bradycardia, include _____ and _____.

3. Nitrous oxide is also called _____.

4. Hypersensitivity to amide local anesthetics is _____.

Critical Thinking

A 65-year-old man is going under local anesthesia for two dental implants. His medical history is satisfactory, but he is taking three different medications: Zocor® 10 mg and niacin 1,000 mg (for hypercholesterolemia), and Allegra® 180 mg (for allergies).

1. What would be the best type of local anesthesia for this patient?

2. If his dentist is using the preferred local anesthesia for this procedure, would there be any drug interactions with the medications that the patient is taking?

3. What may be the adverse effects for local anesthesia used in this procedure?

Drug Therapy for the Musculoskeletal System

OBJECTIVES

After completing this chapter, the reader should be able to:

1. Discuss skeletal muscle relaxants.
2. Discuss neuromuscular blocking agents.
3. Explain the goals of pharmacotherapy with skeletal muscle relaxants.
4. Define centrally acting skeletal muscle relaxants.
5. Explain the major side effect of dantrolene (direct-acting skeletal muscle relaxant).
6. Discuss drugs used to treat gout.
7. Explain the mechanism of action of corticosteroids.
8. Explain gold compounds and their indications.
9. Define drugs for gouty arthritis and drugs commonly used for treatment.

GLOSSARY

Articular – related to the joints of the body

Contusion – an injury to body part or tissue without a break in the skin

Exfoliative dermatitis – a skin disorder characterized by reddening and scaling of 100% of the skin; erythroderma

Gout – a disease caused by a congenital disorder of uric acid metabolism; metabolic arthritis

Hematoma – blood that has seeped from a blood vessel and collects in tissue, organs, or space

Laceration – cut or break in the skin

Periosteum – a thick, fibrous membrane covering the entire surface of a bone except its articular cartilage and where it attaches to tendons and ligaments

Osteoarthritis (OA) – arthritis characterized by erosion of articular cartilage that mainly affects weight-bearing joints in older adults

Rheumatoid arthritis (RA) – a chronic and progressive condition that affects more women than men, focusing mainly on the joints of the hands and feet, and leading to deformity and disability

Spasticity – a type of increase in muscle tone at rest, characterized by increase resistance of the muscles to stretching

Sprain – injury to supporting ligaments of a joint

Strain – injury resulting from overstretching a muscle, results in tear of muscle or muscle and tendon

Synapse – a specialized junction at which a nerve cell communicates with a target cell

OVERVIEW

Muscle spasms, spasticity, and joint disorders are some of the most common disorders in humans of any age. Medications used to treat these conditions may be classified in two broad categories: skeletal muscle relaxants and nonsteroidal anti-inflammatory drugs (NSAIDs). In this chapter, we will focus on drugs such as skeletal muscle relaxants (for disorders such as muscular spasticity due to neurological disorders), gold salts (for arthritis), and agents used to treat gout. NSAIDs will be discussed with more depth in Chapter 21.

ANATOMY REVIEW

- The musculoskeletal system consists of several separate body systems: the skeletal system, the muscular system, and the articular system (Figure 10-1).

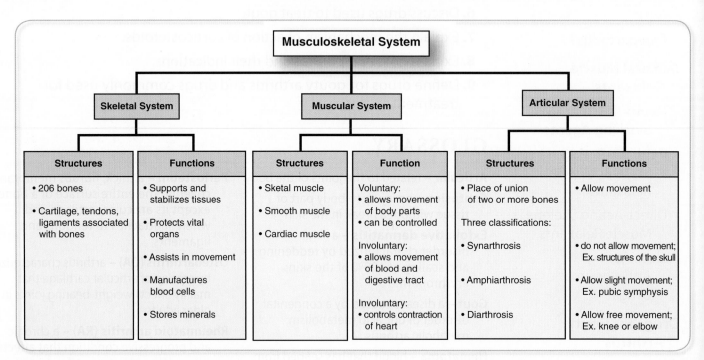

Figure 10-1 The musculoskeletal system.

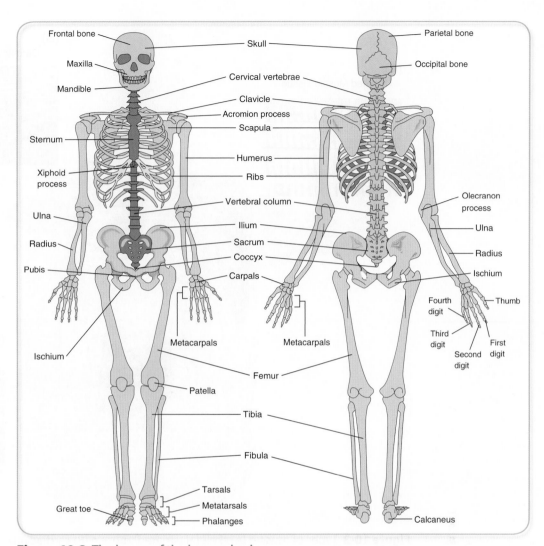

Figure 10-2 The bones of the human body.

- The skeletal system consists of 206 bones as well as the cartilage, ligaments, and tendons associated with the bones (Figure 10-2).

- Functions of the skeletal system include: support and stabilization, protection of organs, assistance with movement, manufacture of blood cells, and storage of minerals.

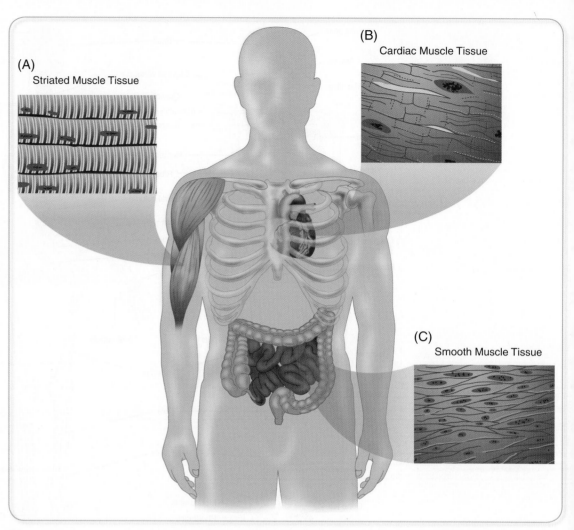

(A)
Striated Muscle Tissue

(B)
Cardiac Muscle Tissue

(C)
Smooth Muscle Tissue

Figure 10-3 Types of muscle (A) skeletal (striated) muscle (B) cardiac muscle (C) smooth muscle.

- The muscular system consists of three types of muscle: skeletal, smooth, and cardiac (Figure 10-3).
- Skeletal muscle allows voluntary movement such as flexion and extension of the legs. Smooth muscle allows involuntary movement in particular body organs such as movement of the nutrients through the digestive tract. Cardiac muscle is found only in the heart and controls the involuntary contractions of the heart.
- The **articular** system consists of three types of joints: synarthrosis, amphiarthrosis, and diarthrosis (Figure 10-4).
- Synarthrosis joints, such as the sutures in the skull, do not allow movement.
- Amphiarthrosis joints such as the pubic symphysis allow slight movement.
- Diarthrosis joints allow free range of motion such as the movements around the shoulder girdle.

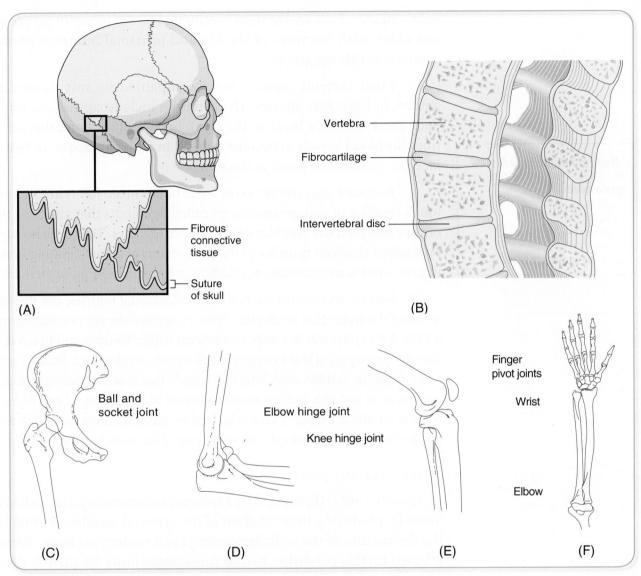

Figure 10-4 Types of joints: (A) synarthrosis (B) amphiarthrosis (C–F) diarthrosis.

MUSCULOSKELETAL DISORDERS

The musculoskeletal system is subject to a large number of disorders. These disorders affect persons of all age groups and occupations. They are a major cause of pain and disability.

Injury and Trauma of the Musculoskeletal System

A broad spectrum of musculoskeletal injuries results from numerous physical forces, including blunt tissue trauma, disruption of tendons and ligaments, and fractures of bony structures. Many of the forces that cause injury to the musculoskeletal system are typical for a particular environmental setting, activity, or age group. Trauma resulting from high-speed motor accidents is a common cause of injury in adults younger than 45. The most common causes of childhood injuries are falls, bicycle-related injuries, and

sports injuries. Falls are the most common causes of injury in people 65 years and older, with fractures of the hip and proximal humerus particularly common in this age group.

Most skeletal injuries are accompanied by soft tissue (muscle, tendon, or ligament) injuries. These injuries include **contusions** (injuries of body parts without a break in the skin), **hematomas** (blood that has seeped from the blood vessels to become trapped in an organ, space, or tissue), and **lacerations** (a cut or break in the skin).

Joints are sites where two or more bones meet. Joints are supported by tough bundles of collagenous fibers called ligaments that attach to the joint capsule and bind the articular ends of bones together. They are also supported by tendons that join muscles to the periosteum of an articulating bone. Joint injuries involve mechanical overloading or forcible twisting or stretching.

Sprains and strains are both musculoskeletal injuries, but they differ in terms of the tissue that is affected. **Sprains** involve the supporting ligaments of a joint. A complete tear in a muscle or tendon is described as a rupture. A **strain** is a stretching or a partial tear in a muscle or a muscle-tendon unit. Strains commonly result from the sudden stretching of a muscle that is actively contracting. Strains can occur at any age, but are more common in middle-aged and older adults. Muscle strains are usually characterized by pain, stiffness, swelling, and local tenderness. Pain is increased with stretching of the muscle group.

Rheumatoid Arthritis

Rheumatoid arthritis (RA) is a systemic inflammatory disease that attacks joints by producing inflammation of the synovial membranes that leads to the destruction of the articular cartilage and underlying bone. Women are affected by this condition two to three times more frequently than men. Although the disease occurs in all age groups, its prevalence increases with age. The peak incidence among women is between the ages of 40 and 60 years, with the onset at 30 to 50 years of age.

The cause of RA has not been established. However, evidence points to a genetic predisposition and the development of joint inflammation that is immunologically mediated.

Joint involvement usually is systemic and involves more than one joint. The patient may complain of joint pain and stiffness that lasts for 30 minutes or longer, and frequently for several hours. The most commonly affected joints initially are the fingers, hands, wrists, knees, and feet. Later, other joints may become involved. Spinal involvement usually is limited to the cervical region.

Gout

Gout is actually a group of diseases known as the gout syndrome. It includes acute gouty arthritis with recurrent attacks of severe joint inflammation, and the accumulation of crystalline deposits in joint surfaces, bones, soft tissue,

---

Medical Terminology Review
periosteum
peri- = *around*
oste- = *bone*
-um = *suffix identifying a singular noun*
structure around the bone

and cartilage. Gout also may cause gouty nephropathy or renal impairment, and uric acid kidney stones.

Uric acid is a waste product of purine metabolism, normally excreted through the kidneys. A sudden increase in serum uric acid levels usually precipitates an attack of gout. Gout often affects a single joint, such as in the big toe. When acute inflammation develops from uric acid deposits, the joint cartilage is damaged. The inflammation causes redness and swelling of the joint, accompanied by severe pain.

Osteoarthritis

Osteoarthritis is by far the most common form of arthritis among the elderly. It is the greatest cause of disability and limitation of activity in older adults. It has been suggested that osteoarthritis begins at a very young age, expressing itself in the elderly only after a long period of latency. Osteoarthritis presents a major management problem, but there is much that can be done to help lessen its effects. Self-control, by maintaining a positive attitude and a sense of self-esteem, is a frequent coping strategy. Treatment of osteoarthritis in the elderly focuses on relief of pain and improvement of functional status.

SKELETAL MUSCLE RELAXANTS

Most muscle strains and spasms are self-limited and respond to rest, physical therapy, and short-term use of aspirin and other analgesics. However, **spasticity** (a form of muscular contraction), as the result of closed head injuries, stroke, cerebral palsy, multiple sclerosis, spinal cord injury, and other neurologic conditions, requires long-term use of muscle relaxants. The skeletal muscles are voluntary muscles. They are under control of the central nervous system (CNS). Skeletal muscle relaxants work by blocking somatic motor nerve impulses through depression of the neurons within the CNS. Transmission of an impulse from the motor nerve to each muscle cell occurs across a space known as the neuromuscular junction (see Figure 10-5). This space is sensitive to chemical changes in its immediate environment. Therefore, the somatic motor nerve impulses cannot be generated. This mechanism may also decrease the availability of calcium ions to the myofibrillar contractile system. Discontinuity of certain afferent reflex pathways by local anesthesia may also effect relaxation of limited muscle groups; local anesthetic block of efferent somatic motor outflow also is used occasionally to relieve localized skeletal muscle spasms.

Neuromuscular Blocking Agents

Neuromuscular blocking agents are chemical substances that interfere locally with the transmission or reception of impulses from motor nerves to skeletal muscles. Table 10-1 shows some popular neuromuscular blocking agents.

Medical Terminology Review

neuromuscular
neuro = of the nerves or nervous system
muscular = of the muscles or muscular system
nerves affecting the muscles of the body

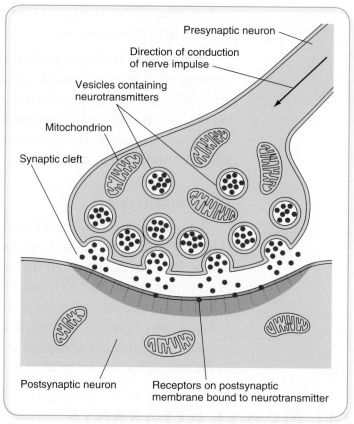

Figure 10-5 The neuromuscular junction.

TABLE 10-1   Neuromuscular Blocking Agents

Generic Name	Trade Name	Route of Administration	Average Adult Dosage
Short Duration			
succinylcholine chloride	Anectine®, Quelicin®	IM, IV	IV: 0.3–1.1 mg/kg; IM: 2.5–4 mg/kg
Intermediate Duration			
atracurium besylate	Tracrium®	IV	0.4–0.5 mg/kg initial; then 0.08–0.1 mg/kg
cisatracurium besylate	Nimbex®	IV	0.15–0.20 mg/kg
rocuronium bromide	Zemuron®	IV	0.6 mg/kg
Extended Duration			
doxacurium chloride	Nuromax®	IV	0.025–0.05 mg/kg initial; then 0.005–0.01 mg/kg
mivacurium chloride	Mivacron®	IV	0.15–0.25 mg/kg
pancuronium bromide	Pavulon®	IV	0.06–0.1 mg/kg

Mechanism of Action

Neuromuscular blocking agents prevent somatic motor nerve impulses, which affect the skeletal muscles. Some agents occupy receptor sites on the motor end plate and are able to block the action of acetylcholine. These agents are called competitive neuromuscular blocking agents. The action of other neuromuscular blocking agents resembles that of acetylcholine by depolarizing the muscle fiber. These agents are not immediately destroyed by cholinesterase. Therefore, their action is more prolonged than that of acetylcholine. Examples of these agents include succinylcholine, atracurium, and doxacurium.

Indications

The principal use of neuromuscular blocking drugs is to provide adequate skeletal muscular relaxation during surgery, controlled respiration, and orthopedic manipulations. The short-acting drugs are used to relax the laryngeal muscles during endotracheal intubation and bronchoscopy. They may also be used to decrease the severity of muscle contractions during electroconvulsive treatment. Neuromuscular blocking agents have been used in the management of tetanus and for various spastic disorders, but the results usually have been dissatisfying. Neuromuscular blocking agents are not effective for rigidity and spasticity of muscles caused by neurological disease or trauma.

Adverse Effects

The most commonly reported adverse effects of neuromuscular blocking agents include drowsiness, increased occurrence of seizures in patients with epilepsy, dry mouth, loss of strength, hypotension, muscle weakness, occasional hepatitis, and cardiac arrhythmias.

Contraindications and Precautions

Neuromuscular blocking agents are contraindicated in patients with hypersensitivity to these drugs or a family history of malignant hyperthermia. Atracurium is contraindicated in patients with myasthenia gravis. Neuromuscular blocking drugs are not safe during pregnancy (category C), lactation, or in children younger than two years.

These agents should be used cautiously in infants and patients with asthma, significant cardiovascular disease, impaired pulmonary function, dehydration, acid-base imbalance, and lactation.

Drug Interactions

Neuromuscular blocking agents play an important role in severe adverse reactions occurring during anesthesia. Most reactions to these agents are of immunological origin, and tests for possible hypersensitivity to these drugs must be conducted before administration of anesthesia. Neuromuscular blocking agents should not be used with muscle relaxants such as succinylcholine, volatile, intravenous, or local anesthetics, antibiotics,

TABLE 10-2 Centrally Acting Skeletal Muscle Relaxants

Generic Name	Trade Name	Route of Administration	Average Adult Dosage
baclofen	Lioresal®	PO	5 mg tid
carisoprodol	Soma®, Rela®	PO	350 mg tid
chlorphenesin carbamate	Maolate®	PO	800 mg tid until effective; reduce to 400 mg qid or less
chlorzoxazone	Paraflex®, Parafon Forte®	PO	250–500 mg tid
cyclobenzaprine hydrochloride	Flexeril®, Cycoflex®	PO	10–15 mg tid
diazepam	Valium®, Valrelease®	PO, IM, IV	PO: 2–10 mg bid-qid; IM/IV: 5–10 mg up to 30 mg
methocarbamol	Robaxin®	PO	1.5 g qid for 2–3 days then reduce to 1 g qid
orphenadrine citrate	Norflex®, Banflex®, Myolin®	PO, IM, IV	PO: 100 mg bid; IM/IV: 60 mg

anticonvulsants, magnesium, diuretics, corticosteroids, or acetylcholine esterase inhibitors (reversal drugs).

Centrally Acting Skeletal Muscle Relaxants

Skeletal muscles are voluntarily controlled by impulses originating in the CNS. Impulses are conducted through the spinal cord in somatic neurons that eventually **synapse** with the muscle in a neuromuscular junction. Table 10-2 shows some examples of the centrally acting skeletal muscle relaxants.

Mechanism of Action

The exact mechanism of centrally acting muscle relaxants is unknown. The neurotransmitter acetylcholine (ACh) is released to combine with ACh receptors on the muscle cell membrane. When an adequate number of ACh receptors are bound, the cell then experiences sodium ion influx, causing an impulse to travel over the cell, which causes a contraction. Relaxation occurs when ACh is broken down by acetylcholinesterase. They may act in the CNS at various levels to depress polysynaptic reflexes; sedative effects may be responsible for relaxation of muscle spasms.

Indications

Use of the centrally acting muscle relaxants is uncertain, owing to their limited selectivity. Involuntary movement of skeletal muscles, such as that which is seen in palsies, chorea, or Parkinsonism, is mostly the result of impairment of feedback control within the brain. These agents may be used to reduce muscle spasms in patients with cerebral palsy, multiple sclerosis, and spinal cord injury.

Adverse Effects

Common adverse effects of centrally acting agents include weakness, fatigue, drowsiness, and dizziness. Baclofen is often the drug of first choice because of its wide safety margin.

Contraindications and Precautions

Centrally acting skeletal muscle relaxants are contraindicated in patients with hypersensitivity to these agents. Cyclobenzaprine should be avoided in the acute recovery phase of myocardial infarction, cardiac arrhythmias, and hyperthyroidism. Centrally acting skeletal muscle relaxants are contraindicated during pregnancy (category B or C), lactation, and in children younger than five years.

These agents should be used cautiously in patients with liver or kidney impairment, bipolar disorder, seizure disorders, stroke, cerebral palsy, depression, head trauma, and diabetes mellitus.

Medical Terminology Review

hyperpyretic

hyper = over, excessive
pyr/o = fire, heat
tic = pertaining to
pertaining to overheating

Drug Interactions

Alcohol, phenothiazines, or CNS depressants may cause additive sedation if they are used with centrally acting skeletal muscle relaxants. Cyclobenzaprine should not be used within two weeks of an MAOI because hyperpyretic crisis and convulsions may occur.

Direct-Acting Skeletal Muscle Relaxants

Medical Terminology Review

spastic

spas = spasms
tic = condition of
the presence of spasms

These agents directly relax the spastic muscle. Direct-acting skeletal muscle relaxants produce about a 50% decrease in contractility of skeletal muscles, but they have no effect on smooth or cardiac muscles. Examples of direct-acting antispasmodic drugs are botulinum toxin type A and B, dantrolene, and quinine sulfate (see Table 10-3).

TABLE 10-3 Direct-Acting Antispasmodic Agents

Generic Name	Trade Name	Route of Administration	Average Adult Dosage
botulinum toxin type A	Botox®, Dysport®	IM	20–50 units injected directly into target muscle
botulinum toxin type B	Myoblock®	IM	2,500–5,000 units / dose injected directly into target muscle
dantrolene sodium	Dantrium®	PO	25 mg / day; increased to 25 mg bid-qid; may increase q4–7 days up to 100 mg bid-tid
quinine sulfate	Quinamm®, Quiphile®	PO	260–300 mg at bedtime

Mechanism of Action

Direct-acting skeletal muscle relaxants do not interfere with neuromuscular transmission or the electrical excitability of muscles. They inhibit the release of calcium ions from storage areas inside skeletal muscle cells. This action makes the muscle less responsive to nerve impulses. Dantrolene is an example of a direct-acting skeletal muscle relaxant that will be discussed in detail.

Indications

Dantrolene is used to treat spasticity resulting from upper motor neuron lesions such as those in spinal cord injury, stroke, multiple sclerosis, and cerebral palsy, but not spasticity resulting from musculoskeletal injury, lumbago, or rheumatoid disorders. The drug is also used to treat malignant hyperthermia.

Adverse Effects

The major adverse effects of dantrolene include muscle weakness, drowsiness, dizziness, nausea, diarrhea, seizures, tachycardia, erratic blood pressure, and pericarditis.

Contraindications and Precautions

Dantrolene is contraindicated in patients with liver disease and respiratory muscle weakness. It may color the urine orange to red. Safe use during pregnancy (category C), lactation, or in children younger than five years is not established.

Dantrolene should be used cautiously in patients with impaired cardiac or pulmonary function, or in patients younger than 35 years (especially women).

Drug Interactions

The use of dantrolene with alcohol and other CNS depressants causes increased CNS depression. Estrogen increases the risk of hepatotoxicity in women younger than 35 years. The use of intravenous dantrolene with verapamil and other calcium channel blockers increases the risk of ventricular fibrillation and cardiovascular collapse.

Slow-Acting Anti-Rheumatic Drugs

Slow-acting anti-rheumatic drugs may be prescribed for patients with rheumatoid arthritis that progresses to deformity, requiring more than an anti-inflammatory agent. Altering the disease course is attempted initially with methotrexate, gold compounds, penicillamine, sulfasalazine, and hydroxychloroquine. Table 10-4 shows second-line agents for rheumatoid arthritis.

Mechanism of Action

Gold compounds (auranofin and gold sodium thiomalate) suppress or prevent inflammation in the acute forms of arthritis, but do not cure the disease. The exact mechanisms of action of slow-acting anti-rheumatic drugs are not known.

Key Concept

Quinine sulfate is an antimalarial drug that is used for nocturnal leg cramps or congenital tonic spasms.

Medical Terminology Review

arthritis
arthr = joint
itis = inflammation
inflammation of the joint

TABLE 10-4 Second-Line Agents for Rheumatoid Arthritis

Generic Name	Trade Name	Route of Administration	Average Adult Dosage
auranofin	Ridaura®	PO	3 mg bid
gold sodium thiomalate	Aurolate®	IM	10 mg week 1; 1.25 mg week 2; then 25–50 mg/wk
methotrexate sodium	Mexate®	PO	15–30 mg/day for 5 days, repeat each 12 wk for 3–5 courses
hydrochloroquine	Plaquenil®	PO	200–600 mg/day
penicillamine	Depen®	PO	125–250 mg/day, may increase after several months
sulfasalazine	Azulfidine®	PO	1–3 g/day

Penicillamine is a chelating drug that is a metabolite of penicillin. It is also classified as an anti-inflammatory drug. The mechanism of action of penicillamine and hydrochloroquine is unknown.

Indications

Slow-acting anti-rheumatic drugs may be prescribed for advanced states of some rheumatoid disorders. The oral gold compound is available as auranofin, whereas the parenteral preparations are aurothioglucose and gold sodium thiomalate. Gold compounds that retard destruction of bone and joints by an unknown mechanism are long-latency drugs used in more advanced stages of some rheumatoid diseases. Gold sodium thiomalate is administered intramuscularly, and auranofin is administered orally.

Corticosteroids are used in severe, progressive rheumatoid arthritis. Prednisone may afford some degree of control, but corticosteroids are usually recognized as agents of last resort. Corticosteroids do not alter the course of rheumatoid arthritis. They may be occasionally used for elderly patients as alternatives to avoid the risks of second-line agents, for patients who cannot tolerate NSAIDs, and for patients with significant systemic manifestations of rheumatoid arthritis.

Adverse Effects

Common adverse effects of gold compounds and penicillamine include GI disturbances, dermatitis, and lesions of mucous membranes. Less common side effects include aplastic anemia and nephritic syndrome. It is important to note that, except for diarrhea, serious toxicity occurs most commonly when parenteral therapy is used. If toxicity occurs gold therapy should be stopped immediately.

Long-term administration of corticosteroids may cause GI bleeding, poor wound healing, hyperglycemia, hypertension, and osteoporosis.

Medical Terminology Review

corticosteroids

cortico = (adrenal) cortex
steroids = hormones
hormones produced in the adrenal cortex

Contraindications and Precautions

These preparations are contraindicated in patients with a history of gold-induced necrotizing enterocolitis, renal disease, **exfoliative dermatitis**, or bone marrow aplasia, in patients who have recently received radiation therapy, and in those with a history of severe toxicity from previous exposure to gold or other heavy metals. Safety during pregnancy (various categories) or lactation and in children is not established.

These agents must be used with caution in patients who have inflammatory bowel disease, rash, liver disease, a history of bone marrow depression, diabetes mellitus, congestive heart failure, and in older adults.

Drug Interactions

Gold compounds may have drug interactions with antimalarials and immunosuppressants. Penicillamine and phenylbutazone increase the risk of blood dyscrasias. Methotrexate with alcohol, azathioprine, and sulfasalazine increase risk of hepatotoxicity. Chloramphenicol, salicylates, NSAIDs, sulfonamides, phenylbutazone, phenytoin, tetracyclines, penicillin, and probenecid may increase methotrexate levels with increased toxicity. Folic acid may alter response to methotrexate.

The combination of penicillamine with antimalarials and gold therapy may potentiate hematological and renal adverse effects. Iron may decrease penicillamine absorption. Iron and antibiotics may alter sulfasalazine absorption.

DRUGS FOR GOUTY ARTHRITIS

There are two types of clinical gouty arthritis: acute and chronic. The initial attack for acute gout is abrupt, usually occurring at night or in the early morning as synovial fluid is reabsorbed. The most common site of the initial attack is the big toe. Other sites that may be affected include the ankle, heel, knee, wrist, elbow, and fingers. There are two choices for therapy: general therapeutic drugs and specific drugs. In acute gout, immobilization of the affected joint is essential. Anti-inflammatory drug therapy should begin immediately, and urate-lowering drugs should not be given until the acute attack is controlled. Specific drugs include colchicines, NSAIDs (see Chapter 21), and corticosteroids. Colchicine and allopurinol are detailed below selectively.

> **Medical Terminology Review**
>
> **antimitotic**
>
> *anti* = opposing
> *mitotic* = development
> *of chromosomes*
> development of chromosomes
> in opposition to one another

Colchicine

Colchicine is a gout suppressant with antimitotic and indirect anti-inflammatory properties.

Mechanism of Action

Colchicine is not an analgesic, and its precise mechanism of action is not known. The drug is well-absorbed after oral administration. It is often combined with probenecid to improve prophylactic therapy of chronic gouty arthritis. Both urinary and fecal routes eliminate colchicine.

Indications

Colchicine is the traditional drug of choice for relieving pain and inflammation and ending the acute gout attack. It is most effective when initiated 12 to 36 hours after symptoms begin. It is also used in combination with either phenylbutazone or allopurinol in the management of acute gout.

Adverse Effects

The drug is very toxic, and it should be stopped at the first symptom of toxicity, such as nausea, vomiting, diarrhea, and abdominal pain. Adverse effects of oral colchicine include nausea, abdominal cramps, and diarrhea.

Contraindications and Precautions

Colchicine is contraindicated in patients with peptic ulcers. Local pain and necrosis can occur with administration of intravenous colchicines.

Drug Interactions

Colchicine may decrease intestinal absorption of vitamin B_{12}.

Medical Terminology Review

uricosuric
urico = related to uric acid
suric = increasing excretion
increased excretion of uric acid

Allopurinol

Allopurinol is a xanthine oxidase inhibitor uricosuric agent.

Mechanism of Action

This drug is not analgesic, but it relieves gouty pain because it blocks the formation of or enhances the excretion of uric acid.

Indications

Allopurinol is used in the treatment of gout, primary or secondary uric acid nephropathy, uric acid stone formation, and renal calculi.

Adverse Effects

Adverse effects of allopurinol include: drowsiness, headache, vertigo, nausea, vomiting, diarrhea, abdominal discomfort, indigestion, malaise, thrombocytopenia, urticaria or pruritus, pruritic maculopapular rash, toxic epidermal necrolysis, hepatotoxicity, and renal insufficiency. In rare cases, allopurinol may cause agranulocytosis, aplastic anemia, and bone marrow depression.

Medical Terminology Review

hyperuricemia
hyper = over; above; beyond
uric = uric acid
emia = blood condition
excessive uric acid in the blood

Contraindications and Precautions

Allopurinol is contraindicated in children, except those with hyperuricemia secondary to cancer. It should not be used by nursing mothers, or by patients who develop a severe reaction to the drug.

Drug Interactions

Alcohol may inhibit renal excretion of uric acid. Ampicillin and amoxicillin increase the risk of skin rash. Allopurinol enhances anticoagulant effects of warfarin. Toxicity from azathioprine, mercaptopurine, cyclophosphamide, and cyclosporin increase with allopurinol.

SUMMARY

Skeletal muscle relaxants and non-narcotic analgesics may be classified in two broad categories: skeletal muscle relaxants and NSAIDs (discussed in Chapter 21). Most muscle strains and spasms are self-limited and respond to rest, physical therapy, and aspirin. Spasticity resulting from closed head injuries, stroke, cerebral palsy, and others require long-term use of muscle relaxants. Neuromuscular blocking agents prevent somatic motor nerve impulses which affect the skeletal muscles. Gold compounds can suppress or prevent inflammation in acute forms of rheumatoid arthritis. The drug of choice for acute gouty arthritis is colchicine.

EXPLORING THE WEB

Visit *www.drugs.com*

• Search for "skeletal muscle relaxants." Review the material presented to gain a better understanding of the drugs that fall within this category.

Visit *www.medicinenet.com* or *www.nlm.nih.gov*

• Search by the disorders or drugs discussed in this chapter to enhance your understanding of the reading.

REVIEW QUESTIONS

Multiple Choice

1. The type of muscle which attaches to bones and joints by connective tissue is which of the following?

   A. smooth
   B. skeletal
   C. myocardium
   D. tendon

2. Which of the following refers to disease of the joints?

   A. bursa
   B. osteoporosis
   C. arthritis
   D. connective

3. Skeletal muscles are voluntary muscles which are under the control of the

   A. central nervous system
   B. peripheral nervous system
   C. environment
   D. calcium ions

4. One of the principal uses of neuromuscular blocking agents is to provide adequate skeletal muscular relaxation during

    A. surgery
    B. rest
    C. epileptic seizures
    D. exercise

5. The abbreviation ACh stands for

    A. ache
    B. aluminum chloride
    C. acetylcholine
    D. acetaminophen

6. A centrally acting skeletal muscle relaxant commonly used to alleviate signs and symptoms of spasticity from multiple sclerosis is

    A. carisoprodol
    B. baclofen
    C. barbiturate
    D. codeine

7. Which of the following drugs may cause urine discoloration from orange to purple-red?

    A. dantrolene
    B. diazepam
    C. chlorzoxazone
    D. cortisol

8. A muscle relaxant which may worsen schizophrenic symptoms when mixed with propoxyphene is

    A. opium
    B. orphenadrine
    C. dantrolene sodium
    D. calcium

9. Pain-relieving drugs are also known as

    A. anaphylactics
    B. antiemetics
    C. analgesics
    D. antitoxins

10. Which of the following is a xanthine oxidase inhibitor agent?

    A. auranofin
    B. allopurinol
    C. acetaminophen
    D. colchicine

11. Gold compounds are indicated in which of the following?

    A. exfoliative dermatitis
    B. rheumatoid arthritis
    C. bone marrow aplasia
    D. exposure to heavy metals

12. The trade name of botulinum toxin type B is

    A. Botox
    B. Dantrium
    C. Dysport
    D. Myobloc

13. Allopurinol is used in the treatment of all of the following disorders, except

    A. temporary relief of mild to moderate pain
    B. secondary uric acid nephropathy
    C. uric acid stone formation
    D. gout

14. Which of the following is an example of a direct-acting antispasmodic drug?

    A. Soma
    B. Robaxin
    C. Dantrium
    D. Flexeril

15. Slow-acting antirheumatic drugs may be prescribed for patients with rheumatoid arthritis that

    A. causes muscle cramps
    B. causes numbness
    C. exists along with palpitations
    D. progresses to deformity

Fill in the Blank

1. Skeletal muscle relaxants work by blocking _____ nerve impulses.

2. Neuromuscular blocking drugs are not safe during pregnancy because they are in category _____.

3. Baclofen is often the drug of first choice as a centrally acting skeletal muscle relaxant because of its wide _____.

4. Name three anti-inflammatory drugs that are classified as slow-acting anti-rheumatic drugs:

    A. _____
    B. _____
    C. _____

5. Name five adverse effects of long-term administration of corticosteroids:

    A. _____
    B. _____
    C. _____
    D. _____
    E. _____

6. The precise mechanism of action of *colchicine* is _____.

7. The most common site of the initial attack of gout is the _____ metatarsophalangeal _____.

Critical Thinking

A 48-year-old woman has been diagnosed with gouty arthritis. She also has a history of hypertension and a chronic peptic ulcer.

1. Though it should be used cautiously, which of the medications for gouty arthritis discussed in this chapter should be prescribed?

2. What would be the treatment choices for acute gouty arthritis?

3. If she received the drug of choice for acute gouty arthritis, what would be the most common adverse effects?

Drug Therapy for Cardiovascular Disorders

OBJECTIVES

After completing this chapter, the reader should be able to:

1. Describe normal cardiac function related to contractility and blood flow.
2. Explain the pathophysiology of angina pectoris.
3. Explain the different types of coronary vasodilators.
4. Explain the common adverse effects associated with each antianginal drug class.
5. Identify the various types of antiarrhythmics and their adverse effects.
6. Describe myocardial infarction and three steps that should be taken to limit myocardial necrosis.
7. List medications that are used in congestive heart failure.
8. Describe vasoconstrictors and their purpose.
9. Discuss the action of digitalis and its side effects.
10. Explain the consequences of congestive heart failure to the cardiovascular system.

GLOSSARY

Angina pectoris – an episodic, reversible oxygen insufficiency

Arrhythmias – deviations from the normal pattern of the heartbeat; also called "dysrhythmias"

Arteriosclerosis – degenerative changes in small arteries, commonly occurring in older individuals and diabetics; walls of arteries lose elasticity and become thick and hard

Atherosclerosis – disease of the arteries characterized by the presence of

atheromas (plaques consisting of lipids, cells, and cell debris, often with attached thrombi, which form inside the walls of large arteries)

Atheromas – plaques consisting of lipids, cells, and cell debris, often with attached thrombi, which form inside the walls of large arteries

Beta-adrenergic blockers – drugs used to reverse sympathetic heart action caused by exercise, stress, or physical exertion

Calcium channel blockers – drugs used to treat stable angina

Congestive heart failure (CHF) – condition in which the heart is not able to pump enough blood to meet the body's metabolic demands

Coronary arterial bypass graft (CABG) – a procedure wherein a vein graft is surgically implanted to bypass the part of the occlusion in the coronary artery

Coronary artery disease (CAD) – a condition in which there is an insufficient supply of oxygen to the myocardium (cardiac muscle); also referred to as "coronary heart disease" and "ischemic heart disease"

Myocardial infarction (MI) – an area of dead cardiac muscle tissue, with or without hemorrhage

Nitrates – drugs used for the treatment of angina

Percutaneous transluminal coronary angioplasty (PTCA) – reduces obstruction by means of invasive procedures requiring cardiac catheterization; the catheter contains an inflatable balloon that flattens the obstruction

Silent angina – a condition that occurs in the absence of angina pain

Vasospastic angina – decubitus angina; characterized by periodic attacks of cardiac pain that occur when a person is lying down

OVERVIEW

Cardiovascular disorders are among the most common causes of death in the United States. There are many factors that contribute to heart disease, such as age, genetics, and lifestyle. Proper diet, exercise, avoiding cigarette smoking, and getting enough rest can do a lot to keep the heart functioning for a long time. Heart disease may also be caused by other conditions or disorders such as high blood pressure, high blood cholesterol levels, obesity, and diabetes. A pharmacy technician should be familiar with the most common disorders of the cardiovascular system and the most effective agents used in the treatment of each of them.

ANATOMY REVIEW

- The cardiovascular system consists of the heart, blood vessels, blood, and lymph (Figure 11-1).

- The heart is a hollow muscular organ consisting of the myocardium, pericardium, and endocardium. Four valves control blood flow into and out of the heart (Figure 11-2).

- Coronary arteries provide blood flow and nutrients to the heart muscle itself (Figure 11-3).

- The largest of the blood vessels are the arteries, which carry oxygenated blood away from the heart to the capillaries. The pulmonary arteries are the exceptions; they carry deoxygenated blood from the heart to the lungs.

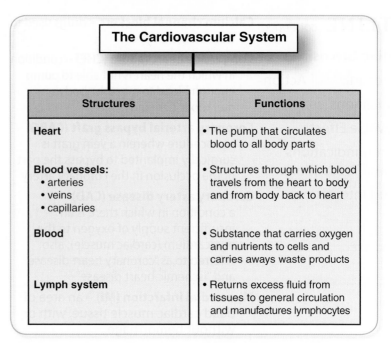

Figure 11-1 The cardiovascular system.

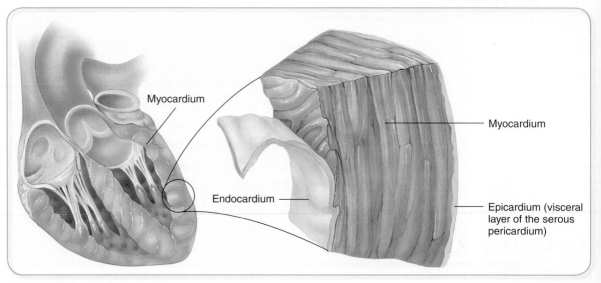

Figure 11-2 The walls and valves of the heart.

- The capillaries are the smallest of the blood vessels. They are the sites of oxygen and nutrient exchange between the blood and the organs of the body.

- The veins carry deoxygenated blood away from the capillaries to the heart.

- There are two circuits for blood flow: the left side of the heart pumps blood to the systemic circuit, while the right side of the heart pumps blood through the pulmonary circuit (Figure 11-4).

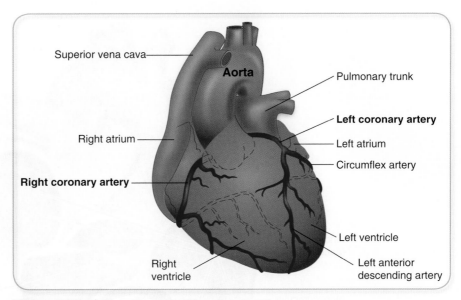

Figure 11-3 The coronary arteries.

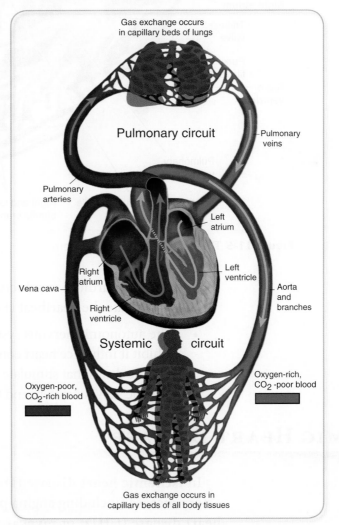

Figure 11-4 The left side of the heart pumps blood to the entire systemic circuit, while the right side pumps blood to the pulmonary circuit.

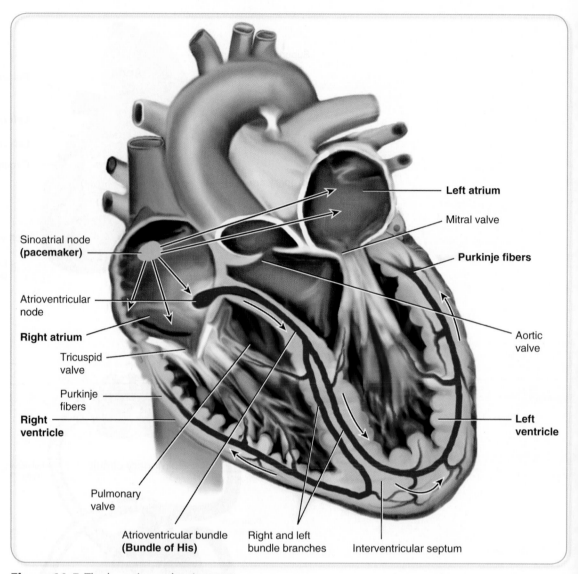

Figure 11-5 The heart's conduction system.

- The myocardium conducts its own electrical impulse, which serves to regulate the heartbeat (Figure 11-5).

- The autonomic nervous system (ANS) and the drugs that stimulate or inhibit it influence heart contractions. The sympathetic nervous system and the drugs that stimulate it *increase* heart rate, whereas the parasympathetic nervous system and the drugs that stimulate it *decrease* heart rate.

ISCHEMIC HEART DISEASE

In **ischemic heart disease (IHD)**—[most commonly called **coronary artery disease** (including angina pectoris), and also referred to as **coronary heart disease (CHD)** or **myocardial infarction** (heart attack)]—, part of the heart muscle is damaged because of obstruction in an artery. The basic problem is insufficient oxygen for the needs of the heart muscle.

A common cause of disability and death, coronary artery disease may ultimately lead to heart failure, serious arrhythmias, or sudden death. There are several factors that may affect functions that control myocardial oxygen demand (see Table 11-1). It is the leading cause of death in men and women in the United States.

Medical Terminology Review

myocardial

my/o- = muscle
cardi/a = heart
-al = pertaining to
the heart muscle

TABLE 11-1 Factors Affecting Cardiac Parameters that Control Myocardial Oxygen Demand

Factors	Heart Rate	Blood Pressure
β-Blockers	Decrease	Decrease
Cold	Increase	Increase
Exercise	Increase	Increase
Nitroglycerin	Increase	Decrease
Smoking	Increase	Increase

Key Concept

Every health care professional should be certified in CPR because heart disease is the number-one cause of death in the United States. It is vital that CPR be applied correctly to patients with suspected heart attacks in order to save their lives.

Arteriosclerosis and Atherosclerosis

Arteriosclerosis is the term used to describe degenerative changes in small arteries, commonly occurring in older individuals and diabetics. Elasticity is lost, and the walls become thick and hard. The lumen gradually narrows and may become obscured. This leads to diffuse ischemia and death in various tissues, such as those of the heart, kidneys, or brain.

Medical Terminology Review

arteriosclerosis

arteri/o = artery
sclera/o = hard
-sis = condition
hardening of the arteries

Atherosclerosis is differentiated by the presence of **atheromas** (plaques consisting of lipids, cells, and cell debris, often with attached thrombi, which form inside the walls of large arteries). Atheromas form primarily in large arteries such as the aorta and the coronary arteries. Figure 11-6 illustrates accumulation of lipids in blood vessels causing occlusion.

Key Concept

Having a buildup of calcium plaque in the arteries means an increased risk of heart attacks and death in multiple ethnic groups, according to recent research.

Angina Pectoris

Angina pectoris is an episodic, reversible oxygen insufficiency. This condition is the most common form of IHD. Angina pectoris is applied to varying forms of transient chest pain that are attributable to insufficient myocardial oxygen. Atherosclerotic lesions that produce a narrowing of the coronary arteries are the major cause of angina. However, tachycardia (increased heart rate), anemia, hyperthyroidism, and hypotension can cause an oxygen imbalance. According to the American Heart Association, angina occurs more commonly in women than men. There are several types of angina: stable (classic), unstable, decubitus (nocturnal), and silent angina. The most common form is classic angina that may occur, with predictable frequency, from exertion (often from exercising), emotional stress, or a heavy meal. Classic angina is relieved by rest, nitroglycerin, or both.

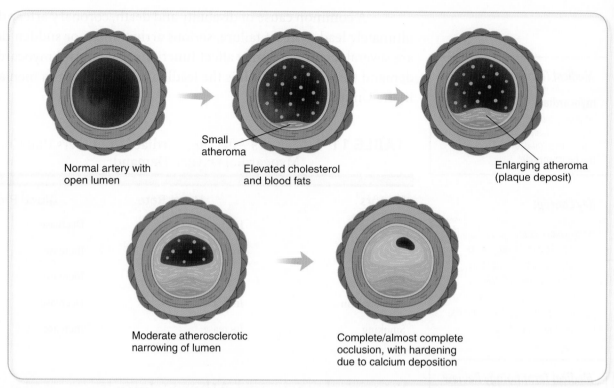

Small atheroma

Normal artery with open lumen

Elevated cholesterol and blood fats

Enlarging atheroma (plaque deposit)

Moderate atherosclerotic narrowing of lumen

Complete/almost complete occlusion, with hardening due to calcium deposition

Figure 11-6 Atherosclerosis showing narrowing of the arteries from plaque buildup.

Unstable angina is a medical emergency, and the patient must be treated in a hospital. It typically has a sudden onset, sudden worsening, and stuttering reoccurrence over days and weeks, and carries a more severe short-term prognosis than stable chronic angina. Unstable angina occurs during periods of rest. Signs of unstable angina include changes in blood pressure, transient heart murmur, and arrhythmias.

Decubitus angina is a condition characterized by periodic attacks of cardiac pain that occur when a person is lying down. It is also known as **vasospastic angina**. Decubitus angina occurs when the decreased myocardial blood flow is caused by spasms of the coronary arteries.

Silent angina is a condition that occurs in the absence of angina pain. One or more coronary arteries are occluded, but the individual remains asymptomatic.

Nocturnal angina is caused by coronary artery spasms and can be treated by calcium channel blockers and nitrates. It occurs during the REM period of sleep.

Treatment goals for angina include:

- Reducing the risk of sudden death

- Preventing myocardial infarction (MI)

- Increasing myocardial oxygen supply

- Reducing pain and anxiety associated with an angina attack

Medical Terminology Review

angioplasty

angio = blood and lymph vessel
plasty = molding or forming surgically
a procedure involving the molding or forming of a blood vessel surgically

Treatment for angina includes surgery and drug therapy. If the coronary arteries are significantly occluded or blocked, **coronary arterial bypass graft (CABG)** or **percutaneous transluminal coronary angioplasty (PTCA)** are performed. CABG is a procedure wherein a vein graft is surgically implanted to bypass the part of the occlusion in the coronary artery. PTCA reduces obstruction by means of invasive procedures requiring cardiac catheterization. The catheter contains an inflatable balloon that flattens the obstruction. Newer techniques use laser angioplasty.

ANTIANGINAL DRUG THERAPY

There are three groups of medications that may meet the treatment goals for angina pectoris.

1. Nitrates
2. β-Adrenergic Blockers
3. Calcium Channel Blockers

Nitrates

Nitrates were the first agents used to relieve angina. This group of drugs reduces myocardial ischemia, but may cause hypotension. Nitrates are still an important part of antianginal therapy. Table 11-2 shows nitrates commonly used in the treatment of angina.

TABLE 11-2 Commonly Used Combination Drugs for Angina and Myocardial Infarction

Generic Name	Trade Name	Route of Administration	Average Adult Dosage
Beta-adrenergic blockers			
atenolol	Tenormin®	PO	25–50 mg/day (max: 100 mg/day)
metoprolol tartrate	Lopressor®, Toprol-XL®	PO	100 mg bid (max: 400 mg/day)
propranolol hydrochloride	Inderal®, Inderal LA®	PO	10–20 mg bid-tid (max: 320 mg/day)
timolol maleate	Betimol®, Blocadren®	PO	15–45 mg tid (max: 60 mg/day)
Calcium channel blockers			
amlodipine	Norvasc®	PO	5–10 mg/day (max: 10 mg/day)
bepridil	Vascor®	PO	200 mg/day (max: 360 mg/day)

(continues)

TABLE 11-2 Commonly Used Combination Drugs for Angina and Myocardial Infarction—*continued*

Generic Name	Trade Name	Route of Administration	Average Adult Dosage
diltiazem hydrochloride	Cardizem®, Dilacor XR®	PO	30 mg qid (max: 360 mg/day)
nicardipine hydrochloride	Cardene®	PO	20–40 mg tid or 30–60 mg SR bid (max: 120 mg/day)
nifedipine	Adalat®, Procardia®	PO	10–20 mg tid (max: 180 mg/day)
verapamil hydrochloride	Calan®, Covera-HS®	PO	80 mg tid-qid (max: 480 mg/day) taken at bedtime
Organic nitrates			
amyl nitrate	(generic only)	Inhalation	1 ampule (0.18–0.3 mL) PRN
isosorbide dinitrate	Iso-Bid®, Isordil®	PO	2.5–30 mg qid
isosorbide mononitrate	Imdur®, ISMO®	PO	20 mg bid
nitroglycerin	Nitrostat®, Nitrocap®,	SL	1 tablet (0.3–0.6 mg) or 1 spray (0.4–0.8 mg) q3–5 min (max: 3 doses in 15 min)
	Nitro-Dur®	Topical	applied transdermally daily

Mechanism of Action

Nitrates primarily are effective in the venous circulation by relaxing vascular smooth muscle and reducing the left ventricle's work. These agents are administered to dilate the blood vessels and stop attacks of angina (see Figure 11-7).

Indications

Nitrates are used in the treatment of angina as coronary vasodilators. Nitrate preparations should be based on onset of action, duration of action, and patient compliance. Nitrate preparations are available in sublingual tablets, nitroglycerin spray bottles, topical nitroglycerin ointments, and transdermal patches. The sublingual route is the most common route of administration for nitroglycerin. This agent begins to work rapidly and lasts for about an hour. This is an ideal preparation for acute anginal pain. Administration should begin as soon as the pain begins, and should not be delayed until the pain is severe. If one tablet is not sufficient, one or two additional tablets should be taken at five-minute intervals. For persistent pain, the patient should see a physician, because he or she may have signs of a myocardial infarction. The shelf life of nitroglycerin is longer in a dark, tightly closed container. After the container is opened, the drug is effective

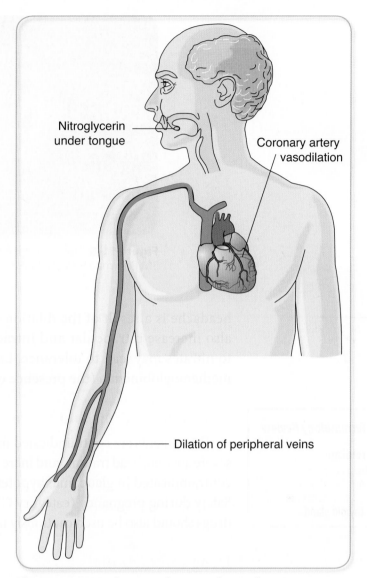

Figure 11-7 Mechanism of action of nitroglycerin.

for approximately 30 days, and the date on which it was opened should be written on the container. Thirty days after the container is opened, the medication should be discarded and replaced with a new bottle.

Transdermal patches contain a reservoir of nitroglycerin. This agent is slowly released for absorption through the skin (see Figure 11-8). The patches are slow in onset and are not effective for an ongoing anginal attack. The application site of the patch should be rotated daily to prevent irritation.

Topical ointment can also be used on the skin by using an applicator, and covering it with plastic wrap held in place with adhesive tape. The sites should be rotated to prevent local irritation.

Adverse Effects

Abrupt discontinuation of long-acting nitroglycerin preparations may cause angina. Vasodilation can lead to orthostatic hypotension, tachycardia, headache, dizziness, weakness, syncope, and blushing. Nitrate-induced

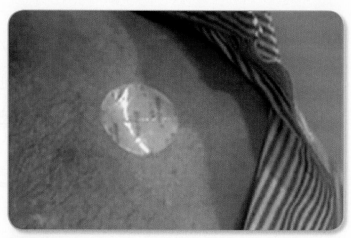

Figure 11-8 Transdermal nitroglycerin patch (Courtesy of 3M Pharmaceuticals, St. Paul, MN).

headache is a result of the dilation of cerebral blood vessels. Nitrates may also increase intraocular and intracranial pressure. Continuous exposure to nitrates may lead to tolerance. Large doses of nitrate drugs can produce methemoglobinemia (the presence of methemoglobin in the blood).

Contraindications and Precautions

These agents are contraindicated in patients with hypersensitivity to nitrates, severe anemia, head trauma, and increased intracranial pressure. Nitrates are also contraindicated in glaucoma, hypotension, hyperthyroidism, and alcoholism. Safety during pregnancy (category C) and lactation is not established. Nitrate drugs should also be used cautiously in severe liver or kidney disease.

Drug Interactions

A combination of nitrates and sildenafil (Viagra) can cause prolonged and potentially life-threatening hypotension. Sildenafil therapy should therefore be contraindicated in patients who use nitrates. Beta-blockers, calcium channel blockers, vasodilators, and alcohol can enhance the hypotensive effect of nitrates. IV nitroglycerin may antagonize the effects of heparin.

Beta-adrenergic Blockers

Beta-adrenergic blockers *(β-blockers)* block the beta 1 receptor site. Beta-blockers decrease the effects of the sympathetic nervous system by blocking the release of the catecholamines epinephrine and norepinephrine, thereby decreasing the heart rate and blood pressure. (They are listed in both Tables 11-2 and 11-4.)

Mechanism of Action

Beta blockers reduce oxygen demand, both at rest and during exertion, in the myocardium, and prevent myocardial infarction (IM).

> ### *Medical Terminology Review*
>
> **hyperthyroidism**
> *hyper* = over; above; beyond
> *thyroid* = the thyroid gland
> *ism* = action; process; practice
> overactive thyroid gland

Indications

The beta-blockers reduce the frequency and severity of exertional angina that is not controlled by nitrates. Therefore, these are an important part of therapy for angina pectoris. Combined therapy with nitrates is often preferred in the treatment of angina pectoris, because of a decrease in the side effects of both agents.

Adverse Effects

Beta-blockers have few adverse effects on the respiratory and cardiovascular systems. Common adverse effects of these drugs include dyspnea, bronchospasm, hypotension, bradycardia, and hypoglycemia. These agents may also cause insomnia and depression.

Contraindications and Precautions

β-blockers are contraindicated in patients with a known hypersensitivity to these agents. β-blockers are also contraindicated for use in patients with asthma, congestive heart failure, heart block, bradycardia, and diabetes mellitus. These drugs should be avoided in patients with cardiogenic shock, pulmonary edema, and peripheral vascular disease.

β-adrenergic blockers should be used with caution in patients prone to non-allergenic bronchospasm (e.g., chronic bronchitis, emphysema), major surgery, stroke, renal disease, or hepatic disease. β-blockers are used cautiously in elderly patients, patients with diabetes mellitus, and in patients prone to hypoglycemia.

Drug Interactions

These agents may interact with atropine and other anticholinergics, NSAIDs, insulin, sulfonylureas, lidocaine, verapamil, prazosin, and terazosin.

Calcium Channel Blockers

Calcium channel blockers are considered third-choice agents in the treatment of stable angina, certain dysrhythmias, and hypertension. Calcium channel blockers are also listed in Table 11-2.

Mechanism of Action

Calcium channel blockers are a type of drug that block the entry of calcium into smooth muscle cells as well as myocytes. They produce arterial vasodilation and thereby reduce arterial blood pressure. They also reduce myocardial contractility, resulting in reduction of myocardial oxygen consumption.

Indications

Calcium channel blockers are used to treat exertional angina that is not controlled by nitrates, and in combination with beta-blockers. This

combination provides the most effective therapy. They are considered the drug of choice in the treatment of angina at rest. Diltiazem and verapamil will reduce the heart rate. Nifedipine, amlodipine, and felodipine are among the most potent calcium-blocking agents. β-blockers are recommended as the first-line treatment of angina pectoris, but if they are not tolerated, calcium channel blockers can be administered. Diltiazem and verapamil can be used, but they have the disadvantage of depressing contractility more than dihydropyridines do. The therapeutic goal in medication use is to reduce the frequency and intensity of anginal attacks without suppressing the cardiac action too much.

Adverse Effects

Common adverse effects related to the use of calcium channel blockers include: flushing, headaches, dizziness, hypotension, ankle edema, constipation, and palpitations. Combinations of nitrates, β-blockers, and calcium channel blockers are often preferred for treatment of angina pectoris, because these agents have fewer adverse effects.

Contraindications and Precautions

Calcium channel blockers are contraindicated in patients with a history of hypersensitivity to these drugs, hypotension, or cardiogenic shock. The major contraindications to combination therapy are associated with the use of β-blockers and calcium channel blockers, which may cause excessive cardiac depression. Calcium channel blockers should be used with caution during pregnancy (category C) and lactation, and in patients with congestive heart failure, hepatic or renal dysfunction, and hypotension.

Drug Interactions

Calcium channel blockers increase risk of orthostatic hypotension with prazosin. Increased blood pressure may occur with aspirin, bismuth subsalicylate, or magnesium salicylate. Some calcium channel blockers increase serum levels and toxicity of cyclosporine.

MYOCARDIAL INFARCTION

Myocardial infarction (MI) is an area of dead cardiac muscle tissue, with or without hemorrhage. Myocardial infarction is produced by an obstruction of the coronary artery, which results in a lack of oxygen to the tissue. Coronary heart disease is the primary cause of death in American males and females as well as a major cause of disability. For those who survive an MI, there is a notably greater risk of a second MI, congestive heart failure, or a stroke occurring within a short time.

A myocardial infarction, or heart attack, occurs when a coronary artery is totally obstructed, leading to prolonged ischemia (reduction of blood supply to the heart) and cell death, or infarction, of the heart wall (see Figure 11-9).

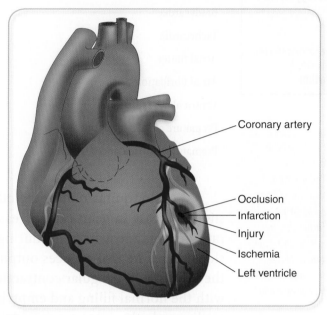

Coronary artery

Occlusion

Infarction

Injury

Ischemia

Left ventricle

Figure 11-9 Myocardial infarction.

After myocardial infarction, there are three goals that should be achieved expeditiously and simultaneously to limit myocardial necrosis and mortality:

- Relief of pain

- Confirmation of diagnosis by electrocardiogram (ECG) and measurements of serum markers

- Assessment and treatment of hemodynamic abnormalities

Pain relief is best achieved with oxygen (2 L/min by nasal cannula), nitroglycerin, and morphine sulfate. The rationale for reperfusion therapy (thrombolytic therapy) is based on the high prevalence of occlusive thrombus in early treatment. The greatest benefit is seen when this therapy is performed within the first four hours of the onset of pain. Antithrombotic agents should be considered for all patients with an acute myocardial infarction. Antithrombotic medications include: unfractionated heparin, low molecular weight heparin, warfarin, aspirin, and antiplatelets (see Chapter 13).

Key Concept

During acute myocardial infarction, women are less likely to experience chest pain than men. Common acute symptoms in women include dyspnea, weakness, fatigue, nausea or vomiting, palpitations, and indigestion.

CARDIAC ARRHYTHMIAS

Arrhythmias (dysrhythmias) are deviations from the normal cardiac rate or rhythm. They may result from damage to the heart's conduction system or from systemic causes such as electrolyte abnormalities, fever, hypoxia, stress, and drug toxicity.

Key Concept

According to a recent study, patients who are diagnosed for the first time with atrial fibrillation have a significantly greater early risk of dying compared with those who do not have this condition. Factors that are strongly associated with death in atrial fibrillation patients include a faster heart rate at diagnosis, being thin, a history of chronic kidney disease, and malignancy.

TABLE 11-3 Various Cardiac Arrhythmias

Type of Arrhythmia	Beats per Minute
Bradycardia	Less than 60
Tachycardia	150 to 250
Atrial flutter	200 to 350
Atrial fibrillation	More than 350
Ventricular fibrillation	Variable
Premature atrial contraction	Variable
Premature ventricular contraction	Variable

Arrhythmias reduce the efficiency of the heart's pumping cycle. A slight increase in heart rate increases cardiac output, but a very rapid heart rate prevents adequate filling during diastole, reducing cardiac output. A very slow heart rate also reduces output to the tissues, including the brain and the heart itself. Irregular contractions are inefficient because they interfere with the normal filling and emptying cycle. Table 11-3 summarizes various cardiac arrhythmias.

ANTIARRHYTHMIC DRUGS

Antiarrhythmic agents do not cure the dysrhythmia, but the goal of treatment is to restore normal cardiac function. These agents are classified in four distinct groups, according to their effects: Class I (sodium channel blockers), which are subclassified into three groups, Class IA, IB, and IC (see Table 11-4); Class II (β-adrenergic blockers); Class III (which interfere with potassium outflow); and Class IV (calcium channel blockers). There are also other agents that may be used for the treatment of arrhythmias, such as digoxin, atropine, and magnesium.

Mechanism of Action

Class I – Fast (sodium) channel blockers decrease the fast sodium influx to the cardiac cells. These drugs decrease conduction velocity in the cardiac tissue, suppress automaticity, and increase recovery time (repolarization). There are three subgroups of fast channel blockers: IA slows conduction and prolongs repolarization (e.g., quinidine, procainamide, disopyramide); IB slows conduction and shortens repolarization (e.g., lidocaine, mexiletine, tocainide); and IC prolongs conduction with little to no effect on repolarization (e.g., flecainide).

Class II – Beta-adrenergic blockers inhibit adrenergic stimulation of the heart, and depress myocardial excitability and contractility. Therefore, they decrease conduction velocity in cardiac tissue. Major beta-adrenergic blockers are listed in Tables 11-2 and 11-4.

TABLE 11-4 Classifications of Antiarrhythmic Drugs

Generic Name	Trade Name	Route of Administration	Average Adult Dosage
Class IA (sodium channel blockers)			
disopyramide phosphate	Norpace®	PO	100–200 mg q6h or 300 mg sust. release cap. q12h
procainamide hydrochloride	Procan®, Procanbid, Pronestyl®	PO, IM, IV	PO: 50 mg/kg/day in divided doses; IM: 0.5–1g q4–8h; IV: 100 mg q5 min at a rate of 25–50 mg/min until arrhythmia is controlled
quinidine gluconate	Quinaglute®	PO	200–300 mg q3–4h for 4 or more doses until arrhythmia terminates
Class IB			
lidocaine hydrochloride	Xylocaine®	IV	50–100 mg bolus at 20–50 mg/min, may repeat in 5 min, then start infusion of 1–4 mg/min immed. after 1st bolus
mexiletine	Mexitil®	PO	200–300 mg q8h (max: 1200 mg/day)
phenytoin	Dilantin®	IV	50–100 mg q10–15 min until dysrhythmia is terminated
Class IC			
flecainide acetate	Tambocor®	PO	100 mg q12h, may increase 50 mg bid q4d (max: 400 mg/day)
moricizine hydrochloride	Ethmozine®	PO	600–900 mg/day
propafenone	Rythmol®	PO	150–300 mg/tid; increase dosage slowly, prn, (max: 900 mg/day)
Class II (β-adrenergic blockers)			
acebutolol	Sectral®	PO	200–600 mg bid increased to 1200 mg/day
atenolol	Tenormin®	PO	25–50 mg/day, may increase to 100 mg/day
esmolol hydrochloride	Brevibloc®	IV	50 mcg/kg/min (max: 200 mcg/kg/min)
nadolol	Corgard®	PO	40 mg once/day, increase to 240–320 mg/day in 1–2 div. doses
propranolol hydrochloride	Inderal®	PO	10–30 mg tid or qid

(continues)

TABLE 11-4   Classifications of Antiarrhythmic Drugs—*continued*

Generic Name	Trade Name	Route of Administration	Average Adult Dosage
Class III (potassium channel blockers)			
amiodarone hydrochloride	Cordarone®	PO	PO: 400–1600 mg/day in 1–3 div. doses
bretylium tosylate	Bretylol®	IV	Rapid injection (5–10 mg/kg), or 1–2 mg/min as continuous infusion
dofetilide	Tikosyn®	PO	125–500 mcg bid
ibutilide fumarate	Corvert®	IV	1 mg infused over 10 min
Class IV (calcium channel blockers)			
diltiazem	Cardizem®	IV	0.25–15 mg/kg bolus over 2 min, may repeat in 15 min with 0.35 mg/kg
verapamil hydrochloride	Calan®	IV	2.5–5 mg initial dose, then 5–10 mg after 15–30 min
Others			
atropine	Atropisol®	IM, IV	0.5–1 mg q1–2h prn (max: 2 mg)
digoxin	Lanoxin®	PO, IV	PO: 0.75–1.5 mg/kg; IV: 0.5–1 mg/kg

Class III – Antiarrhythmics interfere with potassium outflow during repolarization. They prolong the action potential duration and effective refractory period. The prolonged period decreases the frequency of heart rate. Amiodarone decreases automaticity, prolongs atrioventricular conduction, and may even block the exchange of sodium and potassium.

Class IV – Antiarrhythmics selectively block slow calcium channels. Therefore, these agents can prolong nodal conduction and effective refractory period. These calcium antagonists may also decrease the ability of the heart to produce forceful contractions, leading to congestive heart failure. These drugs also relax smooth muscle and cause vasodilation. Verapamil works on the SA node to decrease its activity, thus decreasing the heart rate. It also decreases AV node conduction and is used for AV node dysrhythmias.

Indications

Quinidine is used to treat supraventricular arrhythmias, such as atrial flutter and atrial fibrillation, acute ventricular dysrhythmias, and life-threatening ventricular dysrhythmias. This agent also exhibits antimalarial, antipyretic, and oxytocic actions. Procainamide is safer to use intravenously and has fewer gastrointestinal (GI) adverse effects. Disopyramide has been approved for the treatment of ventricular arrhythmias. Generally, it is reserved

for patients who are intolerant of quinidine or procainamide. Lidocaine doses must be adjusted in patients with congestive heart failure or hepatic disease. Mexiletine is used primarily for chronic treatment of ventricular arrhythmias associated with previous myocardial infarction. Tocainide is useful for the treatment of ventricular tachyarrhythmias. Phenytoin is an antiepileptic drug that has proved to be useful in treating digitalis-induced tachyarrhythmias. β-adrenergic blockers are useful for treating tachyarrhythmias due to increased sympathetic activity, and also are used for a variety of other arrhythmias, atrial flutter, and atrial fibrillation. These are sometimes used for digitalis toxicity. Propranolol is the most common β-blocker that is used as an antiarrhythmic. Amiodarone is useful for severe refractory supraventricular and ventricular tachyarrhythmias. Amiodarone also possesses antianginal effects. Calcium channel blockers are useful for angina and for hypertension. Verapamil is useful for reentrant supraventricular tachycardia. Digitalis drugs are the principal medications for the treatment of congestive heart failure and certain arrhythmias. Digoxin is the drug most often prescribed because it can be administered orally and parenterally. It has an intermediate duration of action. The process of establishing the correct therapeutic dose of digitalis for maintaining optimal functioning of the heart without toxic effects is referred to as digitalization. The margin between effective therapy and dangerous toxicity is very narrow. Careful monitoring of the cardiac rate and rhythm with an ECG, cardiac function, adverse effects, and the blood digitalis level is required to determine the therapeutic maintenance dose.

Adverse Effects

Quinidine can lead to skeletal muscle weakness, especially in patients with myasthenia gravis. Rapid infusion of quinidine may cause severe hypotension and shock. It can produce ringing of the ears, dizziness, diarrhea, thrombocytopenia, and ventricular arrhythmias.

A high incidence of adverse reactions to procainamide is seen with chronic use. Severe or irreversible heart failure has been produced more frequently by procainamide than by quinidine. Procainamide also often causes drug-induced lupus syndrome.

Disopyramide drug may cause dry mouth, blurred vision, constipation, and urinary retention.

High doses of lidocaine can cause cardiovascular depression, confusion, and light-headedness. Otherwise, there is a low level of cardiotoxicity with the use of lidocaine. The most common side effects are neurologic, in contrast to quinidine and procainamide. Lidocaine has little effect on the autonomic nervous system. The common adverse effects of phenytoin use are nystagmus, blurred vision, vertigo, and hyperplasia of the gums.

Adverse effects of the use of beta-adrenergic blockers include bronchospasm. Bradycardia and myocardial depression may occur. Atropine

---

Medical Terminology Review

bradycardia
brady = *slow*
cardia = *heart action*
slow heart rate

or isoproterenol may be used to alleviate bradycardia. The most frequent cardiovascular adverse effects due to the use of propranolol are hypertension and bradycardia. It may also cause mental confusion and skin rashes.

Contraindications and Precautions

Class I antidysrhythmic agents are contraindicated in patients with hypersensitivity to these drugs, pregnancy (category B or C), and lactation. They should be avoided in patients with complete AV block, thyrotoxicosis, acute rheumatic fever, extensive myocardial damage, hypotensive states, myasthenia gravis, and digitalis intoxication. Quinidine should be used cautiously in patients with incomplete heart block, impaired kidney or liver function, bronchial asthma, myasthenia gravis, and potassium imbalance. Procainamide is used with caution in patients with hypotension, cardiac enlargement, congestive heart failure, heart attack, coronary occlusion, and hepatic or renal insufficiency.

Class II antidysrhythmic drugs (e.g., propranolol and others) are contraindicated in patients with congestive heart failure, right ventricular failure secondary to pulmonary hypertension, ventricular dysfunction, sinus bradycardia, bronchial asthma or bronchospasm, pulmonary edema, and allergic rhinitis during pollen season. Beta-adrenergic blockers are used cautiously in elderly patients and patients prone to non-allergic bronchospasm (e.g., chronic bronchitis, emphysema), stroke, major surgery, renal or hepatic disease, and diabetes mellitus.

Class III antiarrhythmic drugs (e.g., bretylium) have no contraindications for use in life-threatening ventricular arrhythmias. Safety during pregnancy (category C), lactation, or in children is not established. Amiodarone is contraindicated in patients with hypersensitivity to this agent. Amiodarone should be avoided in cardiogenic shock, severe sinus bradycardia, severe liver disease, and children. Safety during pregnancy (category D) or lactation is not established. Amiodarone is given to patients cautiously if they have cirrhosis of the liver, goiter, hypersensitivity to iodine, electrolyte imbalance, hypokalemia, hypovolemia, and open-heart surgery. It also must be used with caution in elderly patients. Bretylium is used with caution in patients with severe aortic stenosis or severe pulmonary hypertension, and angina pectoris.

Class IV antiarrythmic drugs (calcium channel blockers) are contraindicated in patients with severe hypotension, cardiogenic shock, cardiomegaly, digitalis toxicity, atrial flutter and fibrillation, and severe CHF. Safe use of these agents during pregnancy (category C) or lactation, and in children, is not established. Calcium channel blockers are used cautiously in those individuals with hepatic and renal impairment, heart attack by coronary occlusion, and aortic stenosis.

Drug Interactions

Two antiarrhythmic agents may cause additive effects and may increase the risk for drug toxicity. If quinidine and procainamide are given with digitalis, the

risk of digitalis toxicity may be increased. Quinidine may interact with cimetidine or barbiturates, with quinidine blood levels being increased. Quinidine that is given concurrently with verapamil increases the risk of hypotension. Lidocaine and procainamide may interact and cause additive cardiodepressant effects. Inderal may also increase the risk of lidocaine toxicity.

CONGESTIVE HEART FAILURE

Congestive heart failure (CHF) is one of the most common cardiovascular disorders. This condition occurs when the heart is not able to pump enough blood to meet the body's metabolic demands. Heart failure may be caused by any disorder that affects the heart's ability to receive or eject blood.

Because there is no cure for heart failure, the treatment goals are to prevent, treat, or remove the underlying causes when possible. Drugs can relieve the symptoms of heart failure by a number of different mechanisms, including slowing the heart rate, increasing contractility, and reducing its workload. Drugs used for heart failure include ACE inhibitors, diuretics, vasodilators, and cardiac glycosides. In this section, cardiac glycosides will be discussed in detail. The other drugs also used for heart failure are discussed in Chapter 12.

CARDIAC GLYCOSIDES

Cardiac glycosides are one of the oldest drugs used in the treatment of heart diseases (over 2,000 years). A number of plants contain cardiac glycosides. Digoxin is extracted from the leaves of the purple foxglove (*Digitalis purpurea*). In fact, the generic term digitalis is often used to represent all cardiac glycosides used in the clinical setting.

Cardiac glycosides increase the speed of myocardial contractions in both normal and failing hearts. Under normal cardiac conditions, digitalis treatment results in an increase in systemic vascular resistance and the constriction of smooth muscles in veins (cardiac output may decrease). In heart failure, digitalis increases the force of myocardial contractions, slows the heart rate, and slows the conduction of electrical impulses. The increased force of contractions improves the efficiency of the heart without increasing oxygen consumption. Normal blood circulation is restored and the kidney function is increased. The most common cardiac glycosides are digoxin and digitoxin. The major active ingredients found in digitalis plants are collectively referred to as digitalis. Cardiac glycosides are able to affect the congested heartbeats more forcefully within a shorter period of time. This force increases the amount of blood pumped from the heart and improves blood circulation, thus decreasing the congestion found with heart failure.

Digitalis drugs are principal medications for the treatment of congestive heart failure and certain arrhythmias (atrial fibrillation, flutter, and paroxysmal atrial tachycardias). Digoxin is prescribed the most frequently

because it can be administered orally and parenterally. It has an intermediate duration of action. The process of establishing the correct therapeutic dose of digitalis for maintaining optimal functioning of the heart without toxic effects is referred to as digitalization. There is a very narrow margin between effective therapy and dangerous toxicity. Careful monitoring of the cardiac rate and rhythm with an ECG, cardiac function, side effects, and blood digitalis level is required to determine the therapeutic maintenance dose.

Mechanism of Action

Cardiac glycosides act by increasing the force and velocity of myocardial systolic contraction (positive inotropic effect). They also decrease conduction velocity through the atrioventricular node.

Indications

Cardiac glycosides are used principally in the prophylactic management and treatment of heart failure, and to control the ventricular rate in patients with atrial fibrillation or flutter. These drugs are also used to treat and prevent recurrent atrial tachycardia, cardiogenic shock, and angina pectoris.

Since individual cardiac glycosides have similar pharmacologic and therapeutic properties, the choice of a preparation depends on the onset of action required, desired route of administration, and duration of action. Digoxin is the most commonly used cardiac glycoside, primarily because it may be administered by various routes, and it has an intermediate duration of action.

Adverse Effects

The most dangerous adverse effect of digoxin is its ability to cause dysrhythmias, particularly in patients who have hypokalemia. Common adverse effects of digoxin therapy include nausea, vomiting, anorexia, and abnormalities of the nervous system such as headache, blurred vision (yellow-green halos), diplopia, photophobia, drowsiness, fatigue, and confusion.

Contraindications and Precautions

Cardiac glycosides are contraindicated in patients with known hypersensitivity to these agents, ventricular tachycardia, and ventricular failure, and in the presence of digitalis toxicity.

Cardiotonics are used cautiously in patients with renal insufficiency, hypokalemia, advanced heart disease, acute MI, severe lung disease, hypothyroidism, pregnancy (category A), and lactation. Fetal toxicity and neonatal death have been reported from maternal digoxin overdosage.

Drug Interactions

Cardiotonics react with many different drugs, including antacids, cholestyramine, and diuretics. Colestipol decreases digoxin absorption.

SUMMARY

Diseases of the cardiovascular system are among the leading causes of death in the United States. There are varieties of medications, some of which are effective on the myocardium itself, while some others affect the blood vessels of the vascular system. Vasodilators, such as nitrates, increase the size of blood vessels to improve circulation of the blood for the management of angina pectoris. Cardiac glycosides come from digitalis and are used to increase the force of myocardial contractions in congestive heart failure. Antidysrhythmics are used to treat disorders of the cardiac rhythm. These disorders may occur from coronary artery disease, electrolyte imbalances, cardiac conduction abnormalities, or even from endocrine disease (thyroid disorders).

EXPLORING THE WEB

Visit *www.intelihealth.com*

- Search for "cardiac drugs." Read some of the related articles on disorders of the heart and cardiovascular system and the drug therapies used to treat them.

Visit *www.americanheart.org*

- Research the diseases and conditions discussed within this chapter for further understanding of them.

REVIEW QUESTIONS

Multiple Choice

1. Which of the following antianginal drugs are also used as antihypertensives and antiarrhythmics?

   A. nitrates
   B. vasoconstrictors
   C. diuretics
   D. beta-adrenergic blockers

2. Which of the following drugs is the class of calcium channel blockers?

   A. propranolol
   B. isosorbid
   C. verapamil
   D. atenolol

3. Early signs of toxicity of digitalis include:

   A. mental disorders
   B. nausea and vomiting
   C. tachycardia
   D. seizures

4. Which of the following medications is not used for dysrhythmia?

   A. beta-adrenergic blockers
   B. digoxin
   C. heparin
   D. atropine

5. A combination of nitrates and sildenafil (Viagra) can cause:

   A. stroke
   B. hypotension
   C. heart murmur
   D. hypertension

6. An example of a class II antidysrhythmic drug is:

   A. propranolol
   B. digoxin
   C. bretylium
   D. quinidine

7. Which of the following are common adverse effects of antidysrhythmic drugs?

   A. fatigue, diarrhea, hypertension
   B. dizziness, hypotension, and weakness
   C. anorexia, fatigue, and constipation
   D. fatigue, hypertension, and headache

8. An antidysrhythmic drug may cause:

   A. increased hepatic insufficiency
   B. decreased cardiac output
   C. increased cardiac output
   D. increased renal insufficiency

9. Which of the following administration routes for nitroglycerin is the most common?

   A. sublingual
   B. transdermal patch
   C. topical ointment
   D. parenteral

10. Combined therapy with nitrates is often preferred in treatment of angina pectoris because it results in which of the following?

   A. better toleration
   B. less adverse effects
   C. less expense
   D. increased blood volume

Fill in the Blank

1. Beta-blockers reduce the frequency and severity of exertional angina that is not controlled by _____.

2. Class I antiarrhythmic drugs are also called _____.

3. Calcium channel blockers are in Class _____ of the antiarrhythmic drugs.

4. Common side effects of phenytoin use are _____, _____, _____, and _____.

5. Cardiac glycosides act by increasing the force and velocity of _____.

Matching

_____ 1. Subclass IA (fast channel blockers)

_____ 2. Subclass IB

_____ 3. Subclass IC

_____ 4. Class III (agents that interfere with potassium outflow)

_____ 5. Class IV (calcium channel blockers)

A. verapamil (Calan)

B. lidocaine (Xylocaine)

C. bretylium (Bretylol)

D. procainamide (Pronestyl)

E. flecainide (Tambocor)

Critical Thinking

A man who is 57 years old is experiencing severe chest pains. He arrives at the emergency room of his local hospital with cool and clammy skin, blood pressure of 92/60, and a weak, irregular pulse of 90. He is given oxygen and an ECG machine is set up to monitor him. After blood tests, he is initially diagnosed with MI of the left ventricle. His wife tells the doctors that he is a heavy cigarette smoker, loves fried foods and meat, and often complains of indigestion and stomach pain. He is very busy at work and often feels fatigued at night. His father died of a heart attack, and he is fearful of the same thing happening to him. The doctors suspect generalized atherosclerosis.

1. List the elements of this patient's history that are high-risk factors for atherosclerosis.

2. How does atherosclerosis cause an MI?

3. If his reported indigestion was actually angina, explain how this pain might have occurred.

Websites:

www.americanheart.org

www.cardiologychannel.com/angina/index.shtml

CHAPTER 12

Antihypertensive Agents and Hyperlipidemia

OBJECTIVES

After completing this chapter, the reader should be able to:

1. Describe the major physiological factors that regulate blood pressure.
2. Define the three forms of hypertension.
3. Describe the effects of cardiac output, peripheral resistance, and blood volume on blood pressure.
4. Identify the major risk factor associated with hypertension.
5. Explain the role of the kidneys and renin-angiotensin-aldosterone system in blood pressure regulation.
6. Describe the classification of antihypertensives.
7. Identify different types of diuretics.
8. Describe the mechanisms of action of all drug groups used in the treatment of hypertension.
9. State common adverse effects of the antihypertensive drug groups.
10. Discuss the angiotensin-converting enzyme (ACE).
11. Describe hyperlipidemia and the importance of cholesterol and triglycerides.
12. Describe combination drug therapy for hyperlipidemia.

GLOSSARY

Angiotensin-converting enzyme inhibitors – drugs that competitively inhibit conversion of angiotensin I to angiotensin II, a potent vasoconstrictor, through the angiotensin-converting enzyme activity, with resultant lower levels of angiotensin II

Angiotensin II receptor antagonists – drugs that block the binding of angiotensin II to the angiotensin II type 1 receptor

Cardiac output – the amount of blood the heart pumps to the body in one minute

Diastolic blood pressure – the pressure measured at the moment the ventricles relax

Diuretics – drugs that increase sodium excretion and lower blood volume

Essential hypertension – idiopathic (occurring spontaneously from an unknown cause); also known as primary hypertension

Hyperlipidemia – an increase in triglycerides and cholesterol

Hypertension – an abnormal increase in arterial blood pressure

Lipoprotein – a class of blood chemicals whose molecules are comprised of a lipid portion and a protein portion

Malignant hypertension – an uncontrollable, severe, and rapidly progressive form of hypertension with many complications

Niacin – vitamin B_3, nicotinic acid

Primary hypertension – idiopathic (occurring spontaneously from an unknown cause); also known as essential hypertension

Rhabdomyolysis – a potentially fatal destruction of skeletal muscle, characterized by the presence of myoglobin in the urine; it is also associated with acute renal failure in heatstroke

Sclerotic – hardening, toughening

Secondary hypertension – results from renal (e.g., nephrosclerosis) or endocrine (e.g., hyperaldosteronism) disease, or pheochromocytoma, a benign tumor of the adrenal medulla; in this type of hypertension, the underlying problem must be resolved

Statins – a class of drugs that inhibits the activity of an enzyme that forms cholesterol in the body; so named because all of their generic names end with "-statin" (e.g., lovastatin)

Steatorrhea – elimination of large amounts of fat in the stool

Stroke volume – the volume of blood pumped with each heartbeat

Sympatholytic drugs – a group of drugs that blocks or inhibits the effects of epinephrine or norepinephrine on the cells that normally react to them

Systolic blood pressure – the pressure measured at the moment the heart contracts

Vasodilators – drugs used to relax or dilate vessels throughout the body

OVERVIEW

Hypertension (high blood pressure) is the most common cardiovascular disease. The prevalence varies with age, race, education, and many other variables. Sustained arterial hypertension damages blood vessels in the kidneys, heart, and brain, leading to an increased incidence of cardiac failure, coronary diseases, stroke, and renal failure. Effective pharmacologic lowering of blood pressure has been shown to prevent damage to blood vessels and to substantially reduce morbidity and mortality rates.

A number of metabolic disorders that involve elevation in levels of any of the **lipoproteins** (a class of blood chemicals whose molecules are comprised of a lipid portion and a protein portion) are termed **hyperlipidemias**. The term *hyperlipidemia* denotes increased levels of triglycerides and cholesterol in the plasma. Analysis of serum lipids includes assessment of all of the

Medical Terminology Review

hyperlipidemia

hyper = over; above; beyond
lipid = fat
emia = blood condition
condition in which there are increased levels of fat in the blood

subgroups (total cholesterol, triglycerides, low-density lipoproteins, and high-density lipoproteins), because the proportions in which these groups are found in the blood indicate the risk factors for the individual. The danger of elevated cholesterol levels is that cholesterol collects on blood vessel walls and calcifies. This hardening of the arteries causes the vessels to narrow, lose resiliency, and become rough enough to damage passing blood cells. Damaged blood cells trigger clotting, which can result in stroke or myocardial infarction.

BLOOD PRESSURE

Key Concept

The main factors determining blood pressure are cardiac output and systemic vascular resistance (the total amount of resistance the blood has to overcome to travel throughout the body). Blood pressure is regulated by an interaction between the nervous, humoral, and renal systems.

Blood pressure is a measurement of the pressure exerted on the walls of arteries as the heart pumps. The pressure measured at the moment the heart contracts is called **systolic blood pressure**. The pressure measured at the moment the ventricles relax is called **diastolic blood pressure**. The arteries closest to the heart maintain the highest pressures. Pressure decreases in the arteries the farther the arteries are from the heart.

Blood pressure is determined by **cardiac output** and **stroke volume**. The amount of blood the heart pumps to the body in one minute is the cardiac output. The stroke volume is the volume of the blood pumped with each heart beat. Cardiac output is dependent upon stroke volume and the rate at which the heart beats. Therefore, cardiac output can be increased by increasing the heart rate, increasing the stroke volume, or increasing both factors.

HYPERTENSION

Hypertension is defined as an abnormal increase in arterial blood pressure, the incidence of which increases with age. According to the American Heart Association, in approximately 90% of cases, the cause is unknown, and more than a third of those affected have no idea that they have hypertension. Risk factors for hypertension include family history, stress, obesity, smoking, lifestyle, diabetes mellitus, and excessive lipid blood levels. Hypertension must be diagnosed in early stages (see Table 12-1). When it is not properly treated, the risk of stroke, coronary artery disease, congestive heart failure, and renal failure increases.

There are three classifications of hypertension:

1. **Primary** or **essential hypertension** is idiopathic (occurring spontaneously from an unknown cause) and is the form discussed in this section.

2. **Secondary hypertension** results from renal (e.g., nephrosclerosis) or endocrine (e.g., hyperaldosteronism) disease, or pheochromocytoma,

TABLE 12-1   Blood Pressure and Hypertension

Classification	Systolic (mm Hg)	Diastolic (mm Hg)
Normal	Less than 120	Less than 80
Prehypertension	120–139	80–89
Stage I hypertension	140–159	90–99
Stage II hypertension	160 or higher	100 or higher

a benign tumor of the adrenal medulla. In this type of hypertension, the underlying problem must be resolved.

3. **Malignant hypertension**, the third type, is an uncontrollable, severe, and rapidly progressive form of hypertension with many complications.

Hypertension is sometimes classified as systolic or diastolic depending on the measurement that is elevated. For example, elderly persons with loss of elasticity in the arteries frequently have high systolic pressure and a low diastolic value.

Essential hypertension develops when the blood pressure is consistently above 140/90. This figure may be adjusted for the individual's age. The diastolic pressure is important because it indicates the degree of peripheral resistance and the increased workload of the left ventricle. The condition may be mild, moderate, or severe.

In essential hypertension, there is an increase in arteriolar vasoconstriction, which is attributed variously to increased susceptibility to stimuli or increased stimulation, or perhaps a combination of factors. A very slight decrease in the diameter of the arterioles causes a major increase in peripheral resistance, reduces the capacity of the system, and increases the diastolic pressure. Frequently, vasoconstriction leads to decreased blood flow through the kidneys, leading to increased renin, angiotensin, and aldosterone secretion. These substances increase vasoconstriction and blood volume, further increasing blood pressure. Figure 12-1 illustrates the development of hypertension. If this cycle is not broken, blood pressure can continue to increase. Renal failure is increased during hypertension because the flow of the blood through the kidneys is reduced. Kidneys are very important in maintaining electrolyte balances, especially those of sodium and water.

The increased blood pressure causes damage to the arterial walls, which become hard and thick (**sclerotic**), narrowing the lumen. Blood supply to the involved area is reduced, leading to ischemia and necrosis with loss of function. The areas most commonly damaged are the kidneys, brain, and retinas.

Key Concept

Atherosclerosis, myocardial infarction, heart failure, renal failure, stroke, impaired mobility, and generalized edema are all associated with chronic hypertension.

Medical Terminology Review

vasoconstriction

vaso = blood vessel
constriction = narrowing
narrowing of the blood vessels

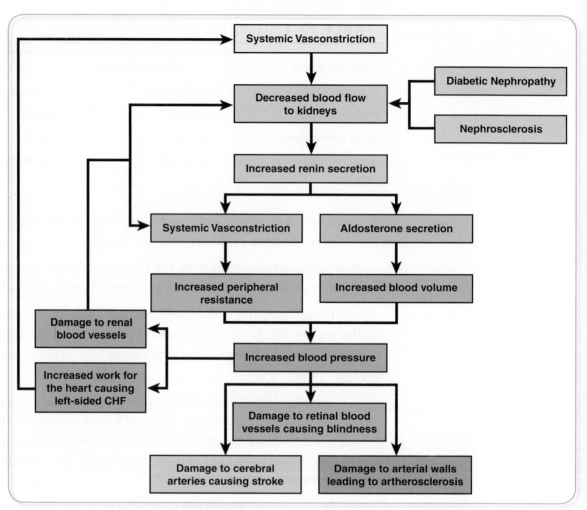

Figure 12-1 Development of hypertension.

Antihypertensive Therapy

In primary hypertension, long-term therapy is necessary to prevent the morbidity and mortality associated with uncontrolled hypertension. Treatment primarily aims to lower the blood pressure toward "normal" with minimal side effects, and to prevent or reverse organ damage. Antihypertensive drugs do not cure hypertension. They only control it. After withdrawal of the drug, the blood pressure will return to levels similar to those before treatment with medication, if all other factors remain the same. There are numerous antihypertensive drugs in the treatment and management of all degrees of hypertension. In mild cases of hypertension, the initial treatment regimen usually includes diet modification (reducing salt), weight reduction, mild exercise programs, smoking cessation, and stress reduction. Drugs prescribed to lower blood pressure act in various ways. The drug of choice varies according to the degree of hypertension (mild, moderate, or severe). Antihypertensives are sometimes combined for greater effectiveness and to reduce side effects. There are five groups

of drugs which act to lower blood pressure in the following manner: (1) angiotensin-converting enzyme inhibitors, (2) angiotensin II receptor antagonists, (3) adrenergic blockers, centrally and peripherally acting blockers (sympatholytics), (4) peripheral vasodilators, and (5) diuretics. They are explained below in more detail.

Angiotensin-converting Enzyme Inhibitors

Angiotensin-converting enzyme inhibitors (ACE inhibitors) competitively inhibit conversion of angiotensin I to angiotensin II, a potent vasoconstrictor, through the angiotensin-converting enzyme activity, with resultant lower levels of angiotensin II. Lower angiotensin II levels increase plasma renin activity and reduce aldosterone secretion.

Mechanism of Action

Angiotensin-converting enzyme (ACE) inhibitors slow the formation of angiotensin II, which reduces vascular resistance, blood volume, and blood pressure. Renin is an enzyme that is released by the kidneys in response to reduced renal blood circulation or hyponatremia. This enzyme acts in the plasma angiotensinogen to produce angiotensin I. Then, angiotensin I is converted to angiotensin II, mostly in the lungs. Angiotensin II is a vasoconstricting agent. It causes sodium retention via the release of aldosterone. In the adrenal gland, angiotensin II is converted to angiotensin III. Both angiotensin II and III stimulate the release of aldosterone. Angiotensin I is inactive in the cardiovascular system. Angiotensin II has several cardiovascular-renal actions. The most important site of the angiotensin-converting enzyme (ACE) is in the lungs, but ACE also is found in the kidneys, central nervous system, and elsewhere. Figure 12-2 shows the renin-angiotensin system. Examples of ACE inhibitors are shown in Table 12-2.

Indications

ACE inhibitors are becoming the drugs of choice in the first-line treatment of essential hypertension.

Adverse Effects

Although ACE inhibitors as a group are relatively free of side effects or toxicities in most patients, they do occur, and some can be life-threatening. The adverse effects of ACE inhibitors may include: dizziness, angioedema, loss of taste, photosensitivity, severe hypotension, dry cough, hyperkalemia, blood dyscrasias, and renal impairment.

Contraindications and Precautions

ACE inhibitors are contraindicated in patients with hypersensitivity to these agents, kidney damage, heart failure, hepatic impairment, and diabetes mellitus. ACE inhibitors are avoided during pregnancy (category D). Safety during lactation or in children is not established.

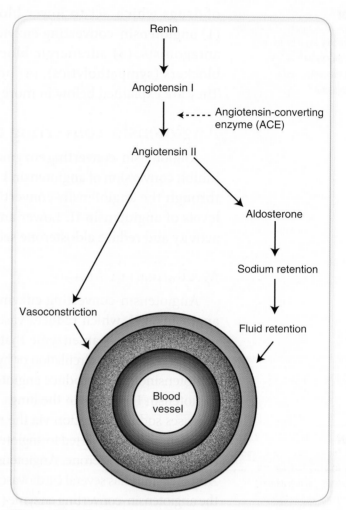

Figure 12-2 Renin-angiotensin system.

ACE inhibitors should be used cautiously in patients with renal impairment or hypovolemia, or who are receiving diuretics or undergoing dialysis. These drugs are used with caution in patients with congestive heart failure, hepatic impairment, and diabetes mellitus.

Drug Interactions

ACE inhibitors increase risk of hypersensitivity reactions with allopurinol. They decrease antihypertensive effects with indomethacin. ACE inhibitors also increase captopril effects with probenecid. Some ACE inhibitors may increase coughing if combined with capsaicin. Fosinopril increases the risk of potassium levels if taken with potassium-sparing diuretics. Quinapril may increase digoxin levels and decrease tetracycline absorption.

Angiotensin II Receptor Antagonists

Angiotensin II receptor antagonists block the binding of angiotensin II to the angiotensin I receptor. Angiotensin II receptor antagonists have

TABLE 12-2 Examples of ACE Inhibitors

Generic Name	Trade Name	Route of Administration	Average Adult Dosage
benazepril hydrochloride	Lotensin®	PO	10–40 mg/day in 1–2 divided doses
captopril	Capoten®	PO	6.25–25 mg t.i.d.; may increase to 50 mg t.i.d.
enalapril maleate	Vasotec®	PO	5–40 mg/day
fosinopril	Monopril®	PO	5–40 mg/day (max: 80 mg/day)
lisinopril	Prinivil®, Zestril®	PO	10–40 mg/day (max: 80 mg/day)
moexipril hydrochloride	Univase®	PO	7.5–30 mg/day
perindopril erbumine	Aceon®	PO	4 mg once per day; may increase to 8 mg/day
quinapril hydrochloride	Accupril®	PO	10–20 mg q.d., may increase up to 80 mg/day in 1–2 div. doses
trandolapril	Mavik®	PO	1–4 mg/day
ramipril	Altace®	PO	2.5–5 mg/day

beneficial effects on the symptoms and hemodynamics of patients with congestive heart failure.

Mechanism of Action

Angiotensin II receptor antagonist drugs work by blocking the binding of angiotensin II to the angiotensin I receptors. By blocking the receptor site, these agents inhibit the vasoconstrictor effects of angiotensin II as well as preventing the release of aldosterone due to angiotensin II from the adrenal glands.

Indications

This class of drugs has been one of the most rapidly growing groups of drugs for the treatment of hypertension. Currently, six agents are available and include candesartan cilexetil, eprosartan, irbesartan, losartan, telmisartan, and valsartan (see Table 12-3).

Adverse Effects

Angiotensin receptor blockers should not be used in special hypertensive populations, such as diabetics with nephropathy or congestive heart failure, unless the patient cannot tolerate an ACE inhibitor.

Key Concept

Postural hypotension is a common adverse effect of antihypertensive drugs. Abrupt withdrawal of treatment may lead to rebound hypertension.

TABLE 12-3 Angiotensin II Receptor Antagonists

Generic Name	Trade Name	Route of Administration	Average Adult Dosage
candesartan cilexetil	Atacand®	PO	8–32 mg/day
eprosartan mesylate	Teveten®	PO	400–800 mg/day
irbesartan	Avapro®	PO	150–300 mg/day
losartan potassium	Cozaar®	PO	25–50 mg/day
olmesartan medoxomil	Benicar®	PO	20–40 mg/day
telmisartan	Micardis®	PO	40–80 mg/day
valsartan	Diovan®	PO	80–160 mg/day

Contraindications and Precautions

Angiotensin II receptor antagonists are contraindicated in patients with a known hypersensitivity to these agents. These drugs are also contraindicated in pregnancy (category C, first trimester; category D, second and third trimesters) and lactation.

Angiotensin II receptor antagonists are used cautiously in patients with concurrent administration of high-dose diuretics, potassium-sparing diuretics, or potassium salt substitutes, and in diabetes or lactation. Angiotensin II receptor antagonists should be used with caution in patients with hepatic or renal impairment, or in elderly patients.

Drug Interactions

Some of these drugs, such as losartan, decrease serum levels and effectiveness if taken concurrently with phenobarbital. Losartan is converted to an active metabolite by cytochrome P450, which may decrease the antihypertensive effects of losartan. Telmisartan increases serum levels and risk of toxicity of digoxin if combined.

Adrenergic Blockers, Centrally and Peripherally Acting Blockers (Sympatholytics)

The **sympatholytic** drugs include groups of medications beta-adrenergic blocking agents, centrally acting alpha-antagonists, postganglionic adrenergic blockers, and alpha-adrenergic blocking agents. These drugs are summarized in Table 12-4.

Mechanism of Action

Beta blockers reduce peripheral resistance and inhibit cardiac function. They also block renin secretion. Centrally acting antiadrenergic blockers act

Key Concept

The beta-blockers, calcium channel antagonists, angiotensin II antagonists, combined α- and β-antagonists, and centrally acting sympathetic depressants lower both cardiac output and systemic vascular resistance.

TABLE 12-4   Sympatholytic Agents

Generic Name	Trade Name	Route of Administration	Average Adult Dosage
α/β-Blockers			
labetalol hydrochloride	Trandate®	PO, IV	Initial: 100 mg b.i.d.; maint: 200–400 mg b.i.d., IV 20 mg slowly over 2 min with 40–80 mg over 10 min if needed
β-Blockers			
acebutolol hydrochloride	Sectral®	PO	200–800 mg/day in 2 div. doses
atenolol	Tenormin®	PO	25–100 mg once/day
betaxolol hydrochloride	Kerlone®	PO	5–10 mg/day (max: 20 mg/day)
bisoprolol fumarate	Zebeta®	PO	2.5–20 mg/day
carteolol hydrochloride	Cartrol®	PO	2.5–10 mg/day
metoprolol tartrate	Lopressor®	PO, IV	PO: 50–450 mg/day; IV: 40–320 mg/day
nadolol	Corgard®	PO	40 mg once per day; may increase to 240–320 mg/day
penbutolol	Levatol®	PO	10–20 mg/day; may increase to 40–80 mg/day
propranolol hydrochloride	Inderal®	PO	40–60 mg b.i.d.; usually requires 160–480 mg/day
timolol maleate	Blocadren®	PO	10 mg b.i.d.; may increase to 60 mg/day
Centrally Acting Blockers			
clonidine hydrochloride	Catapres®	PO or Transdermal system	Initial: 0.1 mg b.i.d.; maint: 0.1–0.2 mg/day
guanabenz acetate	Wytensin®	PO	Initial: 4 mg b.i.d.; max. 32 mg b.i.d.
guanfacine hydrochloride	Tenex®	PO	1–3 mg/day
methyldopa	Aldomet®	PO, IV	Initial: 250 mg b.i.d.; maint: 500 mg to 3 g/day in 2–4 doses

(continues)

TABLE 12-4 Sympatholytic Agents—*continued*

Generic Name	Trade Name	Route of Administration	Average Adult Dosage
Peripherally Acting Blockers			
doxazosin mesylate	Cardura®	PO	Initial: 1 mg/day; maint: 2–16 mg qd
guanadrel	Hylorel®	PO	Initial: 10 mg/day; most require 20–75 mg/day
guanethidine	Ismelin®	PO	Initial: 10 mg/day; average 25–50 mg/day
prazosin hydrochloride	Minipress®	PO	First dose limited to 1 mg h.s.; then 1 mg b.i.d.-t.i.d.; may increase to 20 mg/day
reserpine	Serpalan/Serpasil®	PO	0.1–0.25 mg/day
terazosin	Hytrin®	PO	Initial: 1 mg h.s., then 1–5 mg/day

primarily within the central nervous system on alpha 2 receptors to decrease sympathetic outflow to the cardiovascular system. Methyldopa decreases total peripheral resistance while having little effect on cardiac output or heart rate (except in older patients). Clonidine stimulates alpha 2 receptors centrally, and decreases vasomotor tone and heart rate. Guanabenz and guanfacine are centrally acting alpha2-adrenergic agonists that have actions similar to clonidine.

Peripherally acting adrenergic inhibitors are powerful antihypertensives that may interfere with the release of norepinephrine from nerve endings or may block receptors in the vascular smooth muscle. This class of antihypertensive drug is best avoided unless it is necessary to treat severe hypertension that is unresponsive to all other medications, because agents in this class are poorly tolerated by most patients. Guanethidine is one of the most potent antihypertensive drugs currently in clinical use. Guanethidine acts in peripheral neurons, where it first produces a sympathetic blockade. Guanadrel is chemically and pharmacologically similar to guanethidine.

Indications

Beta-blockers are used for the initial treatment of hypertension. These medications can be used for angina, acute myocardial infarctions, and hypertension. Propranolol was the first beta-blocking agent shown to block both beta 1 and beta 2 receptors. It is available as both a fast-acting product and a long-acting product. Nadolol was the first beta-blocker that allowed once-daily dosing.

It blocks both beta 1 and 2 receptors. Timolol was the first beta-blocker shown to be effective after an acute myocardial infarction to prevent sudden death.

Alpha and beta blockers are drugs available for hypertensive patients who have not responded to initial antihypertensive therapy. These agents are similar to beta-blockers.

Centrally acting antiadrenergic drugs have been used in the past as alternatives to initial antihypertensives, but their use in mild to moderate hypertension has been reduced primarily due to other available drugs. Clonidine is effective in patients with renal impairment, although they may require a reduced dose or a longer dosing interval. Clonidine is also available as a transdermal patch (Clonidine-TTS), which releases the drug slowly over seven days. Guanabenz and guanfacine are recommended as adjunctive therapy with other antihypertensives for additive effects when initial therapy has failed.

Adverse Effects

Beta-blockers are not totally safe in patients with bronchospastic diseases such as asthma and chronic obstructive pulmonary disease (COPD). Suddenly stopping beta-blocker therapy puts the patient at risk for a withdrawal syndrome.

The adverse effects of alpha and beta blockers include postural hypotension, nausea, dizziness, headache, and bronchospasm.

The use of methyldopa is limited because it may produce sedation and must be administered 2 to 4 times daily. Other less common adverse effects include hemolytic anemia, hypotension and drowsiness, nausea, vomiting, sore tongue, sexual dysfunction, nasal congestion, and hepatic dysfunction. Sedation and dry mouth are common with use of clonidine but usually disappear with continued therapy. Clonidine has a tendency to cause or worsen depression. Its action is apparent within 30 to 60 minutes after administration of an oral dose. Adverse effects of guanabenz and guanfacine include sedation, dry mouth, dizziness, and reduced heart rate.

Reserpine is derived from the *Rauwolfia serpentina* plant. Because of the high incidence of adverse effects, other drugs are usually chosen first. When used, reserpine is given in low doses and in conjunction with other antihypertensive agents. Common adverse effects include drowsiness, dizziness, weakness, lethargy, memory impairment, sleep disturbances, and weight gain. Postural and exercise hypotension, fluid retention, and sexual dysfunction are common side effects when using guanethidine. Guanadrel should be avoided in patients with congestive heart failure, angina, and stroke. Adverse effects include fainting, orthostatic hypotension, and diarrhea.

Contraindications and Precautions

Beta-blockers are contraindicated in patients with a known hypersensitivity to the individual agents. Use of beta-blockers should be avoided in patients

Key Concept

The control of malignant hypertension is usually achieved using direct-acting peripheral vasodilators, in particular, sodium nitroprusside.

with uncompensated heart failure, cardiogenic shock, hypotension, and pulmonary edema. Safety of these drugs during pregnancy (category B) or lactation is not established.

Alpha/beta blockers are contraindicated in bronchial asthma, uncontrolled cardiac failure, cardiogenic shock, and severe bradycardia. Safe use during pregnancy (category C), lactation, or in children is not established. Centrally acting blockers (e.g., clonidine patch) are contraindicated in patients with collagen diseases (such as systemic lupus erythematosus) and during pregnancy (category C).

Beta-blockers should be used with caution in patients with hepatic or renal impairment, diabetes mellitus, and bronchospastic disease (asthma, emphysema), and patients undergoing major surgery involving general anesthesia. Abrupt withdrawal of beta blockers should be avoided, since sudden withdrawal may result in rebound hypertension, angina, and heart attack. This drug dose should be tapered over several weeks.

Drug Interactions

Patients taking guanethidine should avoid over-the-counter preparations that contain adrenergic substances such as cold medicines, because the combination may potentiate an acute hypertensive effect.

Peripheral Vasodilators

Vasodilators are used to relax or dilate vessels throughout the body. Some work on either veins or arteries; others work on both. Vasodilators are prescribed as second-line agents to initial therapy in patients taking diuretics, beta-blockers, ACE inhibitors, calcium-channel blockers, alpha-adrenergic blockers, or alpha/beta-adrenergic blockers.

Mechanism of Action

Vasodilators block the movement of calcium into the smooth muscle of the blood vessels to cause relaxation of the smooth muscle, and dilation of the resistance vessels.

Indications

Vasodilator agents are reducers of hypertension. A peripheral vasodilator is frequently used in the treatment of moderate to severe hypertension.

Hydralazine and minoxidil may be used in the treatment of moderate essential or early malignant hypertension and hypertensive emergencies, virtually always in conjunction with other antihypertensive drugs. However, mainly because of side effects, they are generally not used until other, safer therapy has failed. Because they increase renal blood flow, they are often used to treat toxemia of pregnancy. They are sometimes

---

Medical Terminology Review

vasodilator

vaso = blood vessel
dilator = agent that causes expansion
a substance that causes dilation of the blood vessel

Key Concept

All vasodilators should be discontinued slowly to avoid paradoxical hypertensive effects.

TABLE 12-5 Vasodilators

Generic Name	Trade Name	Route of Administration	Average Adult Dosage
diazoxide	Hyperstat®, Proglycem®	IV	1–3 mg/kg up to 150 mg, repeat at 5–15 min intervals p.r.n.
fenoldopam mesylate	Corlopam®	IV	0.025–0.3 mcg/kg/min by continuous infusion for up to 48 hours
hydralazine hydrochloride	Apresoline®	PO, IM, IV	PO: 10–50 mg q.i.d.; IM: 10–50 mg q4–6h; IV: 10–20 mg q4–6h, may increase to 40 mg
minoxidil	Rogaine®	PO	5 mg/day, increased q3–5 days up to 40 mg/day in single or div. doses p.r.n. (max: 100 mg/day)
nitroprusside sodium	Nipride®, Nitropress®	IV	0.3–0.5 mcg/kg/min (max: 10 mcg/kg/min)
prazosin hydrochloride	Minipress®	PO	1 mg b.i.d.-t.i.d. up to 20 mg/day

used in acute congestive heart failure or after myocardial infarction (see Table 12-5).

Adverse Effects

Toxic effects of hydralazine are syndromes resembling rheumatoid arthritis or lupus erythematosus, the appearance of which necessitates the withdrawal of the drug. Common adverse effects of vasodilator drugs include headache, dizziness, tachycardia, palpitations, anxiety, nausea, vomiting, disorientation, depression, edema, impotence, and allergic reactions.

Contraindications and Precautions

Vasodilators are contraindicated in patients with coronary artery disease, mitral valvular rheumatic heart disease, atriovenous shunt, and myocardial infarction. Safe use of vasodilators during pregnancy (category C) or lactation is not established.

Medical Terminology Review

hyponatremia

hypo = below; beneath; under
natr = sodium
emia = blood condition
low sodium levels in the blood

TABLE 12-6   Diuretics Used to Treat Hypertension

Generic Name	Trade Name	Route of Administration	Average Adult Dosage
amiloride hydrochloride	Midamor®	PO	5 mg/day; may increase to 20 mg/day in 1–2 divided doses
chlorothiazide sodium	Diuril®	PO	250-500 mg–1 g in 1–2 div. doses
chlorthalidone	Thalitone®, Hygroton®	PO	12.5–25 mg/day (max: 100 mg/day)
furosemide	Lasix®	PO	20–80 mg b.i.d. (max: 600 mg/day)
hydrochlorothiazide	HydroDIURIL®, HCTZ®	PO	12.5–100 mg in 1–2 div. doses
indapamide	Lozol®	PO	2.5 mg once per day; may increase to 5 mg/day
spironolactone	Aldactone®	PO	25–100 mg/day
torsemide	Demadex®	PO, IV	10–20 mg/day, up to 200 mg/day
triamterene	Dyrenium®	PO	100 mg b.i.d. (max: 300 mg/day)

Vasodilators are used cautiously in patients with stroke, hepatic insufficiency, advanced renal impairment, hyponatremia, and in the elderly.

Drug Interactions

Hydralazine should be used with caution in patients receiving MAOIs. Profound hypotensive episodes may occur when hydralazine is used along with diazoxide injections.

Diuretics

Diuretics increase sodium excretion and lower blood volume. Diuretics are divided into four categories according to their action: thiazide diuretics, loop diuretics, potassium-sparing diuretics, and osmotic diuretics. The type of diuretic used is determined by the condition being treated. For example, carbonic anhydrase inhibitors, such as acetazolamide (Diamox) are used to lower intraocular pressure. This agent is known as a diuretic compound. The most common diuretics that are used for hypertension are listed in Table 12-6.

Mechanism of Action

Thiazide agents are the most commonly used type of diuretic, increasing excretion of water, sodium, chloride, and potassium.

Key Concept

Sodium nitroprusside and diazoxide can be administered only parenterally. Hydralazine and minoxidil are orally administered agents, most suitable for effective long-term outpatient therapy.

Loop diuretics inhibit sodium and chloride reabsorption. They are the most effective diuretics available. Potent diuretics such as furosemide (Lasix), bumetanide (Bumex), and ethacrynic acid (Edecrin) are not thiazides but act in a similar way to increase excretion of water, sodium, chloride, and potassium. Their action is more rapid and effective than that of thiazides, with a greater diuresis.

Potassium-sparing diuretics achieve their diuretic effects differently and less potently than the thiazides and loop diuretics. Their most pertinent shared feature is that they promote potassium retention.

Traditionally, substances that increase urine formation, where the excess appears in the urine accompanied by an increased volume of water, are called osmotic diuretics.

Indications

Thiazides may be prescribed for the treatment of edema caused by heart failure or cirrhosis, as well as hypertension.

Loop diuretics are not prescribed routinely for hypertension, but are used when diuresis is required. Loop diuretics are used in the treatment of edema associated with impaired renal kidney function or liver disease. They are also commonly prescribed for the treatment of congestive heart failure, pulmonary edema, and ascites caused by malignancy or cirrhosis. If thiazides are ineffective in the treatment of hypertension, loop diuretics such as furosemide or ethacrynic acid are sometimes used in combination with other antihypertensives.

Potassium-sparing diuretics include spironolactone, triamterene, and amiloride, and are sometimes administered under conditions in which potassium depletion can be dangerous. Spironolactone is a specific competitive inhibitor of aldosterone at the receptor site level. It is effective only when aldosterone is present. Triamterene and amiloride exert their effect independent of the presence or absence of aldosterone. The potassium-sparing agents are used in the management of edema associated with congestive heart failure, hepatic cirrhosis with ascites, the nephrotic syndrome, and idiopathic edema. Because these diuretics have little antihypertensive action of their own they are used mainly in combination with other drugs in the management of hypertension, and to correct hypokalemia often caused by other diuretic agents. Spironolactone also is used in primary hyperaldosteronism.

Mannitol has been shown to increase renal plasma flow and glomerular hydrostatic pressure. Mannitol and urea are most commonly used to reduce intracranial or intraocular pressure. Mannitol has also been used to prevent and treat acute renal failure or during certain cardiovascular surgery. Mannitol is also used alone or with other diuretics to promote excretions of toxins in cases of drug poisoning.

Medical Terminology Review

hyperuricemia

hyper = over; above; beyond
uric = relating to uric acid or urine
emia = blood condition
excess blood in the urine

Adverse Effects

Adverse effects of thiazides include: hypokalemia, hypochloremia, muscle weakness (spasm), postural hypotension, vertigo, headache, fatigue, lethargy, hyperuricemia, and hyperglycemia.

Adverse effects of loop diuretics include fluid and electrolyte imbalance with dehydration, hypotension, collapse, hypokalemia, nausea, vomiting, anorexia, diarrhea, hyperglycemia, blurred vision, and hearing impairment.

Adverse effects resulting from use of potassium-sparing diuretics are hyperkalemia (which may lead to cardiac arrhythmias), dehydration, weakness, fatigue, lethargy, weight loss, nausea, vomiting, diarrhea, and hypotension. Gynecomastia and carcinoma of the breast have been reported after using spironolactone.

The major toxic effect of osmotic diuretics is related to the amount of solute administered and its effect on the volume and distribution of body fluids. Adverse effects include: fluid and electrolyte imbalance, headache, mental confusion, nausea, vomiting, tachycardia, hypertension, hypotension, allergic reactions, and severe pulmonary edema.

Contraindications and Precautions

Thiazide diuretics are contraindicated for patients with diabetes, severe renal failure, impaired liver function, and a history of gout.

Loop diuretics should be avoided in patients with liver disease, kidney impairment, diabetes, pregnancy (category C), and lactation. Loop diuretics are also contraindicated in dehydrated patients and children under 18 years of age.

Potassium-sparing diuretics are contraindicated in patients with anuria, acute renal insufficiency, impaired renal function, or hyperkalemia.

Osmotic diuretics are contraindicated in kidney failure, severe pulmonary edema, pregnancy, lactation, and cardiovascular disease.

Diuretics are used cautiously in patients with hepatic or renal dysfunction, electrolyte imbalance, diabetes, pregnant women, lactation, and in children. ACE inhibitors should be used with caution in patients with sodium depletion, hypovolemia, and coronary insufficiency.

Drug Interactions

Many drugs can interact with the antihypertensive agents and decrease their effectiveness. These drugs include: antidepressants, antihistamines, and beta-adrenergic bronchodilators. Absorption of the ACE inhibitors may be decreased when given with antacids. The effect of angiotensin II receptor agonists may be decreased if NSAIDs or phenobarbital are given with them.

Hyperlipidemia

Lipids or fats, which are usually transported in various combinations with proteins (lipoproteins), play a key role in cardiovascular disorders. Lipids, including cholesterol and triglycerides, are essential elements in the body. They are synthesized in the liver; therefore, they can never be eliminated from the body.

Dietary or drug therapy of elevated plasma cholesterol levels can reduce the risk of atherosclerosis, and subsequent cardiovascular disease. A patient with high serum cholesterol and increased low-density lipoprotein (LDL) is at risk of atherosclerotic coronary disease and myocardial infarction. Atherosclerosis is a disorder in which lipid subgroups [total cholesterol, triglycerides, low-density lipoproteins (LDL), and high-density lipoproteins (HDL)] in various proportions indicate risk factors for the individual. Comparison of HDL and LDL is shown in Figure 12-3. Table 12-7 shows an analysis of cholesterol and triglycerides.

Analysis of serum lipids includes assessment of all the deposits that accumulate on the lining of the blood vessels, resulting in degenerative changes and obstruction of blood flow (see Figure 12-4). Obstructions may be partial or complete, and emboli are common. Factors such as genetic conditions, high cholesterol diet, elevated serum LDL levels, and elevated blood pressure predispose patients to development of this condition.

Diseases of plasma lipids can be manifested as an elevation in triglycerides (hyperlipidemia), or as an elevation in cholesterol. Elevated triglycerides can produce life-threatening pancreatitis.

Medical Terminology Review

atherosclerosis
athero = deposit
sclero = hard or hardened
sis = state or condition
a condition of hardened deposits in the arteries

Medical Terminology Review

hyperlipidemia
hyper = over; above; beyond
lipid = fat
emia = blood condition
excess fat in the blood

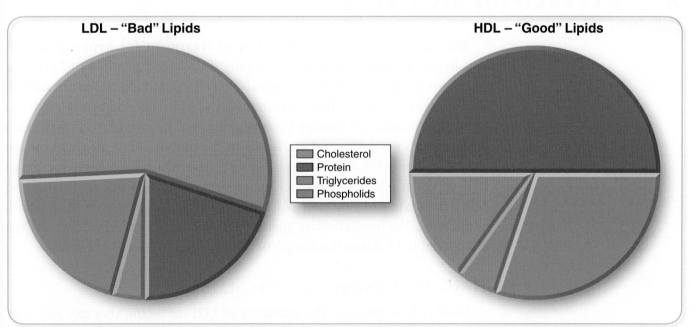

Figure 12-3 Comparison of HDL to LDL.

TABLE 12-7 Normal Values of Cholesterol and Triglyceride Levels

Cholesterol Level	Cholesterol Category
Less than 200 mg/dL	Desirable
200–239 mg/dL	Borderline
> 240 mg/dL	High
HDL Cholesterol Level	**HDL Cholesterol Category**
Less than 40 mg/dL (for men) and less than 50 mg/dL (for women)	Low HDL cholesterol. A major risk factor for heart disease.
60 mg/dL and above	High HDL cholesterol. An HDL of 60 mg/dL and above is considered protective against heart disease.
LDL Cholesterol Level	**LDL Cholesterol Category**
Less than 100 mg/dL	Optimal
100–129 mg/dL	Above optimal
130–159 mg/dL	Borderline high
160–189 mg/dL	High
$\geq$ 190 mg/dL	Very high
Triglyceride Level	**Triglyceride Category**
Less than 150 mg/dL	Normal
150–199 mg/dL	Borderline high
200–499 mg/dL	High
500 mg/dL and above	Very high

ANTIHYPERLIPIDEMIC DRUGS

Key Concept

Torcetrafib is a new drug that, when combined with Lipitor, raises HDL ("good cholesterol") levels.

Medications are not the first line of treatment for hyperlipidemia. Antihyperlipidemic drugs are used only if diet modification and exercise programs fail to lower LDL to normal levels. When medications are started, diet therapy must continue. Antihyperlipidemics are the group of drugs prescribed in adjuvant therapy to reduce elevated cholesterol levels in patients with high cholesterol and LDL levels in the blood. These medications are used to decrease the risk of arteriosclerosis. The major drugs for reduction of LDL cholesterol levels are bile acid sequestrants and nicotinic acid. The fibric acid derivatives and clofibrate (Atromid-S) are less effective in reducing LDL cholesterol. The most effective agents for reducing plasma LDL levels are the statins. Table 12-8 lists the drugs commonly used to lower lipid levels.

HMG-CoA Reductase (The Statins)

Statins have become the mainstay of LDL-reducing therapy, and they are the most effective agents for reducing plasma LDL levels. The statins

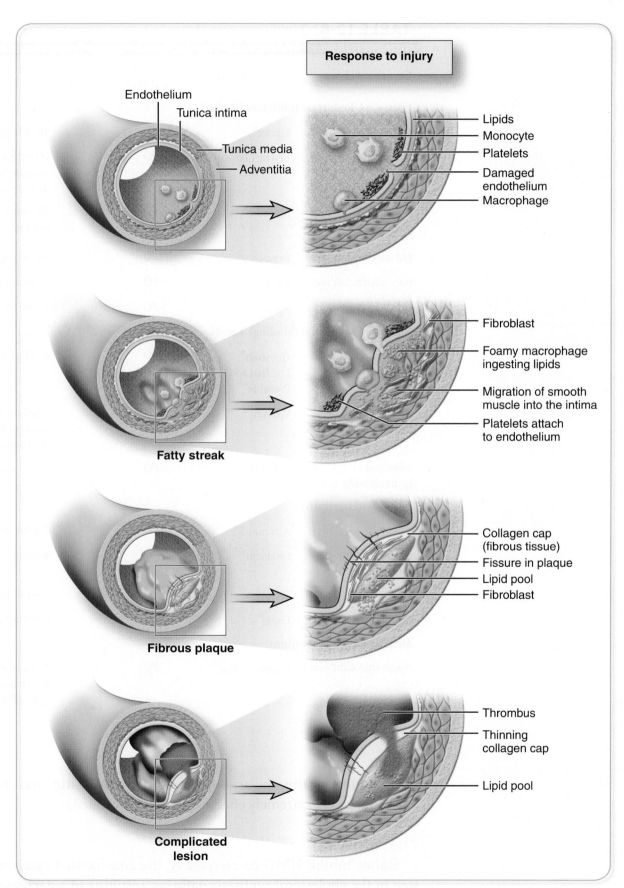

Figure 12-4 Development of atherosclerosis.

TABLE 12-8   Lipid-lowering Drugs

Generic Name	Trade Name	Route of Administration	Average Adult Dosage
HMG-CoA Reductase Inhibitors (Statins)			
atorvastatin calcium	Lipitor®	PO	10–80 mg/day
fluvastatin sodium	Lescol®, Lescol XL®	PO	20 mg h.s.; may increase to 80 mg/day in 1–2 divided doses
lovastatin	Mevacor®, Altoprev®	PO	20–40 mg 1–2 times per day
pravastatin sodium	Pravachol®	PO	10–80 mg/day
rosuvastatin calcium	Crestor®	PO	5–40 mg/day
simvastatin	Zocor®	PO	10–80 mg/day
Bile Acid Sequestrant (binding) Agents			
cholestyramine resin	Questran®, LoCHOLEST®, Prevalite®	PO	4–24 g b.i.d.-q.i.d.
colesevelam hydrochloride	Welchol®	PO	3 tablets b.i.d. with meals or 6 tablets q.d. with a meal
colestipol hydrochloride	Colestid®	PO	15–30 g b.i.d.
Fibric Acid Derivatives			
clofibrate	Atromid-S®	PO	2 g/day in div. doses
dextrothyroxine sodium	Choloxin®	PO	4–8 mg/day
fenofibrate	Tricor®	PO	54–160 mg/day
gemfibrozil	Lopid®	PO	600 mg b.i.d.
Miscellaneous Preparations			
niacin (nicotinic acid)	Niaspan®, Niac®	PO	1–3 g in div. doses or extended release: 500–2000 mg/day

include: atorvastatin, fluvastatin, lovastatin, pravastatin, and simvastatin. These statins are extremely effective and well-tolerated.

Mechanism of Action

Statins inhibit HMG co-enzyme A, the enzyme that catalyzes the first step in the cholesterol synthesis pathway, resulting in a decrease in serum cholesterol and serum LDLs.

Key Concept

*HMG-CoA reductase inhibitors are usually well-tolerated. A rare but serious adverse effect is **rhabdomyolysis** (destruction of skeletal muscle).*

Indications

The statin drugs are used as adjuncts to diet in treatment of elevated total cholesterol, serum triglycerides, and LDL cholesterol in patients with primary hypercholesterolemia.

Adverse Effects

HMG-CoA reductase inhibitors may cause headache, flatulence, abdominal pain, cramps, constipation, nausea, and heartburn. They have an impressively low frequency of serious adverse effects. The most important side effects are transaminase elevation and acute myositis.

Contraindications and Precautions

HMG-CoA reductase inhibitors are contraindicated in patients with hypersensitivity to these agents, serious liver disorders, and during pregnancy (category X) and lactation. HMG-CoA reductase inhibitors should be used with caution in patients with acute infection, visual disturbances, hypotension, endocrine disorders, and a history of alcoholism.

Drug Interactions

HMG-CoA reductase inhibitors may have decreased effects if taken with rifamycin. There is possible severe myopathy (disorders of the striated muscles) or rhabdomyolysis if taken with cyclosporine, erythromycin, gemfibrozil, niacin, and other statins. When the HMG-CoA reductase inhibitors are given with oral anticoagulants, the effect of the anticoagulants will be increased.

Bile Acid Sequestrants

Bile acid sequestrants are a group of drugs that chemically combine with bile acids in the intestine, causing these bile acids to be eliminated from the body. Bile acid sequestrants are prescribed to lower blood cholesterol and other blood lipid levels. Cholestyramine (Questran) and colestipol (Colestid) are examples of bile acid sequestrants.

Mechanism of Action

Bile acid sequestrant drugs bind to bile acids to form an insoluble substance that cannot be absorbed by the intestine. Therefore, it is excreted in the feces. This action increases loss of bile acids, and the liver uses cholesterol to manufacture more bile. This leads to lowered serum cholesterol levels.

Indications

Bile acid sequestrants are used as adjuncts to diet therapy in management of patients with primary hypercholesterolemia with a significant risk of atherosclerotic heart disease and MI. These agents may also be prescribed to relieve pruritus associated with partial biliary obstruction.

Adverse Effects

Constipation is a common problem associated with bile acid sequestrants. Other adverse effects are fecal impaction, hemorrhoids, nausea, and abdominal pain. Additional adverse effects include weight loss or gain, vitamin A, D, and K deficiencies (from poor absorption), and bleeding tendencies caused by depletion of vitamin K.

Contraindications and Precautions

Bile acid sequestrants are contraindicated in patients with a known hypersensitivity to the medications. Bile acid sequestrants are avoided in those with complete biliary obstruction, pregnancy (category C), and lactation. Safe use of these drugs in children younger than 16 years is not established.

Bile acid sequestrants should be used cautiously in patients with bleeding disorders, hemorrhoids, peptic ulcer, and malabsorption states (e.g., **steatorrhea**). These agents are used with caution in patients with a liver or kidney impairment, and during pregnancy or lactation.

Drug Interactions

Bile acid sequestrants decrease the absorption of oral anticoagulants, digoxin, tetracyclines, penicillins, and phenobarbital. Therefore, bile acid sequestrants should be given alone and other drugs administered at least 1 hour before or 4 hours later.

Fibric Acid Derivatives

These agents reduce hepatic synthesis of cholesterol and result in a reduction in the plasma concentration of very-low-density lipoprotein (VLDL) and triglycerides. Because more successful medications are on the market, clofibrate is no longer the hypolipidemic drug of choice, although it is still used for patients who may not respond to other medications.

Mechanism of Action

Fibric acid derivatives stimulate the liver to increase breakdown of VLDL to LDL, and decrease liver synthesis of VLDL by inhibiting cholesterol formation.

Indications

Primary indication of clofibrate is for hyperlipidemia that does not respond to diet. Clofibrate is also prescribed for patients with very high serum triglycerides with abdominal pain and pancreatitis that does not respond to diet.

Adverse Effects

Adverse effects of fibric acid derivatives include angina, arrhythmias, swelling, phlebitis, and pulmonary emboli. These agents also cause nausea,

vomiting, diarrhea, flatulence, gastritis, and gall stones (with long-term therapy). Clofibrate may produce impotence, dysuria, hematuria, leukopenia, and anemia.

Contraindications and Precautions

Fibric acid derivatives are contraindicated in patients with hypersensitivity to these agents, impaired renal or hepatic function, primary biliary cirrhosis, pregnancy (category C), and lactation. Safe use of fibric acid derivatives in children younger than 14 years is not established.

Fibric acid derivatives are used cautiously in patients with a history of jaundice or hepatic disease, gallstones, peptic ulcer, hypothyroidism, and cardiovascular disease.

Drug Interactions

Fibric acid derivatives may increase anticoagulant effects by lowering plasma protein binding. They increase the effect of antidiabetics, and exaggerate diuretic response to furosemide. Clofibrate increases the effects of insulin. With probenecid, the therapeutic and toxic effects of clofibrate are increased. With ursodiol, there is increased risk of gallstone formation.

Niacin

Niacin (vitamin B_3, nicotinic acid) can exert cholesterol- and triglyceride-lowering effects at high concentrations, resulting in a decrease of LDL and VLDL levels, and an increase in HDL levels, but its use is limited by its side effects.

Mechanism of Action

Nicotinic acid may partially inhibit the release of free fatty acids from adipose tissue and increase lipoprotein activity, which could increase the rate of triglyceride removal from plasma. These actions reduce the total LDL (bad cholesterol) and triglycerides, resulting in increased HDL (good cholesterol).

Indications

Niacin may be prescribed as an adjunct to diet for treatment of adults with very high serum triglyceride levels who present a risk of pancreatitis, and who do not respond adequately to dietary control.

Adverse Effects

Nicotinic acid may cause headache, anxiety, hypotension, flushing or burning feelings in the skin, dry skin, peptic ulcer, or abnormal liver function tests. Other adverse effects of this agent include hyperuricemia, glucose intolerance, nausea, vomiting, diarrhea, hyperglycemia, and elevated plasma uric acid.

Contraindications and Precautions

Niacin is contraindicated in patients with hypersensitivity to this agent, hepatic impairment, severe hypotension, or arterial bleeding. Niacin also is contraindicated in patients with active peptic ulcer, pregnancy (category C), lactation, and children younger than 16 years.

Niacin is used cautiously in individuals with history of gallbladder disease, liver impairment, and peptic ulcer. This agent should be used with caution in glaucoma, angina, coronary artery disease, and diabetes mellitus.

Drug Interactions

Niacin can increase the effectiveness of antihypertensives or vasoactive drugs. It also increases the risk of bleeding with anticoagulants. Niacin decreases absorption with bile acid sequestrants and separate doses must be at least 4 to 6 hours apart.

Combination Drug Therapy

Certain combinations of medications can be useful in treating markedly elevated LDL cholesterol levels. Combination therapy can maximize the reduction in LDL levels. It can also allow the limiting of dosages of individual LDL-reducing drugs, thus limiting side effects. For patients with elevations in both triglycerides and LDL, the addition of nicotinic acid or a fibric acid derivative to control triglyceride levels can allow the use of a bile acid sequestrant to help reduce LDL levels. The following are the most effective combinations for lowering LDL:

- A statin plus a bile acid sequestrant
- A statin plus nicotinic acid
- Nicotinic acid plus a bile acid sequestrant
- A statin plus a bile acid sequestrant plus nicotinic acid

The combination of a fibric acid derivative with a statin should usually be avoided because of an increased risk of myopathy.

SUMMARY

Antihypertensive drugs include diuretics (to lower blood volume), ACE inhibitors, beta-blockers, and vasodilators. In some cases, calcium channel blockers must be used with care for the elderly. Medications are used only when lifestyle changes have not adequately lowered elevated blood pressure.

To reduce the circulating hyperlipidemia, medications may be required. The statins reduce the enzyme necessary for cholesterol production. Nicotinic acid reduces LDL and VLDL levels. The fibric acid derivatives decrease triglyceride and VLDL levels while raising HDL levels. These medications for hyperlipidemia are long-term therapy.

EXPLORING THE WEB

Visit *http://www.americanheart.org*

- Search for information on management of hypertension and hyperlipidemia.

Visit *http://www.hearthealthywomen.org*

- What are some of the challenges related to managing cardiovascular health for women that are different than for men?

Visit *www.cvphysiology.com*

- Click on "hypertension" and review additional information to further your understanding of hypertension.

Visit *www.hypertension-facts.org*

- For additional resources and information on hypertension.

Visit *www.medicinenet.com* or *www.nlm.nih.gov/medlineplus*

- Search for the disorders or drugs discussed in this chapter. What additional information can you find?

REVIEW QUESTIONS

Multiple Choice

1. Which of the following antianginal drugs are also used as antihypertensives?

   A. nitrates
   B. vasoconstrictors
   C. diuretics
   D. beta-adrenergic blockers

2. Thiazides are contraindicated in all of the following patients, except those with:

   A. impaired liver function
   B. edema caused by heart failure
   C. diabetes
   D. a history of gout

3. Hydralazine (Apresoline) is a(n):

   A. vasodilator
   B. vasoconstrictor
   C. anticoagulant
   D. antiarrhythmic

4. An example of a angiotensin-converting enzyme (ACE) inhibitor is:

   A. captopril (Capoten)
   B. acebutolol (Sectral)
   C. lidocaine (Xylocaine)
   D. procainamide (Pronestyl)

5. Hypertension with an unknown etiology is referred to as:

   A. secondary hypertension
   B. malignant hypertension
   C. familial hypertension
   D. primary hypertension

6. The trade names of clonidine include which of the following?

   A. Corgard
   B. Catapres
   C. Aldomet
   D. Lopressor

7. Which of the following agents have become the mainstay of LDL-reducing therapy?

   A. calcium channel blockers
   B. cardiac glycosides
   C. angiotensin II receptor antagonists
   D. HMG-CoA reductase inhibitors

8. Which of the following is the initial treatment of hypertension?

   A. beta-blockers
   B. antiarrhythmic drugs
   C. antihyperlipidemic drugs
   D. cardiac glycosides

9. Which of the following is the generic name of Aramine?

   A. dopamine
   B. metaraminol
   C. ephedrine
   D. epinephrine

10. Which of the following may be caused as a result of ACE inhibitor therapy?

    A. hyperglycemia
    B. hypercalcemia
    C. hyperkalemia
    D. hypernatremia

11. Which of the following type of antihypertensive drugs may affect the renin-angiotensin system to increase urine?

    A. vasodilators
    B. ACE inhibitors
    C. direct-acting vasodilators
    D. adrenergic blockers

12. An example of a potassium-sparing diuretic is:

    A. chlorothiazide (Diuril)
    B. acetazolamide (Diamox)
    C. furosemide (Lasix)
    D. spironolactone (Aldactone)

13. Which of the following is a common adverse effect of a bile acid sequestrant?

    A. double vision
    B. constipation
    C. insomnia
    D. hypotension

14. Which of the following is the first drug of choice to lower hyperlipidemia?

    A. statins
    B. fibric acids
    C. bile acids
    D. nicotinic acids

15. Which of the following is a potent vasoconstrictor?

    A. renin
    B. angiotensin I
    C. angiotensin II
    D. aldosterone

Matching

Generic Name	Trade Name
_____ **1.** simvastatin	**A.** Welchol
_____ **2.** gemfibrozil	**B.** Lipitor
_____ **3.** fenofibrate	**C.** Pravachol
_____ **4.** pravastatin	**D.** Tricor
_____ **5.** cholestyramine	**E.** Questran
_____ **6.** atorvastatin	**F.** Lopid
_____ **7.** colesevelam	**G.** Zocor

Critical Thinking

A 48-year-old woman who was diagnosed with essential hypertension 5 years ago has avoided taking her medication for the last 4 months because she claims that she feels fine without it. She has decreased her regular exercise due to taking care of her new home business, and has noticed occasional nosebleeds, blurred vision, dizziness, and overall tiredness. Her doctor examines her and finds her blood pressure to be 185/115. He also hears crackling noises (rales) when he listens to her lungs, and notices that she has ruptures in the capillaries of the retinas in her eyes. He prescribes blood pressure medication, urinary tests to check her kidneys, rest and relaxation, and instructs her to see a nutritionist.

1. What is the pathophysiology of essential hypertension?

2. Since the patient has high diastolic pressure, what possible problems may be associated with her condition?

3. The doctor suspects mild congestive heart failure. Explain how this can develop as a result of hypertension.

Anticoagulant Drugs

OBJECTIVES

After completing this chapter, the reader should be able to:

1. Explain the terms *hemostasis*, *aggregation*, and *thrombophlebitis*.
2. Describe the mechanism of action of heparin.
3. Discuss the uses and adverse effects of anticoagulant.
4. Explain factors that usually predispose the development of a thrombus.
5. List three common coagulation disorders.
6. Describe the mechanism of action of thrombolytic drugs.
7. Explain the indications of antiplatelet drugs.
8. Identify oral anticoagulant agents and their indications.
9. Explain thrombocytopenia and thrombolytics.
10. Discuss the role of vitamin K in the process of clotting.

GLOSSARY

Aggregation – the clumping together of platelets to form a clot

Alopecia – loss of hair from anywhere on the body, sometimes until complete baldness is reached

Anticoagulants – agents used to prevent the formation of a blood clot

Antiplatelet agents – drugs that inhibit normal platelet function, usually by reducing their ability to aggregate and inappropriately form blood clots

Blood coagulation – the process by which blood clots

Embolism – obstruction or occlusion of a vessel

Fibrin – gel-like threads

Fibrinogen – a plasma protein

Fibrinolysis – the breakdown of fibrin

Hemostasis – a process that stops bleeding in a blood vessel

Heparin – a potent anticoagulant naturally obtained from the liver and lungs of domestic animals; in humans, it is usually found in basophils or mast cells

Mast cells – large cells found in connective tissue that contain many biochemicals, including histamine; mast cells are involved in inflammation secondary to injuries and infections, and are sometimes implicated in allergic reactions

Phlebothrombosis – clotting in a vein without primary inflammation

Placebo – an inert substance given to a patient instead of an active medicine

Prothrombin – a glycoprotein formed and stored in the parenchymal cells of the liver and present in the blood; a deficiency of prothrombin leads to impaired blood coagulation

Thrombin – enzyme occurring in blood during the clotting process

Thrombocytopenia – decrease in the number of platelets in circulating blood

Thrombogenic – substances causing blood clots

Thrombolytics – drugs designed to dissolve blood clots that have already formed within a blood vessel

Thrombophlebitis – venous inflammation with thrombus formation

Thromboplastin – substance to cause clotting

Thrombosis – the formation of a clot

Thrombus – a clot in the cardiovascular system formed during life from constituents of blood

Venous stasis – injury to the veins causing loss of proper function of the vein and impairing the ability of blood flow to return to the heart

OVERVIEW

The ability of blood to clot in response to injury is essential to protection of the body from unnecessary blood loss. Clotting disorders impair this ability of the body to protect itself. Excessive blood loss can lead to shock and ultimately death if left untreated. In this circumstance, drugs may be administered to aid the clotting process.

There are other instances in which clots may form and travel through the venous system, becoming lodged in a vessel and causing a blockage of blood flow. This can cause tissue damage and may also cause the death of the individual if the blockage occurs in the vessels of the lungs or the heart. Drugs that can dissolve or prevent clots from forming may be given to alleviate or prevent this type of event.

BLOOD COAGULATION

Blood coagulation (clotting) is of the utmost importance in the protection of the body from undue blood loss. It is well known that people with blood-clotting disorders, such as hemophilia, lead precarious lives, which can be terminated abruptly by a minor injury, such as slight bruising. In a healthy person, such injuries would often pass unnoticed.

On the other end of the spectrum, many individuals suffer from problems of intravascular clots (thrombi) being formed. This can lead to blockage of the smaller blood vessels in the body and, consequently, tissue ischemia. A common cause of this is **venous stasis** (injury to the veins causing loss of proper function of the vein and impairing the ability of blood flow to return to the heart), due to inactivity such as that which can occur in prolonged bedrest.

Related to a **thrombus** is a blood embolus, which is a fragment of a blood clot that occludes a vessel. The clot may have been formed due to procedures such as surgery. In this case, a fragment of a natural clot escapes into the circulation and blocks a major vessel. For example, blockage of one of the pulmonary arteries results in a pulmonary embolism.

Hemostasis is the spontaneous arrest of bleeding from a damaged blood vessel. The normal vascular endothelial cells and circulating blood platelets are not **thrombogenic** (causing blood clots) unless blood vessels or platelets are damaged by cuts or injury. Hemostasis or blood clotting occurs as a result of the following steps:

- The immediate response of a blood vessel to injury is vasoconstriction or vascular spasm due to the release of serotonin. In small blood vessels, this decreases blood flow and allows a platelet plug to form.

- Blood platelets release **thromboplastin** (substance to cause clotting) at the site of the injury. Thromboplastin and calcium react with **prothrombin** (a plasma protein produced by the liver) to create **thrombin**.

- The thrombin then changes **fibrinogen** (a plasma protein) into **fibrin** (gel-like threads) which layers over the site of the injury like mesh. This fibrin sheath traps blood cells and plasma and forms a clot (Figure 13-1).

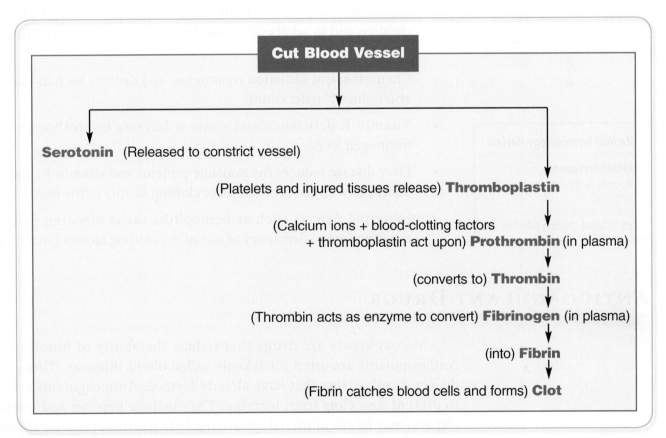

Figure 13-1 Blood clotting process.

COAGULATION DISORDERS

Thrombophlebitis refers to the development of a thrombus in a vein where inflammation is present. The platelets adhere to the inflamed site, and a thrombus develops. In **phlebothrombosis**, a thrombus forms spontaneously in a vein without prior inflammation, although inflammation may develop secondarily in response to **thrombosis**. The clot is less firmly attached in this case, and its development is asymptomatic or silent. Several factors usually predispose the development of a thrombus:

- The first group of factors involves stasis of blood or sluggish blood flow, which is often present in people who are immobile.

- The endothelial lining of the blood vessels is injured, which may have arisen from trauma, chemical injury, intravenous injection, or inflammation.

- The third factor involves increased blood coagulability, which may result from dehydration, cancer, pregnancy, or increased platelet adhesion.

Spontaneous bleeding or excessive bleeding following minor tissue trauma often indicates a blood-clotting disorder. Excessive bleeding has many causes:

- **Thrombocytopenia** may be caused by acute viral infections in children and in adults when platelets are destroyed by HIV infection and certain drugs.

- Chemotherapy, radiation treatments, and cancers such as leukemia also reduce platelet count.

- Vitamin K deficiency may cause a decrease in prothrombin and fibrinogen levels.

- Liver disease reduces the available proteins and vitamin K, and thus, interferes with the production of clotting factors in the liver.

- Inherited defects such as hemophilia cause bleeding disorders resulting from a deficiency of one of the clotting factors (factor VIII).

> ### Medical Terminology Review
>
> **thrombophlebitis**
> *thrombo = blood clot; blood clotting*
> *phleb = vein*
> *itis = inflammation; disease of*
> blood clot within the vein resulting from inflammation
>
> **phlebothrombosis**
> *phlebo = vein*
> *thromb = blood clot; blood clotting*
> *osis = diseased or abnormal condition*
> abnormal formation of a blood clot within a vein

> ### Medical Terminology Review
>
> **thrombocytopenia**
> *thrombo = blood clot; blood clotting*
> *cyto = cell*
> *penia = lack; deficiency*
> lack of blood-clotting platelets

ANTICOAGULANT DRUGS

Anticoagulants are drugs that reduce the ability of blood to clot. Anticoagulants are often mistakenly called blood thinners. These drugs do not dissolve clots that have already formed. Anticoagulants are used to prevent new clots from forming. They include heparin and warfarin. Heparin may be administered intravenously to patients at risk for thrombus formation and warfarin is given orally.

Medical Terminology Review

anticoagulant
anti = opposite; not
coagulant = agent that causes clotting
agent that will prevent clotting

TABLE 13-1 Anticoagulants

Generic Name	Trade Name	Route of Administration	Average Adult Dosage
anisindione	Miradon®	PO	25–250 mg/day
argatroban	Acova®, Novastan®	IV	2–10 mcg/kg/min
bivalirudin	Angiomax®	IV	0.75 mg/kg bolus followed by 1.75 mg/kg/hr for 4h
heparin sodium	Hep-Lock®	IV	Infusion 5,000–40,000 units/day subcutaneously; 15,000–20,000 units/b.i.d.
lepirudin	Refludan®	IV	0.4 mg/kg bolus followed by 0.15–16.5 mg/kg/hr for 2–10 days
pentoxifylline	Trental®	PO	400 mg t.i.d.
warfarin sodium	Coumadin®	PO, IV	Usual dose: 2–10 mg/day
Low molecular weight (fractionated) heparins (lmwhs)			
dalteparin sodium	Fragmin®	SC	For the first 30 days, give 200 units/kg once daily (max: 18,000 units/day); Months 2–6: give 150 units/kg once daily
enoxaparin	Lovenox®	SC	30 mg b.i.d. for 10–14 days
tinzaparin sodium	Innohep®	SC	175 units/kg daily for at least 6 days

Heparin

Heparin is a potent anticoagulant naturally obtained from the liver and lungs of domestic animals. In humans, it is usually found in basophils or **mast cells**. Heparin preparations are available as heparin sodium and the low- and high-molecular weight heparins (fractionated heparins). Examples of anticoagulants are listed in Table 13-1.

Mechanism of Action

Heparin prevents the conversion of fibrinogen to fibrin, and inactivates several of the factors needed for blood clotting. Heparin can be inactivated by hydrochloric acid in the stomach, and must not be administered orally. Therefore, it is given either subcutaneously or through IV infusion. The onset of action for IV heparin is immediate, whereas subcutaneous heparin may take up to an hour for maximum therapeutic effect.

Indications

Heparin and heparin substitutes are used prophylactically for deep vein thrombosis, pulmonary embolism, or atrial embolism. Heparin is also indicated in patients with atrial fibrillation and heart valve replacement surgery. Low molecular weight heparins (LMWHs) have become the drugs of choice for many clotting disorders such as coronary occlusion, acute myocardial infarction, and peripheral arterial embolism. After the initiation of anticoagulant therapy with heparin, oral anticoagulants can be started immediately. After about 48 hours, the heparin can be withdrawn, as the oral anticoagulants take this time to exert their effect.

Adverse Effects

Spontaneous bleeding is the major complication of heparin administration. Skin rashes, pruritus, burning sensations of the feet, hypertension, fever, chills, headache, and chest pain are seen in some patients. Hypersensitivity reactions may cause bronchospasms and an anaphylactic reaction. The LMWHs may produce fewer adverse effects than other types of heparin.

Contraindications and Precautions

Heparin preparations are contraindicated in patients with a history of hypersensitivity to this agent, active bleeding hemophilia, open wounds, or severe thrombocytopenia. LMWHs should be avoided in patients with a hypersensitivity to the drug and in those patients with thrombocytopenia or active bleeding. Heparin preparations are used with caution in patients with alcoholism or history of allergy (asthma, hives, hay fever, eczema); during menstruation, pregnancy (category C), especially the last trimester, and the immediate postpartum period. Heparin therapy requires caution in the elderly, patients in hazardous occupations, and those with cerebral embolism.

Drug Interactions

Use of heparin with other anticoagulants may increase anticoagulant effects to a dangerous level. Use with caution with salicylates such as aspirin.

Warfarin

Warfarin is the mainstay of long-term anticoagulant therapy, and is one of the original drugs of the coumarin group.

Mechanism of Action

Warfarin is structurally similar to vitamin K, which is involved in the synthesis of prothrombin in the liver. Therefore, warfarin indirectly interferes with blood clotting by depressing hepatic synthesis of vitamin K-dependant coagulation factors II, VII, IX, and X.

Indications

Warfarin is used as a prophylaxis and for the treatment of deep vein thrombosis, pulmonary embolism, treatment of atrial fibrillation with embolism. Warfarin is also prescribed as an adjunct in the treatment of coronary occlusion, cerebral transient ischemic attacks (TIAs), and as a prophylactic in patients with prosthetic cardiac valves.

Adverse Effects

In the correct and individualized dosage, warfarin is almost devoid of adverse effects not related to its anticoagulant action. **Alopecia** and sustained erection are the only ones of any consequence, but these are rare. Adverse effects such as nausea and dizziness occur with similar frequency to those caused by a **placebo**.

Contraindications and Precautions

Warfarin is contraindicated in patients with a known hypersensitivity to this drug, bleeding tendencies, vitamin C or K deficiency, hemophilia, clotting factor deficiency, active bleeding, open wounds and active peptic ulcer. Warfarin should be avoided in patients with severe hepatic and renal disease, pericarditis with acute myocardial infarction, recent surgery of brain, spinal cord, or eye.

Warfarin is used cautiously in debilitated patients, older adults, and patients with alcoholism, allergic disorders, or psychosis. Warfarin should be used with caution in patients with hepatic and renal insufficiency, diarrhea, fever, and pancreatic disorders.

Drug Interactions

Cholestyramine can decrease warfarin absorption, thus reducing its effects. Colestipol and sucralfate have also been reported to interfere with warfarin absorption, but only to a minor degree.

Acetohexamide, acetaminophen, and allopurinol may enhance the anticoagulant effects of warfarin.

ANTIPLATELET DRUGS

Platelets play a key role in hemostasis and thrombus formation. Platelets adhere to thrombin, collagen, and various other substances. Antiplatelet agents are prescribed to suppress aggregation (clumping) of platelets. A number of drugs may be used for stopping thrombi in arteries rather than anticoagulants in veins. The most commonly used antiplatelet drug is aspirin. It has been proven effective for preventing myocardial infarctions and strokes. Other medications may be used as antiplatelet drugs, including glycoprotein antagonists, ticlopidine, and abciximab (Table 13-2).

TABLE 13-2   Antiplatelet Drugs

Generic Name	Trade Name	Route of Administration	Average Adult Dosage
aspirin	ASA®(acetylsalicylic acid)	PO	80 mg daily–650 mg b.i.d.
dipyridamole	Persantine®	PO	75–100 mg/q.i.d.
ADP receptor blockers			
clopidogrel bisulfate	Plavix®	PO	75 mg daily
ticlopidine	Ticlid®	PO	250 mg b.i.d.
Glycoprotein IIB/IIIA receptor blockers			
abciximab	ReoPro®	IV	0.25 mg/kg initial bolus over 5 min; then 10 mcg/min for 12 hours
eptifibatide	Integrilin®	IV	180 mcg/kg initial bolus over 1–2 min; then 2 mcg/kg/min for 24–72 hours
tirofiban hydrochloride	Aggrastat®	IV	0.4 mcg/kg/min for 30 min; then 0.1 mcg/kg/min for 12–24 hours

Mechanism of Action

Eptifibatide and tirofiban are two of the newest glycoprotein antagonists used to delay clotting by altering platelet aggregation that have received approval by the Food and Drug Administration. These agents are prescribed in conjunction with heparin and aspirin. Other antiplatelet agents have the same mechanism of action as these new drugs.

Indications

Ticlopidine prevents platelet aggregation, which reduces risk of thrombotic stroke in patients who have experienced stroke precursors. Abciximab is an antiplatelet drug used with heparin and aspirin to prevent coronary vessel occlusion in patients undergoing percutaneous transluminal coronary angioplasty or atherectomy. Clopidogrel is an antiplatelet agent used in patients who have recently had myocardial infarction or stroke.

Adverse Effects

The primary side effects associated with glycoprotein antagonists are bleeding and thrombocytopenia (a decrease in blood platelet levels). Adverse effects of ticlopidine include neutropenia (a decrease in white blood cells), thrombocytopenia, and bleeding. The adverse effects of clopidogral include fatigue, arthralgic pain, headache, dizziness, hypertension, edema, and risk of bleeding.

Key Concept

Garlic is an herb that has been shown to decrease the aggregation (stickiness) of platelets, thus producing an anticoagulant effect.

Contraindications and Precautions

Antiplatelet drugs are contraindicated in patients with hypersensitivity to these drugs or those who have neutropenia, thrombocytopenia, bleeding ulcer, and uncontrolled hypertension. Antiplatelets should be avoided in patients with recent major surgery or trauma, intracranial bleeding within six months, renal dialysis, and aneurysm.

Antiplatelet drugs are used cautiously in patients with severe liver and renal impairment. These agents should be given with caution to patients at risk for bleeding from trauma, surgery, or GI bleeding, and pregnancy (category B).

Drug Interactions

Aspirin has drug interactions with anticoagulants, hypoglycemic agents, uricosuric agents, spironolactone, alcohol, corticosteroids, pyrazolone derivatives, NSAIDs, urinary alkalinizers, phenobarbital, phenytoin, and propranolol. Ticlopidine potentiates the effect of aspirin and NSAIDs; it also should not be used along with antacids, cimetidine, digoxin, theophylline, phenobarbital, phenytoin, or propranolol. There is no direct drug information as yet available about eptifibatide, however, its adverse effects on the body are well documented. Tirofiban, when used in combination with heparin and aspirin, has been associated with an increase in bleeding. Formal drug interaction studies with abciximab have not been conducted, although an increase in bleeding when abciximab is used concurrently with heparin, other anticoagulants, thrombolytics, and antiplatelet agents has been documented. Use of clopidogrel with NSAIDs has caused increased GI blood loss, and it should be used with aspirin, heparin, or warfarin with caution.

THROMBOLYTIC DRUGS

Thrombolytics are agents that dissolve existing clots. Administration of thrombolytic agents such as tissue plasminogen activator, urokinase, or streptokinase is capable of dissolving an arterial clot, such as a clot in a coronary artery in a patient with an acute myocardial infarction. These agents are able to dissolve clots in various access devices.

The body normally regulates **fibrinolysis** such that unwanted fibrin clots are removed, whereas fibrin present in wounds is left to maintain hemostasis. The steps of fibrinolysis are shown in Figure 13-2.

Mechanism of Action

Thrombolytic agents break down fibrin clots by converting plasminogen to plasmin (fibrinolysis). Plasmin is an enzyme that breaks down the fibrin of a blood clot.

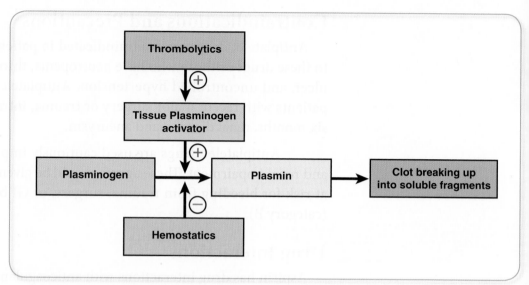

Figure 13-2 Process of fibrinolysis.

Indications

Thrombolytic drugs are used to treat acute myocardial infarction, pulmonary embolism, acute ischemic cerebrovascular accident (CVA), deep vein thrombosis, and coronary thrombosis, and to clear clots in arteriovenous cannulas and blocked IV catheters. Table 13-3 lists the major thrombolytic drugs.

Adverse Effects

Bleeding is the most common adverse effect of thrombolytic drugs, often because of percutaneous trauma or spontaneous bleeding from GI

TABLE 13-3 Thrombolytic Drugs

Generic Name	Trade Name	Route of Administration	Average Adult Dosage
alteplase recombinant	Activase®	IV	Begin with 60 mg and then infuse 20 mg/hour over next 2 hours
anistreplase	Eminase®	IV	30 units over 2–5 min
reteplase recombinant	Retavase®	IV	10 units over 2 min; repeat dose in 30 min
streptokinase	Streptase®	IV	250,000–1.5 million units over a short period of time
tenecteplase	TNKase®	IV	30–50 mg infused over 5sec
urokinase	Abbokinase®	IV	4,400–6,000 units administered over several minutes to 12 hours

tract. Other adverse effects include unstable blood pressure, ventricular dysrhythmias, itching, and nausea.

Contraindications and Precautions

Thrombolytic drugs are contraindicated in patients with a known hypersensitivity, active bleeding, a history of recent trauma, recent intracranial surgery, and a history of stroke. The patient must be monitored carefully for signs of bleeding every 15 minutes for the first hour of therapy and every 30 minutes thereafter.

Thrombolytic drugs should be used cautiously in patients who have recently undergone major surgery, or those who have hypertension and diabetic retinopathy. Thrombolytic drugs are used with caution in pregnancy (category C) with the exception of urokinase (category B).

Drug Interactions

Thrombolytic drugs along with aspirin, dipyridamole, or an anticoagulant may increase the risk of bleeding.

Key Concept

Alteplase with herbal supplements (ginkgo) may increase thrombolytic effects.

SUMMARY

Anticoagulants are used to treat deep venous thrombosis by disrupting the coagulation process and the formation of fibrin. The most potent anticoagulants include heparin and warfarin. Antiplatelet agents suppress clumping of platelets to stop thrombi from forming in arteries. Thrombolytics dissolve existing clots by breaking down fibrin and converting plasminogen to plasmin. All of these agents are important to help avoid blood clotting problems in the body, which can lead to a variety of conditions, including tissue ischemia, various embolisms, and stroke.

EXPLORING THE WEB

Visit *www.americanheart.org*

- Search for "anticoagulants" review-related articles to further enhance your understanding of these drugs.

Visit *www.medicinenet.com*

- Choose a disorder or drug type discussed in this chapter, and search for it. What additional information or research is available related to this topic?

Visit *www.webmd.com*

- From the health A-Z index choose Heart Disease, then click on "All Heat Disease topics." Look for articles related to the topics covered in this chapter. What additional information is available?

REVIEW QUESTIONS

Multiple Choice

1. Anticoagulants are used prophylactically for all of the following conditions or disorders, except

   A. prevention of thrombus in pulmonary embolus
   B. hypothyroidism
   C. deep vein thrombosis
   D. atrial fibrillation

2. Which of the following is an antagonist of warfarin?

   A. vitamin D
   B. vitamin A
   C. vitamin K
   D. niacin

3. The spontaneous arrest of bleeding from a damaged blood vessel is called

    A. hematoma
    B. hemosiderosis
    C. hemostasis
    D. hemostatic

4. The onset of action for intravenous heparin is

    A. immediate
    B. an hour
    C. three days
    D. one week

5. Which of the following is a major complication of heparin administration?

    A. hypertension
    B. hypersensitivity reaction
    C. bronchospasms
    D. bleeding

6. Ticlid (ticlopidine) is a drug that includes which of the following groups of drugs?

    A. thrombolytics
    B. anticoagulants
    C. antiplatelets
    D. hemostatics

7. Which of the following anticoagulants have become the drugs of choice for many clotting disorders?

    A. low molecular weight heparins
    B. high molecular weight heparins
    C. warfarins
    D. vitamin K

8. Which of the following agents is used to suppress aggregation of platelets?

    A. heparin
    B. aspirin
    C. warfarin
    D. protamine sulfate

9. Which of the following is an example of thrombolytic drugs?

    A. protamine sulfate
    B. plasminogen activator
    C. warfarin
    D. heparin

10. Which of the following is the most common adverse effect of thrombolytics?

    A. constipation
    B. hypertension
    C. vomiting
    D. bleeding

Fill in the Blank

1. Thrombophlebitis refers to the development of a clot in a vein where _____.

2. Anticoagulants are drugs that reduce the ability of _____.

3. After initiation of anticoagulant therapy with heparin, _____ can be started immediately.

4. The major complication for heparin administration is _____.

5. Warfarin is structurally similar to _____.

6. The most commonly used antiplatelet drug is _____.

Matching

Match the first column (generic names) of LMWHs with the second column (trade names):

_____ 1. tinzaparin   **A.** Normiflo

_____ 2. danaparoid   **B.** Fragmin

_____ 3. dalteparin   **C.** Orgaran

_____ 4. adeparin   **D.** Innohep

Critical Thinking

George is 99 years old. He has had multiple disorders and taken many different medications in his life. His skin is very thin, and only a little pressure to his skin can cause bleeding. Some of his regular medications include antidepressants, antihypertensive drugs, and baby aspirin for his heart condition.

1. What do you think are the causes of bleeding from the skin?

2. What can George's physician suggest to prevent his bleeding?

3. What medications should George stop taking because they may increase the likelihood of bleeding?

Drug Therapy for Allergies and Respiratory Disorders

OUTLINE

OBJECTIVES

After completing this chapter, the reader should be able to:

1. Identify basic anatomical structures of the respiratory system.

2. Compare histamines and antihistamines.

3. Be able to list three popular asthma medications.

4. Discuss the uses and general drug actions of the bronchodilators in asthma.

5. Discuss different types of mucolytics and expectorants.

6. Explain how decongestants work and identify serious adverse effects.

7. Identify the chemical mediators that are important in asthma.

8. Discuss drugs used for smoking cessation.

9. Explain the indication of mast cell stabilizers and the mechanism of action.

10. Discuss chemical mediators.

GLOSSARY

Allergic rhinitis – inflammation of the nasal mucosa that is due to the sensitivity of the nasal tissue to an allergen

Allergy – a state of hypersensitivity induced by exposure to a particular antigen

Anaphylactic shock – a severe and sometimes fatal allergic reaction

Antigen – a substance that is introduced into the body and induces the formation of antibodies

Antihistamines – drugs that counteract the action of histamine

Antitussives – agents that relieve or prevent coughing

Asthma – a chronic inflammatory disorder of the airways of the respiratory system

Bronchiectasis – a destruction and widening of the large airways

Bronchodilators – agents that relax the smooth muscle of the bronchial tubes

OUTLINE *(continued)*

Chemical mediators – substances released by mast cells and platelets into interstitial fluid and blood; these substances include histamines, leukotrienes, serotonin, and prostaglandins

Chronic obstructive pulmonary disease (COPD) – a group of common chronic respiratory disorders that are characterized by progressive tissue damage and obstruction in the airways of the lungs

Cystic fibrosis – a genetic disorder affecting the exocrine glands, causing thick mucus to obstruct the bronchioles in the lungs

Dry powder inhaler (DPI) – a device used to deliver medication in the form of micronized powder into the lungs

Emphysema – the destruction of the alveolar walls and septae, which leads to large, permanently inflated alveolar air space

Expectorants – agents that promote the removal of mucus secretions from the lung, bronchi, and trachea, usually by coughing

Glucocorticoids – the most potent and consistently effective anti-inflammatory agents that are currently available for relief of respiratory conditions

Histamine – a chemical substance naturally found in all body tissues that protects the body from factors in the environment that produce allergic and inflammatory reactions

Leukotriene modifiers – a relatively new class of drugs designed to prevent asthma and allergic reactions before they occur by either inhibiting leukotriene production, or preventing leukotrienes from binding to cellular receptors

Leukotrienes – substances that contribute to the inflammation associated with asthma

Mast cell stabilizers – substances that work to prevent allergy cells (called mast cells) from breaking open and releasing chemicals that help cause inflammation; they work slowly over time

Metered dose inhaler (MDI) – a hand-held pressurized device used to deliver medications for inhalations

Mucolytic – destroying or dissolving the active agents that make up mucus

Septae – walls of the bronchioles

Xanthine derivatives – a substance that is effective for relief of bronchospasm in asthma, chronic bronchitis, and emphysema

OVERVIEW

The respiratory system provides the mechanisms for transporting oxygen from the air into the blood, and for removing carbon dioxide from the blood. Oxygen is essential for cell metabolism, and the respiratory system is the only means of acquiring oxygen. Carbon dioxide is a waste material resulting from cell metabolism.

The respiratory system consists of two anatomic areas: the upper and lower respiratory tracts. In addition, the pulmonary circulation, the muscles required for ventilation, and the nervous system (which plays a role in controlling respiratory function) are integral to the function of the respiratory system.

ANATOMY REVIEW

- The upper respiratory system consists of the nasal cavity, sinuses, and pharynx. The lower respiratory system consists of the larynx, trachea, bronchi, bronchioles, alveoli, and lungs (Figure 14-1).

- The respiratory system exchanges oxygen and carbon dioxide in the body through respiration.

- There are three types of respiration: external respiration is breathing or ventilation, internal respiration is the exchange of oxygen and carbon dioxide between the cells and lymph, and cellular respiration is the use of oxygen to release energy stored in nutrient molecules (Figure 14-2).

- Figure 14-3 outlines the functions of each of the structures that make up the respiratory system.

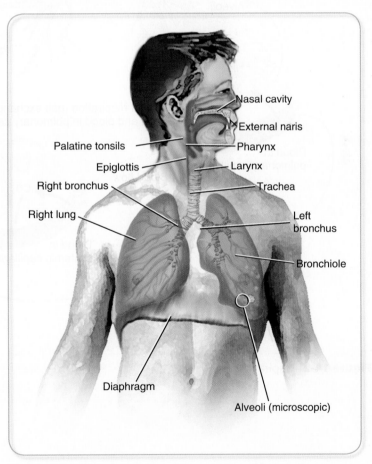

Figure 14-1 The structures of the upper and lower airways.

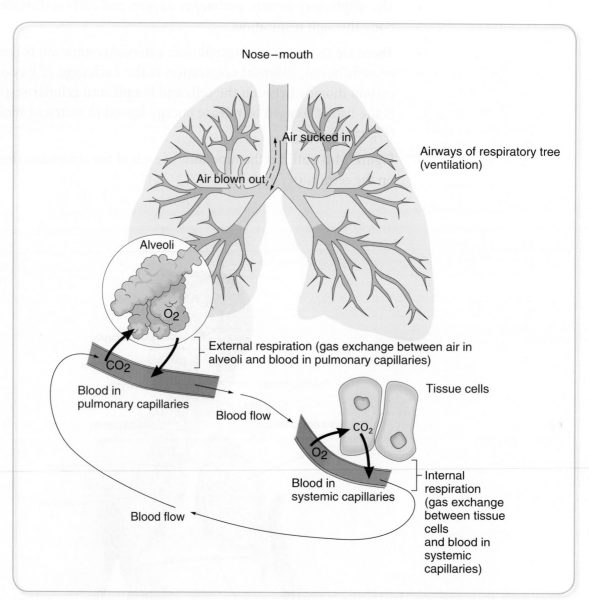

Nose—mouth

Air sucked in

Air blown out

Airways of respiratory tree (ventilation)

Alveoli

O_2

CO_2

External respiration (gas exchange between air in alveoli and blood in pulmonary capillaries)

Blood in pulmonary capillaries

Blood flow

Tissue cells

CO_2

O_2

Blood in systemic capillaries

Internal respiration (gas exchange between tissue cells and blood in systemic capillaries)

Blood flow

Figure 14-2 Respiration.

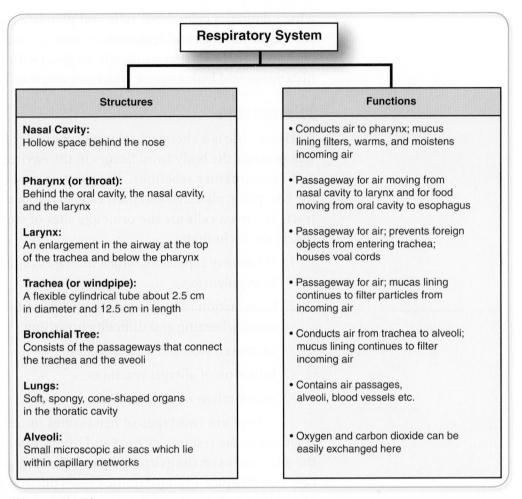

Figure 14-3 The respiratory system.

ALLERGIES

An **allergy** is a state of hypersensitivity induced by exposure to a particular **antigen** (a substance that is introduced into the body and induces the formation of antibodies), resulting in harmful immunologic reactions on subsequent exposures. The term is usually used to refer to hypersensitivity to an environmental antigen. There are varieties of allergic reactions such as allergic rhinitis, allergic conjunctivitis, allergic asthma, and allergic dermatitis. This chapter focuses on respiratory disorders and drug therapy, with allergic rhinitis and allergic asthma being discussed.

CHEMICAL MEDIATORS

Allergies result in an inflammatory process in the nasal passages and airways. The inflammatory process is basically the same regardless of the cause of the allergic response. The severity of the inflammation may vary with the specific situation. The inflammation may result in tissue injury,

which damages cells. Mast cells and platelets release **chemical mediators**, such as histamines and leukotrienes into the interstitial fluid and blood. The chemical mediators that are mostly involved with allergies and asthma include histamines and leukotrienes, which are discussed below.

Histamines

Histamine is a chemical substance naturally found in all the body tissues that protects the body from factors in the environment that produce allergic and inflammatory reactions. The greatest concentration of histamine is in the basophils, platelets, and mast cells in the skin, lungs, and gastrointestinal tract. The mast cells are the principle sites of storage. Histamine has several functions, including:

1. Dilation of capillaries, which increases capillary permeability and results in hypotension.
2. Contraction of most smooth muscle of the bronchial tree, which may cause wheezing and difficulty breathing.
3. Increased stomach acid secretion.
4. Initiation of allergic reactions.
5. Acceleration of the heart rate.

There are two types of histamines in our body. One causes allergic reactions in the respiratory tract and interacts with H_1 receptors on cells, and the other works on the gastrointestinal tract and interacts with H_2 receptors on cells (see Chapter 15). Histamine causes dilation and increased permeability of capillaries. It is one of the first mediators of an inflammatory response. Antihistamine drugs inhibit this immediate, transient response. Both H_1 and H_2 receptors mediate the contraction of vascular smooth muscle. Histamine has also been postulated to be a neurotransmitter in the central nervous system. The H_1 receptor may be blocked with antihistamine drugs.

Leukotrienes

Leukotrienes contribute to the inflammation associated with asthma. They are broncho-constrictive substances released during asthma and inflammation. Leukotrienes (slow-reacting substances of anaphylaxis [SRS-A]) are substances that produce effects similar to those of histamine. These substances cause smooth muscle contraction and increased vascular permeability. Leukotrienes appear to be important in the later stages of the inflammation associated with asthma. They stimulate slower and more prolonged responses than do histamines.

ALLERGIC REACTION

An allergic reaction occurs when the immune system reacts to a foreign substance. The body attempts to get rid of the substance, be it an allergen from the environment or a medication. In the case of an allergic reaction

to a medication, the body's response is harmful and may cause serious symptoms. Common allergic reactions include nausea, diarrhea, vomiting, headache, and lightheadedness. Other symptoms include anxiety, hives, palpitations, shortness of breath, rash, swelling, and wheezing. The most common allergies caused by natural environmental allergies include dust, pollen, and pet dander. The most common medications that cause allergic reactions include anticonvulsants, barbiturates, iodine, anesthetics, and antibiotics (including sulfa medications).

Anaphylactic Shock

Anaphylactic shock is an allergic reaction that may be life threatening. Its onset is sudden, severe, and involves the entire body. Anaphylactic shock causes a massive release of histamine and other substances, which cause airway constriction (making breathing very difficult), abdominal cramping, vomiting, and diarrhea. Common causes of anaphylactic shock include foods, medications, insect stings, and allergies to latex. Foods which are most likely to cause this condition include nuts, fish, milk, and eggs. Individuals who have food allergies or asthma are believed to be more likely to develop anaphylactic reactions. The most common insect stings in the United States include bees, yellow jackets, hornets, wasps, and ants. Anaphylactic reactions often begin with tingling sensations, itching, metallic taste sensation, hives, sensation of warmth, symptoms of asthma, swelling of the mouth and throat, a drop in blood pressure, or loss of consciousness. These types of reactions are usually treated with epinephrine, followed by antihistamines and steroids.

Allergic Rhinitis

Allergic rhinitis is the inflammation of the mucus membranes in the nose, throat, and airways that is due to the sensitivity of the tissue to an antigen, also called an allergen. The nasal mucosa is rich with mast cells (large cells that contain a wide variety of biochemicals, including histamine). These cells, along with basophils (a type of white blood cell), recognize environmental agents as they try to enter the body. Individuals with allergic rhinitis contain numerous mast cells. Allergic rhinitis is usually associated with watery nasal discharge and itching of the nose and eyes, caused by a localized sensitivity reaction to house dust, animal dander, or an antigen, commonly pollen. The condition may be seasonal. It is commonly known as "hay fever." Allergic rhinitis is caused by histamine release, while non-allergic rhinitis is often a symptom of the common cold.

> **Medical Terminology Review**
>
> **rhinitis**
>
> *rhin = nose*
> *itis = inflammation*
> inflammation of the nose

ANTI-ALLERGIC AGENTS

The therapeutic goals of treating allergic rhinitis are to prevent its occurrence and to relieve symptoms. Drugs used to prevent or treat allergic rhinitis include antihistamines (H_1-receptor antagonists), intranasal steroids, and mast cell stabilizers. Antihistamines and common OTC antihistamine

TABLE 14-1 First- and Second-generation H$_1$-receptor Antagonists

Generic Name	Trade Name	Route of Administration	Average Adult Dosage
First-generation Agents			
azatadine	Optimine®	PO	1–2 mg b.i.d.-t.i.d. prn
azelastine hydrochloride	Astelin®	Intranasal	2 sprays per nostril b.i.d.
brompheniramine maleate	Veltane®	PO	4–8 mg t.i.d.-q.i.d. (max: 40 mg/day)
chlorpheniramine maleate	Chlor-Trimeton®	PO	2–4 mg t.i.d.-q.i.d. (max: 24 mg/day)
clemastine fumarate	Tavist®	PO	1.34 mg b.i.d. (max: 8.04 mg/day)
cyproheptadine hydrochloride	Periactin®	PO	4 mg t.i.d. or q.i.d. (max: 0.5 mg/kg/day)
dexbrompheniramine maleate	Drixoral®	PO	6 mg b.i.d.
dexchlorpheniramine maleate	Dexchlor®	PO	2 mg q4–6 h (max: 12 mg/day)
diphenhydramine hydrochloride	Benadryl(R)	PO	25–50 mg 3–4 times/day (max: 300 mg/day)
promethazine hydrochloride	Phenergan®	PO	12.5 mg/day (max: 50 mg/day)
tripelennamine hydrochloride	PBZ-SR®	PO	25–50 mg q4–6 h (max: 600 mg/day)
triprolidine hydrochloride	Actidil®	PO	2.5 mg b.i.d. or t.i.d.
Second-generation Agents			
cetirizine hydrochloride	Zyrtec®	PO	5–10 mg/day
desloratadine	Clarinex®	PO	5 mg/day
fexofenadine hydrochloride	Allegra®	PO	60 mg b.i.d. or 180 mg once per day
loratadine	Claritin®	PO	10 mg/day

combinations will be focused on here. Mast cell stabilizers and steroids are discussed later in this chapter.

H$_1$-receptor Antagonists

H$_1$-receptor antagonists (**antihistamines**) are commonly used for the treatment of allergies. These drugs relieve the symptoms of runny nose, sneezing, and itching of the eyes, nose, and throat as seen in allergic rhinitis. Table 14-1 shows various H$_1$-receptor antagonists. Antihistamines are

TABLE 14-2 OTC Combination Antihistamine Drugs

Antihistamine	Decongestant	Trade Name
chlorpheniramine	phenylephrine	Actifed® Cold and Allergy tablets
chlorpheniramine	pseudoephedrine	Actifed® Cold and Sinus caplets
diphenhydramine	phenylephrine	Benadryl® Allergy/Cold caplets
chlorpheniramine	pseudoephedrine	Chlor-Trimeton® Allergy-Decongestant tablets
brompheniramine	phenylephrine	Dimetapp® Cold and Allergy Elixir
dexbrompheniramine	pseudoephedrine	Drixoral® Allergy and Sinus Extended Release tablets
chlorpheniramine	pseudoephedrine	Sinutab® Sinus Allergy tablets
diphenhydramine	phenylephrine	Sudafed® PE Nighttime
chlorpheniramine	pseudoephedrine	Triaminic® Cold/Allergy
chlorpheniramine	pseudoephedrine	Tylenol® Allergy Sinus caplets

often combined with decongestants and antitussives in OTC sinus and cold medicines. Table 14-2 shows examples of combination OTC drugs.

Mechanism of Action

The primary action of antihistamines is to block the effect of histamine at H_1-receptors, thus blocking histamine release.

Indications

H_1-receptor antagonists are used to treat minor symptoms of various allergic conditions and the common cold, such as runny nose, sneezing, and for the prevention of motion sickness, vertigo, and reactions to blood or plasma in susceptible patients.

Adverse Effects

Common adverse effects of H_1-receptor antagonists include dry mouth, dizziness, headache, urinary retention, nausea, vomiting, sedation, hypotension, and a decrease in the number of white blood cells.

Contraindications and Precautions

H_1-receptor antagonists are contraindicated in patients with hypersensitivity to these agents, prostatic hypertrophy, glaucoma, and GI obstructions. H_1-receptor antagonists should be used cautiously in patients with asthma or hyperthyroidism.

Drug Interactions

Use of H_1-receptor antagonists with CNS depressants such as opioids or alcohol will cause increased sedation. Some OTC cold preparations (for

example, diphenhydramine) may increase anticholinergic adverse effects. MAOIs may cause a hypertensive crisis.

ASTHMA

Asthma is defined as a chronic inflammatory disorder of the airways of the respiratory system (see Figure 14-4). It is a condition with wheezing and shortness of breath due to constriction of the bronchioles. Asthma is most commonly classified as allergic, exercise-induced, or caused by infections of the respiratory tract. Symptoms include breathlessness, cough, wheezing, and chest tightness. The airway becomes inflamed with edema and mucus plugs, and hyperactivity of the bronchial tree adds to the symptoms.

During asthmatic attacks, when bronchiole constriction and increased secretions are present, bronchodilators are used for relief. Anti-inflammatory drugs, such as glucocorticoids, leukotriene inhibitors, and cromolyn, may be

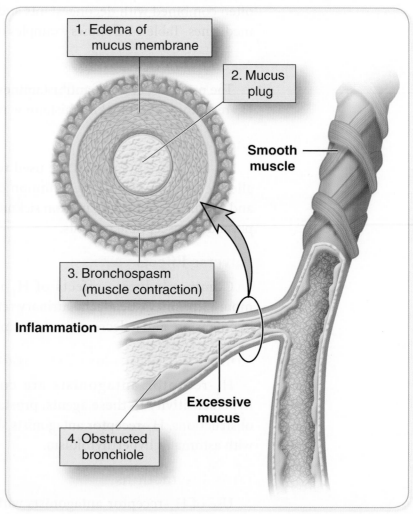

1. Edema of mucus membrane

2. Mucus plug

Smooth muscle

3. Bronchospasm (muscle contraction)

Inflammation

Excessive mucus

4. Obstructed bronchiole

Figure 14-4 Acute asthmatic episode.

prescribed for relief of symptoms. The majority of medications for asthma are administered by inhalation. Anti-asthma medications can be divided into two categories: long-term control and quick-relief medications.

For safety, asthmatic patients should learn how to manage their disease and its complications, as well as limit exposure to irritants that will trigger asthma attacks. Since symptoms alone are not always sufficient to measure respiratory status, patients learn how to use peak flow meters. These meters measure the peak expiratory flow rate (PEFR) from a patient's lungs. They should be used two times per day with the results of each usage written down so that results over time can be discussed with the patient's physician.

> **Medical Terminology Review**
>
> **bronchiole**
> *bronchi* = air tube
> *ole* = small; little; minute
> small tube in the airway

ANTI-ASTHMA AGENTS

There are various groups of medications used in the treatment of asthma, including bronchodilators, anti-inflammatory drugs, leukotriene modifiers (antagonists), and mast cell stabilizers.

Bronchodilators

Bronchodilators are agents that widen the diameter of the bronchial tubes, and are used to rapidly relieve the acute bronchospasm of asthmatic attack. Bronchodilators include beta-adrenergic agonists and xanthenes (theophylline). Beta-adrenergic drugs are the most commonly prescribed bronchodilators. Table 14-3 lists bronchodilators for asthma.

Beta-adrenergic Drugs

Beta-adrenergic drugs work as both cardiac and respiratory agonists. They are commonly referred to simply as beta-blockers. These drugs or hormones act through the sympathetic nervous system. Their effects include

TABLE 14-3 Drugs Used as Bronchodilators to Treat Asthma

Generic Name	Trade Name	Route of Administration	Average Adult Dosage
Anticholinergics			
ipratropium bromide	Atroven®	PO	2 inhalations by MDI q.i.d. (max: 12 inhalations/day)
ipratropium bromide and albuterol sulfate	Combivent®	PO	2 inhalations q6 h (max: 12 inhalations/day)
tiotropium bromide	Spiriva®	PO	1 capsule inhaled/day by Handihaler device
Beta-Agonists/Sympathomimetics			
albuterol	Proventil®, Ventolin®	PO	2–4 mg t.i.d.-q.i.d.

(continues)

TABLE 14-3   Drugs Used as Bronchodilators to Treat Asthma—
continued

Generic Name	Trade Name	Route of Administration	Average Adult Dosage
bitolterol mesylate	Tornalate®	PO	2 inhalations by MDI t.i.d.-q.i.d.
epinephrine bitartrate	AsthmaHaler®, Bronkaid Mist suspension®	PO	0.1–0.5 mL or 1:1000 q20 by MDI min-4 h inhalation prn
formoterol fumarate	Foradil®	PO	1–2 inhalations by DPI q4 h up to 5 days
isoproterenol hydrochloride	Isuprel®	PO, IV	0.01–0.02 mg prn
levalbuterol hydrochloride	Xopenex®	Nebulizer	0.63 mg t.i.d.-q.i.d.
metaproterenol sulfate	Alupent®	PO	MDI: 2–3 inhalations q3–4 h (max: 12 inhalations/day); PO: 20 mg q6–8 h
pirbuterol acetate	Maxair®	PO	2 inhalations by MDI q.i.d. (max: 12 inhalations/day)
salmeterol xinafoate	Serevent®	PO	2 inhalations of aerosol by MDI b.i.d.
terbutaline sulfate	Brethaire®, Brethine®	PO	2.5–5 mg t.i.d. (2 inhalations by MDI q4–6 h)
Methylxanthines			
aminophylline	Truphylline®	IV	6 mg/kg over 30 minutes
theophylline	Elixophyllin®	PO, IV	PO: 5 mg/kg in divided doses, q6 h; IV: Loading dose: 5 mg/kg

increased heart rate, dilation of bronchial tubes in the lungs, and reduction of the force and rate of uterine contractions during labor.

Drugs with primary beta-1 agonist activity act mainly on the heart, increasing heart rate and raising blood pressure. The primary beta-2 agonist activity acts mainly on the lungs and uterus. Consequently, drugs that stimulate the beta-2 receptors produce bronchodilation. They are used to treat asthma and premature labor. Epinephrine (which is normally secreted from the adrenal gland) and isoproterenol are two potent beta-receptor stimulators.

Mechanism of Action.   The main action is on the smooth muscle of the bronchial tree and on the heart. A typical medication is isoproterenol,

which may be taken orally or by injection. Beta-2 receptor drugs are the most effective medications to reduce acute bronchospasms and exercise-induced asthma. These agents provide bronchodilation by stimulating the beta-2 receptors in the smooth muscle of the lung. Epinephrine and ephedrine are nonselective adrenergic agents, and naturally occurring catecholamine may be obtained from animal adrenal glands or prepared synthetically.

Indications. Epinephrine is used for the temporary relief of bronchospasm. These agents are used in acute asthmatic attacks and congestion. Salmeterol is preferred for prophylaxis and maintenance therapy for asthma or bronchospasm. Salmeterol is the only agent of this class available in the U.S., and is indicated for long-term prevention of asthma symptoms and the prevention of exercise-induced bronchospasm. Salmeterol should not be used in place of anti-inflammatory therapy or to treat acute bronchospasm.

Adverse Effects. Adverse effects of beta-2 agonists include dizziness, headache, tremor, palpitations, and sinus tachycardia. Common adverse effects of epinephrine and ephedrine include insomnia, tachycardia, nervousness, and anorexia. The cardiotoxic effects have led to the discovery and use of more specific respiratory agents that do not cause tachycardia or nervousness.

Contraindications and Precautions. Beta-2 adrenergic agents are contraindicated in patients with hypersensitivity to these drugs, or during pregnancy (category C) and lactation.

Drug Interactions. Salmeterol generally does not interact with other drugs. Other beta-2 agonists may have drug interactions with anesthetics, digitalis, ergotamine, and MAOIs.

Xanthine Derivatives

This group of drugs is chemically related to caffeine, which dilates bronchioles in the lungs. **Xanthine** derivatives are effective for the relief of bronchospasm in several diseases (see Table 14-3).

Mechanism of Action. Xanthine derivatives relax the smooth muscles of the bronchial tree and stimulate cardiac muscle and the CNS. Methylxanthine is the base of xanthine derivatives that must be converted to theophylline. Theophylline has a narrow therapeutic range, and is not used as commonly today. Instead, the beta-2 adrenergic agents are safer and more effective. Theophylline provides mild bronchodilation in asthmatics. This drug may also have important anti-inflammatory properties and enhance mucociliary clearance. Theophylline is available for oral administration in standard or sustained-release formulas with forms that last up to 24 hours. Theophylline has a small therapeutic range and beta-2 agonists are safer and more effective. Therefore, the xanthenes are not used as commonly today.

Medical Terminology Review

bronchospasm
broncho = air tube
spasm = narrowing; contraction
narrowing of the bronchioles or airways

Indications. These xanthine agents are used for the prevention and treatment of bronchial asthma and for the treatment of emphysema and bronchitis.

Adverse Effects. Adverse effects include tachycardia, insomnia, nervousness, headache, and nausea. Patients with hyperthyroidism, acute pulmonary edema, convulsive disorders, and heart disease cannot use xanthine derivatives. Adverse effects of theophylline at therapeutic doses include insomnia, upset stomach, aggravation of dyspepsia, and urination difficulties in elderly men with prostatism. Dose-related toxicities are common and include nausea, vomiting, tachyarrhythmias, headache, seizures, hyperglycemia, and hypokalemia.

Contraindications and Precautions. Xanthine derivatives are contraindicated in individuals with known hypersensitivity, seizure disorders, uncontrolled arrhythmias, peptic ulcers, and hyperthyroidism. Xanthine derivatives should be used cautiously in patients older than 60 years or those who have cardiac disease, hypertension, congestive heart failure, hypoxemia, and liver dysfunctions. These agents are used during pregnancy (category C) and lactation with caution.

Drug Interactions. Xanthine drugs can produce drug interactions with caffeine, cimetidine, fluoroquinolones, antibiotics, rifampin, phenobarbital, and phenytoin.

Anti-inflammatory Drugs

Many anti-inflammatory agents are used to reduce the incidence of asthma attacks. Glucocorticoids, leukotriene inhibitors, and mast cell stabilizers are commonly used. See Table 14-4.

> **Key Concept**
>
> *Observe and report early signs of possible toxicity from xanthine derivatives, which may include: anorexia, nausea, vomiting, dizziness, shakiness, restlessness, abdominal discomfort, and marked hypotension.*

TABLE 14-4 Anti-inflammatory Medications for Treatment of Asthma

Generic Name	Trade Name	Route of Administration	Average Adult Dosage
Glucocorticoids			
beclomethasone dipropionate	Beconase AQ®, Vancenase®	PO	1–2 inhalations by MDI t.i.d.-q.i.d.
budesonide	Pulmicort Turbuhaler®	PO	1–2 inhalations by MDI (200 mcg/inhalation)
flunisolide	AeroBid®	PO	2–3 inhalations by MDI b.i.d.-t.i.d.
fluticasone propionate	Flonase®, Flovent®	PO	2 inhalations by MDI (44 mcg ea.) b.i.d.
triamcinolone acetonide	Azmacort®	PO	2 inhalations by MDI t.i.d.-q.i.d.

(continues)

TABLE 14-4 Anti-inflammatory Medications for Treatment of Asthma—*continued*

Generic Name	Trade Name	Route of Administration	Average Adult Dosage
Leukotriene Modifiers			
montelukast	Singulair®	PO	10 mg/day in the evening
zafirlukast	Accolate®	PO	20 mg b.i.d. 1 h before or 2 h after meals
zileuton	Zyflo®	PO	600 mg q.i.d.
Mast Cell Stabilizers			
cromolyn sodium	Intal®	PO	1 inhalation by MDI q.i.d.
nedocromil sodium	Tilade®	PO	2 inhalations by MDI q.i.d.

Glucocorticoids

Glucocorticoids are the most potent and consistently effective anti-inflammatories that are currently available. There are three commonly used devices for inhalation administration: metered dose inhalers, nebulizers, and dry powder inhalers. Drug administration with a **metered dose inhaler (MDI)** is often accomplished with one or two puffs from a hand-held pressurized device (See Figure 14-5).

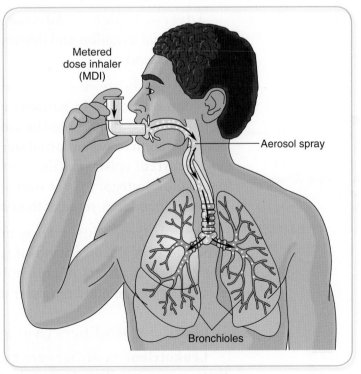

Figure 14-5 Use of metered dose inhaler.

Dry powder inhalers (DPIs) deliver medication in the form of micronized powder into the lungs. An example of a medication that is available in DPI form is albuterol. DPIs are breath-activated and are easier to use than MDIs. A nebulizer uses a small machine that converts a solution into a mist. The mist droplets are inhaled through either a facemask or a mouthpiece.

Quick-relief asthma medicines are also referred to as "rescue inhalers." They are usually given via nebulizers or MDIs. Examples of these medicines include Proventil and Atrovent. Also, certain oral steroids such as prednisone and prednisolone are utilized in rescue inhalers.

Systemic glucocorticoids are used to treat status asthmaticus and inhaled glucocorticoids are used for maintenance therapy. Inhaled glucocorticoids are the most effective means of controlling asthma. Combined preparations containing a glucocorticoid and a long-acting bronchodilator are considered useful in limiting the amount of the glucocorticoid needed to control asthma.

Mechanism of Action. They enter target cells where they have anti-inflammatory, immunosuppressive, and salt-retaining effects.

Indications. Inhaled glucocorticoids are preferred for the long-term control of asthma and are first-line agents for patients with persistent asthma. Dosages for inhaled glucocorticoids vary depending on the specific agent and delivery device. Systemic glucocorticoids are most effective for long-term asthma therapy. Long-term use of inhaled glucocorticoids in children is not recommended because these agents may suppress growth and suppress the adrenal glands for production of hormones.

Adverse Effects. Adverse reactions to corticosteroid inhalation include nasal irritation and dryness, headache, nausea, epistaxis, dizziness, hoarseness, and cough.

Contraindications and Precautions. Local (inhaled) glucocorticoids are contraindicated in patients with hypersensitivity to the drugs and lactation. These drugs should be used cautiously in patients with concomitant administration of systemic oral steroids, active tuberculosis, viral infections, and recurrent epistaxis. Glucocorticoids should be used with caution in pregnancy (category C for oral and category B for inhaled). Safety and efficacy for children younger than six years is not established.

Drug Interactions. Drug interactions increase the therapeutic and toxic effects of glucocorticoids if taken concurrently with troleandomycin. They decrease effects of anticholinesterases if taken concurrently with corticotropin; profound muscular depression is possible.

Leukotriene Modifiers (Antagonists)

Leukotriene modifiers are a class of biologically active compounds that occur naturally in leukocytes and produce allergic and inflammatory reactions similar to those of histamine. They are thought to play a role in the

---

Key Concept

Inhaled glucocorticoids may cause bronchospasm, requiring their use to be discontinued and an alternate treatment started.

development of allergic and autoallergic diseases such as asthma, rheumatoid arthritis, inflammatory bowel disease, and psoriasis.

Mechanism of Action.   Leukotriene antagonists such as zafirlukast (Accolate) block the bronchoconstriction, mucus production, and inflammation that occur with asthma. Zafirlukast was the first medication in this new anti-inflammatory class. A newer drug is called zileuton (Zyflo). It is rapidly absorbed via oral administration. Montelukast (Singulair) is the latest addition to this class of drugs. Montelukast acts as a bronchodilator, respiratory stimulant, and leukotriene receptor antagonist. This medication should be given at night for maximum effectiveness.

Indications.   Leukotriene modifiers are used for prophylaxis and chronic asthma in adults and children older than 12 years. Zafirlukast is prescribed as maintenance therapy for patients with chronic asthma. Montelukast is prescribed prophylactically for asthma attacks (see Table 14-4).

Adverse Effects.   Zafirlukast is a safer drug and has few adverse effects. Adverse effects of zileuton include liver toxicity and dyspepsia. The main adverse effects of montelukast are headaches and GI symptoms.

Contraindications and Precautions.   The leukotriene modifiers are contraindicated in patients with history of hypersensitivity to these medications. Montelukast is contraindicated in severe asthma attacks, bronchoconstriction due to asthma, or status asthmaticus. Montelukast should be avoided during lactation. Zileuton and zafirlukast are contraindicated in patients with active liver disease and during lactation and pregnancy. The leukotriene modifiers should be used cautiously in hepatic insufficiency. Safety and effectiveness in children younger than 12 years are not established.

Drug Interactions.   Leukotriene modifiers may double theophylline levels and increase toxicity. They increase the hypoprothrombinemic effects of warfarin. These agents may increase levels of beta-blockers (especially propranolol) and lead to hypotension and bradycardia.

Mast Cell Stabilizers

The two mast cell inhibitors that are available for the prophylaxis of asthma include cromolyn sodium and nedocromil. They are used to prevent asthma symptoms and improve airway function in patients with mild persistent asthma or exercise-induced asthma (see Table 14-4).

Mechanism of Action.   Mast cell stabilizers suppress the release of substances that cause bronchoconstriction and inflammation from the mast cells in the respiratory tract.

Indications.   Cromolyn is the drug of choice as a prophylactic for moderate allergic asthma, especially in children, because of its safety and efficacy. It is also used to reduce the symptoms of seasonal allergic attacks. Mast cell stabilizers are used in combination with other drugs in the treatment of allergic disorders and in the prevention of exercise-induced bronchospasm.

Adverse Effects. Adverse effects of mast cell stabilizers include nausea, fatigue, headache, dizziness, hypotension, and an unpleasant taste.

Contraindications and Precautions. Mast cell stabilizers are contraindicated in patients with a known hypersensitivity, coronary artery disease or history of arrhythmias, dyspnea, and acute asthma, and during pregnancy (category B) and lactation. Safe use in children younger than six years is not determined. Mast cell stabilizers should be used cautiously in patients with renal or hepatic dysfunction.

Drug Interactions. There are no clinically important drug interactions with cromolyn.

DECONGESTANTS

Key Concept

Chicken soup may actually help you fight off a cold. The heat, fluid, and salt found in chicken soup may help you fight off the viral infection that is a cold.

The common cold generally involves a runny nose, sneezing, nasal congestion, coughing, sore throat, headache, and many other symptoms. There are over one billion colds in the U.S. every year. Colds occur mostly during the winter or during rainy seasons. People are most contagious during the first two to three days of the cold, and usually not contagious at all by days seven to ten. Certain cold viruses can also cause the patient to experience muscle aches, postnasal drip, and decreased appetite. Complications of the common cold include: bronchitis, pneumonia, ear infection, sinusitis, and aggravation of asthma.

Nasal congestion and a runny nose are primarily associated with the first stage of inflammation, vasodilation, and increased capillary permeability. Decongestants cause vasoconstriction of nasal mucosa and reduce congestion or swelling. These agents are available in both oral and nasal preparations. Table 14-5 shows decongestant agents.

Mechanism of Action

The most effective way of alleviating the symptoms of nasal congestion is to induce vasoconstriction through stimulation of alpha-receptors of the sympathetic nervous system that is affiliated with the nasal vasculature. Therefore, decongestants are alpha agonists.

Indications

The most common uses for decongestants are the relief of nasal congestion due to infection or allergy, and inflammation in the eyes. They are also used to relieve respiratory distress of bronchial asthma, chronic bronchitis, and emphysema.

Adverse Effects

Decongestants should only be used by order of a physician for those patients with glaucoma, prostate cancer, and heart disease. Decongestants may increase blood sugar levels in patients with diabetes mellitus. Warnings

TABLE 14-5 Drugs Used to Treat Nasal Congestion

Generic Name	Trade Name	Route of Administration	Average Adult Dosage
Anticholinergic			
ipratropium bromide	Atrovent®	Nasal	2 sprays in each nostril 3–4 times/day for only 4 days
Sympathomimetics			
ephedrine hydrochloride	Efedron®	Intranasal	2–4 drops t.i.d.-q.i.d.
naphazoline hydrochloride	Privine®	Intranasal	2 drops q3–6 h
oxymetazoline	Afrin®, Neo-Synephrine®	Intranasal	2–3 sprays b.i.d. for up to 3–5 days
pseudoephedrine hydrochloride	Sudafed®	PO	60 mg q4–6 h
tetrahydrozoline hydrochloride	Tyzine®	Intranasal	2–4 drops or sprays q3 h
xylometazoline	Otrivin®	Intranasal	1–2 sprays b.i.d.

on the labels of OTC preparations instruct patients with hypertension, diabetes mellitus, ischemic heart disease, and hyperthyroidism about possible adverse effects involved in the use of decongestants. They may cause tachycardia, insomnia, nervousness, restlessness, blurred vision, and nausea or vomiting. Ephedrine is on the way out of the market due to its toxicities. It is still legal in many applications except dietary supplements. The purchasing of ephedrine or pseudoephedrine is currently limited and monitored, and regulations vary between states.

Contraindications and Precautions

Decongestants are contraindicated in patients with hypersensitivity to these agents, glaucoma, hypertrophy of prostate, certain types of heart disease, or diabetes mellitus. Decongestants should be avoided in patients with hyperthyroidism and hemorrhagic stroke.

Decongestants are used cautiously in patients with ischemic heart disease. The safe use of decongestants during pregnancy (category C) and lactation is not established.

Drug Interactions

Nasal decongestants such as ephedrine or pseudoephedrine may cause severe hypertension with MAOIs such as furazolidone. They may also decrease vasopressor response with reserpine, methyldopa, and urinary acidifiers.

ANTITUSSIVES, EXPECTORANTS, AND MUCOLYTICS

Antitussives suppress coughing. Coughing is a reflex response to irritation of the bronchial mucosal layer, such as that seen in inflammatory conditions. The cough reflex has an important role in clearing the lungs of excessive mucus and other secretions. **Expectorants** are agents that promote the removal of mucus secretions from the lungs, bronchi, and trachea, usually by coughing. These medications are available OTC and by prescription. Expectorant and mucolytic drugs include acetylcysteine, guaifenesin, and dornase alfa (see Table 14-6).

Mechanism of Action

Expectorants are also **mucolytic** (destroying or dissolving the active agents which make up mucus). In many cases, expectorants are added to other drugs, such as antitussives, decongestants, and antihistamines, to help remove mucus. Acetylcysteine is a mucolytic agent that decreases the viscosity of mucus. It is also an antidote to acetaminophen hepatotoxicity. Guaifenesin is safer and more effective.

Indications

There are specific expectorants indicated for the treatment of cystic fibrosis, including acetylcysteine and dornase alfa. These agents are able to

> **Medical Terminology Review**
>
> **mucolytic**
>
> *muco = mucus*
> *lytic = breaking down*
> **agent to break down mucus**

TABLE 14-6 Antitussive, Expectorant, and Mucolytic Drugs

Generic Name	Trade Name	Route of Administration	Average Adult Dosage
Opioid Antitussives			
codeine	(generic only)	PO	10–20 mg q4–6 h p.r.n. (max: 120 mg/24 h)
hydrocodone bitartrate	Hycodan®, others	PO	5–10 mg q4–6 h p.r.n. (max: 15 mg/dose)
Nonopioid Antitussives			
benzonatate	Tessalon®	PO	100 mg t.i.d. p.r.n. up to 600 mg/day
dextromethorphan	Benylin®	PO	10–20 mg q4 h or 30 mg q6–8h
Expectorant			
guaifenesin	Robitussin®, others	PO	200–400 mg q4 h (max: 2.4g/day)
Mucolytic			
acetylcysteine	Mucomyst®	PO	Inhalation by MDI: 1–10 mL of 20% solution q4–6 h or 2–20 mL of 10% solution q4–6 h

reduce the risk of respiratory infections. The drug works within 3 to 7 days of starting the medication.

Adverse Effects

The common adverse effects of antitussives include dizziness, drowsiness, nausea, and vomiting. Acetylcysteine may cause bronchospasm and a burning sensation in the upper respiratory passage.

Contraindications and Precautions

The contraindications and precautions for these agents are not significant.

Drug Interactions

By inhibiting platelet function, guaifenesin may increase the risk of hemorrhage in patients receiving heparin therapy. There are no significant drug interactions listed for acetylcysteine or dornase alfa.

CHRONIC OBSTRUCTIVE PULMONARY DISEASE

Chronic obstructive pulmonary disease (COPD) is a group of common chronic respiratory disorders that are characterized by progressive tissue damage and obstruction in the airways of the lungs. Emphysema, chronic bronchitis, and chronic asthma are some examples. Other conditions, such as **cystic fibrosis** (a genetic disorder affecting the exocrine glands, causing thick mucus to obstruct the bronchioles in the lungs), and **bronchiectasis** may lead to similar obstructive effects. Table 14-7 compares the characteristics of emphysema and chronic bronchitis.

Emphysema

Emphysema is the destruction of the alveolar walls and **septae**, which leads to large, permanently inflated alveolar air space (see Figure 14-6). Cigarette

TABLE 14-7 Comparisons between Emphysema and Chronic Bronchitis

Characteristic	Emphysema	Chronic Bronchitis
Etiology (cause)	Smoking, genetics	Smoking, air pollution
Location	Alveoli	Bronchi
Cough and Dyspnea	Some coughing, marked dyspnea	Early, constant cough; some dyspnea
Cyanosis (bluish skin)	No	Yes
Sputum	Little	Large amounts

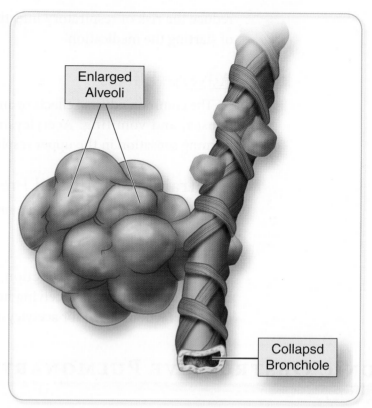

Figure 14-6 Alveoli and bronchioles affected by emphysema.

smoking is implicated in most cases of emphysema. However, a genetic factor contributes to the early development of the disease in non-smokers.

Avoidance of respiratory irritants and cessation of smoking may slow the progress of emphysema. Immunization against influenza and pneumonia is essential.

Chronic Bronchitis

Chronic bronchitis involves significant changes in the bronchi resulting from constant irritation from smoking or exposure to industrial pollution. The effects are irreversible and progressive.

Individuals with chronic bronchitis usually have a history of cigarette smoking or of living in an urban or industrial area, particularly in geographic locations where smog is common. In some cases, asthma is an associated condition.

DRUGS FOR SMOKING CESSATION

Cigarettes contains chemical compounds that affect most of the organs of the human body. Cigarette smoking causes cancers of the mouth, pharynx, larynx, lungs, esophagus, pancreas, kidney, bladder, and cervix. It also may

TABLE 14-8 Drugs for the Stoppage of Smoking Tobacco

Generic Name	Trade Name	Route of Administration	Average Adult Dosage
bupropion hydrochloride	Zyban®	PO	75–100 mg t.i.d.
nicotine polacrilex	Nicorette Gum®	PO	2–4 mg q1–2 h p.r.n. (max: 24 pieces/day)
nicotine polacrilex	Nicotrol Inhaler®	Nasal	Inhalation: 4 mg p.r.n. (max: 64 mg/day)
nicotine polacrilex	Commit lozenge®	PO	4 mg q1–2 h p.r.n.
nicotine polacrilex	Nicotrol NS®	Nasal	1–2 sprays per nostril/h (max: 40 sprays per nostril/day)
nicotine polacrilex	Nicotrol®, Nicoderm CQ®	Topical	7–21 mg/day (transdermal patch)

cause leukemia and may increase the risk of heart disease, lung disease, or stroke. Cigarette smoking can cause the lungs to develop emphysema, chronic bronchitis, and bacterial pneumonia.

The benefits of smoking cessation include better health and a longer life. The most commonly used drugs for smoking cessation are listed in Table 14-8.

Bupropion is an antidepressant for which the dosage form for smoking cessation varies. For example, bupropion (Zyban) is used as a tablet. Habitrol, Nicoderm, Nicotrol, and Prostep are available as transdermal patches. Nicorette is used as a gum, and Nicotrol NS must be used as a spray. Zyban is the first non-nicotine drug for smoking cessation. It can be used alone or with the nicotine patch. Some nicotine inhalers may be used in combination with fluoxetine for smoking cessation. It is suspected that certain antidepressants such as fluoxetine, when added to nicotine replacement therapy (NRT), might improve abstinence rates. NRT products are intended to help patients stop smoking while dealing with withdrawal symptoms and cravings that result from ceasing the habit. NRT is thought to be useful and beneficial for tobacco users who want to quit their addiction. For most people, it is considered to be completely safe. According to the Cochrane review, former smokers using nicotine replacement therapy are 1.5 to 2 times more likely to stop smoking than patients who try to stop using any other methods.

Mechanism of Action

The neurochemical mechanism of the antidepressant effect of bupropion is not understood; it is chemically unrelated to other antidepressant agents. It is a weak blocker of neuronal uptake of serotonin and norepinephrine, and inhibits the reuptake of dopamine to some extent.

Indications

Bupropion is used for treatment of depression. It also aids in smoking cessation.

Adverse Effects

Adverse effects of nicotine, nicotine polacrilex, and nicotine transdermal systems include headache, dizziness, lightheadedness, insomnia, irritability, tachycardia, palpitations, hypertension, nausea, salivation, vomiting, cough, hiccups, and hoarseness.

Contraindications and Precautions

Products containing nicotine are contraindicated during pregnancy or lactation, in patients with known hypersensitivity, heart or blood vessel disease, high blood pressure, diabetes, overactive thyroid, skin rash or irritation, stomach ulcers, pheochromocytoma, dental problems, mouth sores, sore throat, jaw pain, or temporomandibular joint disorder. Precautions include the regular monitoring of the patient's health by his or her physician during use of smoking cessation drugs, and keeping these products away from children and pets because they can cause severe harm if ingested.

Drug Interactions

Bupropion may increase the risk of adverse effects with levodopa and toxicity with MAOIs. It also increases the risk of seizures with drugs that lower seizure threshold, including alcohol.

SUMMARY

The exchange of oxygen and carbon dioxide in the lungs is one of the most important tasks of physiology, as it supplies oxygen at the cell level in body tissue. Oxygen is essential to sustain life. Therefore, the respiratory tract is necessary for the inspiration of oxygen and the expiration of carbon dioxide. Respiratory system disorders such as allergic asthma and chronic obstructive pulmonary disease (COPD) are common in the U.S. Antihistamines are used to relieve allergic reactions throughout the body, but they are also used commonly in patients with respiratory tract disorders to relieve rhinorrhea and allergic bronchitis. Cough-suppressing preparations are indicated for nonproductive coughs. If the cough is productive, suppression is not available, and an expectorant may be used to assist in expelling the secretions.

Bronchodilators induce smooth muscle relaxation, which eases breathing. They are used to treat asthma, COPD, and chronic bronchitis. Epinephrine and beta-2 agonists are indicated in acute asthma. Leukotriene agonists (new on the market), such as albuterol and mast cell stabilizer (cromolyn), are used for exercise-induced asthma. Glucocorticoids are administered by inhalation.

EXPLORING THE WEB

Visit **http://familydoctor.org**

- Search for "decongestants." What information is available to further aid in your understanding of this type of drug?

Visit **www.aafa.org**, **www.nhlbi.nih.gov**, and **www.lumgusa.com**

- Review information on the different types of asthma and allergies. Do a search for some of the other disorders covered in this chapter at the American Lung Association Web site. Bookmark these sites for future reference.

REVIEW QUESTIONS

Multiple Choice

1. Which of the following substances may cause allergic rhinitis?

   A. epinephrine
   B. chlorpheniramine
   C. hydrocodone
   D. histamine

2. Adverse reactions to corticosteroid inhalation include:

   A. cough, hoarseness, and headache
   B. cough, diarrhea, and dyspepsia

    C. pulmonary edema, convulsive disorders, and hypothyroidism

    D. pulmonary edema, convulsive disorders, and hyperthyroidism

3. Which of the following drugs is an expectorant?

    A. ephedrine

    B. adrenaline

    C. acetylcysteine

    D. bupropion

4. The trade name for guaifenesin is:

    A. Tussionex

    B. Robitussin

    C. Benadryl

    D. Tessalon

5. Which of the following is indicated for cessation of smoking tobacco?

    A. bupropion

    B. diazepam

    C. salmeterol

    D. albuterol

6. Which of the following is the brand name of bupropion?

    A. Habitrol

    B. Zyban

    C. Nicotrol

    D. Prostep

7. Dextromethorphan is classified as:

    A. an opioid cough suppressant

    B. a xanthine derivative

    C. a non-steroid contraceptive

    D. a nonopioid cough suppressant

8. Another name for allergic rhinitis is:

    A. contact dermatitis

    B. hay fever

    C. yellow fever

    D. photosensitivity

9. Which of the following is/are considered to be the drug(s) of choice for chronic asthma?

    A. theophylline

    B. albuterol

    C. antihistamines

    D. glucocorticoids

10. The initial stimulus for cough probably arises from which of the following parts of the respiratory system?

    A. bronchial mucosa

    B. pharynx

    C. mouth

    D. nasal cavities

11. The trade name of fluticasone includes which of the following?

    A. Flonase
    B. Pulmicort
    C. Singulair
    D. Tilade

12. Which of the following agents is known as an opioid?

    A. guaifenesin
    B. hydrocodone
    C. albuterol
    D. aminophylline

13. Leukotrienes are part of a class of biologically active compounds that occur naturally in which of the following body cells?

    A. white blood cells
    B. red blood cells
    C. platelets
    D. mast cells

14. Which of the following agents would increase bronchial secretions?

    A. theophylline
    B. cromolyn
    C. hydrocodone
    D. acetylcysteine

Fill in the Blank

1. Cromolyn is one of the mast cell stabilizers and the drug of choice as a prophylactic for moderate _____, especially in _____.

2. The leukotriene modifiers are used for prophylaxis and chronic asthma in _____.

3. Xanthine derivatives are indicated for treatment of:

    a. _____
    b. _____
    c. _____

4. Zileuton is one of the leukotriene modifiers that may cause _____.

5. Anaphylactic shock causes a massive release of _____.

Matching

Generic Name	Trade Name
_____ 1. terbutaline	A. Serevent
_____ 2. pirbuterol	B. AsthmaHaler
_____ 3. ephedrine bitartrate	C. Proventil
_____ 4. albuterol	D. Maxair
_____ 5. salmeterol	E. Brethaire

Critical Thinking

A 75-year-old man went to the emergency room for shortness of breath, coughing, sputum production, and fever. The E.R. physician ordered a chest x-ray and blood tests. The patient had a history of cigarette smoking for 30 years. After the various tests, the physician diagnosed this patient with emphysema and pneumonia.

1. Name the major predisposing factors for emphysema and pneumonia at this patient's age.

2. With this patient's history of cigarette smoking, what other complications may this patient have?

3. If the patient was advised to stop smoking, name the available drugs that help a person to stop smoking.

Drug Therapy for Gastrointestinal Disorders

OBJECTIVES

After completing this chapter, the reader should be able to:

1. Explain the mechanisms of action and therapeutic effects of antacids.
2. Identify the major classes of drugs used to treat peptic ulcers.
3. Describe the use of H$_2$-receptor antagonists in the treatment of peptic ulcers.
4. Define proton pump inhibitor agents and their indications.
5. Explain the treatment for the bacterium *Helicobacter pylori*.
6. Identify the common adverse effects of major laxative, antidiarrheal, and antiemetic drugs.
7. Name the five major classifications of laxatives.
8. Identify the most effective antidiarrheal agents.
9. Explain adsorbent agents and their indications.
10. Describe the mechanism of action of bulk-forming agents.

GLOSSARY

Adsorbent agents – drugs with the ability to adsorb gases, toxins, and bacteria

Antacids – neutralize hydrochloric acid and raise gastric pH, thus inhibiting pepsin (a gastric enzyme)

Antiemetic – a drug that stops vomiting

Bulk-forming laxatives – natural or synthetic polysaccharide derivatives that absorb water to soften the stool and increase bulk to stimulate peristalsis

Calcium carbonate – a substance that causes acid rebound, which may delay ulcer-related pain relief and ulcer healing

Chemical digestion – the alteration of food into different forms through chemicals and enzymes

Emetic – a drug that induces vomiting

Emollient laxatives – substances that act as surfactants by allowing absorption of water into the stool

Helicobacter pylori – a bacterial species that is associated with several gastroduodenal diseases

Histamine H$_2$-receptor antagonists – drugs that block the action of histamine on parietal cells in the stomach, decreasing acid production

Lubricant laxative – a substance, such as mineral oil, that works by increasing water retention in the stool to soften it

Mechanical digestion – the breakdown of large food particles into smaller pieces by physical means

Peptic ulcer – a lesion located in either the stomach (gastric ulcer) or in the duodenum (small intestine)

Saline laxatives – substances that create an osmotic effect to increase water content and stool volume

Stimulant laxatives – substances that stimulate bowel mobility and increase secretion of fluids in the bowel

Stool softeners – substances that decrease the consistency of stool by reducing surface tension

Zollinger-Ellison syndrome – peptic ulceration with gastric hypersecretion and tumor of the pancreatic islets

OVERVIEW

The digestive system, sometimes called the gastrointestinal tract, alimentary tract, or gut, consists of a long hollow tubule. The digestive tract secretes substances used in the process of digestion into the canal. The growth of the body depends upon the consumption, absorption, and metabolism of food. This system also involves the elimination of waste. The digestive system is subject to many disorders, some of which are very common. Numerous drugs are used to treat these varying conditions.

ANATOMY REVIEW

- The digestive system consists of the mouth, pharynx, esophagus, stomach, small intestine, large intestine, rectum, and anus (Figures 15-1 and 15-2).

- There are several accessory organs of the digestive system these include the salivary glands, liver, gallbladder, and pancreas (Figure 15-1).

- The role of the digestive tract is to change food into forms the body can use and to eliminate waste.

- There are two forms of digestion: **Mechanical digestion** breaks large food particles into smaller pieces such as by chewing. **Chemical digestion** is the alteration of the smaller food particles by substances such as digestive enzymes, bile, and acids.

- Nutrients from the digestive tract are absorbed into the blood stream by moving across the lining of the digestive tract.

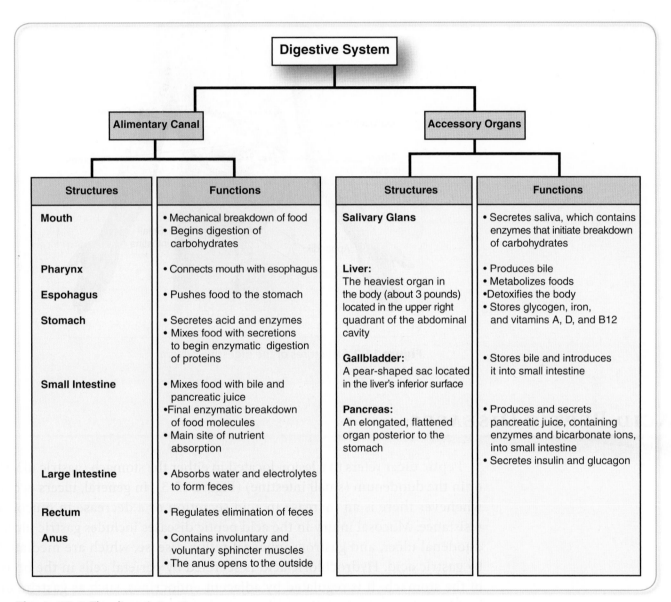

Figure 15-1 The digestive system.

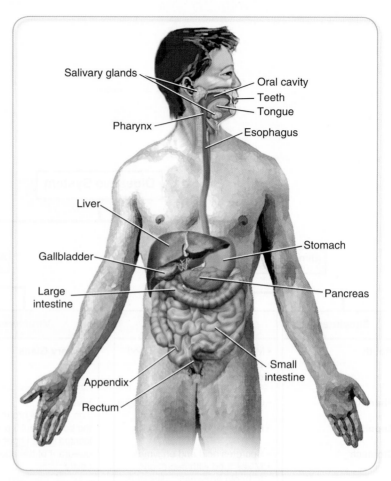

Figure 15-2 Structures of the digestive system.

ACID PEPTIC DISEASES

Peptic ulcer refers to a lesion located in either the stomach (gastric ulcer) or in the duodenum (small intestine) (Figure 15-3). In general, ulcers occur whenever there is an increase in acid secretion or a decrease in mucosal resistance. Mucosal injury in the acid peptic diseases includes gastric ulcer, duodenal ulcer, and gastroesophageal reflux disease, which are mediated by gastric acid. Hydrochloric acid is secreted by parietal cells in the body of the stomach. It is regulated by adjacent endocrines, such as gastrin, or by histamine, somatostatin, and prostaglandin E_2. Gastrin is a relatively weak stimulant of the parietal cells. It acts primarily to cause the release of histamine, which is the most potent stimulus of acid secretion, and acts as the common mediator. Histamine antagonists inhibit acid secretion that is stimulated by gastrin and acetylcholine, as well as histamine. There are a number of causes of peptic ulcer, including:

- Family history
- Smoking tobacco
- Alcohol

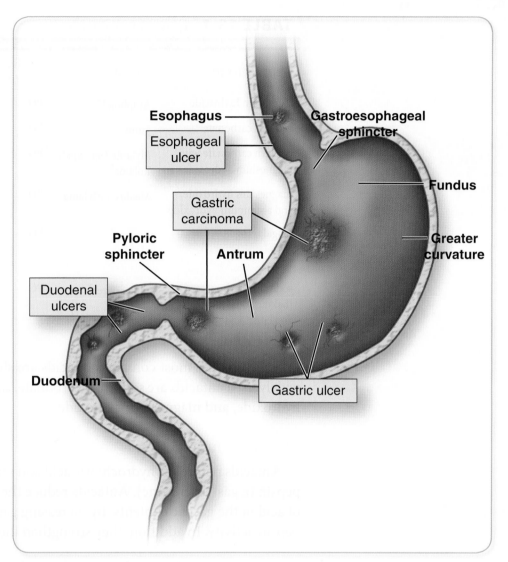

Figure 15-3 Sites of peptic ulcers.

- Coffee
- Stress
- Infection with *Helicobacter pylori* (H. pylori)
- Blood group O
- Anti-inflammatory drugs (aspirin, NSAIDs, and glucocorticoids)

A wide variety of prescription and OTC medications are available for the treatment of peptic ulcer. These drugs include: antacids, H_2-receptor antagonists, proton pump inhibitors, and antibiotics. Antibiotics treat peptic ulcers caused by *Helicobacter pylori.*

Antacids

There are differences in the types of **antacids**, in terms of their contents, neutralizing capacity, duration of action, side effects, and cost. These must be considered when choosing an antacid for therapeutic use. Antacids are

TABLE 15-1 Common Antacids

Generic Name	Trade Name	Route of Administration	Average Adult Dosage
aluminum hydroxide	Amphojel®	PO	600 mg t.i.d.-q.i.d.
calcium carbonate	Tums®	PO	0.5–2 g b.i.d.-t.i.d.
calcium carbonate with magnesium hydroxide	Mylanta Gel-caps®, Rolaids®	PO	2–4 capsules or tablets p.r.n.
magnesium hydroxide and aluminum hydroxide	Maalox®, Mylanta	PO	5–15 mL liquid or 2–4 tablets
magaldrate	Riopan®	PO	480–1080 mg (5–10 mL) or 1–2 tablets daily
sodium bicarbonate (baking soda); aspirin, and citric acid	Alka Seltzer®	PO	300 mg–2 g/day

OTC drugs. The most common antacids are shown in Table 15-1. The most widely used antacids are sodium bicarbonate, **calcium carbonate**, aluminum hydroxide, and magnesium hydroxide.

Mechanism of Action

Antacids neutralize hydrochloric acid and raise gastric pH, thus inhibiting pepsin (a gastric enzyme). Antacids reduce the concentration and total load of acid in the gastric contents. By increasing gastric pH, antacids also inhibit pepsin activity. In addition, they strengthen the gastric mucosal barrier.

Indications

These agents are used widely for the relief of heartburn, dyspepsia, and medical treatment of peptic ulcer. The primary role of antacids in the management of acid-peptic disorders is the relief of pain. Nonsystemic antacids (magnesium or aluminum substances) are preferred to systemic antacids such as sodium bicarbonate for intensive ulcer therapy because they avoid the risk of alkalosis. Liquid antacid forms have a greater buffering capacity than tablets. However, tablets are more convenient to carry. Antacid mixtures such as aluminum hydroxide with magnesium hydroxide provide more even, sustained action than single-agent antacids, and permit a lower dosage of each compound.

Adverse Effects

Constipation can occur in patients using calcium carbonate and aluminum-containing antacids. Diarrhea is a common adverse effect of magnesium- and sodium-containing antacids. If diarrhea occurs, the patient may alternate the antacid mixture with aluminum hydroxide. Hypophosphatemia and osteomalacia can occur with long-term use of aluminum hydroxide, but

---

Medical Terminology Review

hypophosphatemia

hypo = under, below, less than normal
phosphat = phosphate
emia = blood condition
having lower than normal phosphate levels in the blood

osteomalacia

osteo = bone
malacia = softening
softening of the bone

hypercalcemia

hyper = over, above, more than normal
calc = calcium
emia = blood condition
having excess amounts of calcium in the blood

these conditions can also occur with short-term use in severely malnourished patients, such as alcoholics. Calcium carbonate usually is avoided because it causes acid rebound, hypercalcemia, vomiting, metabolic alkalosis, confusion, and renal calculi. It may also delay pain relief and ulcer healing.

Contraindications and Precautions

Antacids are contraindicated in patients with severe abdominal pain of unknown cause, and during lactation. Sodium bicarbonate is contraindicated in patients with hypertension, congestive heart failure (CHF), severe renal disease, and edema. It should not be used for ulcer therapy. All antacids should be used cautiously in elderly patients and renally impaired patients. Chronic administration of calcium carbonate-containing antacids should be avoided because of hypercalcemia. Calcium carbonate and magnesium-containing antacids should be used cautiously in patients with severe renal disease.

Drug Interactions

Because antacids alter gastric pH and affect absorption of ingested substances, they have a high potential for drug interactions. To ensure consistent absorption and therapeutic efficacy, orally administered drugs should be given 30 to 60 minutes before antacids. These agents bind with tetracycline and inhibit its absorption, reducing its therapeutic efficacy. Antacids may destroy the coating of enteric-coated drugs, leading to premature drug dissolution in the stomach. Antacids may interfere with the absorption of many drugs, including cimetidine, ranitidine, digoxin, isoniazid, iron products, anticholinergics, and phenothiazines.

Histamine H_2-Receptor Antagonists

There are two types of histamine receptors: histamine (H_1) and histamine (H_2). The second of these mediates the acid secretion from gastric parietal cells and is inhibited by the H_2-receptor-blocking drugs. These drugs may be preferred to other antiulcer agents because of their convenience and lack of effect on GI motility. H_2-receptor antagonists are listed in Table 15-2.

Mechanism of Action

Cimetidine was the first H_2-receptor antagonist approved for clinical use. It blocks the H_2 receptor on the parietal cells of the stomach, thus decreasing gastric acid secretion.

Indications

H_2-receptor antagonists are used to promote healing of gastric and duodenal ulcers, and hypersecretory states such as **Zollinger-Ellison syndrome**. Prototypes of H_2-receptor antagonists include cimetidine, famotidine, nizatidine, and ranitidine. They are a remarkably safe group of drugs.

TABLE 15-2 H$_2$-receptor Antagonists

Generic Name	Trade Name	Route of Administration	Average Adult Dosage
cimetidine	Tagamet®	PO	300–400 mg 1 to 2 times per day
famotidine	Pepcid®, Pepcid AC®	PO	40 mg at bedtime
nizatidine	Axid®, Axid AR®	PO	150 mg b.i.d. or 300 mg h.s.
ranitidine hydrochloride	Zantac®	PO, IV	PO: 100–150 mg b.i.d. or 300 mg at bedtime; IV: 50 mg q6–8 h; 150–300 mg/24 h by continuous infusion

Cimetidine is available OTC for the treatment of acute gastric ulcer, duodenal ulcer, and gastroesophageal reflux. It is also used in the treatment of Zollinger-Ellison syndrome.

Famotidine is the most potent H$_2$-receptor antagonist. After a 40-mg dose, mean nocturnal gastric acid secretion is reduced by 94 percent for up to 10 hours. It is recommended for the short-term treatment of mucosal ulcers of the GI tract. Famotidine is absorbed incompletely. It should be used in a lower dosage and at longer dosing intervals in patients with severe renal insufficiency.

The newest H$_2$-receptor antagonist, nizatidine, may be used to treat and prevent recurrence of duodenal ulcers. It is also used for gastric ulcers, and gastroesophageal reflux. More than 90 percent of an oral dose is excreted in the urine within 12 hours, and 60 percent as unchanged drug. Therefore, it should be used in reduced dosage in patients with severe renal insufficiency.

Ranitidine is a more potent drug. It is five to ten times more potent than cimetidine. Ranitidine requires a less frequent dosing schedule than cimetidine. It is an H$_2$-receptor antagonist indicated for the short-term treatment of duodenal ulcers and the management of hypersecretory conditions such as Zollinger-Ellison syndrome. The pharmacokinetic profile of ranitidine is similar to that of cimetidine.

Adverse Effects

The list of adverse reactions is long, but the incidence is low. Among the adverse effects associated with all four drugs are headache, dizziness, malaise, myalgia, nausea, diarrhea, constipation, rashes, pruritus, and impotence. Adverse effects, such as unusual bleeding, fever, sore throat, hallucinations, or skin rash should be reported promptly, and the therapy must be discontinued.

Contraindications and Precautions

Histamine H$_2$ antagonists should be avoided in patients with a known hypersensitivity, and during lactation or pregnancy. These agents are used cautiously in patients with hepatic or renal dysfunction. Cimetidine is used

with caution in patients with diabetes mellitus. Histamine H_2 antagonists are used cautiously in elderly patients because they may cause confusion, and a dosage reduction may be needed. Cimetidine, famotidine, and ranitidine are pregnancy category B drugs, while nizatidine is a pregnancy category C drug. All of these drugs should be used cautiously during pregnancy and lactation.

Drug Interactions

Cimetidine increases the risk of decreased white blood cell counts with antimetabolites and alkylating agents. It also increases serum levels and risk of toxicity of warfarin-type anticoagulants, phenytoin, beta-adrenergic blocking agents, alcohol, quinidine, lidocaine, theophylline, chloroquine, and diazepam.

Nizatidine increases serum salicylate levels with aspirin. Ranitidine also increases the effects of warfarin and toxicity of lidocaine. Ranitidine decreases the effectiveness of diazepam and its clearance.

Proton Pump Inhibitors

The final common pathway in gastric acid secretion is the proton pump adenosine triphosphatase. The physiological essence of this enzyme is the exchange of hydrogen ions for potassium ions. Thus, hydrogen is secreted by the parietal cell into the gastric lumen in exchange for potassium. Proton pump inhibitors should be taken prior to meals, because these drugs are more potent when taken orally prior to meals. They are also absorbed more effectively in the morning.

Mechanism of Action

Proton pump inhibitors or gastric pump inhibitors inhibit H^+ and K^+ ions, which generate gastric acids.

Indications

Proton pump inhibitors are widely used in the short-term therapy of duodenal and gastric ulcers. Proton pump inhibitor agents are also used in the treatment of gastroesophageal reflux disease, gastric ulcer, and for long-term treatment of pathologic hypersecretory conditions such as Zollinger-Ellison syndrome. Examples of proton pump inhibitors are shown in Table 15-3.

Omeprazole is used in the treatment of acid peptic disorders. It is approved for the short-term treatment of duodenal ulcers, severe gastroesophageal reflux, and hypersecretory conditions. It is also effective in the prevention of NSAID ulcers and their complications. The antisecretory effect of omeprazole occurs within one hour, with maximum effect occurring within two hours.

Lansoprazole suppresses gastric acid formation in the stomach. Lansoprazole is indicated for the short-term treatment of acute duodenal ulcer, gastric ulcer, and erosive esophagitis. It is most effective given 30 to 60 minutes prior to a meal. Like other proton pump inhibitors, it is very effective in healing acid peptic disease.

Key Concept

Goals of drug therapy for peptic ulcer include the relief of symptoms, promotion of ulcer healing, and prevention of reoccurrences.

TABLE 15-3   Proton Pump Inhibitors

Generic Name	Trade Name	Route of Administration	Average Adult Dosage
esomeprazole magnesium	Nexium®	PO	20–40 mg/day
lansoprazole	Prevacid®	PO	15–60 mg/day for 4 weeks
omeprazole	Prilosec®	PO	20 mg once per day for 4–8 weeks
pantoprazole sodium	Protonix®	PO	40 mg/day
rabeprazole sodium	AcipHex®	PO	20 mg/day for 4 weeks

Adverse Effects

There are numerous adverse effects of the proton pump inhibitors, but they occur infrequently. Headache, diarrhea, abdominal pain, dizziness, rash, and constipation are seen with nearly the same frequency as is seen with the H_2-blockers.

Adverse reactions to omeprazole include headache, diarrhea, abdominal pain, nausea, dizziness, vomiting, and constipation. It is contraindicated for long-term use in patients with gastroesophageal reflux disease, duodenal ulcers, and in lactating women.

Adverse effects of lansoprazole are fatigue, dizziness, headache, nausea, diarrhea, constipation, anorexia, or increased appetite.

Contraindications and Precautions

Proton pump inhibitors are contraindicated in long-term use for gastroesophageal reflux disease (GERD) and duodenal ulcers. They are also contraindicated in patients with hypersensitivity to these agents and children younger than two years, and during pregnancy (categories B and C). Lansoprazole should be avoided in patients with severe hepatic impairment.

Proton pump inhibitors are used with caution in patients with dysphasia, metabolic or respiratory alkalosis, and hepatic disease, and during pregnancy. Safety and efficacy in children under the age of 18 years are not established.

Drug Interactions

Omeprazole increases serum levels and potentially increases the toxicity of benzodiazepines, phenytoin, and warfarin. This agent shows decreased absorption with sucralfate (these drugs should be given at least 30 minutes apart).

Lansoprazole decreases serum levels if taken concurrently with sucralfate. It decreases serum levels of ketoconazole and theophylline.

Key Concept

Gastroesophageal reflux disease (GERD) involves the periodic flow of gastric contents into the esophagus.

Rabeprazole increases serum levels and potentially increases the toxicity of benzodiazepines when taken concurrently.

Treatment for *Helicobacter pylori* with Ulcer

Peptic ulcer disease is believed to be caused by high gastric secretion. *Helicobacter pylori* is found in 75 percent of duodenal ulcers. In chronic peptic ulcer, it has been found that eradication of the bacterium prevents ulcer relapse in about 95 percent of the cases. There is also a relationship between *Helicobacter* infection and adenocarcinoma of the stomach. Treatments for peptic ulcer patients usually include antacids, H₂-receptor antagonists, or proton pump inhibitors, but other drugs are added as necessary. For the eradication of *H. pylori* and healing of duodenal and gastric ulcers in drug therapy, special antibiotics must be added. These antibiotics include amoxicillin (Amoxil), clarithromycin (Biaxin), tetracycline (Achromycin), and metronidazole (Flagyl). Bismuth products must also be added, such as bismuth subsalicylate (Pepto-Bismol) and ranitidine bismuth citrate. Bismuth compounds are highly effective when combined with proton pump inhibitors and/or antibiotics. Eradication rates with these combinations are greater than 80 percent. Adverse effects of bismuth products include neurotoxicity, dark stools and tongue, headache, diarrhea, and abdominal pain. For the treatment of *Helicobacter pylori* with ulcer, antisecretory agents (proton pump inhibitors) should be included. Therefore, combination drugs for *H. pylori* infections should be used as follows:

Helidac (bismuth, metronidazole, tetracycline)

Prevpac (amoxicillin, clarithromycin, lansoprazole)

Tritec (bismuth, ranitidine)

Key Concept

Peptic ulcers are most commonly caused by the use of NSAIDs or are due to a Helicobacter pylori infection.

The goals of treatment of active *H. pylori*–associated ulcers are to relieve dyspeptic symptoms, to promote ulcer healing, and to eradicate *H. pylori* infection.

PANCREATIC DISORDERS

The pancreas plays an extremely important role in digestion and secretes digestive enzymes. The main pancreatic enzymes include lipase, amylase, chymotrypin, and trypsin. These enzymes aid in the digestion of fats, carbohydrates, and proteins. Fat digestion is compromised if pancreatic enzyme secretions are insufficient. The most common cause of pancreatic insufficiency is chronic pancreatitis.

Pancreatic Enzyme Replacement Therapy

Pancreatic enzyme replacements include pancreatin and pancrelipase (see Table 15-4). These agents may be obtained from beef or pork pancreas, which

TABLE 15-4 Pancreatic Enzyme Replacements

Generic Name	Trade Name	Route of Administration	Average Adult Dosage
pancreatin	Entozyme®	PO	1–3 capsules w/each meal, and 1 capsule w/each snack as directed by physician; may be swallowed whole w/ or without fluid, or contents may be sprinkled into food or drink
pancrelipase	Cotazym®, Pancrease®, Viokase®	PO	1–3 capsules or tablets, or 1–2 packets of powder 1–2 h before, during, or 1 h after meals, w/ an extra dose taken w/ any food eaten between meals

contains the necessary enzymes to digest fats, proteins, and carbohydrates. Pancrelipase is preferred because it has more enzyme activity.

Mechanism of Action

Pancreatic enzyme replacement therapy works similarly to the way pancreatin and pancrelipase work normally in the body. These enzymes hydrolyze triglycerides to fatty acids and glycerol, proteins to oligopeptides, and starches to oligosaccharides and maltose.

Indications

Pancrelipase is used as replacement therapy in the symptomatic treatment of malabsorption syndrome due to cystic fibrosis, chronic pancreatitis, pancreatectomy, GI bypass surgery, and cancer of the pancreas.

Adverse Effects

In the recommended dosage, pancrelipase is free of adverse effects. Serious adverse effects of replacement therapy of pancreatic enzymes are rare. Common adverse effects include nausea, vomiting, anorexia, diarrhea, cramping, and hyperuricemia.

Contraindications and Precautions

Pancreatic enzyme replacement therapy is contraindicated in patients with a known history of allergy to hog protein or enzymes. These agents

should be avoided in patients suffering from esophageal strictures, in those with pancreatitis, and during pregnancy (category C). Pancreatic enzyme replacement therapy should be used in lactating women with caution.

Drug Interactions

Pancreatic enzyme replacement therapy may decrease the absorption of iron.

GALLSTONE-SOLUBILIZING AGENTS

The gallbladder is a hollow organ located next to the liver that acts as the storage place for bile. Bile is formed in the liver to aid in digestion. The bile is then stored in the gallbladder to be released into the intestines as food passes.

A gallstone is a solid mass that forms in the gallbladder or the bile duct (Figure 15-4). Gallstones are usually formed by the combination of cholesterol and calcium compounds. They can produce intense pain when they block the bile duct. Gallstone-solubilizing agents include ursodiol and chenodiol. Only ursodiol is sold in the U.S.

Mechanism of Action

Ursodiol is a naturally occurring bile acid that is made by the liver and secreted in bile. It blocks the liver enzyme that produces cholesterol, and thereby decreases production of cholesterol by the liver and the amount of cholesterol in bile. It also reduces the absorption of cholesterol from the intestine. By decreasing the concentration of cholesterol in bile, it prevents the formation and promotes the dissolution of cholesterol-containing gallstones.

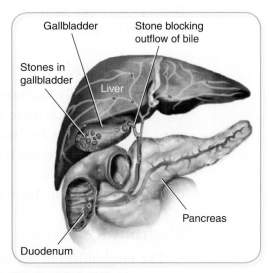

Figure 15-4 Gallstones.

Indications

Ursodiol is used to prevent cholesterol gallstones from forming during rapid loss of weight. It is also used to dissolve cholesterol gallstones that do not contain calcium and are less than 2 cm in diameter. It is also used to treat primary biliary cirrhosis.

Adverse Effects

The most common adverse effects are rash, itching, nausea, vomiting, stomach pain, back pain, constipation, and diarrhea.

Contraindications and Precautions

Contraindications include hypersensitivity to ursodiol, bile acids, or any component of the formulation, high cholesterol, radiopaque substances, bile pigment stones, stones greater than 20 mm in diameter, and allergy to bile acids.

Gallstone-solubilizing agents should be used with caution in patients with a non-visualizing gallbladder and those with chronic liver disease. Ursodiol is not recommended for use in children.

Drug Interactions

Aluminum-containing antacids, cholestyramine, and colestipol reduce the absorption of ursodiol and therefore reduce its action.

DIARRHEA

Diarrhea is the manifestation of many illnesses. Its etiology includes infections (bacterial, viral, fungal, and parasitic), irritable bowel syndrome, inflammatory bowel disease (ulcerative colitis and Crohn's disease), toxins (food poisoning), drugs, and other causes. Treatment should be directed to the underlying cause.

Antidiarrheals

It is occasionally necessary to use antidiarrheals for convenience, or for conditions for which there is no primary treatment. The most commonly used antidiarrheals are anticholinergics, opioid narcotics, meperidine congeners (diphenoxylate), and loperamide. Opioid antidiarrheals are the most effective drugs for controlling diarrhea. Selected agents used to treat diarrhea are shown in Table 15-5.

Mechanism of Action

The mechanism of action for anticholinergics and opioid narcotics is discussed in Chapters 6 and 21.

TABLE 15-5 Drugs Used to Treat Diarrhea

Generic Name	Trade Name	Route of Administration	Average Adult Dosage
bismuth subsalicylate	Pepto-Bismol®	PO	2 tablets q.i.d. with 2 additional antibiotics for 10–14 days
camphorated opium tincture (schedule iii)	Paregoric®	PO	5–10 mL after loose stool, q2 h up to q.i.d. prn
difenoxin with atropine	Motofen®	PO	1–8 mg/day
diphenoxylate with atropine	Lomotil®	PO	1–2 tablets or 5–10 mL t.i.d.-q.i.d.
loperamide	Imodium®	PO	4 mg as a single dose, then 2 mg after each diarrhea episode

Indications

Antidiarrheal agents are used to treat diarrhea, a symptom of bowel disorders, and not the disorder itself. The management of diarrhea depends on finding the underlying cause, replacing water and electrolytes as needed, reducing cramping, and reducing the passage of stools. Diarrhea is usually self-limiting and resolves without further effects. Diarrhea in children may become a medical emergency in as little as 24 hours because of the loss of electrolytes.

Adverse Effects

Adverse effects of antidiarrheal drugs commonly include nausea, vomiting, anorexia, constipation, drowsiness, sedation, euphoria, headache, dizziness, drowsiness, and rash. Diphenoxylate is a narcotic-related agent that has no analgesic activity, but causes sedation and euphoria. Generally, this drug is combined with atropine (an anticholinergic drug), which may produce dry mouth.

Contraindications and Precautions

Antidiarrheal drugs are contraindicated in patients with pseudomembranous colitis, abdominal pain of unknown origin, or obstructive jaundice. These agents should be avoided in children younger than two years.

Antidiarrheals are used with caution in patients with severe liver impairment or inflammatory bowel disease. They should be used cautiously in pregnant women (category B).

Drug Interactions

Concurrent use of antidiarrheals with an MAOI increases the risk of a hypertensive crisis. Antidiarrheals may cause an additive CNS depression when given with antihistamines, sedatives, hypnotics, alcohol, and narcotics.

GAS RETENTION

The production of excessive gas necessitates relief of gastric and intestinal distention. Gas retention is caused by air swallowing, peptic ulcer, dyspepsia, irritable bowel disease, and diverticulitis. Other factors for production of gas in the GI tract include gas-forming foods such as beans, onions, and cabbage, or after gastroscopy, and bowel radiography.

Antiflatulents

Medications for excessive gas, or to prevent formation of gas in the GI tract, include some antacids or carminatives (substances which stimulate the expulsion of gas from the GI tract, and also increase muscle tone, thereby stimulating peristalsis), that are available as OTC drugs. Simethicone is the most common active ingredient used, in such trade names as Phazyme, Mylanta, and Gas-X. Simethicone disperses in the GI tract, and prevents the formation of gas pockets in the GI tract.

Mechanism of Action

The actual mechanism of action for antiflatulents is unknown, but the predominant theory is that these agents reduce the surface tension of small air bubbles trapped in the GI tract. This allows them to coalesce into larger bubbles, which are more easily eliminated than the smaller ones.

Indications

Antiflatulents are used to prevent the formation of gas in the GI tract. Gas retention is a problem in conditions of air swallowing, diverticulitis (inflammation of the colon), peptic ulcer, irritable bowel disease, and dyspepsia. Another use of antiflatulents is to relieve gas following gastroscopy and bowel radiography.

Adverse Effects

Antiflatulents are generally safe and have no side effects.

Contraindications and Precautions

Antiflatulents are contraindicated in patients with a known hypersensitivity to any component of these drugs. Charcoal should be used in pregnant women with caution (category C).

Drug Interactions

There are no reported drug interactions with antiflatulents.

CONSTIPATION

Constipation is the difficult or infrequent passage of stool. Normal stool frequency ranges from two to three times daily to two to three times per week. Since constipation is a symptom rather than a disease, medical evaluation should be undertaken in patients who develop constipation.

Laxatives

Laxatives are drugs that either accelerate fecal passage or decrease fecal consistency. They work by promoting one or more of the mechanisms that cause diarrhea. Because of the wide availability and marketing of OTC laxatives, there is a potential that an appropriate diagnosis will not be sought. Table 15-6 shows the most commonly used laxatives.

TABLE 15-6 Commonly Used Laxatives

Generic Name	Trade Name	Route of Administration	Average Adult Dosage
Bulk Forming:			
methylcellulose	Citrucel®	PO	500–6000 mg/day
polycarbophil	Equalactin®, FiberNorm®	PO	1 g q.i.d. prn (max: 6 g/day)
psyllium hydrophilic muciloid	Metamucil®, Perdiem Plain®	PO	1–2 tsp in 8 oz water up to q.i.d.
Fecal Softeners:			
docusate sodium	Colace®, Dialose®, Modane®, Regutol®, Surfak®	PO	50–500 mg/day
Salines and Osmotics:			
glycerin	Fleet Babylax®, Glycerol®	Rectal	1 suppository or 5–15 mL enema (inserted high into rectum and retained for 15 min)
lactulose	Cephulac®	PO	30–60 mL/day prn
magnesium citrate	Citrate of Magnesia®	PO	1000–6000 mg/day
magnesium hydroxide	Phillips' Milk of Magnesia®	PO	15 mL h.s.

(continues)

TABLE 15-6 Commonly Used Laxatives—*continued*

Generic Name	Trade Name	Route of Administration	Average Adult Dosage
Hydroxidemagnesium:			
magnesium sodium phosphate	Fleet Enema®	Rectal	133 mL/day
sorbitol	Sorbitol®	PO, Rectal	30–150 mL/day
Stimulants:			
bisacodyl	Dulcolax®	PO, Rectal	PO: 5–15 mg prn; Rectal: 1 suppository
castor oil	Emulsoil®, Purge®	PO	15–60 mL/day p.r.n.
cascara sagrada	Cascara Sagrada® (fluid extract)	PO	0.5–1.5 mL/day
Lubricants:			
mineral oil	Kondremul®	PO	2–15 teaspoonfuls/day
Stool Softeners:			
docusate calcium	Surfak®	PO, Rectal	50–500 mg/day; Rectal: 50–100 mg added to enema fluid
docusate potassium	Dialose®	PO, Rectal	PO: 1–3 caps/day; Rectal: 1 suppository
docusate sodium	Colace®	PO, Rectal	1–4 tabs or capsules/day

Mechanism of Action

Laxatives are divided into several categories as a function of their mechanisms of action, including: bulk-forming, saline, stimulant, emollient, and lubricant laxatives. Laxatives should not be taken if nausea, vomiting, or abdominal pain is present.

Bulk-forming laxatives are natural or synthetic polysaccharide derivatives that absorb water to soften the stool and increase bulk, which stimulates peristalsis. Bulk-forming laxatives work in both the small and large intestines. The onset of action of these agents is slow, usually occurring between 12 and 72 hours.

Saline laxatives work by creating an osmotic effect that increases the water content and volume of the stool. This increased volume results in distention of the intestinal lumen, causing increased peristalsis and bowel motility. The onset of action varies depending on the effect and dosage form. Rectal formulations such as enemas or suppositories have an onset of action of 5 to 30 minutes, whereas oral preparations work within 3 to 6 hours.

Key Concept

All bulk-forming agents must be given with at least eight ounces of water to minimize the possible constipation experienced by some patients.

Stimulant laxatives work in the small and large intestine to stimulate bowel motility and increase the secretion of fluids into the bowel. The oral preparations usually have an onset of action within 6 to 10 hours. Rectal preparations usually have an onset of action within 30 to 60 minutes.

Emollient laxatives act as surfactants by allowing absorption of water into the stool, which makes the softened stool easier to pass. Emollient laxatives have a slow onset of action (24 to 72 hours), which is why they are not considered the drugs of choice for severe acute constipation. They are more useful for preventing constipation.

Mineral oil, which is a **lubricant laxative**, works in the colon to increase water retention and soften the stool. Mineral oil has an onset of action of between 6 and 8 hours.

Stool softeners decrease the consistency of stools by reducing the surface tension. Stool softeners permit easier penetration and mixing of fats and fluids with the fecal mass. This results in a softer, more easily passed stool. Docusate (Colace) acts as a detergent and stool softener. It usually takes 1 to 3 days to be effective. Stool softeners have a wide margin of safety and few potential adverse reactions. Stool softeners are combined with laxatives in such medications as Peri-Colace and Doxidan to soften stools while enhancing stool evacuation (see Table 15-6).

Indications

Laxatives are used prophylactically in patients who should avoid straining during defecation, and for treatment of constipation associated with hard, dry stools. They are prescribed for short-term relief of constipation. Certain laxatives are indicated to empty the large intestine for rectal and bowel examinations. Laxatives are particularly useful in patients who must avoid straining to pass hard stools, such as those patients who recently had a myocardial infarction or rectal surgery.

Adverse Effects

Stool softeners have a wide margin of safety and few potential adverse reactions. High doses or prolonged use of laxatives may cause diarrhea and a loss of water and electrolytes. Serious adverse effects include abdominal pain, perianal irritation, fainting, and weakness.

Contraindications and Precautions

Laxatives are contraindicated in patients with a known hypersensitivity, acute appendicitis, intestinal obstruction, fecal impaction, and acute hepatitis. Laxatives should be used cautiously in patients with rectal bleeding, in pregnant women (category C), and during lactation. Magnesium hydroxide is used with caution in patients with renal impairment.

Drug Interactions

Mineral oil may impair GI tract absorption of fat-soluble vitamins (A, D, E, and K).

VOMITING

The causes of vomiting include infectious diseases that can directly irritate vomiting centers to inhibit impulses going to the stomach. Certain drugs, radiation, and chemotherapy may irritate the GI tract or stimulate the chemoreceptor trigger zone and vomiting center in the brain (medulla). After surgery, particularly abdominal surgery, nausea and vomiting are common. The main neurotransmitters that produce nausea and vomiting include dopamine, serotonin, and acetylcholine. Persistent vomiting may cause dehydration, imbalance of electrolytes, metabolic alkalosis, and arrhythmias, which in turn, may precipitate further vomiting.

Emetics

An **emetic** is a drug that induces vomiting. Emetics (such as apomorphine, morphine, and digitalis) may act directly by stimulation of the medulla oblongata, or they may act reflexively by irritant action on the GI tract (such as copper sulfate, mustard, sodium chloride, and zinc sulfate).

Mechanism of Action

The emetic known as ipecac induces vomiting by stimulating the chemoreceptors of the vomiting reflex, and by the irritation of the gastric mucosal. Approximately 80 to 90 percent of people taking the medication begin vomiting within 20 to 30 minutes.

In most cases, ipecac is not absorbed because it is removed in vomitus. The effects of ipecac are stopped with activated charcoal.

Indications

Emetics are drugs used to promote vomiting, usually used in cases of poisoning or drug overdose. The nearest poison control center should be called prior to using these medications. Syrup of ipecac is the OTC drug used to bring about vomiting and should be included in any home emergency kit.

Adverse Effects

There are no serious adverse effects to ipecac. The only problem with any emetic is the aspiration of stomach contents.

Contraindications and Precautions

Emetics should not be used in patients who are unconscious or semi-comatose, or in whom coma is expected imminently. These agents should

Key Concept

A nasogastric tube is a safer and more efficient tool for emptying the stomach than the use of emetics.

Key Concept

The administration of ipecac should be followed by a full eight-ounce glass of water to promote vomiting. If vomiting does not occur in 30 minutes, another dose may be given.

Key Concept

The misuse of ipecac syrup has occurred in persons with eating disorders, such as bulimia, which may result in ipecac toxicity (muscle weakness and cardiotoxic effects).

not be used in patients with severe heart disease or advanced pregnancy. They are contraindicated in poisoning caused by corrosive or petroleum products. Safe use in pregnancy has not been established (category C).

Drug Interactions

Drug interactions with emetic drugs are rare. Other medications should not be taken with syrup of ipecac, as the rapid onset of vomiting will not allow enough time for the other medications to be absorbed.

Antiemetics

Antiemetics are used to prevent or relieve nausea and vomiting that are associated with many different disorders. Table 15-7 shows the most commonly used antiemetics.

TABLE 15-7 Common Antiemetic Agents

Generic Name	Trade Name	Route of Administration	Average Adult Dosage
Antihistamines and Anticholinergics:			
cyclizine hydrocholoride	Marezine®	PO	50 mg q4–6 h
dimenhydrinate	Calm-x®, Dramamine®	PO	50–100 mg q4–6 h
meclizine hydrochloride	Antrizine®, Bonamine®	PO	25–50 mg/day
scopolamine	Transderm-Scop®, Transderm-V®	Transdermal	1 patch q72 h starting 12 h before anticipated travel
Corticosteroids:			
dexamethasone	Decadron®	PO	0.25–4 mg b.i.d.-q.i.d.
methylprednisolone sodium succinate	Solu-Medrol®	PO	2–60 mg/day in div. doses
Dopamine Antagonists:			
droperidol	Inapsine®	IM, IV	2.5 mg; additional doses of 1.25 may be given
metoclopramide hydrochloride	Reglan®	IM, IV	10–20 mg near end of surgery
promethazine hydrochloride	Phenergan®, Prometh	PO, IM, IV	12.5–25 mg q4-6 h prn

(continues)

TABLE 15-7 Common Antiemetic Agents—*continued*

Generic Name	Trade Name	Route of Administration	Average Adult Dosage
Sedatives:			
diazepam	Diastat®, Valium®	PO, IM, IV	2–30 mg/day
lorazepam	Ativan	IV	1–1.5 mg prior to chemotherapy
Serotonin Receptor Antagonists:			
dolasetron mesylate	Anzemet®	PO	100 mg/day one hour prior to chemotherapy
granisetron	Kytril®	IV	10 mcg/kg 30 min prior to chemotherapy
ondansetron hydrochloride	Zofran®	PO	4 mg t.i.d p.r.n. 0.25 mg 30 min prior to chemotherapy
palonosetron	Aloxi®	IV	0.25 mg infused over 30 seconds (30 minutes prior to chemotherapy)
Neurokinin Receptor Antagonist:			
aprepitant	Emend®	PO	125 mg one hour prior to chemotherapy

Mechanism of Action

The mechanism of action of antiemetics is largely unknown, except that they help to relax the portion of the brain that controls muscles that cause vomiting. Some of these agents, such as prochlorperazine, depress the center of vomiting in the medulla.

Indications

There are several classes of drugs used as antiemetics, which will be discussed in various chapters. These agents are used for the treatment of drug overdose and for certain poisonings. They are also prescribed for certain conditions that are associated with vomiting, such as postchemotherapy, motion sickness, pregnancy, and other conditions.

Phenothiazines are the largest group of drugs used for severe nausea and vomiting. Prochlorperazine is the most commonly prescribed antiemetic medication in this group.

Adverse Effects

Since drowsiness is common to most of the antiemetics, patients should be cautioned not to drive or operate hazardous machinery while taking these drugs. Dose-related anticholinergics adverse effects, such as dry mouth, constipation, and tachycardia, are common.

Contraindications and Precautions

Key Concept

Transdermal scopolamine is a 72-hour patch that is placed behind the ear.

Antiemetics are contraindicated in patients with hypersensitivity to these drugs. They are also contraindicated in children younger than two years of age, and during pregnancy (category C). Antiemetics are used with caution in children, pregnant women, and dehydrated patients.

Drug Interactions

Antiemetics may have differing drug interactions based on their types. For example, serotonin antagonists usually have no drug interactions, while dopamine is affected by antiemetics, which are antagonistic. Prochlorperazine interacts with alcohol to increase CNS depression. Antacids and antidiarrheals inhibit absorption of this agent.

ADSORBENTS

Adsorbent agents have the ability to adsorb gases, toxins, and bacteria. Only certain materials that possess chemical adsorptive properties lend themselves effectively to detoxification and to the adsorption of gases resulting from abnormal intestinal fermentation. Such substances are kaolin and activated charcoal. Many of the nonsystemic antacids may serve as internal protectives and adsorbents. Antacids commonly are combined with kaolin or other adsorbents.

Mechanism of Action

These agents adsorb bacterial toxins that might be implicated in causing diarrhea or adsorb toxic substances swallowed into the GI tract by inhibiting GI adsorption. Adsorbents work by increasing the viscosity of the gut contents, and forming sludge.

Indications

Adsorbents are used for acute treatment of poisoning, primarily as an emergency antidote in many forms of poisoning. It is the emergency treatment of choice for virtually all drugs and chemicals. Charcoal capsules are also used for the relief of flatulence and the discomfort of abdominal gas.

Adverse Effects

Adverse effects include vomiting (related to rapid ingestion of high doses), constipation, diarrhea, and black stools.

Contraindications and Precautions

Adsorbents are contraindicated in patients with suspected obstructive bowel lesion, and pseudomembranous colitis. These agents should not be used for more than two days without medical direction. Safety during pregnancy (category C) or lactation is not established. Adsorbents should be used cautiously in infants or children younger than three years, and in elderly patients.

Drug Interactions

Adsorbents can inactivate syrup of ipecac and laxatives with activated charcoal. Adsorbents decrease the effectiveness of other medications.

SUMMARY

The functions of the GI tract include digestion, storage, food absorption, and waste elimination. There are varieties of drugs that are used to treat disorders of the gastrointestinal system, including antacids, H_2-receptor antagonists, proton pump inhibitors, antidiarrheals, laxatives, antiemetics, and adsorbents. Gastric ulcer, duodenal ulcer, and gastroesophageal reflux disease are accompanied with increased secretion of hydrochloric acid, for which antacids, H_2-receptor antagonists, and proton pump inhibitors should be used. Peptic ulcer, which may be caused by *Helicobacter pylori* bacteria, should be treated with the combination of special antibiotics, bismuth products, and proton pump inhibitor drugs. There are several different laxative drugs that either accelerate fecal passage or decrease fecal consistency. Antiemetics are used to prevent or relieve nausea and vomiting. Adsorbents are used primarily as emergency antidotes in many forms of poisoning.

EXPLORING THE WEB

Visit *http://digestive.niddk.nih.gov*

- Search for additional information about the digestive diseases and disorders discussed in this chapter. Enhance your understanding of the function of the digestive system and the drug therapies used to treat disorders of the digestive system.

Visit *http://familydoctor.org*

- Search for OTC remedies to relieve gastrointestinal symptoms.

Visit *www.medicalnewstoday.com*

- Search for the various types of drugs discussed in this chapter. Is there new information about or research being done on these types of drugs?

REVIEW QUESTIONS

Multiple Choice

1. Gastrin hormones are released from the stomach and act primarily to release:

   A. histamine
   B. pepsin
   C. pancreatic enzymes
   D. all of the above

2. The generic name of Amphojel is:

   A. magaldrate
   B. sodium bicarbonate
   C. aluminum hydroxide
   D. calcium carbonate

3. Sodium bicarbonate is contraindicated in patients with:

   A. congestive heart failure
   B. severe renal disease
   C. hypertension
   D. all of the above

4. Which of the following H$_2$-receptor antagonists was the first drug approved for clinical use?

   A. famotidine
   B. nizatidine
   C. ranitidine
   D. cimetidine

5. The generic name of Axid is:

   A. cimetidine
   B. nizatidine
   C. famotidine
   D. ranitidine

6. Which of the following laxatives is particularly useful in patients who recently had a rectal surgery to avoid straining to pass hard stools?

   A. lubricant
   B. emollient
   C. saline
   D. stimulant

7. Which of the following is the generic name of Dulcolax?

   A. bisacodyl
   B. docusate
   C. senna
   D. cascara sagrada

8. For eradication of *Helicobacter pylori* with ulcer, you should combine:

   A. bismuth products and proton pump inhibitors
   B. antibiotics, bismuth, and proton pump inhibitors
   C. proton pump inhibitors and antibiotics
   D. antibiotics and bismuth products

9. The generic name of Tagamet is:

   A. ranitidine
   B. nizatidine
   C. famotidine
   D. cimetidine

10. Chronic administration of calcium carbonate–containing antacids may cause:

    A. hyperparathyroidism
    B. hypercalcemia
    C. hypertension
    D. hyperglycemia

11. Which of the following is the purpose of the therapeutic uses of activated charcoal?

    A. decreased effectiveness of other medications
    B. decreased blood sugar level
    C. relief of vomiting and diarrhea
    D. relief of flatulence and the discomfort of abdominal gas

12. Which of the following agents is used for treatment of vomiting after chemotherapy?

    A. mineral oil
    B. scopolamine patch
    C. senna
    D. magnesium citrate

13. The trade name of diphenoxylate with atropine is:

    A. Imodium
    B. Furoxone
    C. Lomotil
    D. Motofen

14. Which of the following is an adverse effect of antiflatulents?

    A. coma
    B. vomiting
    C. headache
    D. generally none

Matching

_____ 1. lansoprazole   A. Pepcid

_____ 2. cimetidine   B. Axid

_____ 3. omeprazole   C. AcipHex

_____ 4. ranitidine   D. Tagamet

_____ 5. rabeprazole sodium   E. Prevacid

_____ 6. famotidine   F. Zantac

_____ 7. nizatidine   G. Prilosec

Fill in the Blank

1. What are the indications for antacids?

_____

_____

_____

2. What is the mechanism of action of H$_2$-receptor antagonists?

_____

_____

_____

3. What are the most serious adverse effects of mineral oil laxatives?

_____

_____

_____

Critical Thinking

A 45-year-old male patient was diagnosed with gastritis caused by *H. pylori*. He exhibited symptoms of this disorder for more than 15 months, and did not take any medications or see any physicians before this visit.

1. List medications that may be used to treat this disorder.

2. If this disorder remains untreated, what would the probable consequences be?

3. Explain why *H. pylori* can grow even in the extremely acidic conditions of the stomach.

Hormonal Therapy for Endocrine Gland Disorders

OBJECTIVES

After completing this chapter, the reader should be able to:

1. Explain the location of the major endocrine glands and their hormone secretion.
2. Describe the effect of thyroxine on the body organs.
3. Compare and contrast the roles of calcitonin hormone and parathyroid hormone.
4. Compare and contrast the functions of the pancreatic hormones.
5. Explain diabetes mellitus.
6. Name some risk factors for development of diabetes mellitus in older adults.
7. Identify the different types of insulin.
8. Explain the primary functions of the adrenal cortex.
9. Define the term "hormone" and then list the hormones that are secreted from the anterior pituitary gland.
10. Describe parathyroid hormone and its main functions.

GLOSSARY

Acromegaly – overdevelopment of the bones of the head, face, and feet

Adrenocorticotropic hormone (ACTH) – another hormone from the anterior pituitary gland that stimulates the growth of the adrenal gland cortex and the secretion of corticosteroids

Adrenogenital syndrome – congenital adrenal hyperplasia; a group of disorders involving steroid hormone production in the adrenal glands, leading to a deficiency of cortisol

Androgen – the generic term for any natural or synthetic compound, usually a steroid hormone, that stimulates or controls the development of masculine characteristics by binding to androgen receptors

Antidiuretic hormone (ADH) – released when the body is low on water, and causes the kidneys to conserve water, but not salt, by concentrating the urine and reducing urine volume

Antithyroid drug – a chemical agent that lowers the basal metabolic rate by

OUTLINE (continued)

interfering with the formation, release, or action of thyroid hormones

Calcitonin (CT) – produced primarily by the parafollicular cells of the thyroid gland

Conn's syndrome – a disease of the adrenal glands involving excess production of the hormone *aldosterone*

Cushing's syndrome – a disease caused by the excessive body production of cortisol; it can also be caused by excessive use of cortisol or other steroid hormones

Diabetes mellitus – a complex disorder of carbohydrate, fat, and protein metabolism caused by lack of or inefficient use of insulin in the body; classified as type I (insulin-dependent diabetes mellitus [IDDM]), or type II (non-insulin-dependent diabetes mellitus [NIDDM])

Dwarfism – a condition of lack of growth of the arms and legs in proportion to the head and trunk; it may be caused by over 200 different other conditions, including achondroplasia, kidney disease, genetic conditions, and problems with hormones or metabolism

Epinephrine (adrenaline) – produced by the medulla of adrenal glands, and is a "fight or flight" hormone that is released when danger threatens

Epiphyses – the ends of long bones that are originally separated from the main bone by a layer of cartilage, becoming unified through ossification

Follicle-stimulating hormone (FSH) – a gonadotropin that stimulates the growth and maturation of follicles in the ovary in females and promotes spermatogenesis (the process by which male gametes develop into mature spermatozoa) in males

Gigantism – condition produces excessive growth (a "giant") if the hypersecretion of GH occurs before puberty

Glucagon – an important hormone in carbohydrate metabolism

Glucocorticoids – steroid hormones that can bind with the cortisol receptor and trigger similar effects

Graves' disease – an autoimmune disorder that involves overactivity of the thyroid gland (hyperthyroidism)

Growth hormone (GH) – secreted by the anterior pituitary gland in response to growth hormone-releasing hormone (GHRH)

Hirsuitism – excessive hair growth on the face, abdomen, breasts, and back

Hormone – a chemical messenger that serves as a signal to target cells; are produced by nearly every organ system and type of tissue

Hyperactive – abnormally and easily excitable or exuberant

Hypercalcemia – an excessive amount of calcium in the blood

Hyperpituitarism – a condition that results in the excess secretion of hormones that are secreted from the pituitary gland

Hyperthyroidism – a condition of excessive amounts of thyroxine

Hypoactive – abnormally inactive

Hypothalamus – the part of the brain that lies below the thalamus; it regulates body temperature, certain metabolic processes, and other autonomic activities

Hypothyroidism – a deficiency disease that causes cretinism (mental and physical retardation) in children

Insulin – a hormone secreted by the pancreas that regulates carbohydrate and fat metabolism, especially the conversion of glucose to glycogen

Lugol's solution – Lugol's iodine; a solution of iodine often used as an antiseptic, disinfectant, or starch indicator, to replenish iodine deficiency, to protect the thyroid from radioactive materials, and for emergency disinfection of drinking water

Luteinizing hormone (LH) – secreted by the anterior lobe of the pituitary gland that is necessary for proper reproductive function

Mineralocorticoids – steroid hormones that influence salt and water balance; they are released from the adrenal cortex

Myxedema – condition of thyroid insufficiency or resistance to thyroid hormone

Negative feedback system – method by which regulation of hormones is achieved; released in response to concentration in the blood

Norepinephrine (noradrenaline) – released from the medulla of the adrenal glands, and is also a central nervous system and sympathetic nervous system neurotransmitter

Oxytocin (OT) – also acts as a neurotransmitter in the brain; in women, it is released during labor and lactation

Parathyroid hormone (PTH) – also called parathormone, is secreted by the parathyroid glands and increases the levels of calcium in the blood

Prolactin (PRL) – a hormone that is primarily associated with lactation; it is secreted from the anterior pituitary gland

Spermatogenesis – the process by which male gametes develop into mature spermatozoa

Steroids – numerous naturally occurring or synthetic fat-soluble organic compounds that include sterols, bile acids, adrenal hormones, sex hormones, digitalis compounds, and certain vitamin precursors

Thyroid-stimulating hormone (TSH) – a substance secreted by the anterior lobe of the pituitary gland that controls the release of thyroid hormone and is necessary for the growth and function of the thyroid gland

Thyroxine (T_4) – the major hormone secreted by the follicular cells of the thyroid gland

Tremors – involuntary tremblings or quiverings

OVERVIEW

The endocrine system consists of specialized cell clusters, glands, hormones, and target tissues. The glands and cell clusters secrete hormones and chemical transmitters in response to stimulation from the nervous system and other sites. Together with the nervous system, the endocrine system regulates and integrates the body's metabolic activities, and maintains internal homeostasis. Each target tissue has receptors for specific hormones. Hormones connect with the receptors, and the resulting hormone-receptor complex triggers the target cell's response.

The overactivity or underactivity of a gland is the malfunction that most commonly causes endocrine disease. If a gland secretes an excessive amount of its hormone, it is **hyperactive**. When a gland fails to secrete its hormone or secretes an inadequate amount, it is **hypoactive**.

ANATOMY REVIEW

- The major glands of the endocrine system include: pituitary, pineal, thyroid, parathyroid, thymus, adrenals, pancreas, and the gonads (Figure 16-1).

- Endocrine glands secrete **hormones**, or chemical messengers, directly into the bloodstream. These hormones coordinate and direct activities of specific target cells or organs.

- Each gland releases a specific hormone or hormones and generates specific effects (Table 16-1).

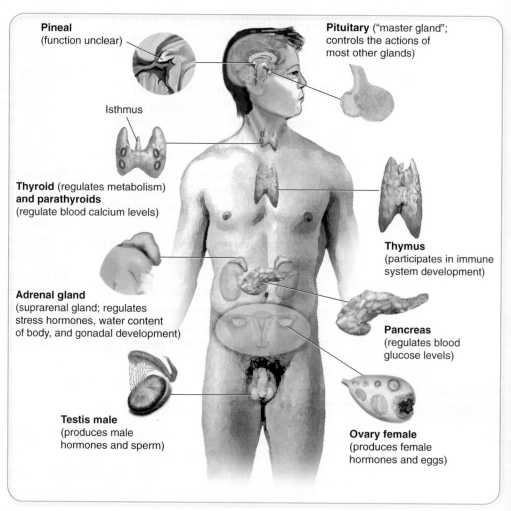

Figure 16-1 Location of the endocrine glands.

TABLE 16-1   Sources and Effects of Major Hormones

Source	Hormone	Primary Effects
Hypothalamus	Hypothalamic-releasing hormones	Stimuli to anterior pituitary to release specific hormone; decrease release of specific hormone by anterior pituitary
Pituitary – anterior lobe (adenohypophysis)	Growth hormone (GH, somatotropin)	Stimulates synthesis of protein
	Adrenocorticotropic hormone (ACTH)	Stimulates secretion of (primarily) cortisol from adrenal cortex
	Thyroid-stimulating hormone (TSH)	Stimulates the thyroid gland
	Follicle-stimulating hormone (FSH)	In women: stimulates ovarian follicle growth and estrogen secretion; in men: stimulates sperm production
	Luteinizing hormone (LH)	In women: stimulates ovum maturation and ovulation; in men: stimulates testosterone secretion

(continues)

TABLE 16-1   Sources and Effects of Major Hormones—*continued*

Source	Hormone	Primary Effects
Pituitary – posterior lobe (neurohypophysis)	Prolactin (PRL)	Stimulates milk production during lactation
	Antidiuretic hormone (ADH, or vasopressin)	Increases kidney reabsorption of water
	Oxytocin	Stimulates uterine contractions after delivery; stimulates milk ejection during lactation
Pancreas – beta cells of islets of Langerhans	Insulin	Transports glucose and other substances into cells; lowers blood glucose levels
Pancreas – alpha cells	Glucagon	Increases blood glucose level; glycogenolysis in the liver
Parathyroid gland	Parathyroid hormone (PTH)	Increases blood calcium levels by stimulating bone demineralization; increases absorption of serum calcium in kidneys and digestive tract
Thyroid gland	Calcitonin	Decreases calcium release from bones to lower blood calcium levels
	Thyroxine (T_4) and triiodothyronine (T_3)	Increase cellular metabolic rates
Adrenal cortex	Aldosterone	Increases water and sodium kidney reabsorption
	Cortisol	Decreases immune response; is anti-inflammatory; has a catabolic effect on tissues; stress response
Adrenal medulla	Norepinephrine	Generalized vasoconstriction
	Epinephrine	Stress response; increases force and rate of heart contraction; bronchodilation; vasodilation in skeletal muscle; visceral and cutaneous vasoconstriction

HORMONAL REGULATION

Hormones are secreted only as needed by the body and organs. When the concentration of a particular hormone in the body reaches a particular level, the gland that secretes the hormone will stop secretion of the hormone until the concentration of the hormone in the body drops below a particular level and it is triggered to release more. For example, insulin is secreted when the blood glucose level rises. This type of control is called a **negative feedback system**.

Role of the Hypothalamus in the Endocrine System

The **hypothalamus** of the brain is the main integrative center for the endocrine and autonomic nervous systems. The hypothalamus helps control some endocrine glands by neural and hormonal pathways. Neural pathways connect the hypothalamus to the posterior pituitary gland. Neural stimulation of the posterior pituitary causes the secretion of two effector hormones: antidiuretic hormone (also known as vasopressin) and oxytocin.

The hypothalamus also exerts hormonal control at the anterior pituitary gland, by releasing and inhibiting hormones and factors, which arrive by a portal system. Hypothalamic hormones stimulate the pituitary glands to synthesize and release trophic hormones. These hormones include corticotropin (also called adreno-corticotropic hormone), thyroid-stimulating hormone, and gonadotropins, such as luteinizing hormone and follicle-stimulating hormone. Secretion of trophic hormones stimulates the adrenal cortex, thyroid gland, and gonads. Hypothalamic hormones also stimulate the pituitary gland to release or inhibit the release of effector hormones, such as growth hormone and prolactin (Figure 16-2).

> ### *Medical Terminology Review*
>
> **hypothalamus**
>
> *hypo = low; under; beneath*
> *thalamus = gray matter deeply situated in the forebrain*
> structure deep to the gray matter of the forebrain
>
> **corticotrophin**
>
> *cortico = stimulating the cortex*
> *tropin = hormone*
> a hormone that stimulates the cortex

Hormones

Hormones are natural chemical substances secreted into the bloodstream from the endocrine glands that regulate and control the activity of an organ or tissues in another part of the body. The synthesis and secretion of many hormones are controlled by other hormones or changes in the concentration of essential chemicals or electrolytes in the blood. Drugs and diseases can modify hormone secretion as well as specific hormone effects at target organs. Some hormones affect nearly all the tissues of the body, but the action of others is restricted to a few tissues or organs. The majority of hormones, such as thyroxine, epinephrine, parathyroid hormone, insulin, and glucagon, are proteins. Several other groups of hormones, such as those produced by the adrenal cortex and the gonads, are **steroids**. A list of major hormones and endocrine glands is provided in Table 16-1. Hormones from the various endocrine glands work together to regulate vital processes of the body that include the following:

1. Secretions in the digestive tract

2. Energy production

3. Composition and volume of extracellular fluid

4. Adaptation and immunity

5. Growth and development

6. Reproduction and lactation

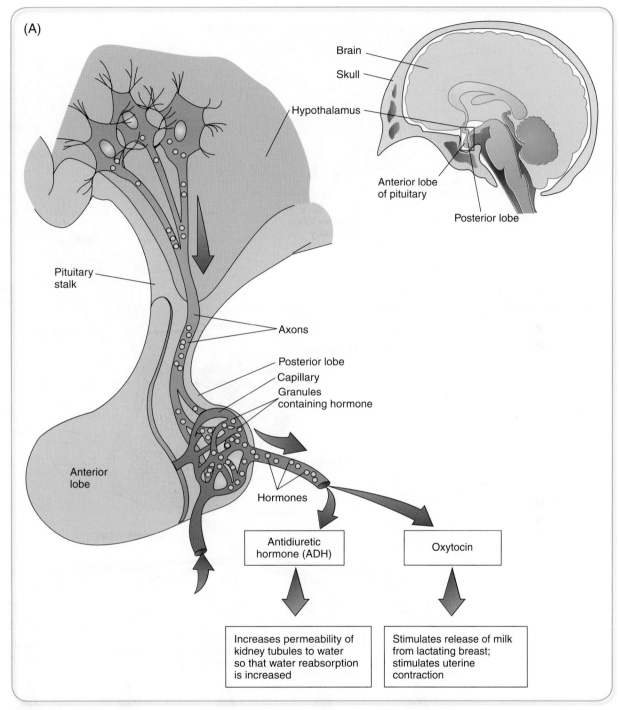

(A)

Brain

Skull

Hypothalamus

Anterior lobe of pituitary

Posterior lobe

Pituitary stalk

Axons

Posterior lobe
Capillary
Granules containing hormone

Anterior lobe

Hormones

Antidiuretic hormone (ADH)

Oxytocin

Increases permeability of kidney tubules to water so that water reabsorption is increased

Stimulates release of milk from lactating breast; stimulates uterine contraction

Figure 16-2A The relationship between the hypothalamus and the (A) posterior lobe of the pituitary gland (B) anterior lobe of the pituitary gland.

The inactivation of hormones occurs enzymatically in the blood, liver, kidneys, or target tissues. Hormones are secreted primarily via the urine and, to a lesser extent, via the bile. In medicine, hormones generally are used in three ways: (1) for replacement therapy; (2) for pharmacologic effects beyond replacement; and (3) for endocrine diagnostic testing.

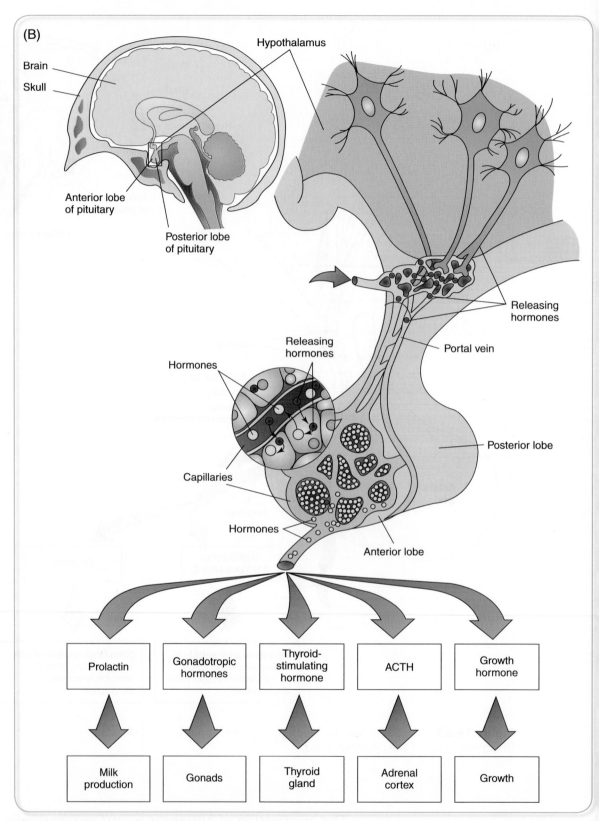

Figure 16-2B The relationship between the hypothalamus and the (A) posterior lobe of the pituitary gland (B) anterior lobe of the pituitary gland.

Growth Hormone

Growth hormone (GH) is secreted by the anterior pituitary gland in response to growth hormone-releasing hormone (GHRH). Its secretion is controlled in part by the hypothalamus. GH promotes protein synthesis in all cells, increases fat mobilization, and the use of fatty acids for energy. Growth effects depend on the presence of thyroid hormone, insulin, and carbohydrates. It is prescribed for **dwarfism**, a condition in which the growth of long bones is abnormally decreased by an inadequate production of growth hormone.

Adrenocorticotropic Hormone

Adrenocorticotropic hormone (ACTH) is another hormone from the anterior pituitary gland that stimulates the growth of the adrenal gland cortex and the secretion of corticosteroids. Under normal conditions, a diurnal rhythm occurs in ACTH secretion, with an increase beginning after the first few hours of sleep and reaching a peak at the time a person awakens. ACTH is used generally for diagnostic testing, and not for therapeutic purposes. The adverse effects include insomnia, delayed wound healing, increased susceptibility to infection, and acne.

Thyroid-stimulating Hormone

Thyroid-stimulating hormone (TSH) is a substance secreted by the anterior lobe of the pituitary gland that controls the release of thyroid hormone and is necessary for the growth and function of the thyroid gland. TSH stimulates the thyroid gland to increase the uptake of iodine and increase the synthesis and release of thyroid hormones. It is prescribed for hypothyroidism and diagnostic tests.

Follicle-stimulating Hormone

Follicle-stimulating hormone (FSH) is a gonadotropin that stimulates the growth and maturation of follicles in the ovary and promotes **spermatogenesis** (the process by which male gametes develop into mature spermatozoa) in the male. It is secreted by the anterior pituitary gland. The ovarian follicle produces estrogen, which reaches a high level before ovulation and suppresses release of FSH. In males, FSH maintains the integrity of the seminiferous tubules and influences all the stages of sperm production. It may be used to treat some conditions. One form is derived from the urine of postmenopausal women.

Luteinizing Hormone

Luteinizing hormone (LH) is secreted by the anterior lobe of the pituitary gland and is necessary for proper reproductive function. In females, an acute rise of LH triggers ovulation. In males, where LH is also called Interstitial Cell Stimulating Hormone (ICSH), it stimulates the production of testosterone.

Prolactin

Prolactin (PRL) is a hormone that is primarily associated with lactation. It is secreted from the anterior pituitary gland. Prolactin release is stimulated by thyrotropin-releasing factor.

Antidiuretic Hormone

Antidiuretic hormone (ADH) is released when the body is low on water, and causes the kidneys to conserve water, but not salt, by concentrating the urine and reducing urine volume. It also raises blood pressure by inducing vasoconstriction. ADH is released from the hypothalamus and stored in the posterior lobe of the pituitary gland.

Oxytocin

Oxytocin (OT) also acts as a neurotransmitter in the brain. In women, it is released during labor and lactation. It is also released by both sexes during orgasm. Oxytocin is mostly manufactured by the hypothalamus.

Thyroxine

Thyroxine (T_4) is the major hormone secreted by the follicular cells of the thyroid gland. It is involved in controlling metabolic body processes and influencing physical development.

Calcitonin

Calcitonin (CT) is produced primarily by the parafollicular cells of the thyroid gland. Calcitonin participates in calcium and phosphorus metabolism. In many ways, it counteracts the effects of parathyroid hormone.

Parathyroid Hormone

Parathyroid hormone (PTH), also called parathormone, is secreted by the parathyroid glands and increases the levels of calcium in the blood. Parathyroid hormone reduces the uptake of phosphate in the proximal tubules of the kidney, meaning that more phosphate is excreted through the urine.

Medical Terminology Review

glucocorticoids
gluco = glucose; glucagon; sugar
corticoids = steroid hormones
steroid hormones released
in response to sugar levels in
the blood

Glucocorticoids

Glucocorticoids are steroid hormones that can bind with the cortisol receptor and trigger similar effects. They are released from the adrenal cortex. Cortisol (hydrocortisone) is the most important human glucocorticoid. It regulates or supports a variety of important cardiovascular, metabolic, immunologic, and homeostatic functions.

Mineralocorticoids

Mineralocorticoids are steroid hormones that influence salt and water balance. They are released from the adrenal cortex. The primary endogenous mineralocorticoid is aldosterone, which acts on the kidneys to provide active reabsorption of sodium and passive reabsorption of water. This eventually results in an increase of blood pressure and blood volume.

Androgens

Androgen is the generic term for any natural or synthetic compound, usually a steroid hormone, which stimulates or controls the development of masculine characteristics by binding to androgen receptors. They are released from the adrenal cortex. Androgens are also the original anabolic steroids. The primary and most well-known androgen is testosterone.

Epinephrine

Epinephrine (adrenaline) is produced by the medulla of adrenal glands, and is a "fight or flight" hormone that is released when danger threatens. It increases heart rate and stroke volume, dilates the pupils, constricts arterioles in the skin and gut, and dilates arterioles in the leg muscles. It is commonly used to treat cardiac arrest and other cardiac dysrhythmias.

Norepinephrine

Norepinephrine (noradrenaline) is released from the medulla of the adrenal glands, and is also a central nervous system and sympathetic nervous system neurotransmitter. It supports the "fight or flight" response, increasing heart rate, triggering the release of glucose, and increasing skeletal muscle readiness.

Glucagon

Glucagon is a hormone that is very important for carbohydrate metabolism. It is synthesized and secreted by the alpha cells of the pancreas. Glucagon helps maintain the level of glucose in the blood by causing the liver to release glucose through a process known as glycogenolysis. This release prevents the development of hypoglycemia.

Insulin

Insulin is a hormone that regulates carbohydrate and fat metabolism. It is synthesized and released by the beta cells of the pancreas. Insulin is used medically to treat some forms of diabetes mellitus. Most insulin produced each day is produced during the digestion of meals. Insulin therapy often requires frequent blood glucose checking by the patient.

Insulin may be administered via syringes, injection pens, insulin pumps, and inhalers. Inhalation insulin uses only short-acting insulin, and is used in combination with a long-acting insulin to treat type 1 diabetes. Short, intermediate, mixed, and long-acting insulins may be injected using syringes and injection pens. Lantus insulin (insulin glargine) is a newer, ultra-long-acting type of insulin, administered by injection once per day. Its activity begins in a little more than one hour, and lasts for about 24 hours, without any peaks in its effectiveness.

ALTERATIONS IN THE FUNCTION OF THE PITUITARY GLAND

Key Concept

Regular monitoring of height, weight, and blood glucose levels is essential for a patient taking somatotropin.

Medical Terminology Review

somatotropin
  somato = body
  tropin = hormone
hormones involved in regulating body functions

Hyperpituitarism can result from damage to the anterior lobe of the pituitary gland or from inadequate secretion of hormones. The most noticeable result of hyperpituitarism is the effect of excessive amounts of GH. The condition produces excessive growth (a "giant") if the hypersecretion of GH occurs before puberty, which is called **gigantism**. If the excessive production of GH occurs after puberty, it can result in **acromegaly** (overdevelopment of the bones of the head, face, and feet). Treatment of these two conditions includes surgery, radiation, and medication therapy. Growth hormone insufficiency during childhood causes **dwarfism**.

Diabetes insipidus is a disease that results from a deficiency of ADH. In the absence of ADH, water is not reabsorbed by the kidneys and is excreted in the urine. Excessive water loss can quickly lead to dehydration. Whenever possible, the underlying cause of diabetes insipidus must be corrected. ADH is used in the treatment of diabetes insipidus.

Growth Hormone Replacement

Growth hormone replacement therapy may be used to treat many different conditions, including Turner syndrome, chronic renal failure, intrauterine growth retardation, and severe idiopathic short stature, to maintain muscle mass in AIDS patients, and for patients with short bowel syndrome.

Mechanism of Action

Although still widely debated, it is believed that the mechanism of action of GH is similar to that of tryptophan, which is released by increased levels of serotonin at night.

Indications

The main indication for replacement of GH is growth failure in children. Treatment is prolonged and may cause a six-inch growth in height. Special agents used for hormone therapy of the pituitary gland are listed in Table 16-2.

TABLE 16-2 Drugs used for Hormone Therapy of the Pituitary Gland

Generic Name	Trade Name	Route of Administration	Average Adult Dosage
Anterior Pituitary Gland			
Growth Hormone			
sermorelin	Geref®	SC	30 mcg/kg/day
somatropin	Humatrope®	SC	0.006 mg/kg/day (0.018 IU/kg/day)
somatrem	Protropin®	IM, SC	0.18 mg/kg/wk, divided into equal doses
Growth Hormone Inhibitor			
octreotide	Sandostatin®	SC, IV	Initial: 50 mcg; 100–600 mcg/day in 2–4 divided doses
Adrenocortical Hormones			
corticotropin	Acthar®, ACTH-80®	IM, SC	IM: 80–120 units/day; SC: 10–25 units in 500 mL D$_5$W infused over 8 h
cosyntropin	Cortrosyn®	IM, IV (diagnostic agent)	0.25 mg
Posterior Pituitary Gland			
desmopressin acetate	DDAVP®, Stimate®	PO, IV, SC, Nasal spray	PO: 0.2–0.4 mg/day; IV/SC: 0.3 mcg/kg/min pre-op, may repeat in 48 h p.r.n.; Nasal spray: 10 mcg b.i.d.
vasopressin	Pitressin®	IM, SC	5–10 units b.i.d. – t.i.d.

Adverse Effects

The side effects of GH therapy include headache, increased blood glucose levels, and muscle weakness. Other adverse effects include swelling at the injection site, myalgia, hypercalciuria, and hyperglycemia.

Contraindications and Precautions

Growth hormones such as somatrem and somatropin are contraindicated in patients with closed **epiphyses** (the ends of long bones that are originally separated from the main bone by a layer of cartilage, becoming unified through ossification), underlying progressive intracranial tumor, and diabetic retinopathy. These hormones should be avoided in patients during chemotherapy, radiation therapy, untreated hypothyroidism, and obesity.

Growth hormones are also contraindicated in pregnancy (category B or category C, depending on the brand).

Growth hormones should be used cautiously in patients with diabetes mellitus or family history of the disease, sleep apnea, lactation, and hypothyroidism.

Drug Interactions

Depending on dosage, anabolic steroids, androgens, estrogens, and thyroid hormones may interact with growth hormones.

ALTERATIONS IN THE FUNCTION OF THE THYROID GLAND

Hypothyroidism is a deficiency disease that causes cretinism (mental and physical retardation) in children. It is usually due to a deficiency of iodine in the mother's diet during pregnancy. Hypothyroidism in adults results from hypothalamic pituitary or thyroid insufficiency or resistance to thyroid hormone, which is called **myxedema.** The disorder can progress to hyposecretion of thyroid hormone. Hypothyroidism is more common in women than in men in the U.S. Hyposecretion of thyroid hormones may also be caused by lack of iodine in the diet, surgical removal of the thyroid, or radiation therapy to the thyroid. It may also be due to pituitary dysfunction. Thyroid hormones are approved for supplement or replacement needs of hypothyroidism. Thyroid hormones are usually initiated in small doses until adequate response is reached. Long-term use of thyroxine may cause osteoporosis or progressive loss of bone mass in postmenopausal women. Thyroxine is contraindicated in patients who have had a myocardial infarction. Table 16-3 shows common drugs used for disorders of the thyroid gland.

TABLE 16-3   Selected Medications Used as Drugs for the Thyroid Gland

Generic Name	Trade Name	Route of Administration	Average Adult Dosage
Natural thyroid replacement			
desiccated thyroid (T_3, T_4)	Armour® Thyroid	PO	None–it is based on natural production of the hormone per patient
Synthetic thyroid replacement			
levothyroxine sodium (T_4)	Levothroid®, Synthroid®	PO	100–400 mcg/day
liothyronine sodium (T_3)	Cytomel®	PO	25–75 mcg/day

(continues)

TABLE 16-3 Selected Medications Used as Drugs for the Thyroid Gland—*continued*

Generic Name	Trade Name	Route of Administration	Average Adult Dosage
liotrix (T_3, T_4)	Thyrolar®	PO	12.5–30 mcg/day
Antithyroid preparations			
potassium iodide	Pima®, Lugol's Solution®	PO	50–250 mg t.i.d. for 10–14 days before surgery
methimazole	Tapazole®	PO	5–15 mg t.i.d.
propylthiouracil (PTU)	generic only	PO	300–450 mg/day divided q8h
Calcitonin			
calcitonin (salmon)	Fortical®, Calcimar®	IM/SC, Nasal spray	IM/SC: 100 IU/day, may decrease to 50–100 IU/day; Nasal spray: 200 IU/day

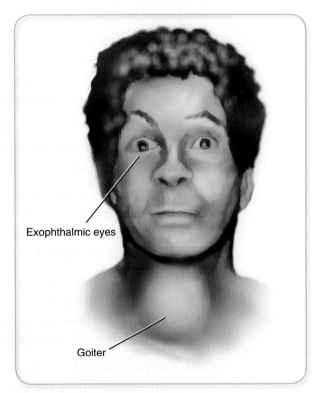

Figure 16-3 Hyperthyroidism.

Hyperthyroidism is a condition of excessive amounts of thyroxine (Figure 16-3). This condition stimulates cellular metabolism and increases respiration and body temperature. Hyperthyroidism causes nervousness and tremors (a shakiness of the hands).

Graves' disease is an example of hyperthyroidism. This disease is far more common in women than in men, and usually affects young women. Graves' disease can sometimes be treated with medication that inhibits the synthesis of thyroxine or by administration of radioactive iodine, which destroys the thyroid gland. Removal of the thyroid gland, however, may be necessary. If the gland is removed, hormonal supplements must be given. With partial removal of the thyroid gland, the remaining portion still secretes hormones.

Antithyroid Agents

An **antithyroid drug** is a chemical agent that lowers the basal metabolic rate by interfering with the formation, release, or action of thyroid hormones. A variety of compounds are known as antithyroid drugs. Iodine thyroid products (iodide ions), radioactive iodine, methimazole, and propylthiouracil are the drugs of choice for antithyroid therapy. These medications can cross the placenta and stop fetal thyroid development. They also pass through breast milk to affect the infant. Selected medication used as drugs for the thyroid gland are shown in Table 16-3.

Radioactive Iodine

Radioactive iodine is a radioactive isotope of iodine used in diagnostic radiology and radiotherapy. It is used particularly for the treatment of some thyroid conditions. Most radioactive iodine is excreted in urine, but small amounts may be found in sputum, perspiration, feces, and vomitus.

Mechanism of Action. Destructive radiation (beta rays) is emitted by the trapped isotope, which effectively destroys thyroid cells without appreciably damaging surrounding tissue.

Indications. Radioactive isotopes of iodine, particularly sodium iodide I^{131} are commonly used for the diagnosis and treatment of hyperthyroidism. When administered orally or intravenously, I^{131} is rapidly taken up and stored by the thyroid gland.

Adverse Effects. The extent of thyroid damage can be predetermined by carefully selecting the proper dose of isotope. Low doses are used diagnostically and pose a minimal risk to thyroid tissue, although high doses can effectively destroy all thyroid function, resulting in hypothyroidism.

Contraindications and Precautions. The antithyroid drugs are contraindicated in the last trimester of pregnancy (category D) and during lactation. These agents are also contraindicated with concurrent administration of sulfonamides or coal tar derivatives such as aminopyrine or antipyrine. Antithyroid agents must be used with caution in patients with infection, bone marrow depression, and impaired liver function. These drugs are also used cautiously in patients with concomitant administration of anticoagulants or other drugs known to cause agranulocytosis.

Drug Interactions. Iodine interacts with selenium and possibly with vanadium. Amiodarone, potassium iodide, or sodium iodide can reverse the efficacy of thyroid hormones.

Iodine Thyroid Products

These drugs have been shown to be useful in treatment of mild hyperthyroidism, particularly in young patients. Prior to the introduction of the thioamides in the 1940s, iodides were major antithyroid agents; today, they are rarely used as sole therapies.

Mechanism of Action. Iodine ion (**Lugol's solution**) inhibits the synthesis of the active thyroid hormones T_3 and T_4 and inhibits the release of these hormones into blood circulation.

Indications. Iodides may be used in several different forms. The most popular are Lugol's solution (strong iodine solution), which contains 5 percent iodine and 10 percent potassium iodide, and saturated solution of potassium iodide (SSKI). Iodides are used as adjunctive therapy with antithyroid drugs in preparation for thyroidectomy, treatment of thyrotoxic crisis, or neonatal thyrotoxicosis.

Adverse Effects. Lugol's solution may cause hypothyroidism, hyperthyroidism, goiter (enlargement of the thyroid), rashes, and swelling of the salivary glands.

Contraindications and Precautions. Potassium iodide is contraindicated in patients with hypersensitivity to iodine. This agent should be avoided in patients with hyperthyroidism, hyperkalemia, and acute bronchitis, and during pregnancy (category D) and lactation.

Potassium iodide should be used cautiously in patients with renal impairment, cardiac disease, pulmonary tuberculosis, and Addison's disease.

Drug Interactions. Lugol's solution can increase the risk of hypothyroidism if taken concurrently with lithium. Potassium-sparing diuretics, potassium supplements, and ACE inhibitors increase the risk of hyperkalemia.

Methimazole

Methimazole is an antithyroid agent that is about ten times more potent than propylthiouracil.

Mechanism of Action. Methimazole inhibits the synthesis of thyroid hormones by the coupling of iodine. This agent crosses the placental barrier and is concentrated by the fetal thyroid.

Indications. Methimazole has emerged as an effective drug for controlling hyperthyroidism. It is also used prior to surgery or radiotherapy of the thyroid.

Adverse Effects.   Observation of patients using methimazole has shown that adverse effects are not common. Some patients may develop a mild skin rash, and agranulocytosis has developed in a small number of patients. In very rare instances, methimazole may affect the central nervous system, causing headache, depression, drowsiness, vertigo, and neuritis.

Contraindications and Precautions.   Methimazole is contraindicated during lactation and pregnancy (category D). This drug should be used cautiously with other drugs known to cause agranulocytosis.

Drug Interactions.   Methimazole increases theophylline clearance and decreases effectiveness if given to hyperthyroid patients. This agent alters the effects of oral anticoagulants. It increases the therapeutic effects and toxicity of digitalis glycoside, metroprolol, and propranolol when hyperthyroid patients become euthyroid.

Propylthiouracil

Propylthiouracil (PTU) is a chemically related antithyroid drug, and is a major drug for the treatment of thyrotoxicosis.

Mechanism of Action.   PTU inhibits the synthesis of thyroid hormones, partially inhibiting the peripheral conversion of T_4 to T_3.

Indications.   PTU is used for treatment of hyperthyroidism, iodine-induced thyrotoxicosis, and hyperthyroidism associated with thyroiditis. Propylthiouracil is also used to establish euthyroidism prior to surgery or radioactive iodine treatment.

Adverse Effects.   PTU may cause neuritis, vertigo, drowsiness, depression, and headache. Other adverse effects of this agent include skin rash, skin pigmentation, loss of hair, nausea, vomiting, loss of taste, hepatitis, or nephritis. The most dangerous complication of propylthiouracil is agranulocytosis, an infrequent but potentially fatal adverse effect.

Contraindications and Precautions.   PTU is contraindicated in the last trimester of pregnancy (category D) and during lactation. PTU should be avoided with concurrent administration of sulfonamides or coal tar derivatives such as aminopyrine or antipyrine. PTU is used cautiously in patients with infection, liver dysfunction, and bone marrow depression.

Drug Interactions.   PTU increases risk of oral bleeding. The other side effects of PTU are similar to methimazole.

Medical Terminology Review

thyroiditis
   thyroid = thyroid gland
   itis = inflammation; disease of
   inflammation of the thyroid gland

Key Concept

The cross-sensitivity between propylthiouracil and methimazole is about 50 percent; therefore, switching drugs in patients with severe reactions is not recommended.

ALTERATIONS IN FUNCTION OF THE PARATHYROID GLAND

A deficiency of PTH may occur in some patients for a variety of reasons, ranging from a congenital absence of the parathyroid glands to surgery involving the thyroid gland. Such a deficiency results in a reduction of serum calcium levels, elevated phosphate levels, and a wide array of symptoms, including increased neuromuscular irritability and psychiatric disorders.

The treatment of hypoparathyroidism focuses on the replenishment of calcium stores to reverse the patient's hypocalcemia. Therefore, administration of calcium salts, particularly calcium chloride and calcium gluconate, is indicated.

Vitamin D is also commonly used in patients with hypoparathyroidism to promote calcium absorption from the gastrointestinal tract and to further stabilize a patient's condition.

An overactive parathyroid gland secretes too much PTH, which raises the level of circulating calcium above normal. This condition is called **hypercalcemia**. Much of the calcium comes from bone resorption and increased absorption of calcium by the kidneys and the gastrointestinal system. As the calcium level rises, the phosphate level falls.

With the loss of calcium bones are weakened. They tend to bend, become deformed, and fracture spontaneously. Excessive amounts of calcium cause the development of kidney stones because calcium forms insoluble compounds. Calcium deposited within the walls of the blood vessels makes them hard. Calcium deposits may also be found in the stomach and lungs.

Therapy for hyperparathyroidism often includes surgery. However, phosphate supplementation and/or potent diuretics, such as furosemide (Lasix), may be administered to promote an increase in the excretion of excess calcium. Calcitonin may also be used for treating hypercalcemia.

ALTERATIONS IN FUNCTION OF THE ADRENAL GLANDS

Overactivity of the adrenal cortex can take different forms, depending on which group of hormones is secreted in excess. **Cushing's syndrome** develops from an excess of glucocorticoids, the hormones that raise the blood sugar level. In excess, they cause hyperglycemia. The patient with Cushing's syndrome retains salt and water, resulting in hypertension and atherosclerosis, which develops as a result of excess circulating lipids.

Conn's syndrome is another form of hyperadrenalism. In this disease, aldosterone is secreted in excess. This causes retention of sodium and water and an abnormal loss of potassium in the urine. Hypertension develops as a result of the salt imbalance and water retention. Muscles become weak to the point of paralysis.

Adrenogenital syndrome is another form of hyperadrenalism, also called adrenal virilism. In this condition, androgens (male hormones) are secreted in excess. If this excessive secretion occurs in children, it stimulates premature sexual development. The sex organs of a male child greatly enlarge, and in a female, the clitoris enlarges, a male distribution of hair develops, and the voice deepens.

Excessive androgen secretion in a woman causes masculinization (adrenal virilism). Hair develops on the face, a condition called **hirsuitism**,

---

Medical Terminology Review

virilism

viril(e) = having male characteristics
ism = state; condition; quality
a condition in which male characteristics develop

and the hairline recedes. The breasts diminish in size, the clitoris enlarges, and ovulation and menstruation cease.

Addison's disease results when the adrenal glands fail to produce corticosteroids and aldosterone. The adrenal glands may be destroyed by cancer or infection, or inhibited by chronic use of steroid hormones, such as prednisone.

With aldosterone deficiency, the patient is unable to retain salt and water. The kidneys are unable to concentrate urine, and eventually dehydration ensues. Severe dehydration can ultimately lead to shock. Cortisol deficiency leads to low blood glucose levels, impaired protein and carbohydrate metabolism, and generalized weakness.

Treatment with Glucocorticoids

Prolonged use of glucocorticoids may suppress the pituitary gland, and the body will not produce its own hormone. If these hormones are used for extended periods of time, they cannot be stopped abruptly, and a step-down dosage should be used to taper gradually the amount of drug the patient is receiving.

Mechanism of Action

Cortisone enters target cells, where it has anti-inflammatory and immunosuppressive effects.

Indications

Adrenal corticosteroids are used for replacement therapy in patients with adrenal insufficiency, such as Addison's disease. In this condition, administration of both mineralocorticoids and glucocorticoids may be required. Glucocorticoids are also used to treat rheumatic, inflammatory, allergic, neoplastic, and other disorders as supportive therapy with other medications. These agents are of value in decreasing some cerebral edemas. Certain skin conditions are often markedly improved with the use of topical or systemic glucocorticoids. Probably the most use of these agents is treatment of arthritic and rheumatic disorders. Table 16-4 lists some steroids and adrenal corticosteroids.

Adverse Effects

Certain side effects may appear during the first week of treatment with glucocorticoids. They include euphoria, suicidal depression, psychoses, anorexia, hyperglycemia, increased susceptibility to infections, and acne. Chronic glucocorticoid therapy may cause additional side effects such as diabetes mellitus, glaucoma, cataracts, osteoporosis, and edema.

Glucocorticoids must be used cautiously in congestive heart failure, hypertension, liver failure, and renal failure.

TABLE 16-4   Steroids and Adrenal Corticosteroids

Generic Name	Trade Name	Route of Administration	Average Adult Dosage
Glucosteroids			
betamethasone acetate	Celestrone®	PO, IM, IV, Topical	PO: 0.6–7.2 mg/day; IM/IV: 0.5–9 mg/day as sodium phosphate; Topical: Apply thin film b.i.d.
cortisone acetate	Cortone®	PO, IM	20–300 mg/day in 1 or more div. doses, try to reduce periodically by 10–25 mg/day to lowest effective dose
dexamethasone	Decadron®, Maxidex®	PO, IM	PO: 0.25–4 mg b.i.d. to q.i.d.; IM: 8–16 mg q1–3wk or 0.8–1.6 mg intralesional q1–3 wk
methylprednisolone	Medrol®	PO	5–60 mg/day in single or divided doses
prednisone	Prelone® Aristocort®	PO	0.1–0.15 mg/kg/day
triamcinolone	Kenacort®	PO, IM, SC	4–48 mg 1–2 times/day

Contraindications and Precautions

Glucocorticoids are contraindicated in patients with emotional instability or psychotic tendencies, hyperlipidemia, diabetes mellitus, hypothyroidism, osteoporosis, and peptic ulcer.

Drug Interactions

Drug interactions include the increased therapeutic and toxic effects of cortisone if taken concurrently with troleandomycin. Cortisone also decreases the effects of anticholinesterases if taken concurrently with corticotropin, and profound muscular depression is possible. Steroid blood levels are decreased if cortisone is taken concurrently with phenytoin, phenobarbital, or rifampin. Decreased serum levels of salicylates are seen if it is taken concurrently with cortisone.

Treatment with Mineralocorticoids

Treatment with the primary mineralocorticoid (aldosterone) corrects the metabolism of sodium and potassium on renal tubular mineralocorticoid retention. This causes sodium reabsorption and potassium loss. Aldosterone is utilized in treating Addison's disease, which is a deficiency of adrenocortical secretions.

Treatment with Androgens

Androgen therapy is used for a variety of conditions, depending on gender. Androgens are primarily used to treat prostate cancer, breast cancer, and menopausal conditions. They are also often used illegally to build muscle mass.

ALTERATIONS IN THE FUNCTION OF THE PANCREAS

The most important disease involving the endocrine pancreas is **diabetes mellitus**, a disorder of carbohydrate metabolism that involves either an insulin deficiency, insulin resistance, or both. Diabetes, if untreated or uncontrolled, leads to hyperglycemia. Severe hyperglycemia and ketoacidosis may produce diabetic coma or unconsciousness, which requires much higher doses of insulin.

Diabetes mellitus is a complex disorder of carbohydrate, fat, and protein metabolism caused by lack of or inefficient use of insulin in the body. The two general classifications for diabetes mellitus are type I, or insulin-dependent diabetes mellitus (IDDM), and type II, or non-insulin-dependent diabetes mellitus (NIDDM). Table 16-5 compares type I and type II diabetes.

Treatment with Insulin

Normally, insulin is used for the treatment of type I diabetics if the pancreas does not produce enough insulin. Insulin needs may vary every

TABLE 16-5 General Differences of Type I and Type II Diabetes

	Type I	Type II
Age at onset	Pre-adolescence (juvenile onset)	After age 30 years (adult onset)
Onset	Acute	Insidious
Body weight	Thin	Obese
Hereditary factors	Family history	Present in immediate family
Treatment	Insulin replacement	Diet or oral hypoglycemic agents or insulin replacement
Hypoglycemia or ketoacidosis	Often	Less common

TABLE 16-6 Insulin Preparations

Preparation	Trade Name	Onset of Action	Duration of Action
Short-acting Insulin			
Insulin (regular)	Novolin®, Humulin R®	30–60 min 15 min	6–8 hrs 6–8 hrs
Prompt insulin zinc suspension	Semilente®	60–90 min	12–16 hrs
Intermediate-acting Insulin			
Isophane insulin (NPH)	Novolin N®, Humulin N®	2 hrs, 2 hrs	18–24 hrs, 18–24 hrs
Insulin zinc suspension (lente)	Humulin L®, Novolin L®	60–150 min 60–150 min	18–24 hrs 18–24 hrs
Long-acting Insulin			
Protamine zinc insulin suspension	PZI®	4–8 hrs	36 hrs
Extended insulin zinc suspension	Ultralente®, Humulin U®	4–8 hrs	36 hrs

6 to 8 hours. Normal fasting insulin levels range from 80 to 100 mg/dL. Insulin preparations are available from three different species, including cows, pigs, and humans. Human insulin now is produced by chemical conversion from porcine insulin and by *Escherichia coli*, into which the human genes for insulin have been inserted. The recombinant product has the same physiological properties as insulin from beef or pork but is much less likely to cause allergic reactions. Insulins are classified based on their time of pharmacological action as short-acting, intermediate-acting, and long-acting. Most diabetic patients require a combination of short- and long-acting insulin. Table 16-6 shows varieties of insulins and their properties.

Special Consideration

Patients who will be using insulin must be instructed on the rotation method of taking their medication. Insulin is absorbed more rapidly in the arm or thigh, especially with exercise. The abdomen is used for a more consistent absorption. Glucose levels should be checked per physician instructions. All insulin should be checked for expiration date and clearness. Insulin should not be given if it appears cloudy. Vials should not be shaken but rotated in between the hands to mix contents.

If regular insulin is to be mixed with NPH or lente insulin, the regular insulin should be drawn into the syringe first. Unopened vials should be stored in the refrigerator and freezing should be avoided. The vial in use can be stored at room temperature. Vials should not be put in glove

Key Concept

The most diagnostic sign of type I diabetes is sustained hyperglycemia. Fasting blood glucose levels of 126 mg/dL or greater on at least two separate occasions is diagnostic for diabetes.

Key Concept

Hypoglycemic reactions may occur at any time, but most commonly occur when insulin is at its peak activity.

compartments, suitcases, or trunks. It is imperative that the physician be called if any adverse reactions to the medications are observed.

Mechanism of Action

The primary action of insulin is to promote the entry of glucose into cells.

Indications

Insulin is used to control hyperglycemia in the diabetic patient, and for the emergency treatment of acute ketoacidosis. It may be administered intravenously or subcutaneously. Regular insulin is also available as Humulin 70/30 (a mixture of 70 percent isophane insulin and 30 percent regular insulin) or as Humulin 50/50 (a mixture of 50 percent of both isophane and regular insulin).

Adverse Effects

The most dangerous adverse effect of insulin therapy is hypoglycemia. The other adverse effects include tachycardia, sweating, drowsiness, and confusion. If severe hypoglycemia is not immediately treated with glucose, convulsions, coma, and death may occur.

Contraindications and Precautions

Insulin is contraindicated in patients with hypersensitivity to insulin animal protein. It is also contraindicated during episodes of hypoglycemia. Insulin should be used with caution in patients with insulin-resistant hyperthyroidism or hypothyroidism, during lactation, in older adults, during pregnancy (category B), and in those with renal or hepatic impairment.

Drug Interactions

Alcohol, anabolic steroids, MAOIs, and salicylates may potentiate hypoglycemic effects. Dextrothyroxine, corticosteroids, and epinephrine may antagonize hypoglycemic effects. Herbals such as garlic and ginseng may potentiate the hypoglycemic effects of insulin.

Oral Antidiabetic Agents

Type II diabetic patients are treated with the oral antidiabetics (oral hypoglycemic medications) and diet. The five classes of oral hypoglycemic medications given for type II diabetes are sulfonylureas, alpha-glucosidase inhibitors, biguanides, meglitinides, and thiazolidinediones. Table 16-7 shows some examples of oral hypoglycemic agents and their duration of action.

Medical Terminology Review

ketoacidosis
keto = *ketone; ketone group*
acid = *having a pH below 7.0*
osis = *condition; process; action*
a condition of metabolic acidosis caused by high concentrations of ketone bodies

TABLE 16-7 Oral Hypoglycemic Agents

Generic Name	Trade Name	Route of Administration	Average Adult Dosage
Sulfonylureas First-generation			
acetohexamide	Dymelor®	PO	250 mg–1.5 g/day
chlorpropamide	Diabinese®	PO	100–250 mg/day (with breakfast)
tolazamide	Tolinase®	PO	100–1000 mg q.d.–b.i.d.
tolbutamide	Orinase®	PO	250 mg to 3 g/day in 1–2 div. doses
Second-generation			
glimepiride	Amaryl®	PO	Initial: 1–2 mg/day with breakfast; may increase to maint. dose of 1–4 mg q.d. (max: 8 mg/day)
glipizide	Glucotrol®, Glucotrol XL®	PO	2.5–5 mg 1–2 times/day
glyburide	DiaBeta®, Glynase®	PO	1.25–5 mg with breakfast
Alpha-glucosidase Inhibitors			
acarbose	Precose®	PO	Start with 25 mg t.i.d. (with meals)
miglitol	Glyset®	PO	25 mg t.i.d. at the start of each meal
Biguanides			
metformin hydrochloride	Glucophage®	PO	500–850 mg/day
Meglitinides			
nateglinide	Starlix®	PO	60–120 mg t.i.d.
repaglinide	Prandin®	PO	0.5–4.0 mg b.i.d.-q.i.d.
Thiazolidinediones			
pioglitazone hydrochloride	Actos®	PO	15–30 mg/day
rosiglitazone maleate	Avandia®	PO	2–4 mg q.d.-b.i.d.
Combination Drugs			
glipizide/metformin	Metaglip	PO	2.5 mg glipizide/250 mg metaformin per day
glyburide/metformin	Glucovance®	PO	1.25 to 5 mg glyburide/250 to 500 mg metformin per dayq.d.-b.i.d.
rosiglitazone maleate/metformin	Avandamet®	PO	1 to 4 mg rosiglitazone maleate/500 mg metformin per day

Mechanism of Action

Oral hypoglycemic agents stimulate the pancreas to secrete more insulin and increase the sensitivity of insulin receptors in target tissues.

Indications

The advantages of using the second-generation agents are that they have a long duration of action and have fewer side effects. First generation drugs are rarely used today. Of the first-generation agents, tolazamide also has advantages similar to those of the second-generation drugs. Oral hypoglycemic agents are indicated for the treatment of uncomplicated type II diabetes in patients whose diabetes cannot be controlled by diet or exercise only.

Adverse Effects

Adverse effects include nausea, vomiting, headache, blurred vision, sedation, confusion, anxiety, nightmares, and tachycardia.

Contraindications and Precautions

Oral hypoglycemic agents are contraindicated in patients who are receiving sulfonamide or thiazide-type diuretics, who are hypersensitive to the agents, and who have acidosis, severe burns, or severe diarrhea. These agents should be used cautiously in patients with high fevers, severe infections, hyperthyroidism, or kidney function impairment.

Drug Interactions

Oral hypoglycemic medications have the potential to interact with a number of drugs; thus, the patient should always consult with a health care practitioner before adding a new medication or herbal supplement. Ingestion of alcohol will result in distressing symptoms that include headache, nausea, abdominal pain, and flushing.

Behavior Modification for Diabetes

Because diabetes is a lifelong disorder, education of the patient and the family is probably the most important obligation of the physician who provides initial care. This disease is markedly affected on a daily basis by fluctuations in environmental stress, exercise, diet, and the presence of infections. Therefore, the best persons to monitor and manage the disease are the patients themselves and their families.

Summary

The endocrine system provides a means of chemical communication between body parts. The anterior pituitary gland controls activities of the thyroid, adrenals, and sex glands. It also stimulates growth, development, and tissue repair. The pituitary is called the master gland for these reasons. Pituitary activity is governed by the hypothalamus in the brain.

Hyperpituitarism causes an excess of growth hormone. This condition, if present before puberty, results in gigantism. In an adult, excessive production of growth hormone leads to acromegaly.

Severe hypopituitarism impedes growth and development in a child, causing dwarfism. Glands that depend on stimulation by the anterior pituitary are the thyroid, adrenal, and sex glands. The posterior pituitary gland releases vasopressin, also called antidiuretic hormone (ADH), and oxytocin. Insufficiency of ADH causes diabetes insipidus.

The rate of metabolism is controlled by the thyroid gland. An enlargement of this gland is called a goiter. Hyperthyroidism, which is an excess of thyroxine, accelerates heart and respiratory activity, increases metabolic rate, and raises body temperature. A congenital lack of thyroxine results in cretinism (mental and physical retardation). Myxedema is a disease of severe hypothyroidism in an adult.

Hormones of the adrenal cortex are essential to life. Aldosterone regulates salt balance and cortisol affects the metabolism of nutrients. The sex hormones estrogen and androgen are also produced by this gland. Hypoactivity of the adrenal cortex is called Addison's disease.

Hyperactivity of the adrenal cortex causes different diseases, depending on which hormones are in excess amounts. Cushing's syndrome results from an excess of cortisol, and Conn's syndrome results from excessive aldosterone. Precocious puberty and adrenal virilism develop from too much androgen secretion.

PTH regulates the level of circulating calcium and phosphate. Hyperactivity of the parathyroid glands causes hypercalcemia. The high level of calcium comes primarily from bone resorption that weakens the bones. Hypoparathyroidism reduces the level of calcium in the blood, which results in tetany. Hormones of the pancreas, insulin, and glucagon control blood sugar level. Lack of insulin causes an increase in blood glucose levels, the condition called diabetes mellitus.

Hypoglycemia, an abnormally low blood glucose level, results from excess insulin. This condition can develop in the diabetic patient from an overdosage of insulin.

With the loss of calcium, the bones are weakened. They tend to bend, become deformed, and fracture spontaneously. Excessive calcium causes the

formation of kidney stones because calcium forms insoluble compounds. Calcium deposited within the walls of the blood vessels makes them hard. It may also be found in the stomach and lungs.

The therapy for hyperparathyroidism often includes surgery. However, phosphate supplementation and/or potent diuretics, such as furosemide (Lasix), may be administered to promote an increase in the excretion of excess calcium. Calcitonin may also be used to treat hypercalcemia.

EXPLORING THE WEB

Visit *www.endocrineweb.com*

- Look for additional readings and information of the various endocrine glands and the disorders that may occur when they malfunction.

Visit *www.nlm.nih.gov/medlineplus*

- Search for articles related to the topics addressed in this chapter.

Visit *www.pituitary.org*

- Review the FAQs and disorders discussed at this site to further your understanding of the function of the pituitary gland.

REVIEW QUESTIONS

Multiple Choice

1. Which of the following is secreted from the pancreas?

   A. prolactin
   B. growth hormone
   C. glucagon
   D. calcitonin

2. Another name for vasopressin is:

   A. testosterone
   B. cortisol
   C. prolactin
   D. antidiuretic hormone

3. FSH and LH are released from which of the following organs?

   A. hypothalamus
   B. pituitary
   C. ovaries
   D. pancreas

4. Which of the following is a protein?

   A. testosterone
   B. androgen
   C. growth hormone
   D. cortisol

5. Which of the following hormones is stored in posterior parts of the pituitary gland?

   A. oxytocin
   B. growth hormone
   C. prolactin
   D. cortisol

6. The glucocorticoid hormones are under the control of:

   A. LH
   B. TSH
   C. ACTH
   D. FSH

7. Which of the following is a side effect of corticosteroids?

   A. delayed healing with infection
   B. hypotension
   C. weight loss
   D. hypertrophy of the adrenal cortex

8. Which of the following is the trade name of methimazole?

   A. Cytomel
   B. Tapazole
   C. Propyl-Thyracil
   D. Celestrone

9. Glucophage is the trade name of:

   A. metformin
   B. miglitol
   C. glimepiride
   D. glipizide

10. Which of the following agents is used for the diagnosis and treatment of hyperthyroidism?

    A. thyroxin
    B. sodium iodide
    C. parathyroid hormone
    D. phenytoin

11. Propylthiouracil (PTU) is chemically related to which of the following drugs?

    A. antineoplastic
    B. antithyroid
    C. antiparathyroid
    D. antidiuretic

12. The mechanism of action of oral hypoglycemic medications is to:

    A. increase insulin production in the pancreas
    B. decrease insulin secretion from the pancreas
    C. release insulin into the bloodstream
    D. stimulate insulin release from the pancreas

13. All of the following include intermediate-acting insulin, except:

    A. NPH (Humulin)
    B. Lente L
    C. Humulin N
    D. Crystalline zinc

14. Which of the following is the trade name of chlorpropamide?

    A. Diabinese
    B. Dymelor
    C. Tolinase
    D. Glucotrol

15. Which of the following is the most serious adverse effect of insulin?

    A. hyperthermia
    B. hyperthyroidism
    C. hyperglycemia
    D. hypoglycemia

Matching

_____ 1. Adrenal cortex   A. Prolactin

_____ 2. Thyroid   B. Glucagon

_____ 3. Neurohypophysis   C. Norepinephrine

_____ 4. Beta cells of pancreas   D. Aldosterone

_____ 5. Alpha cells of pancreas   E. Insulin

_____ 6. Adrenal medulla   F. Oxytocin

_____ 7. Anterior lobe of pituitary   G. Calcitonin

Critical Thinking

A 43-year-old woman is experiencing chills, weight gain, and a general feeling of weakness, as well as an enlarged thyroid gland. Her physician diagnoses her with *hypothyroidism*.

1. List the most common causes of hypothyroidism.

2. Explain the common treatments for this condition.

3. If the patient were to refuse treatment, what would be the consequence?

Hormones of the Reproductive System and Contraceptives

OBJECTIVES

After completing this chapter, the reader should be able to:

1. Explain the relationship between the anterior pituitary gland and the ovaries.
2. Describe the classes of sex hormones in both males and females.
3. Describe four indications for prescribing estrogens.
4. Discuss common adverse effects accompanying the use of estrogens.
5. Describe four indications for progestational drugs.
6. Explain four indications of androgens.
7. Discuss the therapeutic uses of anabolic drugs.
8. Explain the regulation of the menstrual cycle.
9. Describe the contraindications and precautions of oral contraceptives.
10. List five common sexually transmitted diseases and define them.

GLOSSARY

Amenorrhea – the absence of a menstrual period in a woman of reproductive age

Depot-medroxyprogesterone acetate (Depo-Provera®) – a long-acting progestin

Estrogen – substances capable of producing sexual receptivity in female individuals

Follicle-stimulating hormone (FSH) – a hormone synthesized and secreted by gonadotropes in the anterior pituitary gland; in females, it stimulates the maturation of Graafian follicles; in males, it is critical for spermatogenesis

Gonadotropes – cells in the anterior pituitary gland that produce the gonadotropins known as luteinizing hormone and follicle-stimulating hormone

Gonadotropin-releasing hormone (GnRH) – stimulates the release of FSH and LH from the anterior pituitary gland

Graafian follicles – matured and grown ovarian follicles; these egg-containing tubes grown and develop between puberty, sexual maturation, and menopause

Hypogonadism – a condition of little or no production of sex hormones, usually due to poor function or inactivity of either the testes or the ovaries

Hypoprothrombinemic – the amount of prothrombin factor II in the circulating blood

Progesterone – secreted primarily by the ovarian cells in the corpus luteum at the time of ovulation during the female reproductive years

Testosterone – stimulates the development of the male secondary sex characteristics, initiates the production of sperm, and enhances the functional capacity of the penis and accessory sex organs

OVERVIEW

The female and male reproductive systems are controlled by a small number of hormones, particularly those secreted by the hypothalamus and the anterior pituitary glands. These hormones can be produced with natural or synthetic hormones to achieve therapeutic goals ranging from the prevention of pregnancy to milk production or even replacement therapy.

ANATOMY REVIEW

- The female reproductive system is composed of two ovaries, two fallopian tubes, the uterus, and the vagina (Figure 17-1).

- The male reproductive system is composed of two testes, seminal ducts, glands, and the penis (Figure 17-2).

- The functions of the reproductive system are to create new life through reproduction and to manufacture hormones responsible for the development of reproductive organs and secondary sex characteristics (Figure 17-3).

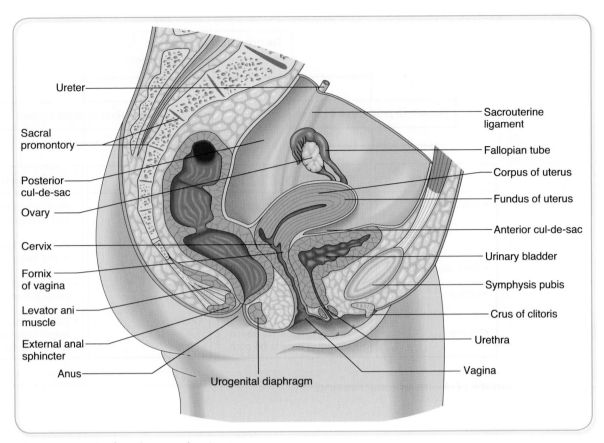

Figure 17-1 The female reproductive system.

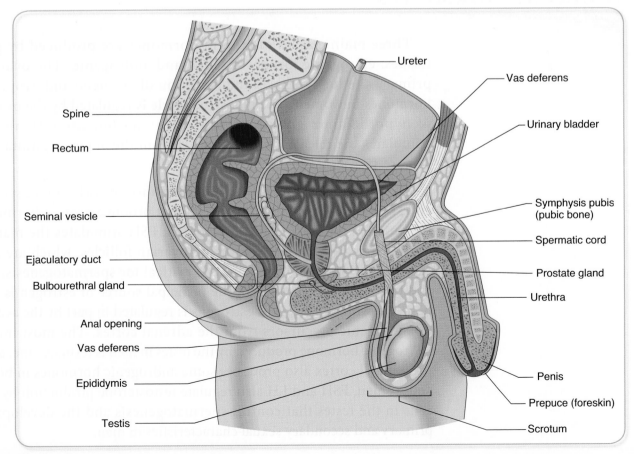

Figure 17-2 The male reproductive system.

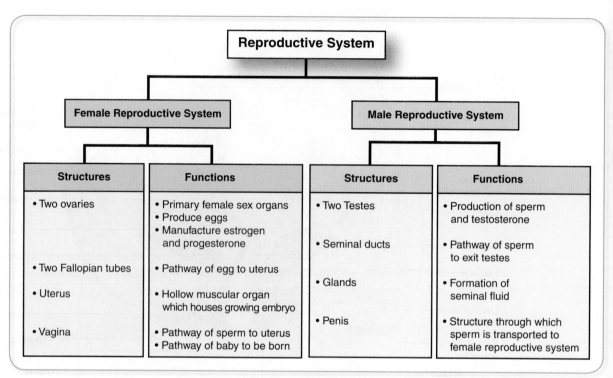

Figure 17-3 The reproductive system.

GONADAL HORMONES

Three main classes of steroid hormones are produced by gonadal tissues: estrogenic, progestational, and androgenic. The ovary is the primary site for synthesis and secretion of **estrogen** and **progesterone** hormones in women. The menstrual cycle is regulated by the production of hypothalamic **gonadotropin-releasing hormone (GnRH)** that stimulates the release of FSH and LH from the anterior pituitary gland (Figure 17-4).

FSH stands for **follicle-stimulating hormone**, a hormone synthesized and secreted by **gonadotropes** (cells that produce protein hormones) in the anterior pituitary gland. In women, FSH stimulates the maturation of the **Graafian follicles** (maturing ovarian follicles, which are actually egg-containing tubes). In men, it is critical for spermatogenesis. In men and postmenopausal women, the principal source of estrogen is adipose tissue, in which the level of estrogens is regulated in part by the availability of androgenic precursors from the adrenal cortex. The most important androgenic hormone produced by the testes in men is **testosterone**, although the adrenal cortex also produces some androgenic hormones in both men and women. FSH and LH also regulate testosterone production by specific cells in the testes that control spermatogenesis and the development of primary and secondary sexual characteristics in men.

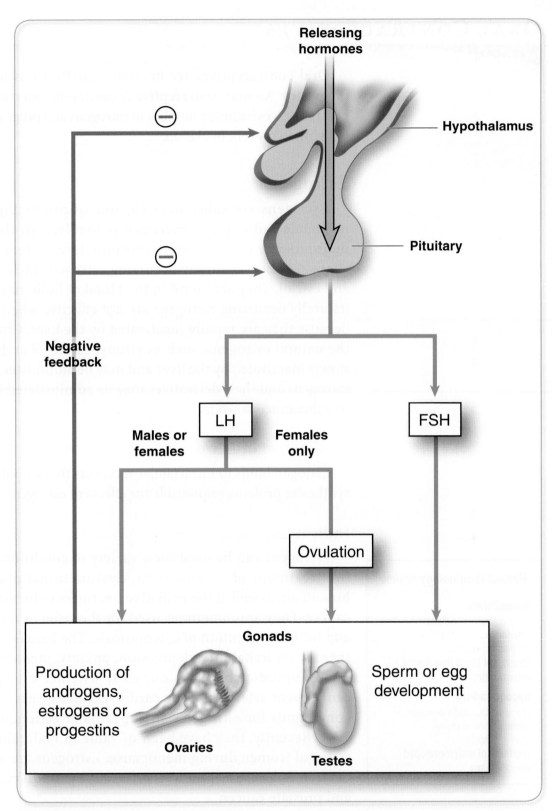

Figure 17-4 Regulation of the hormones of the reproductive system.

ORAL CONTRACEPTIVES

Oral contraceptives are hormone medications for the prevention of pregnancy. An oral contraceptive is commonly referred to as "the pill." Oral contraceptives include a number of estrogens and progestins, or a combination of them, to prevent ovulation.

Estrogens

Estrogens are substances capable of producing sexual receptivity in female individuals. Estrogen is involved in the development and maintenance of the female reproductive system and secondary sex characteristics. Naturally occurring estrogens include estrone, estradiol, and estriol. They are found in the blood of both males and females. Most naturally occurring estrogens are not effective when administered orally, because they are rapidly inactivated by the liver. Chemical derivatives of the natural estrogens, such as ethinyl estradiol and mestranol, are only slowly inactivated by the liver and may be administered orally. The natural estrogens and their derivatives may be administered by the intramuscular or subcutaneous route.

Mechanism of Action

Estrogen binds to intracellular receptors that stimulate DNA and RNA to synthesize proteins responsible for effects of estrogen.

Indications

Estrogens can be used for a variety of conditions. They are used for the treatment of **amenorrhea**, dysfunctional uterine bleeding, and hirsuitism, as well as the palliative treatment of breast cancer and prostate cancer. They are sometimes used for the relief of menopausal symptoms and for the prevention of osteoporosis. The beneficial effects of estrogen therapy on irritability, depression, anxiety, memory, and insomnia are more unpredictable. It is not clear whether estrogen administration can prevent arteriosclerotic cardiovascular disease. There is a choice of compounds for estrogenic therapy. Major estrogens are listed in Table 17-1. Recently, they have been of value in maintaining healthy cardiac status of women during menopause. Estrogens are also used in primary ovarian failure, atrophic vaginitis, **hypogonadism**, atrophic urethritis, and prostate cancer.

Adverse Effects

The most common adverse effects are nausea, vomiting, breast swelling, fluid retention (weight gain), hypertension, and thromboembolic disorders. Other adverse effects include leg cramps, intolerance to contact lenses, spotting, changes in menstrual flow, dysmenorrhea, and amenorrhea.

Medical Terminology Review

amenorrhea

a(-) = absence; lack; not
menorrhea = normal flow of blood during menstruation
absence of blood flow during menstruation

hypogonadism

hypo = slow, under developer
gonad = sexual organs
ism = condition
condition of underdeveloped sexual organs

Medical Terminology Review

thromboembolic

thrombo = blood clot
embolic = condition of a mass in the bloodstream
a blood clot in the bloodstream

TABLE 17-1 Major Estrogens

Generic Name	Trade Name	Route of Administration	Average Adult Dosage
estradiol	Estraderm®, Estrace®	PO, Transdermal patch	Estraderm: 0.45–2 mg twice weekly 0.45–2 mg q.d. in a cyclic regimen (21 days on, 7 days off)
estrogen, conjugated	Premarin®	PO	0.3–1.25 mg q.d. in a cyclic regimen (21 days on, 7 days off)
estropipate	Ogen®, Ortho-Est®	PO	0.75–6 mg q.d. in a cyclic regimen (21 days on, 7 days off)
estradiol cypionate	Dep-Gynogen®, Depogen®	IM	1–5 mg q3–4 weeks
estradiol valerate	Delestrogen®, Duragen-10®, Valergen®	PO	0.45–2 mg/day in a cyclic regimen (21 days on, 7 days off)
ethinyl estradiol	Estinyl®, Feminone®	PO	0.02–0.05 mg q.d. in a cyclic regimen (21 days on, 7 days off)

Contraindications and Precautions

Estrogens should not be used in patients who have a sensitivity to any of the ingredients, are pregnant, or have breast cancer, undiagnosed abnormal uterine bleeding, thrombophlebitis, and thromboembolic disorders.

Drug Interactions

Barbiturates, phenytoin, and rifampin decrease estrogen effects by increasing estrogen metabolism. Oral anticoagulants may decrease **hypoprothrombinemic** (the amount of prothrombin factor II in the circulating blood) effects due to interaction with estrogen. Estrogen may also interfere with the effects of bromocriptine and cause toxicity of cyclosporine.

Progesterone

Progesterone is secreted primarily by the ovarian cells in the corpus luteum at the time of ovulation during the female reproductive years. The corpus luteum secretes progesterone only during the last two weeks of the menstrual cycle. The greatest amount is secreted during the week after ovulation has taken place. Progesterone is responsible for the changes in the uterine endometrium during the second half of the menstrual cycle, the development of the maternal placenta after implantation, and the development of the mammary glands. Progesterone also causes an increase in the viscosity of cervical secretions, which impedes the movement of sperm. Progesterone in high doses suppresses

the pituitary release of LH and the hypothalamic release of GnRH, thus preventing ovulation. Progesterone also decreases uterine motility. A synthetic form of progesterone produced by a chemical modification is needed because the natural type of hormone would be inactivated by the liver. These synthetic preparations are called progestins.

Mechanism of Action

Progesterone changes the uterine lining (endometrium) from a proliferative structure to a secretory one. If fertilization does not take place, the corpus luteum diminishes in size, progesterone and estrogen production drop, and menstruation follows.

Indications

Progesterone is used in irregular uterine bleeding and is combined with estrogen for the treatment of amenorrhea. It is also used in cases of infertility and threatened or habitual abortion. Progesterone is indicated in the treatment of endometriosis and premenstrual syndrome.

Adverse Effects

Common adverse effects include migraine headache, dizziness, lethargy, mental depression, and insomnia. Thromboembolic disorder and pulmonary embolism may occur with administration of progesterone.

Contraindications and Precautions

Progesterone is contraindicated in patients with thrombophlebitis, liver disease, breast cancer, reproductive organ cancer, undiagnosed vaginal bleeding, missed periods, and a hypersensitivity to the medication or any of its ingredients. Use during pregnancy and breastfeeding is not recommended. Progesterone should be used cautiously in patients who suffer from anemia and diabetes mellitus, or have a history of psychic depression. Progesterone should be used with caution in patients with asthma, seizure disorders, and cardiac or kidney dysfunction. This agent must be used cautiously in patients with impaired liver function, previous ectopic pregnancy, venereal disease, and unresolved abnormal Pap smear. Table 17-2 shows the most commonly used progestins.

Drug Interactions

Ketoconazole may inhibit progesterone metabolism. Barbiturates, carbamazepine, phenytoin, and rifampin may alter contraceptive effectiveness.

Estrogen and Progesterone Combinations

Combinations of estrogens and progestins may be used as oral contraceptives in women. This method is nearly 100 percent effective in preventing pregnancy when used as directed. Oral contraceptives contain various amounts of estrogen and progestins. The estrogen inhibits ovulation

---

Key Concept

Progesterone can cause changes in vision, ptosis, diplopia, and retinal vascular lesions.

TABLE 17-2 Most Commonly Used Progestins

Generic Name	Trade Name	Route of Administration	Average Adult Dosage
medroxyprogesterone acetate	Provera®, Depo-Provera®	PO, SC	PO: 5–10 mg/day; SC: one injection every 3 months
norethindrone	Norlutin®	PO	5–20 mg on day 5 through day 25 of menstrual cycle
progesterone	Gesterol®	PO, IM	PO: 400 mg h.s. x 10 days; IM: 5–10 mg for 6–8 consecutive days

by suppressing the normal secretion of FSH. The progestin inhibits pituitary secretion of LH, causes changes in the cervical mucus that makes it unfavorable to penetration by the sperm, and alters the nature of the endometrium.

Mechanism of Action

Fixed combinations of estrogen and progestin produce contraception by preventing ovulation and rendering reproductive tract structures hostile to sperm penetration and zygote implantation.

Indications

The use of estrogen-progestin combinations in a cyclic fashion generally results in the inhibition of conception without preventing menstruation. Most oral contraceptives are taken daily for 20 to 21 days, starting on the fifth day after menstrual bleeding begins. Also available are oral contraceptives with 28-day pill cycles, wherein a pill is taken every day of the cycle so that once started, the pill is not stopped. In the 28-day pill cycle, an inactive pill is taken during the week of menstruation, whereas with the 20- to 21-day pill there is a week without medication, and this is when menstruation takes place. The use of oral contraceptives containing only a progestin has been advocated as a means of reducing some of the risk associated with their use. These products, which are sometimes referred to as "minipills," are generally taken continuously rather than cyclically. Because they contain no estrogen, they do not suppress ovulation. Table 17-3 shows the most commonly used contraceptive agents.

Depot-medroxyprogesterone acetate (Depo-Provera) is a long-acting progestin. It is the injectable long-acting progestin which is approved for contraceptive use in the U.S. There has been extensive worldwide experience with this method over the past three decades. The medication is given as a deep intramuscular injection of 150 mg every three months and has a contraceptive efficacy of 99.7 percent. It has been proven safe and relatively inexpensive. Many women find this method more convenient than the daily oral contraceptives.

TABLE 17-3 Commonly Used Contraceptive Agents

Generic Name	Trade Name	Route of Administration	Average Adult Dosage
Monophasic Agents			
ethinyl estradiol/ drospirenone	Yasmin®	PO	0.03 mg ethinyl estradiol with 3 mg drospirenone taken cyclically (as above)
ethinyl estradiol/ ethynodiol	Zovia®, Demulen®	PO	0.035 mg or 0.05 mg ethynyl estradiol with 1 mg ethynodiol diacetate taken cyclically (as above)
ethinyl estradiol/ levonorgestrel	Alesse®, Nordette®	PO	0.02 mg ethinyl estradiol with 0.10 mg levonorgestrel taken cyclically (as above)
ethinyl estradiol/ norelgestromin	Ortho-Evra®	Transdermal patch	0.75 mg ethinyl estradiol with 6 mg norelgestromin; apply 1 patch for 21 days followed by a 7 day interval with no patch
ethinyl estradiol/ norethindrone (various strengths)	Ovcon®, Loestrin®,	PO	0.035 mg ethinyl estradiol with varying amounts of norethindrone taken cyclically (21 days on, 7 days off)
mestranol/ norethindrone	Necon 1/50®, Ortho-Novum 1/50®	PO	0.05 mg mestranol with 1 mg norethindrone taken cyclically (as above)
Biphasic Agents			
ethinyl estradiol/ norethindrone	Ortho-Novum 10/11®, Nelova 10/11®	PO	First 10 tablets contain 0.035 mg ethinyl estradiol and 0.5 mg norethindrone; the next 11 pills contain 0.035 mg ethinyl estradiol and 1 mg norethindrone; taken cyclically (as above)
Triphasic Agents			
ethinyl estradiol/ levonorgestrel	Triphasil®, Tri-Levlen®	PO	First 6 tablets contain 0.03 mg ethinyl estradiol and 0.05 mg levonorgestrel; the next 5 tablets contain 0.04 mg ethinyl estradiol and 0.075 mg levonorgestrel; the final 10 tablets contain 0.03 mg ethinyl estradiol and 0.125 mg levonorgestrel; taken cyclically (as above)
ethinyl estradiol/ norgestimate	Ortho Tri-cyclin®	PO	In this product, the amount of ethinyl estradiol remains constant at 0.035 mg per tablet, while the norgestimate increases from 0.18 mg per tablet to 0.25 mg; taken cyclically (as above)

(continues)

TABLE 17-3   Commonly Used Contraceptive Agents—*continued*

Generic Name	Trade Name	Route of Administration	Average Adult Dosage
Estrophasic Agents			
ethinyl estradiol/ norethindrone acetate	Estrostep®	PO	In this product, the amount of ethinyl estradiol changes from 0.02 to 0.03 and then to 0.035 mg per tablet, while the norethindrone acetate remains constant at 1 mg per tablet; taken cyclically (as above)
Progestin-only Agents			
norethindrone	Micronor®, Nor-QD®	PO	1 tablet of 0.35 mg/day (each package lasts 28 days with no stoppage in between packages)
norgestrel	Ovrette®	PO	0.75 mg/day
Long-acting Agents			
intrauterine progesterone contraceptive system	Progestasert®	IUD	38 mg IUD inserted by a healthcare professional – lasts for 12 months
medroxyprogesterone	Depo-Provera®	IM	150 mg/mL q13 weeks
medroxyprogesterone with estradiol	Lunelle®	IM	0.5 mL/month; first injection given during first 5 days of menstruation; follow-up injections every 28 to 33 days

Adverse Effects

The classic adverse effects associated with birth control drugs are nausea, weight gain, and breast tenderness, which result from the progesterone they contain. Other adverse effects include fluid retention, irregular vaginal bleeding, and skin discoloration. The most serious adverse effects of oral contraceptives include heart attack, stroke, hypertension, or other forms of thromboembolic disease. Table 17-4 summarizes the dose-related effects of oral contraceptives.

Contraindications and Precautions

Contraceptives are contraindicated in pregnancy (category X), lactation, and missed abortion. These agents should be avoided in individuals with familial or personal history of or existence of breast cancer. Patients with diabetes mellitus, hypertension, or hypercholesterolemia (increased blood cholesterol levels) should not take contraceptive agents. Before the use of any hormonal type of contraception, the patient should have a complete history and physical examination performed. The patient should be informed of the precautions, warnings, and adverse effects.

TABLE 17-4 Dose Related Adverse Effects of Oral Contraceptives

Estrogen excess	Progestin excess
Nausea	Increased appetite
Hypertension	Weight gain
Breast tenderness	Fatigue
Edema	Acne
Migraine headache	Hair loss
	Depression
Estrogen deficiency	**Progestin deficiency**
Early or mid-cycle bleeding	Late breakthrough bleeding
Increased spotting	Amenorrhea
Hypomenorrhea	Hypermenorrhea

Smoking increases the risk of serious adverse effects on the heart and blood vessels from oral contraceptive use. The risk increases with age and heavy smoking (15 or more cigarettes per day), and is quite marked in women older than 35 years of age.

Drug Interactions

Several drugs interact with oral contraceptive agents. Some commonly prescribed drugs in this category are phenytoin, phenobarbital (and other barbiturates), primidone, carbamazepine, and rifampin. Women taking these drugs should use another means of contraception for maximum safety.

DRUGS USED DURING LABOR AND DELIVERY

Generally, two types of medications are used during labor and delivery: uterine stimulants and uterine relaxants.

Uterine Stimulants

Uterine stimulants cause contractions of the myometrium during labor and delivery. Many agents are capable of stimulating the smooth muscle of the uterus, but a few are selective, to be used for the myometrium. These agents are known as oxytocic substances.

Mechanism of Action

Oxytocin injection, by direct action on the myometrium, produces phasic contractions characteristic of normal delivery. It also promotes milk ejection (letdown) reflex in nursing mothers, thereby increasing flow (not volume) of milk.

Indications

Oxytocic agents are used to initiate or improve uterine contraction at term only in carefully selected patients and only after the cervix is dilated and presentation of the fetus has occurred. These agents are also indicated to relieve pain from breast engorgement and control of postpartum hemorrhage and promotion of postpartum uterine involution. Oxytocic agents are often used to induce labor in cases of maternal diabetes, pre-eclampsia, and eclampsia.

Adverse Effects

Oxytocic agents may stimulate contractions of the uterus and cause fetal trauma from rapid pushing (forward) through the pelvis. This can result in fetal death. Adverse effects of these agents may result in anaphylactic reactions, postpartum hemorrhage, edema, fetal bradycardia, maternal cardiac arrhythmias, and hypertensive episodes.

Contraindications and Precautions

Oxytocic agents are contraindicated in patients with hypersensitivity to them. These agents should be avoided in unfavorable fetal position or presentations that are undeliverable without conversion before delivery, and fetal distress in which delivery is not imminent, prematurity, placenta previa, and previous surgery of uterus or cesarean section. Oxytocic drugs should be used with caution in concomitant use of cyclopropane anesthesia or vasoconstrictive drugs.

Key Concept

Herbals such as ephedra and mahuang may interact with oxytocic drugs, causing hypertension.

Drug Interactions

Oxytocic drugs may interact with vasoconstrictors and cause severe hypertension. Oxytocic agents with clopropane anesthesia cause hypotension, maternal bradycardia, and other types of arrhythmias.

Uterine Relaxants

Uterine relaxants are prescribed in the management of preterm labor. These agents decrease uterine contraction and prolong the pregnancy for developing the fetus in full term. Two agents are currently used as uterine relaxants: ritodrine (Yutopar) and terbutaline (Brethine).

Mechanism of Action

Uterine relaxants preferentially stimulate β_2-receptors in uterine smooth muscle, reducing intensity and frequency of uterine contractions.

Indications

Uterine relaxants are used to delay preterm labor in pregnancies of greater than 20 weeks' gestation.

Adverse Effects

Uterine relaxants often alter fetal and maternal heart rates and maternal blood pressure. Common adverse effects of these drugs include nausea, vomiting, nervousness, restlessness, headache, and palpitations.

Contraindications and Precautions

Uterine relaxants are contraindicated in patients with hypersensitivity, and those with antepartum hemorrhage, eclampsia, asthma, and in pregnancies of less than 20 weeks' gestation. Uterine relaxants should be used cautiously in concomitant use of potassium-depleting diuretics and in patients with cardiac disease.

Drug Interactions

Uterine relaxants interact with corticosteroids and may precipitate pulmonary edema. These agents are able to decrease effectiveness when given with a β-adrenergic blocking drug such as propranolol.

DRUGS USED IN THE TREATMENT OF SEXUALLY TRANSMITTED DISEASES

Sexually transmitted diseases (STDs) commonly include gonorrhea, chlamydia, syphilis, genital herpes and warts, and trichomoniasis. All of these diseases are spread by sexual contact. Overall, STDs are on the increase, attributable to more people engaging in premarital sex, higher divorce

TABLE 17-5 Common Sexually Transmitted Diseases

Infection	Cause	Cure or Treatment
Chlamydia	Chlamydia C. trachomatis	Antimicrobial therapy such as azithromycin; to eradicate, retesting is necessary
Genital Herpes	Virus Herpes simplex 2 (HSV-2)	No cure; treatment with antiviral drugs such as oral acyclovir, which reduces activity and shedding
Genital Warts	Virus Human papillomavirus (HPV)	Rarely cured; warts can be removed
Gonorrhea	Bacterium N. gonorrhoeae	Antibacterial drugs such as penicillin or ceftriaxone plus doxycycline; there are some drug-resistant strains; to eradicate, retesting is necessary
Syphilis	Bacterium T. pallidum	Penicillin G (long-acting); to eradicate, retesting is necessary
Trichomoniasis	Protozoa T. vaginalis	Antimicrobial drugs such as metronidazole

rates, and increased numbers of sexual partners. The avoidance of using contraceptive devices is a common factor that leads to STDs being transmitted. Other infections, such as hepatitis B and HIV, can also be spread through sexual contact.

Many STDs are asymptomatic, and a person may be unaware that they are carrying a disease. In addition, certain infections may be transmitted from an infected woman to her fetus or newborn. Recurrent infections due to a lack of immunity to many STDs occur frequently, and an individual may have more than one STD at a given time. See Table 17-5 for a list of common STD infections, their causes, and their treatments.

MALE SEX HORMONES

The hypothalamus, anterior pituitary gland, and testes secrete hormones that control the reproductive functions of males. These hormones initiate and maintain the production of sperm cells, and oversee the development and maintenance of male secondary sex characteristics.

The hypothalamus secretes gonadotropin-releasing hormone, which enters blood vessels that lead to the anterior pituitary gland. LH and FSH are then released. Luteinizing hormone (LH) in males, also called interstitial cell-stimulating hormone (ICSH), promotes development of testicular interstitial cells, which in turn secrete male sex hormones. FSH stimulates the supporting cells of the seminiferous tubules to respond to the effects of the male sex hormone testosterone.

Androgens are secreted mainly in the interstitial tissue of the testes in the male, and secondarily in the adrenal glands of both sexes. Androgens include testosterone and androsterone. Inadequate production of androgens in the male may be due to pituitary malfunction. Testosterone stimulates the development of the male secondary sex characteristics, initiates the production of sperm, and enhances the functional capacity of the penis and accessory sex organs.

Mechanism of Action

Synthetic steroid compound with both androgenic and anabolic activity controls development and maintenance of secondary sexual characteristics (Table 17-6).

Indications

Male sex hormones are used for replacement therapy in androgen deficiency, for the treatment of hypogonadism and cryptorchidism, and for palliative treatment of certain metastatic breast carcinomas in women.

TABLE 17-6 Male Hormones

Generic Name	Trade Name	Route of Administration	Average Adult Dosage
Androgens			
fluoxymesterone	Halotestin®	PO	Males: hypogonadism 2.5–20 mg/day; females: breast cancer, 10–40 mg/day in div. doses
methyltestosterone	Android®	PO	Males: 10–50 mg/day or via buccal tablets, 5–25 mg/day; Females: 50–200 mg/day or via buccal tablets, 25–100 mg/day
testosterone cypionate (in oil)	Depo-Testosterone®	IM	Males: 50–200 mg/dose; Females: 200–400 mg/dose
testosterone enanthate	Delatest®	IM	50–400 mg q2–4 wk
testosterone gel	Androgel®	Topical	5–10 mg/day applied to any area of skin
testosterone transdermal system	Androderm®	Transdermal	One system applied/day
Anabolic Steroids			
nandrolone decanoate	(generic only)	IM	50–200 mg q1–4 wks
oxandrolone	Oxandrin®	PO	2.5 mg b.i.d. – q.i.d. up to 4 weeks (max: 20 mg/day)
oxymetholone	Anadrol-50®	PO	1–5 mg/kg/day
stanozolol	Winstrol®	PO	2 mg t.i.d. to 4 mg q.i.d. for 5 days; may reduce to 2 mg q.d. or q.o.d.
Androgen Hormone Inhibitor			
finasteride	Proscar®	PO	5 mg/day

Adverse Effects

Adverse effects of male hormones in males include gynecomastia, excessive frequency and duration of penile erection, oligospermia, hirsuitism, male pattern baldness, acne, increased or decreased libido, headache, anxiety, and depression. In females, adverse effects include amenorrhea, menstrual irregularities, inhibition of gonadotropin secretion, and virilization (deepening of the voice, clitoral enlargement, increased growth of facial and body hair, and male type baldness).

Contraindications and Precautions

Male hormones are contraindicated in patients with known hypersensitivity to any of its ingredients, in women during pregnancy and lactation, and in men with cancer of the breast or suspected cancer of the prostate. These agents are also contraindicated in patients with pituitary insufficiency, a history of myocardial infarction, hypercalcemia, prostatic hyperplasia, hepatic dysfunction, nephrosis, and in infants and young children. They should be used with caution in elderly patients, in diabetic patients, in those who have hypertension, coronary artery disease, renal disease, hypercholesterolemia and gynecomastia, and in prepubertal males.

Drug Interactions

Testosterone may decrease insulin requirements, and it may interact with oral anticoagulants and potentiate hypoprothrombinemia.

ANABOLIC STEROIDS

A number of compounds derived from or closely related to testosterone may exhibit considerable anabolic effects without causing significant androgenic effects. The anabolic agents, or steroids, are employed to promote weight gain in underweight individuals.

Mechanism of Action

The anabolic steroids are synthetic agents chemically similar to the androgens. These drugs promote tissue-building processes.

Indications

The anabolic steroids are prescribed for management of anemia of renal insufficiency and control of metastatic breast cancer in women.

Adverse Effects

Common adverse effects of anabolic steroids include muscle cramps, nausea, vomiting, diarrhea, anorexia, and abdominal fullness. Jaundice, hepatocellular neoplasms, an increased risk of atherosclerosis, excitation, and insomnia are the most serious adverse effects with prolonged use. Virilization in women is also the most common reaction associated with the use of anabolic steroids, especially when higher doses are used. Acne occurs often in all age groups in both sexes.

Contraindications and Precautions

Anabolic steroids are contraindicated in patients with a known hypersensitivity, serious cardiac disorder, liver impairment, and in men with prostate cancer or enlargement. These agents should not be used during

Key Concept

The use of anabolic steroids by young athletic individuals to promote an increase in muscle mass and strength is a real and dangerous problem. The abuse of anabolic steroids has caused death in young, healthy persons.

pregnancy (category X) and lactation. Anabolic steroids should be used cautiously in benign prostatic hypertrophy and in patients with a history of myocardial infarction.

Drug Interactions

Anabolic steroids may interact with anticoagulants and increase their effects. These agents may decrease insulin and sulfonylurea requirements.

ANDROGEN HORMONE INHIBITORS

Androgen hormone inhibitors such as finasteride (Propecia, Proscar) are synthetic substitutes that are known as antiandrogens.

Mechanism of Action

Finasteride prevents the conversion of testosterone into the potent steroid 5-alpha dihydrotestosterone in the prostate gland.

Indications

Finasteride is used in the treatment of benign prostatic hypertrophy. Androgen inhibitors are also used for the prevention of male pattern baldness in men with early signs of hair loss.

Adverse Effects

The adverse effects of finasteride are usually mild. In some patients, the adverse effects may be impotence, decreased libido, and a decreased volume of ejaculate.

Contraindications and Precautions

Finasteride is contraindicated in patients with hypersensitivity to these agents, in pregnant women (Category X), and during lactation. These agents should be used cautiously in patients with liver dysfunction.

Drug Interactions

Finasteride may antagonize the GI motility effects of metoclopramide.

SUMMARY

In females, the ovaries are the primary sites for synthesis and secretion of estrogen and progesterone hormones in women. These two hormones are under the influence of FSH and LH from the anterior pituitary gland and the hypothalamus. They produce ova and form endocrine secretions that initiate and maintain the secondary female sex characteristics. Estrogens can be used for the treatment of amenorrhea, dysfunctional uterine bleeding, hirsuitism, palliative treatment of breast cancer and prostate cancer, for relief of menopausal symptoms, and for the prevention of osteoporosis. Progesterone is used in irregular uterine bleeding, infertility, threatened or habitual abortion, endometriosis, premenstrual syndrome, and combined with estrogen for the treatment of amenorrhea.

The hypothalamus, anterior pituitary gland, and testes secrete hormones that control the reproductive functions of males. Male sex hormones include testosterone and androsterone. Male sex hormones are used for replacement therapy in androgen deficiency, for the treatment of hypogonadism and cryptorchidism, and for palliative treatment of certain metastatic breast carcinomas in women.

EXPLORING THE WEB

Visit *www.ahealthyme.com*

- Search for information on drugs used during labor.

Visit *www.healthline.com*

- Search for additional information on sex hormones.

Visit *www.healthywomen.org*

- From the health topics menu choose topics discussed in this chapter and research additional information to further your understanding of the chapter topics.

Visit *www.menopause-online.com*

- Click on treatments and look for additional information on pharmacological treatments used in the treatment of menopause.

Visit *www.nlm.nih.gov/medlineplus*

- Search for information on anabolic steroids and/or oral contraceptives. What additional information can you find on these topics?

REVIEW QUESTIONS

Multiple Choice

1. FSH and LH are released from which of the following organs?

   A. hypothalamus
   B. pituitary
   C. ovaries
   D. pancreas

2. Which of the following is the trade name of medroxyprogesterone?

   A. Gesterol
   B. Provera
   C. Norlutate
   D. Norlutin

3. Progesterone is produced in the corpus luteum, which is located in the:

   A. kidneys
   B. ovaries
   C. uterus
   D. testes

4. Which of the following agents is used for the treatment of amenorrhea, dysfunctional uterine bleeding, and hirsuitism?

   A. progesterone
   B. testosterone
   C. oxytocin
   D. estrogen

5. Which of the following hormones is a uterine stimulant?

   A. prolactin
   B. estrogens
   C. oxytocin
   D. insulin

6. Estrogen is contraindicated in which of the following conditions or diseases?

   A. breast cancer
   B. amenorrhea
   C. hirsuitism
   D. prostate cancer

7. Which of the following is the most serious adverse effect of progesterone?

   A. lethargy
   B. mental depression
   C. diplopia
   D. pulmonary embolism

8. All of the following are adverse effects of testosterone in males, except:

   A. penile erection
   B. gynecomastia

C. gigantism

D. oligospermia

9. Which of the following is an indication of anabolic steroids?

A. pernicious anemia

B. megaloblastic anemia

C. renal insufficiency anemia

D. prostatic hypertrophy

10. Which of the following hormones is responsible for the changes in the uterine endometrium during the second half of the menstrual cycle?

A. progesterone

B. estrogen

C. estrogen and progesterone

D. testosterone

11. Which of the following is an example of androgen hormone inhibitor?

A. medroxyprogesterone (Provera)

B. fluoxymesterone (Halotestin)

C. finasteride (Propecia)

D. methyltestosterone (Virilon)

12. Gonadotropin-releasing hormone is secreted from which of the following?

A. ovaries

B. hypothalamus

C. anterior pituitary

D. posterior pituitary

13. All of the following are adverse effects of estrogens, except:

A. weight gain

B. deepening of the voice

C. intolerance to contact lenses

D. amenorrhea

14. Which of the following is a trade name of progesterone?

A. Norlutin

B. Norlutate

C. Provera

D. Gesterol

15. All of the following statements are correct about minipills, except:

A. they contain no estrogen

B. they are taken cyclically

C. they do not suppress ovulation

D. they are taken continuously

Fill in the Blank

1. Young athletes often use anabolic steroids to promote an increase in
_____.

2. Androgens are secreted mainly in the _____ tissue of the testes in the male.

3. Inadequate production of androgens in the male may be due to _____ malfunction.

4. The use of estrogen-progestin combinations in a cyclic fashion generally results in the inhibition of _____ without preventing menstruation.

5. Estrogens are used for the treatment of amenorrhea, dysfunctional uterine bleeding and hirsuitism, as well as the palliative treatment of _____ and _____.

6. FSH is released from the _____ and gonadotropin-releasing hormone (GnRH) is released from the _____.

7. Depo-Provera is a long-acting _____.

Critical Thinking

A 16-year-old male patient has been prescribed testosterone cypionate (Depo-Testosterone) to treat hypogonadism (failure of the sexual organs to develop normally).

1. Why does this patient need this hormone?

2. How should the physician explain the effects of this hormone to the patient?

3. What are the common adverse effects of male hormones such as testosterone cypionate?

Diuretics

OBJECTIVES

After completing this chapter, the reader should be able to:

1. Explain the main function of the urinary system.

2. Identify different sections of the nephron.

3. Describe and compare the five types of diuretics.

4. Explain the mechanisms of drug action and important adverse effects of loop diuretics.

5. Explain the contraindications of thiazide diuretics.

6. Describe the use of osmotic diuretics.

7. Identify the major diuretic groups used in the treatment of different disorders or conditions.

8. Explain the mechanisms of action of the carbonic anhydrase inhibitors.

9. Describe the most important indications for the use of loop diuretics.

10. Explain potassium-sparing diuretics.

GLOSSARY

Anuria – inability to produce urine

Diuretic – a drug that increases the secretion of urine from the kidneys

Gynecomastia – enlargement of breast tissue in males

Hyperkalemia – high blood level of potassium

Hypokalemia – low blood level of potassium

Hyponatremia – low blood level of sodium

Hypotonic – having a lesser osmotic pressure than a reference solution

Impotence – inability to achieve or maintain penile erection

OVERVIEW

The kidneys are the major organs of the body involved with water balance. They have the ability to regulate their output according to the amount of fluid ingested, and the amounts lost from the body by other routes. In conditions such as hypertension, heart failure, liver disorders, or kidney disorders, fluid may accumulate in the body's tissues and diuretics should be used.

Diuretics are mainly used to remove the excess extracellular fluid from the body that can result in edema (abnormal fluid accumulation) of the tissues, and in hypertension. These conditions occur in diseases of the heart, liver, and kidneys. In order to understand the action of diuretics, it is important to have some knowledge of the basic processes that take place in the nephron.

ANATOMY REVIEW

- The structures of the urinary system include two kidneys, two ureters, a bladder, and a urethra (Figures 18-1 and 18-2).

- The urinary system functions to remove waste materials from the body tissues and fluids, to maintain the acid-base balance, and to discharge the waste products from the body.

- The kidneys are the most important of the excretory organs. Kidney failure can result in the buildup of toxic wastes in the body and may lead to death (Figure 18-3).

- The nephron is the basic structural and functional unit of the kidney.

- The renal corpuscle is the site where the process of filtration occurs. In this process, blood pressure forces water and dissolved solutes out of the glomerular capillaries and into a chamber known as the capsular space (Figure 18-4).

- The formation of urine follows this path: blood enters the afferent arteriole → passes through the glomerulus → to Bowman's capsule → now it becomes filtrate (blood minus the red blood cells and plasma proteins) → continues through the proximal convoluted tubule → to the loop of Henle → to the distal convoluted tubule → to the collecting tubule (at this time about 99 percent of the filtrate has been reabsorbed) → approximately 1 mL of urine is formed per minute → the 1 mL of urine goes to the renal pelvis → to the ureter → to the bladder → to the urethra → to the urinary meatus.

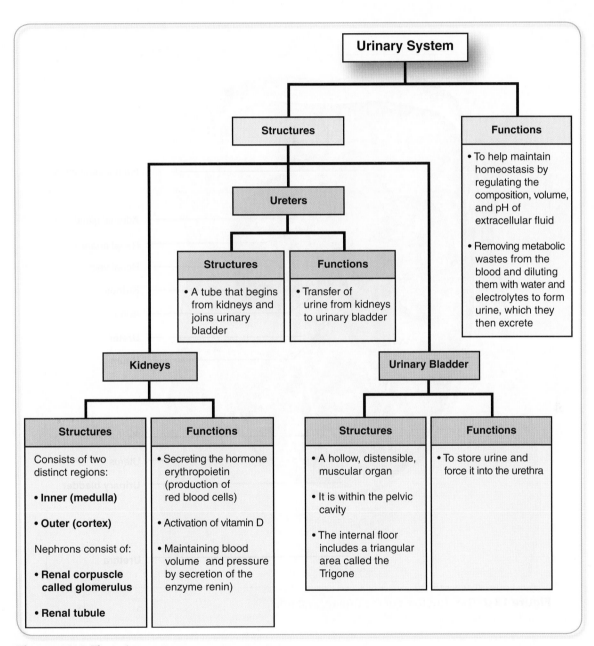

Figure 18-1 The urinary system.

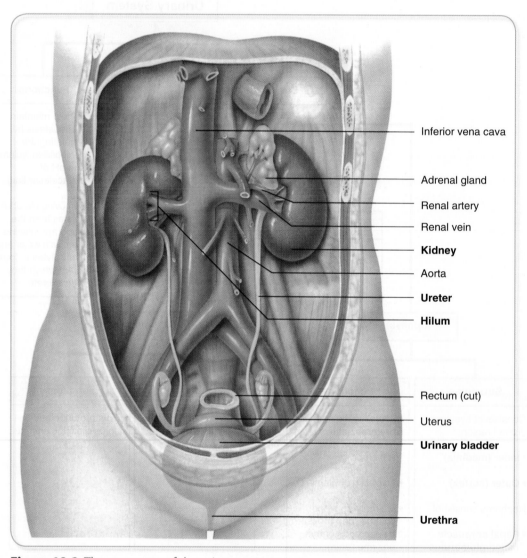

Inferior vena cava

Adrenal gland

Renal artery

Renal vein

Kidney

Aorta

Ureter

Hilum

Rectum (cut)

Uterus

Urinary bladder

Urethra

Figure 18-2 The structures of the urinary system.

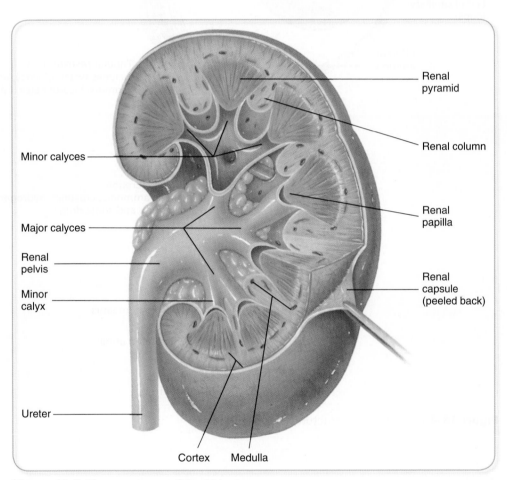

Figure 18-3 The structures of the kidney.

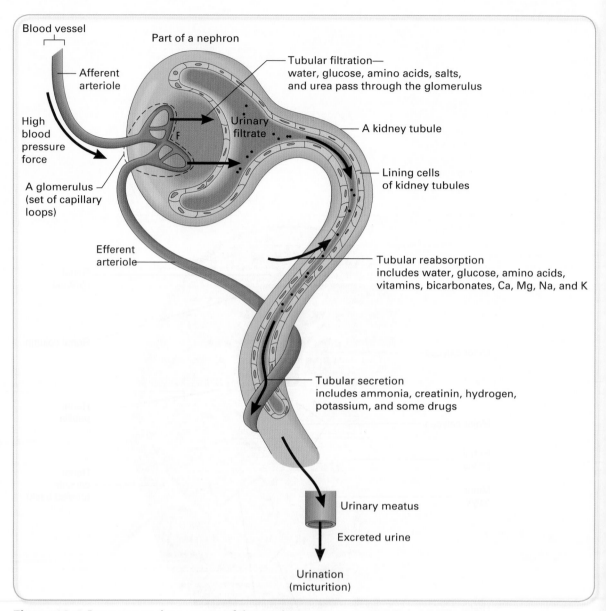

Figure 18-4 Processes and structures of the nephron.

DIURETICS

Diuretics are a group of drugs that promote water loss from the body into the urine. As urine formation takes place in the kidneys, it is not surprising that diuretics have their principal action at the level of the nephron. The action of some diuretics is not confined to their action on the kidneys: they also act elsewhere in the body.

Diuretic drugs are an important part of heart failure management. In heart failure, diuretics are primarily used to clear fluid overload and to sustain normal blood volume. Diuretics are divided into five categories according to their action: loop, thiazide and thiazide-like, potassium-sparing, osmotic, and

TABLE 18-1 Loop Diuretics

Generic Name	Trade Name	Route of Administration	Average Adult Dosage
bumetanide	Bumex®	PO	0.5–2 mg/day
ethacrynic acid	Edecrin®	PO	50–100 mg once or twice/day
furosemide	Lasix®	PO	20–80 mg/day
torsemide	Demadex®	PO, IV	10–20 mg once/day

carbonic anhydrase inhibitors. The type of diuretic used is determined by the condition being treated. For example, carbonic anhydrase inhibitors, such as acetazolamide (Diamox), which is recognized as a diuretic compound, are used to lower intraocular pressure.

Loop Diuretics

Good control of water balance is achieved by alterations in the permeability of the collecting duct system of the kidney to water by the presence of antidiuretic hormone (ADH) from the posterior pituitary gland. This is one of the major control systems for water balance, and slight interference here will completely upset the normal function of the kidney and result in a variation in urine output (Table 18-1).

Mechanism of Action

Loop diuretics act on the medullary part of the ascending limb of the loop (loop of Henle) of the nephron. These drugs inhibit the reabsorption of chloride and sodium ions from the loop into the interstitial fluid. The result is that the interstitial fluid becomes relatively **hypotonic** (having a lower osmotic pressure than water).

Indications

Loop diuretics are used in patients with edematous states and can be given intravenously for immediate action. The most important indications for the use of loop diuretics include acute pulmonary edema, other edematous conditions, and acute hypercalcemia. These agents can also be used in patients with hypertension, but other types of diuretics are probably better in most of these patients. In renal failure, they can also be effective in helping to normalize urine output. Loop diuretics, such as furosemide, are potent but relatively short-acting diuretics used in the management of severe chronic heart failure. They are also useful in the treatment of acute heart failure.

Key Concept

Loop diuretics are the most efficacious diuretic agents available and are rapidly absorbed.

Key Concept

Routine administration of loop diuretics, and probably all diuretics, should be done before late afternoon to avoid severe nocturnal enuresis (bedwetting).

Adverse Effects

A major problem of loop diuretics is the loss of electrolytes from the body. Potassium and sodium are the main ions affected. Potassium loss often leads to hypokalemia, which can result in abnormal cardiac rhythms and even death. Other electrolyte changes can occur, especially with high doses of loop diuretics, and the periodic assessment of blood calcium and magnesium levels is required. Uric acid levels may rise during loop diuretic therapy, which can be problematic for people with gout.

Contraindications and Precautions

Loop diuretics are contraindicated in patients with known hypersensitivity to these drugs. Loop diuretics should be avoided in patients with **anuria** (inability to produce urine), hepatic coma, severe electrolyte deficiency, and during lactation or pregnancy (category C).

Loop diuretics should be used with caution in older adults, cardiac patients, and patients with hepatic cirrhosis, diabetes mellitus, history of gout, and pulmonary edema associated with acute myocardial infarction.

Drug Interactions

Loop diuretics may increase the effectiveness of the anticoagulants or the thrombolytics. Loop diuretics may increase the risk of glycoside toxicity and ototoxicity if taken with an aminoglycoside. Plasma levels of propranolol can increase when the drug is given with furosemide.

Thiazide and Thiazide-like Diuretics

Thiazide diuretics are a group of drugs that are chemically similar and the most commonly prescribed class of diuretics. All of the thiazide diuretics have equivalent effectiveness (Table 18-2).

Mechanism of Action

Thiazide drugs act on the cortical segment of the ascending loop and the distal convoluted tubules of the nephron, and decrease sodium reabsorption. This results in a more concentrated fluid entering the collecting ducts, and therefore decreases water reabsorption and results in a diuresis. Thiazide diuretics have an effect on the peripheral arterioles, which results in vasodilation. This, combined with their diuretic effects, makes them particularly suitable in hypertensive patients (see Chapter 13). This action of these drugs is not completely understood.

Indications

Thiazide diuretics are still considered to be in the front line for the treatment of mild to moderate hypertension either on their own or combined,

---

Medical Terminology Review

hypokalemia
hypo = low
kalemia = blood levels of potassium
low levels of potassium in the blood

Key Concept

The optimum therapeutic effects of thiazide are seen in 15 to 30 minutes when given intravenously. When given orally, thiazide diuretics may take as long as four weeks to be effective.

TABLE 18-2 Thiazide and Thiazide-like Diuretics

Generic Name	Trade Name	Route of Administration	Average Adult Dosage
Thiazide Diuretics			
bendroflumethiazide	Naturetin®	PO	2.5–20 mg, 1–2 times/day
chlorothiazide sodium	Diuril®	PO	250 mg–1 g, 1–2 times/day
hydrochlorothiazide	Esidrix®, HCTZ®	PO	12.5–100 mg, 1–3 times/day
hydroflumethiazide	Diucardin®, Saluron®	PO	25–100 mg, 1–2 times/day
methyclothiazide	Aquatensin®, Enduron®	PO	2.5–10 mg/day
metolazone	Mykrox®	PO	5–20 mg/day
polythiazide	Renese®	PO	1–4 mg/day
trichlormethiazide	Diurese®, Metahydrin®	PO	1–4 mg, 1–2 times/day
Thiazide-like Diuretics			
chlorthalidone	Thalitone®, Hygroton®	PO	50–100 mg/day
indapamide	Lozol®	PO	2.5–5 mg/day

usually with a β-blocker. These drugs are also used to treat edema due to heart failure, liver disease, and corticosteroid or estrogen therapy.

Adverse Effects

Adverse effects of thiazide diuretics, as with loop diuretics, include potassium and sodium loss. Thiazide occasionally causes a rise in blood uric acid levels, which can be problematic in those predisposed to gout. Thiazide can also cause hyperglycemia, which is potentially dangerous in diabetics. Lactation can be suppressed, and thiazides have been used for this purpose. **Impotence** in men can also occur.

Other adverse effects of thiazide diuretics are dehydration, electrolyte imbalances, loss of appetite, dizziness, hypotension, increased sensitivity to sun exposure, and pruritus.

Contraindications and Precautions

Thiazide diuretics are contraindicated in patients with known hypersensitivity to these agents. These drugs are also contraindicated in patients with electrolyte imbalances, anuria, hepatic coma, and renal impairment. Thiazide diuretics should be given with caution during pregnancy (category C) and lactation, in children, and with liver or kidney impairment.

Drug Interactions

If thiazides are used with alcohol, nitrates, or other antihypertensive drugs, they may cause additive hypotensive effects. Anesthetic agents

TABLE 18-3   Potassium-sparing Diuretics

Generic Name	Trade Name	Route of Administration	Average Adult Dosage
amiloride hydrochloride	Midamor®	PO	5 mg/day
spironolactone	Aldactone®	PO	25–200 mg, 1–2 times/day
triamterene	Dyrenium®	PO	100 mg b.i.d.

may increase the effects of thiazides. The effects of anticoagulants may be decreased when given with thiazide diuretics.

Potassium-sparing Diuretics

There are two types of potassium-sparing diuretics, the aldosterone antagonists and those independent of aldosterone. The best-known aldosterone antagonist is spironolactone. These agents are not very powerful as diuretics (see Table 18-3).

Mechanism of Action

Potassium-sparing diuretics (such as spironolactone) inhibit the action of aldosterone on the distal convoluted tubule of the nephron. Aldosterone is the sodium-retaining hormone secreted from the adrenal cortex. If it acts on the distal tubule, the body retains more sodium ions, and water is passively conserved at the same time. When sodium is retained by the nephron at this site, potassium is lost. Therefore, if aldosterone is blocked, potassium is retained and sodium is lost along with a slight increase in diuresis.

> **Key Concept**
>
> *Overall, spironolactone has a rather slow onset of action, requiring several days before full therapeutic effect is achieved.*

Indications

Potassium-sparing diuretics are not usually required for patients who are on loop or thiazide diuretics. Spironolactone has proved to be of tremendous value in the treatment of congestive heart failure.

Adverse Effects

Adverse effects that occur with this type of diuretic are related to their mode of action, and include **hyperkalemia**, acute renal failure, kidney stones, and **hyponatremia**. In men, spironolactone can produce **gynecomastia** due to its estrogenic effect.

Contraindications and Precautions

Potassium-sparing diuretics are contraindicated in patients with hypersensitivity to these drugs, anuria, acute renal insufficiency, and hyperkalemia,

TABLE 18-4 Osmotic Diuretics

Generic Name	Trade Name	Route of Administration	Average Adult Dosage
glycerin	Glycerol®, Osmoglyn®	PO	1–1.8 g/kg given 1–1.5 h before ocular surgery
mannitol	Osmitrol®	IV	100 g as a 10–20% solution over 2–6 h
urea	Ureaphil®	IV	1–1.5 g/kg of 30% solution infused slowly over 1 to 2.5 h

and during pregnancy (category D) or lactation. Potassium-sparing diuretics should be used cautiously in patients with impaired kidney or liver function, history of gouty arthritis, diabetes mellitus, or history of kidney stones.

Drug Interactions

Alcohol, nitrate, and other antihypertensive agents may have increased hypotensive effects when a potassium-sparing diuretic is given. Potassium-sparing diuretics may cause severe hyperkalemia when potassium preparations are also given.

Osmotic Diuretics

Osmotic diuretic drugs are capable of being filtered by the glomerulus, but have a limited capability of being reabsorbed into the bloodstream (see Table 18-4).

Mechanism of Action

Osmotic diuretics work by directly interfering with osmosis. Any substance that enters the body in large enough quantities and is excreted via the kidneys will lead to water being kept in the renal tubules, leading to water loss. This is due to maintenance of a high osmotic pressure in the tubules.

Indications

Osmotic diuretics can be used to reduce increased intracranial pressure and to promote prompt removal of renal toxins. These agents can be used to maintain urine volume and to prevent anuria.

Adverse Effects

Adverse effects of osmotic diuretics include electrolyte imbalance and the potential for dehydration. This potential for dehydration is similar to that which would occur from the drinking of seawater.

Contraindications and Precautions

Osmotic diuretics are contraindicated in patients with known hypersensitivity to these drugs. Osmotic diuretics should be avoided in

patients with severe dehydration, anuria, and electrolyte imbalances. Mannitol is contraindicated in patients with intracranial bleeding.

Osmotic diuretics should be used with caution in patients with electrolyte imbalances or renal impairment. Osmotic diuretics must be given cautiously to pregnant women (category C) and during lactation.

Drug Interactions

Osmotic diuretics increase urinary excretion of lithium, salicylates, barbiturates, potassium, and imipramine.

Carbonic Anhydrase Inhibitors

When a patient is taking carbonic anhydrase inhibitors, it is important that their fluid input, fluid output, glucose levels, and electrolyte levels be monitored. See Table 18-5 for these agents.

Mechanism of Action

Carbonic anhydrase is an enzyme that speeds up the conversion of carbon dioxide into bicarbonate ions and vice versa, according to the following equation:

$$CO_2 + H_2O \leftrightarrow H_2CO_3 \leftrightarrow H^+ + HCO_3^-$$

This reaction occurs in the kidney as well as in other parts of the body. In the kidney, the reaction occurs mainly in the proximal tubule and, as it involves bicarbonate loss, is concerned with acid-base balance. The tubular cells are not very permeable to bicarbonate ions or carbonic acid, but are very permeable to carbon dioxide. Under normal circumstances, carbonic anhydrase in the tubular cell converts the carbonic acid into carbon dioxide and water, which are promptly reabsorbed. If the enzyme is inhibited, there will be a net loss of bicarbonate from the body with a consequent loss of

TABLE 18-5   Carbonic Anhydrase Inhibitors

Generic Name	Trade Name	Route of Administration	Average Adult Dosage
acetazolamide	Diamox®	PO, IM, IV	For glaucoma: PO: 250 mg 1–4 times/day, 500 mg sustained release b.i.d.; IM/IV: 500 mg, may repeat in 2–4 h; For edema: PO: 250–375 mg every AM (5 mg/kg)
dichlorphenamide	Daranide®, Oratrol®	PO	100–200 mg, 1–2 times/day
methazolamide	Neptazane®	PO	50–100 mg b.i.d.-tid

water. The drug acetazolamide is a non-competitive inhibitor of this enzyme, and has been used as a diuretic.

Indications

The carbonic anhydrase inhibitors are used in the treatment of open-angle glaucoma, secondary glaucoma, and preoperative treatment of acute closed-angle glaucoma. These agents are also prescribed in the treatment of edema resulting from congestive heart failure, and drug-induced edema.

Adverse Effects

Carbonic anhydrase inhibitors may cause acidosis (a clinical state where the pH of the blood drops significantly, below 7.35), renal stones, hypokalemia, drowsiness (following large doses), and hypersensitivity reactions.

Contraindications and Precautions

Carbonic anhydrase inhibitors are contraindicated in patients with known hypersensitivity, anuria, severe renal or liver impairment, and imbalance of electrolytes.

Carbonic anhydrase inhibitors should be used cautiously in patients with kidney impairment, and during lactation and pregnancy (category C).

These drugs need to be given with caution in patients with respiratory acidosis, emphysema, or chronic respiratory disease as diuresis can be diminished in the presence of acidotic conditions.

Drug Interactions

Carbonic anhydrase inhibitors interact with renal excretion of amphetamines, ephedrine, quinidine, and procainamide. Carbonic anhydrase inhibitors may decrease the effects of tricyclic antidepressants, thereby enhancing or prolonging their effects. These diuretics also decrease the renal excretion of lithium.

SUMMARY

Diuretics have their principal action at the level of the kidneys' nephrons. These drugs are mainly used to remove the excess extracellular fluid from the body that can result in edema of the tissues and in hypertension. The urinary system has three major functions: excretion, elimination, and homeostatic regulation of the volume of blood plasma.

Diuretic drugs are an important part of heart failure, hypertension, and edema management. These agents are divided into five categories according to their action: loops, thiazide and thiazide-like, potassium-sparing, osmotic, and carbonic anhydrase inhibitors.

Loop diuretics are major controllers for water balance and result in a variation in urine output. Thiazide and thiazide-like diuretics are the most commonly prescribed types of diuretics. The best-known potassium-sparing diuretic is spironolactone, which is an aldosterone antagonist. Osmotic diuretics work by directly interfering with osmosis, which leads the kidneys to keeping water in the renal tubules, resulting in water loss. Carbonic anhydrase is an enzyme that speeds up the conversion of carbon dioxide into bicarbonate ions and vice versa. If the enzyme is inhibited, there will be a net loss of bicarbonate from the body with a consequent loss of water.

EXPLORING THE WEB

Visit *http://nephron.com*

- Explore articles related to the types of diuretics discussed in this chapter.

Visit *www.mayoclinic.com* and *www.medicinenet.com*

- Look for information related to diuretics.

REVIEW QUESTIONS

Multiple Choice

1. Thiazides are contraindicated in patients with all of the following conditions, except:

   A. impaired liver function
   B. edema caused by heart failure
   C. diabetes
   D. a history of gout

2. Which of the following substances may alter the permeability of the collecting duct of the nephron to water?

    A. antidiuretic hormone
    B. insulin
    C. vitamin C
    D. calcitonin

3. Which of the following is the major problem with the loop diuretics?

    A. decrease of uric acid
    B. hyperkalemia
    C. loss of glucose from the kidneys
    D. loss of electrolytes from the body

4. Thiazide drugs act on which of the following segments of the nephron?

    A. descending loop
    B. ascending loop
    C. proximal convoluted tubule
    D. collecting duct

5. Which of the following is an aldosterone antagonist?

    A. mannitol
    B. furosemide
    C. spironolactone
    D. acetazolamide

6. Which of the following is a trade name of acetazolamide?

    A. Osmitrol®
    B. Diamox®
    C. Ureaphil®
    D. Aldactone®

7. Diuretics are mainly used in which of the following?

    A. diabetes
    B. encephalitis
    C. hepatitis B
    D. hypertension

8. Which of the following diuretics are used in the treatment of open-angle glaucoma?

    A. carbonic anhydrase inhibitors
    B. potassium-sparing diuretics
    C. thiazide and thiazide-like diuretics
    D. loop diuretics

9. Which of the following time periods are required for optimum therapeutic effects of orally administered thiazides?

    A. 15 to 30 minutes
    B. 2 to 4 days
    C. 1 to 2 weeks
    D. 3 to 4 weeks

10. The most commonly used osmotic drug is:

    A. ethacrynic acid
    B. furosemide
    C. mannitol
    D. torsemide

11. Carbonic anhydrase inhibitors must be used with caution in pregnant women and are classified as:

    A. category D
    B. category C
    C. category B
    D. category A

12. The mechanism of action of mannitol (a carbonic anhydrase inhibitor) affects which of the following parts of the nephron?

    A. proximal tubule
    B. ascending loop
    C. distal tubule
    D. collecting duct

13. The generic name of Osmoglyn® is which of the following?

    A. isosorbide
    B. mannitol
    C. glycerin
    D. acetazolamide

14. Which of the following organs temporarily stores urine?

    A. kidney
    B. ureter
    C. urethra
    D. bladder

15. A capillary network of renal corpuscles is called:

    A. Bowman's capsule
    B. Henle tubule
    C. proximal convoluted tubule
    D. glomerulus

Matching

_____ **1.** acetazolamide   **A.** Lasix

_____ **2.** mannitol   **B.** Aldactone

_____ **3.** indapamide   **C.** Hygroton

_____ **4.** ethacrynic acid   **D.** Edecrin

_____ **5.** chlorthalidone   **E.** Osmitrol

_____ **6.** furosemide   **F.** Lozol

_____ **7.** spironolactone   **G.** Diamox

Critical Thinking

A 25-year-old male patient is admitted to the intensive care unit (ICU) following a car-train collision. The patient sustained a depressed skull fracture and is on a ventilator. Two days after surgery, there are obvious signs of increasing intracranial pressure. The nurse administers mannitol (Osmitrol®) intravenously over 30 minutes. The patient's wife asks his physician to explain why her husband needs this drug.

1. What explanation should the physician offer?

2. If the patient shows symptoms of intracranial bleeding, what would be the explanation that the physician should give for discontinuing the drug?

Critical Thinking

A 25-year-old male patient is admitted to the intensive care unit (ICU) following a car crash collision. The patient sustained a depressed skull fracture and is on a ventilator. Two days after surgery, there are obvious signs of increasing intracranial pressure. The nurse administers mannitol (Osmitrol) intravenously over 30 minutes. The patient's wife asks his physician to explain why her husband needs this drug.

1. What explanation should the physician offer?

2. If the patient shows symptoms of intracranial bleeding, what would be the explanation that the physician should give for discontinuing the drug?

SECTION III

PHARMACOLOGY FOR DISORDERS AFFECTING MULTI-BODY SYSTEMS

Vitamins, Minerals, and Nutritional Supplements

OBJECTIVES

After completing this chapter, the reader should be able to:

1. Identify characteristics that differentiate vitamins from other nutrients.
2. Describe the functions of common vitamins and minerals.
3. Classify vitamins and minerals.
4. Explain trace elements and their major effects on the body.
5. Describe the role of vitamin and mineral therapies in the treatment of deficiency disorders.
6. Define pharma food.
7. Explain the rationale behind food labeling.
8. Describe the purposes of additives in foods and supplements.
9. Explain the major complication of total parenteral nutrition therapy.
10. Define pernicious anemia, keratomalacia, osteomalacia, and cheilosis.

GLOSSARY

Ascorbic acid – a water-soluble vitamin that is essential for the formation of collagen and fibroid tissue for teeth, bones, cartilage, connective tissue, and skin; also known as vitamin C

Ataxia – loss of the ability to coordinate muscular movement

Beriberi – a deficiency caused by deficiency of thiamine, characterized by neurological symptoms, cardiovascular abnormalities, and edema

Biotin – a water-soluble B complex vitamin that aids in fatty acid production, and in the oxidation of fatty acids and carbohydrates; also known as vitamin B_7

Cachexia – weight loss, wasting of muscle, loss of appetite, and general debility that can occur during a chronic disease

Calciferol – a fat-soluble vitamin chemically related to steroids; calciferol is essential for the normal formation of bones and teeth and important for the absorption of calcium and phosphorus from the GI tract; also known as vitamin D;

Calcium (Ca) – the fifth-most abundant element in the human body, present mainly in the bones

Carotenoids – any of a class of yellow to red pigments, including the carotenes and xanthophylls

Cheilosis – fissures on the lips caused by deficiency of riboflavin

Chloride (Cl) – involved in the maintenance of fluid and the body's acid-base balance

Copper (Cu) – important for the synthesis of hemoglobin because it is part of a co-enzyme involved in its synthesis; also a component of several important enzymes in the body, and essential to good health

Cretinism – arrested physical and mental development with dystrophy of bones and soft tissues due to congenital lack of thyroid secretion

Cyanocobalamin – a water-soluble substance that is the common pharmaceutic form of vitamin B_{12}; involved in the metabolism of protein, fats, and carbohydrates, and also in normal blood formation and neural function

Electrolytes – compounds, particularly salts, that when dissolved in water or another solvent, dissociate into ions and are able to conduct an electric current

Enteral nutrition (EN) – feeding by tube directly into the patient's digestive tract

Fluorine – a chemical element that is used as a diagnostic aid in various tissue scans

Folic acid – essential for cell growth and the reproduction of red blood cells; also known as vitamin B_9

Food additive – any substance that becomes part of a food product

Hemolysis – the destruction or dissolution of red blood cells, with release of hemoglobin

Hypervitaminosis – an abnormal condition resulting from excessive intake of toxic amounts of one or more vitamins, especially over a long period

Hydroxocobalamin – is involved in the metabolism of protein, fats, and carbohydrates, aids in hemoglobin synthesis, is essential for normal functioning of all cells, and is important in energy metabolism; also known as vitamin B_{12}

Hyperalimentation (total parenteral nutrition) – also known as "TPN", this treatment is used to supply complete nutrition to patients when the enteral route cannot be used; all needed nutrients are injected into the body intravenously

Hypomagnesemia – an abnormally low level of magnesium in the blood

Hypovitaminosis – a condition related to the deficiency of one or more vitamins

Intrinsic factor – a substance that is secreted by the gastric mucus membrane and is essential for the absorption of vitamin B_{12} in the intestines

Iodine – an essential micronutrient of the thyroid hormone (thyroxine)

Iron (Fe) – a common metallic element essential for the formation of hemoglobin and myoglobin, as well as the transfer of oxygen to the body tissues

Keratomalacia – a condition, usually in children with vitamin A deficiency, characterized by softening, ulceration, and perforation of the cornea

Magnesium – an important ion for the function of many enzyme systems, and is the second most abundant action of the intracellular fluids in the body

Menadione – a water-soluble injectable form of the product of vitamin K_3

Minerals – inorganic substances occurring naturally in the earth's crust having characteristic chemical compositions

Niacin – contains parts of two enzymes that regulate energy metabolism and is essential for a healthy skin, tongue, and digestive system; also known as vitamin B_3 or nicotinic acid

Nicotinic acid – contains parts of two enzymes that regulate energy metabolism and is essential for a healthy skin, tongue, and digestive system; also known as niacin or vitamin B_3

Osteomalacia – a disease in which the bone softens and becomes brittle

Pantothenic acid – a member of the vitamin B complex widely distributed in plant and animal tissues and that may be an important element in human nutrition; also known as vitamin B_5

Pellagra – a disease caused by a deficiency of niacin and protein in the diet, characterized by skin eruptions, digestive and nervous system disturbances, and eventual mental deterioration

Pharma food – a system of receiving nourishment by breathing in nutritional microparticles

Phosphorus – is essential for the metabolism of protein, calcium, and glucose, aids in building strong bones and teeth, and helps in the regulation of the body's acid-base balance

Potassium – the major electrolyte in intracellular fluids, helping to regulate neuromuscular excitability and muscle contraction

Pyridoxine – a water-soluble vitamin that is part of the B complex and acts as a co-enzyme essential for the synthesis and breakdown of amino acids; also known as vitamin B_6

Retinol – a fat-soluble vitamin essential for skeletal growth, maintenance of normal mucosal epithelium, reproduction, and visual acuity; also known as vitamin A

Riboflavin – one of the heat-stable components of the B complex, it is involved as a co-enzyme in the oxidative processes of carbohydrates, fats, and proteins; also known as vitamin B_2

Rickets – a deficiency disease resulting from a lack of vitamin D or calcium and from insufficient exposure to sunlight, characterized by defective bone growth and occurring mostly in children

Sodium – one of the most important elements in the body; sodium ions are involved in acid-base balance, water balance, transmission of nerve impulses, and contraction of muscles

Sulfur – necessary to all body tissues and is found in all body cells

Thiamine – a water-soluble, crystalline compound of the B complex, essential for normal metabolism and health of the cardiovascular and nervous systems; also known as vitamin B_1

Tocopherol – a fat-soluble vitamin essential for normal reproduction, muscle development, resistance of erythrocytes to hemolysis, and various other biochemical functions; also known as vitamin E

Xerophthalmia – extreme dryness of the conjunctiva resulting from an eye disease or from a systemic deficiency of vitamin A

Vitamins – organic compounds essential in small quantities for physiologic and metabolic functioning of the body

Vitamin A – a fat-soluble vitamin essential for skeletal growth, maintenance of normal mucosal epithelium, reproduction, and visual acuity; also known as retinol

Vitamin B_1 – a water-soluble, crystalline compound of the B complex, essential for normal metabolism and health of the cardiovascular and nervous systems; also known as thiamine

Vitamin B_2 – one of the heat-stable components of the B complex, it is involved as a co-enzyme in the oxidative processes of carbohydrates, fats, and proteins; also known as riboflavin

Vitamin B_3 – contains parts of two enzymes that regulate energy metabolism and is essential for a healthy skin, tongue, and digestive system; also known as niacin or nicotinic acid

Vitamin B_5 – a member of the vitamin B complex widely distributed in plant and animal tissues and that may be an important element in human nutrition; also known as pantothenic acid

Vitamin B_6 – a water-soluble vitamin that is part of the B complex and acts as a co-enzyme essential for the synthesis and breakdown of amino acids; also known as pyridoxine

Vitamin B_7 – a water-soluble B complex vitamin that aids in fatty acid production, and in the oxidation of fatty acids and carbohydrates; also known as biotin

Vitamin B_9 – essential for cell growth and the reproduction of red blood cells; also known as folic acid

Vitamin B_{12} – is involved in the metabolism of protein, fats, and carbohydrates, aids in hemoglobin synthesis, is essential for normal functioning of all cells, and is important in energy metabolism; also known as cyanocobalamin

Vitamin B complex – a pharmaceutical term applied to drug products containing a mixture of the B vitamins, usually B_1 (thiamine), B_2 (riboflavin), B_3 (nicotinamide), and B_6 (pyridoxine)

Vitamin C – a water-soluble vitamin that is essential for the formation of collagen and fibroid tissue for teeth, bones, cartilage, connective tissue, and skin; also known as ascorbic acid

Vitamin D – a fat-soluble vitamin chemically related to steroids that is essential for the normal formation of bones and teeth and important for the absorption of calcium and phosphorus from the GI tract; also known as calciferol

Vitamin E – a fat-soluble vitamin essential for normal reproduction, muscle development, resistance of erythrocytes to hemolysis, and various other biochemical functions; also known as tocopherol

Vitamin K – essential for the synthesis of prothrombin in the liver

Zinc (Zn) – a trace element that is essential several body enzymes, growth, glucose tolerance, wound healing, and taste acuity

OVERVIEW

Vitamins and minerals are required for maintaining normal function and, more important, they are essential for life. The body cannot synthesize vitamins and minerals, and relies on outside sources to provide daily requirements. The vitamins and minerals the body needs come either from the foods we eat or from supplements. Vitamins are considered "natural substances" and food additives rather than drugs. However, niacin and vitamin K are indicated as drugs to affect cholesterol reduction and blood clotting. The vitamin, mineral, and supplement business is a multimillion-dollar industry in the U.S. Some conditions that affect a patient's health are greatly benefited by the use of nutritional supplements. Pharmacy technicians are asked many questions about foods and nutrition, including specific questions about which products or supplements a client may be considering for purchase, and what amount of product to ingest.

VITAMINS

Vitamins are organic compounds essential in small quantities for physiologic and metabolic functioning of the body. With few exceptions, vitamins cannot be synthesized by the body and must be obtained from the diet or dietary supplements. No one food contains all the vitamins. Vitamin deficiency diseases produce specific symptoms that are usually alleviated by the administration of the appropriate vitamin. Vitamins are classified according to their fat or water solubility, their physiological effects, or their chemical structures. They are designated by alphabetic letters and chemical or other specific names. The fat-soluble vitamins are A, D, E, and K; the B complex and C vitamins are water-soluble.

An abnormal condition resulting from excessive intake of toxic amounts of one or more vitamins, especially over a long period, is called **hypervitaminosis**. Serious effects may result from overdoses of fat-soluble vitamins A, D, E, or K, but adverse reactions are less likely with the water-soluble B and C vitamins, except when taken in megadoses. **Hypovitaminosis** may occur due to a deficiency of one or more vitamins. Examples of diseases or conditions caused by hypovitaminosis include avitaminosis, **beriberi**, malnutrition, scurvy, rickets, scorbutus, and moon blindness.

Fat-soluble Vitamins

Each of the fat-soluble vitamins A, D, E, and K has a distinct and separate physiological role. For the most part, they are absorbed with other lipids, and efficient absorption requires the presence of bile and pancreatic juice. They are transported to the liver, and stored in various body tissues. They are not normally excreted in the urine. Table 19-1 provides a summary of the fat-soluble vitamins, sources, functions, and deficiencies or toxicities.

TABLE 19-1 Fat-soluble Vitamins

Name	Food Sources	Functions	Deficiency/Toxicity
Fat-soluble vitamins			
Vitamin A (retinol)	**Animal**	Maintenance of vision in dim light	**Deficiency**
	• Liver	Maintenance of mucous membranes and healthy skin	Night blindness
	• Whole milk	Growth and development of bones	Xerophthalmia
	• Butter	Reproduction	Respiratory infections
	• Cream	Healthy immune system	Bone growth ceases
	• Cod liver oil		
	Plants		**Toxicity**
	• Dark green leafy vegetables		Birth defects Bone pain
	• Deep yellow or orange fruit		Anorexia
	• Fortified margarine		Enlargement of liver
Vitamin D (calciferol)	**Animal**	Regulation of absorption of calcium and phosphorus	**Deficiency**
	• Eggs	Building and maintenance of normal bones and teeth	Rickets
	• Liver	Prevention of tetany	Osteomalacia
	• Fortified milk		Osteoporosis
	• Fortified margarine		Poorly developed teeth and bones
	• Oily fish		Muscle spasms
	Plants		**Toxicity**
	• None		Kidney stones
	Sunlight		Calcification of soft tissues

(continues)

TABLE 19-1 Fat-soluble Vitamins—*continued*

Name	Food Sources	Functions	Deficiency/ Toxicity
Vitamin E (tocopherol)	**Animal**	Antioxidant	**Deficiency**
	• None	Considered essential for protection of cell structure, especially of red blood cells	Destruction of red blood cells
	Plants		**Toxicity**
	• Green and leafy vegetables		No toxicity has been reported
	• Margarines		
	• Salad dressing		
	• Wheat germ and wheat germ oils		
	• Vegetable oils		
	• Nuts		

Vitamin A

Vitamin A (retinol) is one of the fat-soluble vitamins and is essential for skeletal growth, maintenance of normal mucosal epithelium, and visual acuity. Normal stores can last up to one year but are rapidly depleted by stress. Vitamin A has essential roles in the development of vision, bone growth, the maintenance of epithelial tissue, the immunological process, and normal reproduction. Retinol is not found in plant products but fortunately most plants contain a substance called **carotenoids**, which act as provitamins and can be converted into retinol in the intestinal wall and liver. The principal carotenoid in plants is beta-carotene, which gets its name from carrots. Deficiency leads to atrophy of epithelial tissue, resulting in **keratomalacia**, **xerophthalmia**, night blindness, growth retardation (in children), and lessened resistance to infection of the mucous membranes. Plasma vitamin A concentrations are reduced in patients with cystic fibrosis, alcohol-related cirrhosis, hepatic disease, and proteinuria. Plasma vitamin A concentrations are elevated in patients with chronic renal disease.

Toxicity can result from taking only ten times the recommended daily allowance (RDA) for several months. Symptoms of toxicity are varied, and can include excessive peeling of the skin, hyperlipidemia, hypercalcemia, and hepatotoxicity. Ultimately, death can result. An acute dose of about 200 mg can cause immediate toxicity, resulting in increased cerebrospinal pressure. This can cause severe headache, blurring of vision, and the bulging

of the fontanelles in infants. The use of vitamin A is contraindicated in hypervitaminosis A, oral use in malabsorption syndrome, hypersensitivity, and intravenous use.

Vitamin D

Vitamin D (calciferol) is another fat-soluble vitamin that is chemically related to steroids and essential for the normal formation of bones and teeth and for the absorption of calcium and phosphorus from the GI tract. Ultraviolet rays activate a form of cholesterol in an oil of the skin and convert it to a form of the vitamin, which is then absorbed. Vitamin D is considered a hormone. It is used for the prophylaxis and treatment of **rickets**, **osteomalacia**, and other hypocalcemic disorders (tetany) and hypoparathyroidism. Vitamin D_3 is the predominant form of vitamin D of animal origin. It is found in most fish-liver oils, butter, bran, and egg yolks. It is formed in skin exposed to sunlight or ultraviolet rays. Deficiency of the vitamin results in rickets in children, the destruction of bony tissue, and osteoporosis. Hypervitaminosis D produces a toxicity syndrome that may result in hypercalcemia, malabsorption (which can lead to constipation), kidney stones, and calcium deposits on bones. Vitamin D therapy is contraindicated in hypercalcemia, malabsorption syndrome, and renal dysfunction, or if an individual has evidence of vitamin D toxicity or abnormal sensitivity to the effects of vitamin D. Vitamin D_2 is also called ergocalciferol.

Vitamin E

Vitamin E (tocopherol) is a fat-soluble vitamin that is essential for normal reproduction, muscle development, and resistance of erythrocytes to **hemolysis**. It is an intracellular antioxidant and acts to maintain the stability of polyunsaturated fatty acids.

Deficiency of vitamin E is rare, but can lead to anemia in babies, especially if premature. In adults, erythrocytes may have a shortened lifespan, which may result in muscle degeneration of vascular system abnormalities and kidney damage.

Vitamin E is relatively non-toxic, and may cause problems only in the large-dosage range of about 300 mg per day (RDA is only 10 mg per day). At this range, interference with thyroid function and a prolonging of blood clotting time may occur. Sources of vitamin E include vegetable oils such as soybean, corn, cottonseed, and safflower, as well as nuts, seeds, and wheat germ.

Vitamin K

Vitamin K is essential for the synthesis of prothrombin in the liver. The naturally occurring forms, also called quinones, are vitamin K_1 (phylloquinone), which occurs in green plants, and vitamin K_2 (menaquinone), which is

---

Medical Terminology Review

osteoporosis

osteo = bone
poro = cavity; porousness
sis = state; condition
porous state of bones

Key Concept

Inadequate exposure to sunlight and low dietary intake are usually necessary for the development of clinical vitamin D deficiency.

formed as the result of bacterial action in the intestinal tract. Water-soluble forms of vitamins K_1 and K_2 are also available. The fat-soluble synthetic compound, **menadione** (vitamin K_3), is about twice as potent biologically as the naturally occurring vitamins K_1 and K_2, on a weight basis.

In healthy adults, primary vitamin K deficiency is uncommon. Adults are protected from a lack of vitamin K because it is widely distributed in plant and animal tissues, the vitamin K cycle conserves the vitamin, and the microbiologic flora of the normal gut forms menaquinone. However, vitamin K deficiency can occur in adults with marginal dietary intake if they undergo trauma or extensive surgery. Persons with biliary obstruction, malabsorption, or liver disease also have a higher risk of vitamin K deficiency. Certain drugs, including anticonvulsants, anticoagulants, some antibiotics (particularly cephalosporins), salicylates, and megadoses of vitamin A or E can cause vulnerability to vitamin K-related bleeding disease. Vitamin K is used for coagulation disorder and vitamin K deficiency.

It is given prophylactically to infants to prevent hemorrhagic disease of the newborn. Natural vitamin K is stored in the body and is not toxic.

Key Concept

The coumarin group of drugs, such as warfarin, is vitamin K antagonists.

Water-soluble Vitamins

Most of the water-soluble vitamins are components of essential enzyme systems. Many are involved in the reactions supporting energy metabolism. These vitamins are not normally stored in the body in appreciable amounts and are usually excreted in small quantities in the urine; thus, a daily supply is desirable to avoid depletion and interruption of normal physiologic functions.

Vitamin B Complex

Vitamin B complex is a group of water-soluble vitamins that differ from each other structurally and in their biologic effects. Heat and prolonged cooking, especially cooking with water, can destroy B vitamins.

Vitamin B_1.   **Vitamin B_1 (thiamine)** is a water-soluble component of the B vitamin complex that is essential for normal metabolism and the health of the cardiovascular and nervous systems. Thiamine plays a key role in the metabolic breakdown of carbohydrates. It is not stored in the body and must be supplied daily. Rich sources of vitamin B_1 are pork, organ meats, green leafy vegetables, legumes, sweet corn, egg yolks, corn meal, brown rice, yeast, and nuts. Deficiency of thiamine leads to the disease called beriberi, which has neurologic, cardiovascular, and GI symptoms. Thiamine is found in fortified breads, pasta, cereals, whole grains (especially wheat germ), lean meats (especially pork), fish, dried beans, peas, and soybeans. Thiamine toxicity can occur if very large doses are taken for long periods, and this can result in hepatotoxicity.

Key Concept

Thiamine malabsorption commonly occurs in patients with alcoholism, cirrhosis, or gastrointestinal disease.

Alcohol is well-known for its ability to inhibit the absorption of thiamine and folic acid. Alcohol abuse is the most common cause of thiamine deficiency in the U.S.

Vitamin B₂. **Vitamin B₂ (riboflavin)** is one of the heat-stable components of the B vitamin complex. It is essential for certain enzyme systems in the metabolism of fats and proteins. It is sensitive to light. It plays an important role in preventing some visual disorders, especially cataracts.

Riboflavin deficiency is associated with inadequate consumption of milk and other animal products. It is common in patients with chronic diarrhea, liver disease, and chronic alcoholism. Deficiency of riboflavin produces **cheilosis** (fissures on the lips); glossitis (inflammation of the tongue); and seborrheic dermatitis (mainly of the face).

Vitamin B₃. **Vitamin B₃ (niacin or nicotinic acid)** contains parts of two enzymes that regulate energy metabolism. It is essential for a healthy skin, tongue, and digestive system. Severe deficiency results in **pellagra**, mental disturbances, various skin eruptions, and GI disturbances. Pellagra may also occur during prolonged isoniazid therapy, and in cancer patients. Major sources of vitamin B₃ include: lean meats, chicken, eggs, fish, cooked dried beans and peas, liver, nonfat or low-fat milk and cheese, soybeans, and nuts.

In large doses, nicotinic acid can lead to peptic ulcers, diabetes mellitus, cardiac dysrhythmias, and hepatic failure. In view of its potential adverse effects at doses of 100 mg and above, nicotinic acid is being made available only by prescription.

Vitamin B₅. **Vitamin B₅ (pantothenic acid)** is a member of the vitamin B complex. The primary role of pantothenic acid is as a constituent of co-enzyme A and as such it is essential in many areas of cellular metabolism, including fatty acid metabolism, the synthesis of sex hormones, and the functioning of the nervous system and the adrenal glands.

As pantothenic acid is available in many plant and animal sources, it is very rare for individuals to have a deficiency of this vitamin. It is available generally in multivitamin preparations, and a diet rich in fruit, vegetable, cereal, or meat sources would ensure an adequate intake of pantothenic acid.

Vitamin B₆. **Vitamin B₆ (pyridoxine)** is a coenzyme essential for the synthesis and breakdown of amino acids, the conversion of tryptophan to niacin, the breakdown of glycogen to glucose, and the production of antibodies. Therefore, vitamin B₆ is important in the metabolism of blood, CNS, and skin. It is used routinely in patients on isoniazid therapy to prevent the development of neuritis. There has been some success with its use in treating nausea of pregnancy, particularly when given parenterally, and orally in the suppression of lactation. Deficiency of pyridoxine is rare, because most foods contain vitamin B₆. However, deficiency may result from malabsorption, alcoholism, oral contraceptive use, and chemical inactivation by drugs (e.g., hydralazine and penicillamine). Vitamin B₆ deficiency may cause anemia, anorexia, neuritis, nausea, dermatitis, and depressed immunity. The ingestion of megadoses (2 to 6 g/day for 2 to 40 months) of pyridoxine may cause progressive sensory **ataxia**.

Key Concept

Pellagra is characterized by skin and mouth lesions, diarrhea, and loss of memory.

Vitamin B$_7$.   **Vitamin B$_7$ (biotin)** is a water-soluble vitamin that is synthesized by intestinal flora; therefore, deficiency states are rare. Biotin functions in metabolism via biotin-dependent enzymes.

Vitamin B$_9$.   **Vitamin B$_9$ (folic acid)** is essential for cell growth and the reproduction of red blood cells. It functions as a co-enzyme with vitamins B$_{12}$ and C in the breakdown of proteins and in the formation of nucleic acid and hemoglobin. It is also essential for fetal development, particularly of the neural tube. Deficiency causes anemia that may cause spina bifida in a fetus. It is also called folacin.

Vitamin B$_{12}$.   **Vitamin B$_{12}$ (hydroxocobalamin)** is often found as **cyanocobalamin** in pharmaceutical preparations. It is involved in the metabolism of protein, fats, and carbohydrates. It aids in hemoglobin synthesis, is essential for normal functioning of all cells, and is important in energy metabolism. Vitamin B$_{12}$ is available in meat and animal protein foods. Its absorption is complex; it occurs in the terminal portion of the small intestine (ileum) and requires **intrinsic factor** (a secretion of the stomach walls). Deficiency causes pernicious anemia and neurological disorders.

Vitamin B$_{12}$ deficiency is caused by a lack of activated folic acid, which is essential for DNA synthesis and cell division. Lack of vitamin B$_{12}$ can also affect the nervous system, causing numbness in the limbs, mood disturbances, and even hallucinations in severe deficiencies.

Patients who are suffering from vitamin B$_{12}$ deficiency usually respond to massive doses of B$_{12}$ every day, and then need weekly or biweekly intramuscular vitamin B$_{12}$ injections. This vitamin B$_{12}$ therapy must be continued for the remainder of the patient's life.

Vitamin C

Vitamin C (ascorbic acid) is essential for the formation of collagen tissue and for normal intercellular matrices in teeth, bone, cartilage, connective tissues, and skin. This is one of the most controversial vitamins, with some practitioners advocating up to 10 g or more per day. Smokers may need up to 150 mg per day. Anything over that is said merely to produce expensive urine. Ascorbic acid may protect the body against infections and help heal wounds. Therefore, ascorbic acid has multiple functions as either a coenzyme or co-factor. Its role in enhancing absorption of iron is well-recognized. Deficiency causes scurvy, lowered resistance to infections, joint tenderness, dental caries, bleeding gums, delayed wound healing, bruising, hemorrhage, and anemia.

MINERALS AND ELECTROLYTES

Minerals are inorganic substances occurring naturally in the earth's crust that the body needs to help build and maintain body tissues for life functions. They are classified as major and trace elements.

Electrolytes are compounds, particularly salts, that when dissolved in water or another solvent dissociate into ions and are able to conduct an electric current. The concentrations of electrolytes differ in blood plasma and other tissues. Sodium, potassium, and chloride ions are electrolytes. Minerals help keep the body's water and electrolytes in balance.

Major Minerals

The major minerals are defined as those requiring an intake of more than 100 mg/day. The six major minerals are calcium, phosphorus, chloride, sodium, potassium, and magnesium.

Calcium (Ca) is the fifth-most abundant element in the human body and is present mainly in the bones. The body requires calcium ions for the transmission of nerve impulses, muscle contraction, blood coagulation, and cardiac functions. It is a component of extracellular fluid and of soft tissue cells.

Too much calcium will lead to cardiac failure (calcium chloride is included in the lethal injection given in judicial death sentences carried out in certain states of the U.S.). Too little calcium leads to tetany, which, if severe, can result in fatal muscular convulsions. Fortunately, both vitamin D and parathyroid hormone (PTH) can normally keep these levels constant, principally by mobilizing calcium from bone if hypocalcemia is present, and shunting it back into bone in hypercalcemia. Both hypocalcemia and hypercalcemia are due to factors involving either vitamin D or PTH. Benign hypercalcemia due to excessive absorption of calcium may result in calcification of soft tissues and renal damage.

Lack of calcium in the diet results in osteoporosis, in which bone is less dense, and therefore, brittle and weak. The following factors enhance the absorption of calcium: adequate vitamin D, calcitonin, parathyroid hormone, large quantities of calcium and phosphorus in the diet, and the presence of lactose. Abnormally high levels of ionized calcium in the extracellular fluid can produce muscle weakness, lethargy, and coma. Hypocalcemia can cause tetanic seizures and hypertension.

Phosphorus (P) is essential for the metabolism of protein, calcium, and glucose. It aids in building strong bones and teeth, and helps in the regulation of the body's acid-base balance. Nutritional sources are dairy foods, meat, egg yolks, whole grains, and nuts. A nutritional deficiency of phosphorus is rare, and is usually due to secondary factors. Phosphorus deficiency can occur when people abuse antacids containing aluminum compounds. Aluminum compounds combine with phosphates to produce aluminum complexes, which render the phosphates unavailable for absorption. Deficiency of phosphorus can cause weight loss, anemia, abnormal growth, muscular weakness, and bone pains. Anemia, **cachexia**, bronchitis, and necrosis of the mandible bone characterize chronic poisoning by phosphorus. Excessive doses of phosphorus may produce hypocalcemia in some cases.

Key Concept

Soft tissue calcification may occur with intravenous administration of phosphate ions, which is less likely to occur if the infusion is given slowly.

Chloride (Cl) is involved in the maintenance of fluid and the body's acid-base balance. The most common metal chloride is sodium chloride (table salt). Chloride ions are needed for the production of hydrochloric acid in the stomach. Chloride is normally associated with sodium and potassium, which are involved in helping to maintain pressure balances between the various body compartments.

Sodium (Na) is one of the most important elements in the body. Sodium ions are involved in acid-base balance, water balance, transmission of nerve impulses, and contraction of muscles. Major dietary sources of sodium are table salt (sodium chloride), ketchup, mustard, cured meats and fish, cheese, and potato chips. Toxic levels may cause hypertension and renal disease. The kidney is the main regulator of sodium levels in body fluids. In high temperatures and high fever, the body loses sodium through sweat. A dietary deficiency of sodium and chloride ions is unknown.

There is a misconception that during hot weather, the intake of extra sodium as salt tablets is advisable. This may be helpful only in athletes and in people doing strenuous work. In these persons, it is probably better to encourage the consumption of low-fat milk and fruit juices, which contain sodium and potassium together in a more palatable form. Sodium chloride tablets can irritate the stomach.

Potassium (K) is the major electrolyte in intracellular fluids, helping to regulate neuromuscular excitability and muscle contraction. Sources of potassium in the diet are whole grains, meat, legumes, fruit, and vegetables. Potassium is important in glycogen formation, protein synthesis, and the correction of imbalances of acid-base metabolism, especially in association with the action of sodium and hydrogen ions. Potassium salts are very important as therapeutic agents but are extremely dangerous if used improperly. The kidney plays an important role in controlling secretion and absorption of potassium by the body tissues, especially in the muscles and the liver.

Potassium deficiency may result from increased renal excretion, which may be caused by diuretic therapy, large doses of anionic drugs, or renal disorders. Increased GI tract excretion of potassium may occur with the loss of GI fluid through vomiting, diarrhea, surgical drainage, or chronic use of laxatives. Potassium loss through the skin is rare, but can result from perspiration during excessive exercise in a hot environment. Potassium deficiency can cause dysrhythmias, so it is important that patients taking certain diuretics also take some form of potassium supplement. Severe diarrhea can also cause hypokalemia. Potassium chloride is an irritant to the stomach mucosa, so tablets are enteric-coated. Another danger with potassium supplementation is hyperkalemia, which is just as serious as hypokalemia.

Magnesium (Mg) is an important ion for the function of many enzyme systems. Magnesium is the second-most abundant action of the intracellular fluids in the body. It helps to build strong bones and teeth,

Key Concept

Drinking seawater leads to dehydration as the kidneys remove the extra salt by the excretion of essential body water.

Key Concept

If possible, encouraging the patient to consume a high-potassium diet best treats diuretic-induced hypokalemia. Foods that are high in potassium are fruit juices, bananas, wholegrain cereals, and nuts.

and aids in regulating the heartbeat. It is stored in the bone and is excreted mainly by the kidneys. Renal excretion of magnesium increases during diuresis induced by ammonium chloride, glucose, and organic mercurials. Magnesium affects the central nervous, neuromuscular, and cardiovascular systems. Diarrhea, steatorrhea, chronic alcoholism, and diabetes mellitus can produce **hypomagnesemia**. Hypomagnesemia is often treated with administration of parenteral fluids containing magnesium sulfate or magnesium chloride. Excess magnesium (hypermagnesemia) in the body can slow the heartbeat or cause cardiac arrest. Hypermagnesemia is usually caused by renal insufficiency and is manifested by hypotension, muscle weakness, sedation, and confused mental state.

Sulfur (S) is necessary to all body tissues and is found in all body cells. It is necessary for metabolism. Sulfur is a component of some amino acids and is therefore found in protein-rich foods.

Trace Elements

Trace elements are not less important, but occur in very small amounts in the body. They include iron, iodine, zinc, fluorine, and copper. Trace elements are generally defined as those having a required intake of less than 100 mg/day. Trace elements are equally essential for their specific vital tasks.

Iron (Fe) is a common metallic element essential for the formation of hemoglobin and myoglobin. The major role of iron is to transfer oxygen to the body tissues. Inadequate supplies of iron needed to form hemoglobin, poor absorption of iron in the digestive system, or chronic bleeding can cause iron deficiency anemia. Iron exists in two ionic states, depending on its oxidative state: the ferrous (iron II) ion, or Fe^{2+}, and the ferric (iron III) ion, or Fe^{3+}. The ferrous ion is easily oxidized to the ferric ion, and antioxidants such as ascorbic acid help in the absorption of iron from the intestines. Iron is present in most meat, legumes, shellfish, and whole grains. Replacement iron may be supplied by ferrous sulfate (Feosol), preferably the oral form. Iron dextran (Imferon) is an injectable form of iron supplement. Milk and antacids should be avoided with iron consumption.

Iodine (I) is an essential micronutrient of the thyroid hormone (thyroxine). Almost 80 percent of the iodine present in the body is in the thyroid gland. Iodine deficiency can result in goiter or **cretinism**. Iodine is found in seafood, iodized salt, and some dairy products. Deficiencies are common in areas away from the sea, and where water levels are inadequate. Iodine deficiency results in hypothyroidism and goiter. Excessive amounts of iodine can lead to similar conditions. Moderately high amounts of iodine in the diet can be bad for acne, so in areas where there are adequate amounts obtainable in the diet, acne sufferers should avoid iodized salt. Iodine is used as a contrast medium for blood vessels in computed tomography (CT) scans. Radioisotopes of iodine are used in radioisotope-scanning procedures and in palliative treatment of cancer of the thyroid.

Key Concept

Patients should be made aware that iron may turn stools black, but that this effect is harmless.

Iron preparations are best consumed on an empty stomach because this allows for maximum absorption. However, iron may be given with orange juice to assist in decreasing gastrointestinal symptoms.

Key Concept

Iodine poisoning can cause a brownish-colored staining of the mucus membranes.

Zinc (Zn) is essential for several body enzymes, growth, glucose tolerance, wound healing, and taste acuity. Nearly all functional units of the immune system are adversely affected by zinc deficiency. It is also used in numerous pharmaceutics, such as zinc acetate, zinc oxide, zinc permanganate, and zinc stearate. The best sources are protein foods. Zinc deficiency is characterized by abnormal fatigue, decreased alertness, a decrease in taste and odor sensitivity, poor appetite, retarded growth, delayed sexual maturity, prolonged healing of wounds, and susceptibility to infection and injury. Excess zinc supplementation can be dangerous as it can cause an increase in copper excretion, leading to copper deficiency. Other problems with excessive zinc intake are atherosclerosis due to a rise in cholesterol and triglyceride levels, and gastric irritation. Megadoses can result in acute toxicity and can be fatal.

Fluoride (F) is probably the most controversial of the microminerals, as it is added to many of the world's water supplies, and must therefore be consumed whether one wants to or not. There does not seem to be any doubt that, as a mineral, fluoride is an essential nutrient, not just to strengthen tooth enamel, but as a coenzyme for one or more enzyme systems. Unfortunately, many areas of the world have low fluoride concentrations in the soil and drinking water, causing people in these areas to become deficient in the element, resulting in an increase in dental caries. There is also evidence that fluoride can strengthen bones against osteoporosis.

Key Concept

The only food that contains reasonable amounts of fluoride is tea.

Flourine is the gas of which flouride is an ion. Excessive amounts of fluoride are poisonous, and cause mottling of the teeth. Fluoride can also cause warts to become cancerous.

Copper (Cu), like iron, is important for the synthesis of hemoglobin, because it is part of a co-enzyme involved in its synthesis. Copper is also a component of several important enzymes in the body, and is essential to good health. Copper is mostly concentrated in the liver, heart, brain, and kidneys. Good sources of copper are liver, shellfish, nuts, and beans. Copper deficiency is rare. Copper toxicity may be seen in individuals with Wilson's disease (a rare, inherited disorder that causes accumulation of copper in the liver), and in primary biliary cirrhosis. The build-up of copper in the tissue causes widespread tissue toxicity with multiple symptoms. The drug penicillamine (Cuprimine) can bind to copper and remove it from the tissues for excretion.

FOOD LABELING

Food items and supplements must be labeled in the pharmacy. By labeling these items, the technician can understand the importance of nutrition labeling regulations. Labeling of foods and supplements must be accurate and not misleading. The Nutrition Labeling and Education Act of 1990

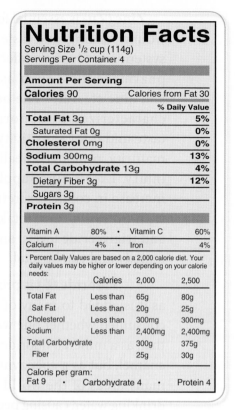

Figure 19-1 Nutrition label.

requires most packaged foods to have a list of a specified set of nutrition facts on the label. Setting of standards and enforcement for nutrition labeling are a responsibility of the Food and Drug Administration (FDA). All the nutrition information on the label is based on the stated serving size. Larger packages, such as cereal boxes, often include additional information not required by law. Figure 19-1 shows an example of a current food label with the minimum required facts.

FOOD ADDITIVES

Any substance that becomes part of a food product is called a **food additive**. Food additives can be added intentionally, such as when salt or cinnamon is added for flavoring, or unintentionally, such as when a pesticide used to treat crops is accidentally incorporated into the plant (or when a drug given to an animal ends up in the food product supplied by the animal). One purpose of food additives is to maintain or improve nutritional value, such as the addition of vitamins and minerals to a food product. The surge in the addition of calcium to juices and other foods is a good example of this function. Another purpose of additives is to maintain freshness in the food. Antioxidants added to foods processed with fat, such as potato chips, help to prevent the fat from becoming rancid, and preservatives help to prevent spoilage and changes in color, texture, and flavor of food. Additives also make food more appealing.

NUTRITIONAL CARE

The proper intake and assimilation of nutrients, especially for the hospitalized patient, is called nutritional care. The nutritional needs of a patient depend on the patient's condition. Nutritional requirements may be provided by regular meals with menus selected from the ordered diet, by tube feeding, or by parenteral hyperalimentation.

Enteral Nutrition

Enteral nutrition (EN) is the delivery of nutrients through a GI tube, or the ingestion of food orally. Enteral tube feeding maintains the structural and functional integrity of the GI tract. It enhances the utilization of nutrients, and provides a safe and economical method of feeding. Enteral tube feedings are contraindicated in patients with the following:

- diffused peritonitis (widespread peritonitis)
- severe diarrhea
- vomiting
- intestinal obstruction that prohibits normal bowel function

Hyperalimentation (Total Parenteral Nutrition)

Hyperalimentation or **total parenteral nutrition (TPN)** is used to meet the patient's nutritional requirements when the enteral route cannot accomplish this. TPN is the treatment of choice for selected patients who are unable to tolerate and maintain adequate enteral intake. TPN is able to supply all the calories, amino acids (proteins), dextrose (carbohydrates), fats, trace elements, vitamins, and other essential nutrients needed for wound healing, immunocompetence, growth, and weight gain. The basic parenteral solution may contain amino acids, carbohydrates, lipids, vitamins, and minerals. Parenteral nutrition (PN) should be undertaken within 1 to 3 days, or in moderation if enteral support is anticipated for more than 5 to 7 days.

PHARMA FOOD

Pharma food is a system of receiving nourishment through breathing. People constantly ingest microparticles that are suspended in the air, such as the dust in every home. The idea behind pharma food is to convert this act, the ingestion of polluting particles (which we are completely accustomed to and takes place in enclosed and outdoor urban areas), into a new form of nourishment. Pharma food is composed of a type of particle that is ingested by breathing and that has beneficial effects on the organism. These particles include (in general) vitamins, amino acids, minerals, or micronutrients, and constitute a volatile muesli that

is released to be inhaled, reaching its destination by the mouth. For the particles to reach the stomach and avoid getting into the lungs, an element called saliva activator has been devised. It activates the salivary glands so that the inhaled particles adhere to saliva and are led to the stomach, where they are assimilated by the digestive system. Often, food products with pharmacological additives designed to improve health by lowering cholesterol or enhancing brain function are inhaled. Because of tough restrictions on advertising, pharma foods are not as popular as they could be, although there are continuing advances in their use. Inhaled lidocaine is now used as a treatment for asthma, which has led to a marked decline in use of steroids, the most popular type of treatment previously. Direct delivery of the lidocaine into the lungs in high concentrations results in minimal systemic exposure and toxicities, but it is not used much anymore. A similar therapy is the use of inhaled reformulated aztreonam to treat cystic fibrosis.

SUMMARY

No single food supplies all the nutrients needed by the body. Therefore, it is important to eat a variety of foods daily to meet all the nutrient needs of the body. Vitamins and minerals are essential in small quantities for physiological and metabolic functioning of the body. Vitamins include water- or fat-soluble substances. Minerals are inorganic substances occurring naturally in the earth's crust that the body needs to help build and maintain body tissues for life functions. Deficiency and toxicity of vitamins or minerals may cause specific conditions or disorders. Pharmacy technicians must be familiar with basic nutrition dietary standards and pathological conditions. In pharmacy practice, there are many questions that clients may ask about foods and nutrition.

EXPLORING THE WEB

Visit *http://ods.od.nih.gov*

- Explore the databases and various research that is being done on substances discussed in this chapter.

Visit *http://win.niddk.nih.gov*

- Look at the publications that are available. Review information and recommendations related to weight loss concerns.

Visit *www.eatright.org*

- Click on Food and Nutrition Information, and review the fact sheets related to vitamins and minerals. What foods provide the beneficial vitamins and minerals discussed in this chapter?

Visit *www.nal.usda.gov*

- Look for information on dietary supplements. What additional information is available?

Visit *www.nlm.nih.gov/medlineplus*

- Search for information on the vitamins and minerals discussed within this chapter.

REVIEW QUESTIONS

Multiple Choice

1. Which of the following vitamins is used for the patient with an overdose of warfarin?

    A. vitamin D
    B. vitamin K
    C. vitamin E
    D. vitamin A

2. Physicians should prescribe vitamin B$_{12}$ for which of the following patients?

   A. inadequate exposure to sunlight
   B. liver disease
   C. hemophilia
   D. pernicious anemia

3. Which of the following minerals should be restricted in patients who are complaining of weakness, dysrhythmias, and hypertension?

   A. magnesium
   B. aluminum
   C. sodium
   D. iron

4. The proper intake and assimilation of nutrients is known as:

   A. nutrient
   B. excretion
   C. nutritional insufficiency
   D. nutritional care

5. Severe deficiency of niacin (vitamin B$_3$) may result in:

   A. beriberi
   B. pellagra
   C. marasmus
   D. pernicious anemia

6. Which of the following types of feeding is more appropriate for when a patient's GI tract is not functioning?

   A. oral
   B. TPN
   C. enteral
   D. enema

7. An essential micronutrient of thyroid hormone (thyroxine) is:

   A. iron
   B. zinc
   C. iodine
   D. copper

8. Calcium deficiency may cause all of the following, except:

   A. rickets
   B. osteoporosis
   C. dwarfism
   D. osteomalacia

9. The Nutrition Labeling and Education Act of 1990 requires most packaged foods to list a specified set of:

   A. vitamin facts on the diet
   B. nutrition facts on the label
   C. mineral and vitamin facts on the diet
   D. nutritional deficiency

10. All of the following are the purposes of food additives, except:

    A. to make food more appealing
    B. to prevent misleading statements on the label
    C. to maintain nutritional value
    D. to main freshness in the food

11. A system of nourishing through breathing is known as:

    A. volatile muesli
    B. immune activator
    C. saliva activator
    D. pharma food

12. Which of the following minerals is able to help in the formation of hemoglobin and the transportation of iron to bone marrow?

    A. fluoride (F)
    B. copper (Cu)
    C. zinc (Zn)
    D. iodine (I)

13. Which of the following vitamins may protect the body against infections or help heal wounds?

    A. vitamin C
    B. vitamin B_{12}
    C. vitamin K
    D. vitamin E

14. All of the nutrition information on the label is based on which of the following?

    A. the amount of cholesterol
    B. the stated calories
    C. the stated serving size
    D. the amount of sodium

15. The purpose of food additives is:

    A. to maintain nutritional value
    B. to improve diets with low cholesterol
    C. to improve diets with high potassium
    D. all of the above

Matching

_____ **1.** vitamin B_2 **A.** folic acid

_____ **2.** vitamin B_3 **B.** nicotinamide

_____ **3.** vitamin B_5 **C.** hydroxocobalamin

_____ **4.** vitamin B_9 **D.** pantothenic acid

_____ **5.** vitamin B_{12} **E.** riboflavin

Fill in the Blank

1. Vitamin K is an antagonist of _____.

2. The only food that contains reasonable amounts of fluoride is _____.

3. The drug penicillamine is able to remove _____ from the tissues for excretion in treatment of _____ disease.

4. Total parenteral nutrition may be administered through a(n) _____ so that nutrition can be precisely monitored.

Critical Thinking

A pharmacy technician named John, who has been working in this position for three years, goes to Seattle to visit his grandmother whom he hasn't seen for nearly ten years. While staying at her house, he notices that she has about 15 different types of vitamins and mineral supplements on her nightstand. He asks her if she takes all of these herself, and she answers, "yes, I take all of them every day—they help me feel younger and give me more energy!" He finds out that she is also taking 3 to 4 different prescribed medications for her hypertension and diabetes.

1. What should John's advice be to his grandmother?

2. Which vitamin or mineral supplements may have potential interactions with diabetes medications?

3. If she were taking vitamin A and vitamin D in excess of the maximum daily requirements, what would be the symptoms of overdosage and toxicity from these vitamins?

Antineoplastic Agents

OBJECTIVES

After completing this chapter, the reader should be able to:

1. Identify the primary causes of cancer.
2. Explain the terms *benign, malignant,* and *neoplasm.*
3. Describe chemotherapy and the types of antineoplastic drugs.
4. Explain hormone therapy as antineoplastic drugs.
5. Describe the first group of antineoplastic agents.
6. List the classes of mitotic inhibitors (plant alkaloids).
7. Explain the mechanism of drug action of antimetabolites and antitumor antibiotics.
8. Explain toxicity of antineoplastic agents.
9. List specific side effects of certain antineoplastic agents on particular organs or systems in the body.
10. Explain different phases of the cell cycle.

GLOSSARY

Alopecia – hair loss

Antineoplastic agents – used to treat cancers or malignant neoplasms

Antimetabolites – prevent cancer cell growth by affecting its DNA production

Benign – cellular growth that is nonprogressive, and non–life-threatening

Carcinogens – any agent directly involved in or related to the promotion of cancer

Heterogeneous – consisting of a diverse range of different items

Malignant – cellular growth that is severe and becomes progressively worse, often becoming life-threatening

Metastasize – to spread from one part of the body to another

Mitotic inhibitors – drugs that block cell growth by stopping cell division

Neoplasm – a tumor; tissue that is composed of cells that grow in an abnormal way

Nitrosoureas – alkylating agents; they act by the process of alkylation to inhibit DNA repair

Palliation – treatment to relieve or reduce intensity of uncomfortable symptoms, but not to produce a cure

Radiation therapy – cancer treatment method whereby drugs are used to treat cancer either before or after surgery

OVERVIEW

A tumor, or **neoplasm**, arises from a single abnormal cell, which continues to divide indefinitely. The lack of growth controls, the ability to invade local tissue, and the ability to spread, or **metastasize**, are characteristics of cancer cells. These properties are not present in normal cells. Tumors are either **benign** (nonprogressive) or **malignant** (spreading). More than 100 different types of malignant neoplasms occur in man. Malignant tumors are also referred to as *cancer*, which is second only to heart disease as a cause of death in the U.S. Common sites for the development of malignant tumors are the skin, lungs, prostate, breasts, and large intestine (colon).

Cancer can be treated surgically or chemically. There are a variety of chemical treatments to consider in the treatment of cancers. The decisions for treatments may be made based upon the type of cancer being treated or the stage of the cancer when diagnosed. This chapter discusses many of the chemotherapeutic treatments used in the treatment of cancer.

CHARACTERISTICS OF CANCER

The proliferation of neoplastic cells leads to the formation of masses called tumors. The terms *neoplasm* and *tumor* are used synonymously. However, it is very important to note that not all neoplasms form tumors. For example, leukemia is a malignant disease of the bone marrow, but the malignant cells are in the blood circulation and thus do not form distinct masses.

Most tumors can be classified clinically as either benign or malignant. Benign tumors have a limited growth potential and a good outcome, whereas malignant tumors grow uncontrollably and eventually kill the host.

Only malignant tumor cells have the capacity to metastasize. Benign tumors never metastasize and always remain localized. Metastasis involves a spread of tumor cells from a primary location to some other site in the body. The spread can occur through three main pathways:

- Through the lymphatics
- Via blood
- By seeding of the surface of body cavities

The Cell Cycle

To understand cancer treatments, normal and malignant cell replication processes should be reviewed. This cell cycle may last between 24 hours to many days. The phases of the cell cycle consist of a first growth phase (G_1), synthesis (S_1), a second growth phase (G_2), mitosis (M), and a resting phase (G_0). See Figure 20-1.

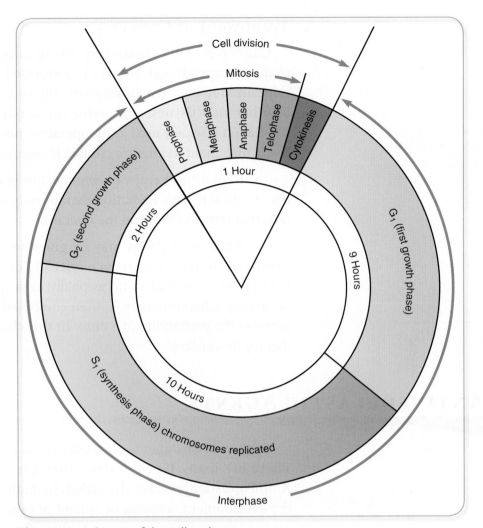

Figure 20-1 Stages of the cell cycle.

Causes of Cancer

The cause of most human cancers is unknown. Nevertheless, many potential agents (**carcinogens**) that result in the development of cancer have been identified, and the sources of many tumors have been explained (see Table 20-1).

TABLE 20-1   Exposure to Carcinogens

Causes	Cancer Sites
Sunlight (UV radiation)	Skin cancer
Human papilloma viruses	Genital warts and cervical cancer
Inhalation carcinogens (3,4-Benzpyrene); cigarette smoking	Lung cancer
Radiation	Thyroid and skin cancer
Metabolic liver carcinogens	Liver cancer
Metabolic excretory carcinogens	Bladder cancer
Metabolic carcinogens; nitrites and nitrates	Intestinal cancer

Treatment of Cancer

Cancer may be treated by using surgery, radiation therapy, and chemotherapy (drugs). Surgery is performed for the removal of a tumor that is localized in one area, or when the tumor is pressing on the airway, nerves, or other vital tissues. It remains the major form of treatment; however, irradiation is widely used as preoperative, postoperative, or primary therapy. Many malignant lesions are curable if detected in the early stage.

Radiation therapy is very effective in destroying tumor cells through non-surgical means. Radiation therapy may follow surgery to kill any cancer cells that remain following the operation.

Anticancer drugs may be given to attempt a cure, for **palliation** (treatment to relieve or reduce intensity of uncomfortable symptoms, but not to produce a cure), or occasionally, as prophylaxis to prevent cancer from occurring. Chemotherapy is often combined with surgery and radiation to increase the probability of a cure. In this chapter, the focus will be on drug therapy for cancers.

ANTINEOPLASTIC AGENTS

Antineoplastic agents are used to treat cancers or malignant neoplasms. There are many types of drug therapies for the treatment of cancer. Antineoplastic agents are also called chemotherapeutic agents. They interrupt the development, growth, or spread of cancer cells. Antineoplastic agents are used for malignant tumors. Antineoplastic agents do not kill tumor cells directly, but interfere with cell replication (Figure 20-2). Each antineoplastic agent is effective at a specific stage in cell replication. It may inhibit DNA, RNA, and protein synthesis of cancer cells. Agents are most commonly given in combinations of two or more at a time. Many antineoplastic medications also have immunosuppressive properties that decrease the patient's ability to produce antibodies to attack infecting organisms. These medications are toxic to the body as a whole because they also destroy normal cells and decrease immunity.

The most common types of antineoplastic agents include: antimetabolites, hormonal agents, special antibiotics, alkylating agents, and mitotic inhibitors (plant alkaloids). Antineoplastic agents require the following special care and handling:

- Preparation only in restricted-access areas under biological safety cabinets

- Syringes and needles must have specialized fittings that are designed for use with these agents (for example, Luer-Lok™ fittings)

- Protective gowns must be worn during preparation

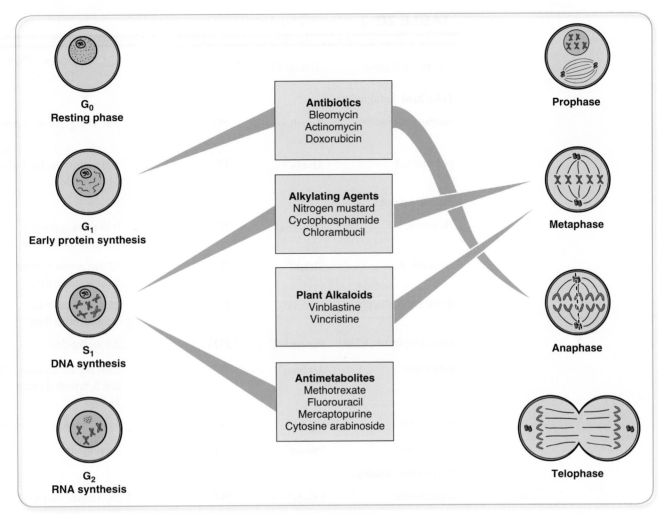

Figure 20-2 The effects of antineoplastic agents on various cell phases.

- Two pairs of protective gloves should be worn, and periodically changed
- A plastic face shield or splash goggles should be worn
- Training classes must be attended by all workers who will be handling antineoplastic agents

Antimetabolites

Antimetabolites prevent cancer cell growth by affecting its DNA production. They are only effective against cells that are actively participating in cell metabolism. The antimetabolite drugs are listed in Table 20-2.

The classes of antimetabolites include:

1. Folic acid antagonists: methotrexate

2. Purine analogs: mercaptopurine

3. Pyrimidine analogs: fluorouracil

TABLE 20-2 Antimetabolites

Generic Name	Trade Name	Route of Administration	Average Adult Dosage
Folic Acid Antagonists			
methotrexate sodium	Amethopterin®, Mexate®	PO	15–30 mg/day for 5 days
pemetrexed	Alimta®	IV	500 mg/m² on day 1 of each 21 day cycle
Purine Analogs			
cladribine	Leustatin®	IV	0.09 mg/kg/day as a continuous infusion
clofarabine	Clolar®	IV	52 mg/m² over 2h for 5 consecutive days
fludarabine phosphate	Fludara®	IV	25 mg/m² daily for 5 consecutive days
mercaptopurine (6 MP)	Purinethol®	PO	2.5 mg/kg/day
nelarabine	Arranon®	IV	1500 mg/m² on days 1, 3, and 5; repeated every 21 days
pentostatin	Nipent®	IV	4 mg/m² every other week
thioguanine	Tabloid®	PO	2 mg/kg/day
Pyrimidine Analogs			
capecitabine	Xeloda®	PO	2500 mg/m²/day for 2 weeks
cytarabine	Depo-Cyt®, Cytosar-U®	IV	200 mg/m² as a continuous infusion over 24 hours
floxuridine	FUDR®	Intra-arterial	0.1–0.6 mg/kg/day as a continuous infusion
fluorouracil (5 FU)	Adrucil®, Carac®	IV	12 mg/kg/day for 4 consecutive days
gemcitabine hydrochloride	Gemzar®	IV	1000 mg/m² q week

Mechanism of Action

Antimetabolites disrupt the metabolic functions of normal cells in the body. They interfere with the activity of enzymes and alter the DNA structure.

Indications

Antimetabolites are used in the treatment of a variety of neoplasms. Methotrexate is effective in the treatment of gestational choriocarcinoma and hydatidiform mole, as well as being immunosuppressant in

kidney transplantation. Methotrexate is also used for acute and subacute leukemias and leukemic meningitis, especially in children. This drug is often indicated to treat severe psoriasis that is non-responsive to other forms of therapy.

Mercaptopurine (6-MP) is used primarily for acute lymphocytic and myelogenous leukemia. Fluorouracil (5-FU) is used systemically as a single agent and in combination with other antineoplastics for palliative treatment of carefully selected patients with inoperable neoplasms of the breast, colon or rectum, stomach, pancreas, urinary bladder, ovary, cervix, and liver.

Adverse Effects

Antimetabolite agents may cause a wide variety of adverse effects. Common adverse effects include anorexia, nausea, vomiting, diarrhea, leukopenia, anemia, and thrombocytopenia. Some adverse effects of antimetabolites are dose-dependent, and may produce impaired liver function, hepatic necrosis, blurred vision, aphasia, and convulsions.

Contraindications and Precautions

Antimetabolite drugs are contraindicated in patients with anemia, thrombocytopenia, and poor nutrition. These agents are also contraindicated in patients with known hypersensitivity to these drugs, renal insufficiency, and during pregnancy (category D) or lactation.

Antimetabolite agents should be used with caution in patients with hepatic or renal impairment, active infection, or other debilitating disorders. These drugs should be avoided in patients with peptic ulcer, ulcerative colitis, and elderly patients.

Drug Interactions

Alcohol and other CNS depressants may enhance CNS depression if taken with antimetabolites. Allopurinol may inhibit metabolism and increase toxicity of mercaptopurine.

Hormonal Agents

Hormonal agents are a class of **heterogeneous** compounds that have various effects on cells. These agents either block hormone production or block hormone action. Their action on malignant cells is highly selective. They are the least toxic of the anticancer medications. The most commonly used hormonal agents in cancer therapy are seen in Table 20-3.

Mechanism of Action

The precise action of hormones on malignant neoplasms is not known. However, these agents are able to counteract the effect of male or female hormones in hormone-dependent tumors.

Medical Terminology Review

leukopenia
leuko = white
penia = (blood cell) decrease
decrease in white blood cells

Key Concept

Antimetabolite and other antineoplastic drugs in older adults may increase the risk of adverse effects. Therefore, a lower dosage is recommended for patients with renal impairment.

TABLE 20-3   Commonly Used Hormonal Agents

Generic Name	Trade Name	Route of Administration	Average Adult Dosage
Hormones			
diethylstilbestrol	DES®, Stilbestrol®	PO	For prostate cancer: 500 mg t.i.d.; for palliation: 1–15 mg/day
ethinyl acetate	Femring®	PO	For breast cancer: 10 mg t.i.d.; for palliation of prostate cancer: 1–2 mg t.i.d.
fluoxymesterone	Halotestin®	PO	10–40 mg t.i.d.
medroxyprogesterone acetate	Provera®, Depo-Provera®	IM	400–1000 mg q week
megestrol acetate	Megace®	PO	40–160 mg b.i.d.-q.i.d.
prednisone	Deltasone®	PO	20–100 mg/m²/day
testolactone	Teslac®	PO	250 mg q.i.d.
testosterone	Andro-Cyp®, Depo-Testosterone®	IM	200–400 mg q2–4 weeks
Hormone Antagonists			
abarelix	Plenaxis®	IM	100 mg on day 1, 15, 29 and q4 weeks thereafter
aminoglutethimide	Cytadren®	PO	250 mg b.i.d.-q.i.d.
anastrozole	Arimidex®	PO	1 mg/day
bicalutamide	Casodex®	PO	50 mg/day
exemestane	Aromasin®	PO	25 mg/day after a meal
flutamide	Eulexin®	PO	250 mg t.i.d.
goserelin acetate	Zoladex®	SC	3.6 mg q28 days
letrozole	Femara®	PO	2.5 mg/day
leuprolide acetate	Lupron®	SC, IM	SC: 1 mg/day; IM: 7.5 mg/month
nilutamide	Nilandron®	PO	300 mg/day for 30 days, then 150 mg/day
tamoxifen citrate	Nolvadex®	PO	10–20 mg b.i.d.
toremifene citrate	Fareston®	PO	60 mg/day

Indications

Hormones and their antagonists have various uses in the treatment of malignant diseases. Steroids are especially useful in treating lymphomas, leukemias, and Hodgkin's disease. They are also used in conjunction with radiation therapy to reduce nausea, weight loss, and tissue inflammation

caused by other antitumor drugs. Gonadal hormones are used in carcinomas of the reproductive tract and advanced breast cancer. For example, estrogen is given to a patient with testicular cancer or carcinoma of the prostate. Estrogen may also be administered to postmenopausal women with breast cancer. Androgens (male hormones) are prescribed in premenopausal women with breast cancer. Antiestrogens, such as tamoxifen, and anti-androgens are used to inhibit hormone production in advanced stages of breast cancer.

Adverse Effects

Major adverse effects include masculization in female patients and feminization in male patient. Estrogen therapy may cause blood clots.

Contraindications and Precautions

Hormonal agents have a wide array of contraindications, including hypersensitivity to the agents. The use of hormonal agents must be avoided in patients with fungal infections, endometrial hyperplasia, thromboembolic disease, and in children. They are ranked in a variety of categories if used during pregnancy and lactation (including categories C, D, and X).

Precautions for the use of hormonal agents include patients with hypertension, gallbladder disease, diabetes mellitus, heart failure, liver or kidney dysfunction, infections, nonspecific ulcerative colitis, diverticulitis, peptic ulcer, osteoporosis, and myasthenia gravis. Hormonal agents must be used with great caution in many other conditions.

Drug Interactions

Hormonal agents may cause drug interactions with many agents, including but not limited to: carbamazepine, phenytoin, rifampin, corticosteroids, oral anticoagulants, barbiturates, amphotericin B, diuretics, ambenonium, neostigmine, and pyridostigmine. Hormonal agents may inhibit antibody response to vaccines and toxoids.

Antitumor Antibiotics

Several antibiotics of microbial origin are very effective in the treatment of certain tumors. They are used only to treat cancer, and are not used to treat infections. These antibiotics include bleomycin, doxorubicin, daunorubicin, idarubicin, mitomycin, and plicamycin (Table 20-4).

Mechanism of Action

The mechanism of action of antitumor antibiotics is the inhibition of DNA and RNA synthesis. Antitumor antibiotics attach to DNA, distorting its structure and preventing normal DNA-to-RNA synthesis.

TABLE 20-4   Antitumor Antibiotics

Generic Name	Trade Name	Route of Administration	Average Adult Dosage
bleomycin sulfate	Blenoxane®	SC, IM, IV	10–20 units/m^2 (1–2 times/week)
dactinomycin	Actinomycin D®, Cosmegan®	IV	500 mcg/day for a max. of 5 days
daunorubicin hydrochloride	Cerubidine®	IV	30–60 mg/m^2/day for 3–5 days
daunorubicin citrate liposomal	DaunoXome®	IV	40 mg/m^2 q2 weeks
doxorubicin hydrochloride	Adriamycin®, Rubex®	IV	60–75 mg/m^2 as a single dose
doxorubicin liposomal	Doxil®	IV	20 mg/m^2 q3 weeks
epirubicin hydrochloride	Ellence®	IV	100–120 mg/m^2 as a single dose
idarubicin	Idamycin PFS®	IV	8–12 mg/m^2/day for 3 days
mitomycin	Mutamycin®	IV	10–20 mg/m^2/day as a single dose
mitoxantrone hydrochloride	Novantrone®	IV	12–14 mg/m^2 q21 days
plicamycin	Mithramycin®, Mithracin®	IV	25–30 mcg/kg/day for 3–4 days
valrubicin	Valstar®	Intrabladder instillation	800 mg q week for 6 weeks

Indications

Antitumor antibiotics are used for treating a few specific types of cancer. For example, plicamycin is used only for treatment of testicular cancer. The only indication for idarubicin is acute leukemia (cancer of the blood).

Adverse Effects

The most serious adverse effects of antitumor antibiotics are low blood cell counts and congestive heart failure. Their common adverse effects include nausea, vomiting, diarrhea, fatigue, headache, and **alopecia** (hair loss). Bleomycin may cause pneumonitis, pulmonary fibrosis, and rash.

Contraindications and Precautions

Antitumor antibiotics are contraindicated in patients with known hypersensitivity, bleeding disorders, coagulation disorders, suppression of bone marrow, electrolyte imbalance, and chickenpox, herpes zoster, and other viral infections; in women of childbearing age; during pregnancy

(various categories, including C and D) and lactation; and in infants less than six months of age.

Precautions for use of antitumor antibiotics include patients with compromised hepatic, renal, or pulmonary function, previous cytotoxic drug or radiation therapy, bone marrow depression, infections, gout, and obesity. There are many other precautions for these agents as well.

Drug Interactions

When bleomycin is given with cisplatin, there is an increased risk of bleomycin toxicity. Mitoxantrone, dactinomycin, mitomycin, and plicamycin increase bone marrow depression. There may be an increased risk of bleeding when plicamycin is used with aspirin, warfarin, heparin, or a nonsteroidal anti-inflammatory drug.

Alkylating Agents

Alkylating agents were the first group of antineoplastic agents. During World War I, chemical warfare was introduced using nitrogen mustard. Alkylating agents came to be used for cancer therapy as a result of observation of the effects of the mustard war gases on cell growth (Table 20-5).

TABLE 20-5 Alkylating Agents

Generic Name	Trade Name	Route of Administration	Average Adult Dosage
Nitrogen Mustards			
chlorambucil	Leukeran®	PO	Initial: 0.1–0.2 mg/kg/day; maint: 4–10 mg/day
cyclophosphamide	Cytoxan®	PO	Initial: 1–5 mg/kg/day; maint: 1–5 mg/kg q7–10 days
estramustine sodium phosphate	Emcyt®	PO	14 mg/kg t.i.d.-q.i.d.
ifosfamide	Ifex®	IV	1.2 g/m²/day for 5 days
mechlorethamine hydrochloride	Mustargen®	IV	6 mg/m² on days 1 and 8 for 28 days
melphalan	Alkeran®	PO	6 mg/day for 2–3 weeks
Nitrosoureas			
carmustine	Gliadel®	IV	150–200 mg/m² q6 weeks
lomustine	CeeNU®	PO	130 mg/m² as a single dose
streptozocin	Zanosar®	IV	500 mg/m² for 5 consecutive day

(continues)

TABLE 20-5 Alkylating Agents—*continued*

Generic Name	Trade Name	Route of Administration	Average Adult Dosage
Miscellaneous Agents			
busulfan	Myleran®	PO	4–8 mg/day
carboplatin	Paraplatin®	IV	360 mg/m² q4 weeks
cisplatin	Platinol®	IV	20 mg/m²/day for 5 days
dacarbazine	DTIC-Dome®	IV	2–4.5 mg/kg/day for 10 days
oxaliplatin	Eloxatin®	IV	85 mg/m² infused over 120 min once q2 weeks
temozolomide	Temodar®	PO	150 mg/m²/day for 5 consecutive days
thiotepa	Thioplex®	IV	0.3–0.4 mg/kg q1–4 week

Mechanism of Action

Most alkylating agents interact with the process of cell division of cancer cells. Antineoplastic or cytotoxic action is primarily due to cross-linking of strands of DNA and RNA as well as inhibition of protein synthesis. These drugs bind with DNA, causing breaks and preventing DNA replication.

Indications

Alkylating agents are used to treat metastatic ovarian, testicular, and bladder cancers. They are also used for the palliative treatment of other cancers. The newer drugs in this category are **nitrosoureas**, lipid-soluble drugs used in treating brain tumors and testicular or ovarian cancers.

Adverse Effects

Major adverse effects of the alkylating agents include nausea, vomiting, anorexia, diarrhea, bone marrow suppression, hepatic and renal toxicity, and dermatitis. Other adverse effects of alkylating drugs include cataracts, anxiety, fever, skin rash, hypertension, tachycardia, dizziness, and insomnia.

Contraindications and Precautions

Alkylating agents are contraindicated in patients with known hypersensitivity, impaired renal function, myelosuppression, impaired hearing, history of gout and urate renal stones, hypomagnesia, concurrent administration with loop diuretics, Raynaud syndrome, and many more conditions, and during pregnancy (various categories) and lactation. Safe use in children is not established for many of these agents.

Precautions include use in patients with previous cytotoxic drug or radiation therapy with other ototoxic and nephrotoxic drugs, hyperuricemia,

---

> **Medical Terminology Review**
>
> **myelosuppression**
> *myelo = bone marrow*
> *suppression = slowing of function*
> slowing of the production and function of the bone marrow

electrolyte imbalances, hepatic impairment, and history of circulatory disorders. There are many other precautions for these agents as well.

Drug Interactions

Drug interactions with alkylating agents include aminoglycosides, amphotericin B, vancomycin, other nephrotoxic drugs, furosemide, barbiturates, phenytoin, chloral hydrate, and corticosteroids. There are other drug interactions with these various agents as well.

Mitotic Inhibitors

Mitotic inhibitors (plant alkaloids) are derived from plants. The primary plant alkaloids are vincristine and vinblastine. Teniposide is a close analog of etoposide and is active against acute leukemias in children. Topotecan is a semisynthetic plant alkaloid used for refractory ovarian cancer that may have activity against small-cell lung cancer. Examples of plant alkaloids are seen in Table 20-6.

Mechanism of Action

Mitotic inhibitors may interfere with cell division, but the antineoplastic mechanism of these agents is unclear.

TABLE 20-6 Mitotic Inhibitors and Other Plant Products

Generic Name	Trade Name	Route of Administration	Average Adult Dosage
Mitotic Inhibitors			
vinblastine sulfate	Velban®	IV	3.7–18.5 mg/m^2 q week
vincristine sulfate	Oncovin®	IV	1.4 mg/m^2 q week (max: 2 mg/m^2)
vinorelbine tartrate	Navelbine®	IV	30 mg/m^2 q week
Taxoids			
docetaxel	Taxotere®	IV	60–100 mg/m^2 q3 weeks
paclitaxel	Taxol®	IV	135–175 mg/m^2 q3 weeks
Topoisomerase Inhibitors			
etoposide	VePesid®	IV	50–100 mg/m^2/day for 5 days
irinotecan hydrochloride	Camptosar®	IV	125 mg/m^2 q week for 4 weeks
teniposide	Vumon®	IV	165 mg/m^2 q3-4 days for 4 weeks
topotecan hydrochloride	Hycamtin®	IV	1.5 mg/m^2/day for 5 days

Indications

Mitotic inhibitor drugs are used in various cancers. For example, docetaxel is prescribed for breast cancer and non–small-cell lung cancer. Vinblastine is indicated for the treatment of Hodgkin's disease, lymphocytic lymphoma, testicular cancer, Kaposi's sarcoma, and breast cancer.

Vincristine is used in acute leukemia and combination therapy for various cancers. Paclitaxel is given to patients for treating ovarian and breast cancers, or for AIDS-related Kaposi's sarcoma.

Adverse Effects

Common adverse effects of mitotic inhibitors include nausea, vomiting, diarrhea, fatigue, mental depression, and alopecia. Infection and peripheral neuropathy are also considered to be unwanted effects of mitotic inhibitors.

Contraindications and Precautions

Mitotic inhibitors are contraindicated in patients with known hypersensitivity to these drugs. Mitotic inhibitors should be avoided in patients with leukopenia or bacterial infection, and during pregnancy (category D) or lactation.

Etoposide is also contraindicated in patients with severe bone marrow depression, and in severe hepatic or renal impairment. Mitotic inhibitors should be used with caution in patients who have impaired kidney or liver function, gout, obstructive jaundice, and idiopathic thrombocytopenic purpura.

Drug Interactions

Mitotic inhibitors may interact with many drugs. For example, vincristine used with asparaginase may cause increased neurotoxicity secondary to decreased liver clearance of vincristine. When mitotic inhibitors are used with calcium channel blockers, they may increase accumulation of these agents in cells.

Summary

A neoplasm is an abnormal cell division of the body. It may be benign or malignant. Only malignant tumors are capable of spreading to other organs or systems of the body. Treatment of the neoplasm depends on the progression of the tumor. Surgery, radiation therapy, chemotherapy, and immunotherapy may be indicated. There are many agents used for this purpose. Many antineoplastic medications also have immunosuppressive properties that decrease the patient's ability to produce antibodies to attack infecting organisms.

Common antineoplastic agents include antimetabolites, hormonal agents, specific antibiotics, alkylating agents, and mitotic inhibitors or plant alkaloids. In some cases, surgery and radiation therapy are also necessary. Toxicity and side effects of chemotherapy and radiation therapy are the major concerns regarding treatment of malignant tumors.

Exploring the Web

Visit the following websites for additional information on drug therapies used to treat cancer:

www.biochemweb.org

www.cancer.org

www.cancer-info.com

www.cdc.gov/niosh

www.mayoclinic.com

Review Questions

Multiple Choice

1. The cell cycle consists of several phases, such as G_0, G_1, S_1, G_2, and M. Which of the following explains the G_0 phase?

   A. resting
   B. synthesis
   C. mitosis
   D. growth

2. Which of the following agents is an antimetabolite?

   A. cyclophosphamide
   B. fluorouracil
   C. mitomycin
   D. nitrogen mustard

3. Which of the following is an example of an antitumor antibiotic?

   A. vinorelbine
   B. topotecan
   C. bleomycin
   D. mercaptopurine

4. Mitotic inhibitors (plant alkaloids) include:

   A. mercaptopurine
   B. testolactone
   C. tamoxifen
   D. vincristine

5. Mercaptopurine may have drug interactions with which of the following agents?

   A. amoxicillin
   B. alcohol
   C. allopurinol
   D. estrogen

6. An adverse effect of methotrexate includes:

   A. bone marrow aplasia
   B. arthritis
   C. hypertension
   D. hyperthyroidism

7. Busulfan has some unusual side effects in addition to its bone marrow suppressive activity. Which of the following side effects are caused by busulfan?

   A. peptic ulcer
   B. testicular cancer
   C. gynecomastia
   D. gastrointestinal bleeding

8. Which of the following is the trade name of doxorubicin?

   A. Mutamycin
   B. Adriamycin
   C. Cosmegan
   D. Blenoxane

9. The route of administration for goserelin is:

   A. oral
   B. intramuscular
   C. intravenous
   D. implant

10. Most plant alkaloids may produce:

    A. nausea and vomiting
    B. internal bleeding
    C. hypertension
    D. gout

11. Which of the following antimetabolic is useful in maintenance therapy of children with acute leukemia?

- **A.** fluorouracil (5-FU)
- **B.** methotrexate (MTX)
- **C.** mercaptopurine (6-MP)
- **D.** vincristine

12. Which of the following is the best drug that may be given to a patient with testicular cancer?

- **A.** tamoxifen
- **B.** estrogen
- **C.** progesterone
- **D.** megestrol

13. The term *metastasize* means to:

- **A.** arise
- **B.** divide
- **C.** spread
- **D.** occur

14. Hycamtin˚ is the trade name of which of the following agents?

- **A.** vincristine
- **B.** vinblastine
- **C.** vinorelbine
- **D.** topotecan

15. The single most active agent against breast cancer is:

- **A.** dactinomycin
- **B.** mitomycin
- **C.** doxorubicin
- **D.** bleomycin

Matching

_____ 1. Resting phase	**A.** G_1	
_____ 2. Cell division	**B.** S_1	
_____ 3. Synthesis	**C.** G_2	
_____ 4. Second growth phase	**D.** M	
_____ 5. First growth phase	**E.** G_0	

Generic Name	Trade Name
_____ 1. vincristine	**A.** VePesid
_____ 2. vinblastine	**B.** Navelbine
_____ 3. vinorelbine	**C.** Oncovin
_____ 4. paclitaxel	**D.** Velban
_____ 5. etoposide	**E.** Taxol

Critical Thinking

A biopsy revealed that a 45-year-old woman had breast cancer. She underwent surgery and her left breast was removed. Her physician ordered radiation therapy and chemotherapy as adjuvant therapies to the surgery.

1. If she were to refuse radiation or chemotherapy, what would be the likely consequence?

2. List the most common adverse effects of chemotherapy.

3. If the physician diagnosed that this patient had metastasis to her bones, which types of treatment should he recommend?

Analgesics

OBJECTIVES

After completing this chapter, the reader should be able to:

1. Differentiate salicylates from nonsalicylate nonsteroid anti-inflammatory drugs.
2. Describe the uses and adverse effects of nonsalicylate analgesics.
3. List the dangers of aspirin use.
4. Explain the contraindications of aspirin.
5. Describe the use of cyclooxygenase-2 inhibitors.
6. Explain the reason behind the use of narcotic analgesics.
7. Outline three narcotic antagonists.
8. Identify the different types of analgesics.
9. Explain the major adverse effects of narcotic analgesics.
10. Describe the opioid receptors.

GLOSSARY

Acute pain – pain that is of sudden onset and brief course; can also mean "severe"

Agonist-antagonists – agents that can initiate or resist actions

Analgesic – a compound that relieves pain by altering perception without producing anesthesia or loss of consciousness

Bradykinin – a polypeptide that mediates inflammation, increases vasodilation, and contracts smooth muscle

Chronic pain – pain that is persistent or long-term; can also mean "low-intensity"

Cyclooxygenase inhibitors – drugs that prevent the action of one of two enzymes that have an essential role in the inflammation process

Intracranial – within the cranium (skull)

Nonsteroidal anti-inflammatory drugs (NSAIDs) – drugs that have analgesic and antipyretic effects

Opioid – a natural or synthetic narcotic substance

Opioid agonists – drugs that can combine with receptors to initiate drug actions

Opioid antagonists – drugs that oppose or resist the action of others

Pain – an unpleasant sensation associated with actual or potential tissue damage

Reye syndrome – an acquired encephalopathy of young children that follows an acute febrile illness; strongly associated with aspirin use

OVERVIEW

Pain is a common problem and an unpleasant sensory experience that is associated with actual damage of tissue. **Pain** is the reaction of the central nervous system to severe harmful stimuli. It may be an early warning system to prevent any further damage to the body. Pain stimuli may be caused by the process of inflammation or tissue injury. Pain may be described as mild, moderate, or severe; acute or chronic; dull or sharp; burning or piercing; and localized or generalized. **Acute pain** is severe pain with a sudden onset. **Chronic pain** lasts a long time or is marked by frequent reoccurrence. During an organ's injury or inflammation, different chemical substances are released. These substances include histamine, prostaglandins (hormone-like substances that control blood pressure, contract smooth muscle, and modulate inflammation), serotonin, and **bradykinin** (a polypeptide that mediates inflammation, increases vasodilation, and contracts smooth muscle). These chemical substances initiate an action potential along a sensory nerve fiber and/or sensitize pain receptors. This chapter provides discussion of the various medicinal products used in the relief of pain.

ANALGESICS

Medical Terminology Review

osteoarthritis
osteo = bone
arthr = joint
itis = inflammation
inflammation of the bones
affecting the joints

Pain-relieving (**analgesic**) drugs are currently available for all levels of painful stimuli. Analgesics may be classified as **opioid** (narcotic) or nonopioid medications. Many of these agents affect pain, fever, and inflammation, depending on their properties. Nonopioid analgesics, antipyretics, and anti-inflammatory drugs are used widely for minor aches and pains, headaches, malaise, rheumatic fever, arthritis, osteoarthritis, gout, and other musculoskeletal disorders. The narcotic (opioid) analgesics are controlled substances used to treat moderate to severe pain.

Salicylates

Salicylates are the oldest of the nonopioid analgesics and nonsteroidal anti-inflammatory drugs (NSAIDs), which are discussed in detail below. They are still often used as analgesics (Table 21-1). The salicylates include aspirin (acetylsalicylic acid), which is the most commonly used. The salicylates may be combined with caffeine to increase their action. Anacin and Excedrin are examples of salicylates that are combined with caffeine. Caffeine can make some of these agents work more quickly or provide additional relief.

Mechanism of Action

The mechanism of action of salicylates is not fully understood. Major actions appear to be associated primarily with inhibiting the formation

TABLE 21-1 Salicylates and Nonsalicylates

Generic Name	Trade Name	Route of Administration	Average Adult Dosage
Salicylates			
aspirin (acetylsalicylic acid)	Bayer®, Ecotrin®	PO, Rectal	PO: 325–650 mg with up to 8 g/day in div. doses;
buffered aspirin	Ascriptin®, Asprimox®	PO, Rectal	PO: 325–650 mg with up to 8 g/day in div. doses;
choline salicylate	Arthropan®	PO	870 mg q3–4 h (max: 6 times/day)
diflusinal	Dolobid®	PO	500–1000 mg/day in 2 div. doses (max dose: 1.5 g/day)
magnesium salicylate	Doan's Pills®, Mobidin®	PO	650 mg t.i.d. or q.i.d. up to 9.6 g/day in div. doses
salsalate	Amigesic®, Artha-G®	PO	325–3000 mg/day in div. doses
sodium salicylate	(generic only)	PO	325–650 mg q4 h
sodium thiosalicylate	Rexolate®	IM	50–150 mg q4–6 h
Nonsalicylates			
acetaminophen	Tempra®, Tylenol®	PO	325–650 mg/day q4–6 h or 1 g 3–4 times/day; max. dose: 4 g/day

of prostaglandins involved in the production of inflammation, pain, and fever.

Indications

Salicylates are also prescribed as NSAIDs for rheumatoid osteoarthritis and often for other inflammatory disorders. Aspirin is absorbed rapidly from the duodenum and stomach. It is used as an antipyretic and analgesic agent in a variety of conditions. Aspirin is indicated for the relief of pain from simple headache, minor muscular aches, and fever. When drug therapy is indicated for the reduction of a fever, it is one of the most effective and safest drugs. Aspirin may be useful in the prevention of coronary thrombosis by prolonging bleeding time, and to prevent blood clots in small arteries.

Adverse Effects

Common adverse effects of high doses of aspirin (in 70 percent of patients) include nausea, vomiting, diarrhea or constipation, dyspepsia, epigastric pain, bleeding, and ulceration in the stomach. Intolerance is relatively common with aspirin and includes rash, bronchospasm, rhinitis, edema, or an anaphylactic reaction with shock, which may be life-threatening. Use of aspirin and other salicylates to control fever during viral infections

---

Medical Terminology Review

antipyretic
anti = not
pyretic = producing fever
fever-reducing

in children and adolescents (influenza, common cold, and chicken pox), is associated with an increased incidence of **Reye syndrome**. Vomiting, hepatic disturbances, and encephalopathy characterize this illness. Salicylates that are combined with caffeine can, in very large doses, cause birth defects to a developing fetus. Caffeine, as used in some of these preparations, can make some kinds of heart disease worse.

Contraindications and Precautions

Salicylates are contraindicated in patients with known hypersensitivity and during pregnancy (category C), but aspirin during pregnancy is category D. The salicylates should be avoided in patients with bleeding disorders or peptic ulcers, or those receiving anticoagulant or antineoplastic drugs. The salicylates, particularly aspirin, are also contraindicated in patients with chicken pox and influenza.

Drug Interactions

Salicylates increase the risk of gastrointestinal ulceration with alcohol and corticosteroids. They also increase the risk of toxicity with carbonic anhydrase inhibitors and valproic acid. Ammonium chloride and other acidifying agents decrease renal elimination and increase the risk of salicylate toxicity. Anticoagulants increase the risk of bleeding. Antacids may decrease the effects of the salicylate. In order to prevent drug interactions, patients must be instructed by their physician and pharmacist about the use of NSAIDs with other OTC analgesics.

Acetaminophen

Another common nonopioid analgesic, acetaminophen is available OTC and is found in most households.

Mechanism of Action

Like aspirin, acetaminophen has analgesic and antipyretic actions. It can be used with relative safety in age groups from young children through older adults. Unlike aspirin, it does not have anti-inflammatory actions. The mechanism of action may be inhibition of prostaglandin in the peripheral nervous system, which makes the sensory neurons less likely to receive the pain signal. Acetaminophen is recommended as a substitute for children with fever of unknown etiology.

Acetaminophen does not displace other drugs from plasma proteins; it causes minimal GI irritation. Acetaminophen has little effect on platelet adhesion and aggregation. It can be substituted for aspirin to treat mild to moderate pain or fever for selected patients who:

- are intolerant to aspirin
- have a history of peptic ulcer or hemophilia

- are using anticoagulants
- are at risk (viral infection) for Reye syndrome

Indications

Acetaminophen is used for fever reduction and the temporary relief of mild to moderate pain. Acetaminophen may be used as a substitute for aspirin when the latter is not tolerated or is contraindicated.

Adverse Effects

Acute acetaminophen poisoning may produce anorexia, nausea, vomiting, dizziness, chills, abdominal pain, diarrhea, hepatotoxicity, hypoglycemia, hepatic coma, and acute renal failure (rare). Chronic ingestion of acetaminophen may cause neutropenia, pancytopenia, leukopenia, and hepatotoxicity in alcoholics, as well as renal damage.

Contraindications and Precautions

Acetaminophen is contraindicated in those with known hypersensitivity to this agent or phenacetin. Acetaminophen should not be used with alcohol.

Precautions include use in children less than three years of age unless directed by a physician, repeated administration to patients with anemia or hepatic disease, with arthritic or rheumatoid conditions affecting children less than twelve years of age, alcoholism, malnutrition, and thrombocytopenia. Safety during pregnancy (category B) or lactation is not established.

Drug Interactions

Cholestyramine may decrease acetaminophen absorption with chronic co-administration. Barbiturates, carbamazepine, phenytoin, and rifampin may increase the potential for chronic hepatotoxicity. Chronic, excessive ingestion of alcohol will increase risk of hepatotoxicity.

Nonsteroidal Anti-inflammatory Drugs

Most of the **nonsteroidal anti-inflammatory drugs (NSAIDs)** have analgesic and antipyretic effects. Little difference is seen between the effects of different NSAIDs, but some patients may respond better to one agent than to another. Anti-inflammatory effects may develop only after several weeks of treatment. Drug selection is generally dictated by the patient's ability to tolerate adverse effects. Aspirin, other salicylates, and newer drugs with diverse structures are referred to as nonsteroidal anti-inflammatory drugs (NSAIDs) to distinguish them from the anti-inflammatory corticosteroids. The number of NSAIDs continues to increase. In addition to salicylate drugs, the NSAIDs available in the U.S. include indomethacin, meclofenamate, piroxicam, sulindac, tolmetin, celecoxib, and many more (Table 21-2).

Medical Terminology Review

anticoagulant
anti = not
coagulant = an agent that causes clotting
an agent that will not cause clotting of the blood

Medical Terminology Review

thrombocytopenia
thrombo = clot
cyto = cell (such as a platelet)
penia = lack of
inability of the blood to clot

TABLE 21-2 Nonsteroidal Anti-inflammatory Drugs (NSAIDs)

Generic Name	Trade Name	Route of Administration	Average Adult Dosage
celecoxib	Celebrex®	PO	100–200 mg b.i.d. p.r.n.
diclofenac sodium	Voltaren®	PO	Osteoarthritis: 100–150 mg/day in div. doses; Rheumatoid arthritis: 150–200 mg/day in div. doses; Ankylosing spondylitis: 100–125 mg/day in div. doses
etodolac	Lodine®, Lodine XL®	PO	Acute pain: 200–400 mg q6–8 h p.r.n.; Osteoarthritis: 600–1200 mg/day in 2–4 div. doses (max: 1200 mg/day or 20 mg/kg for patients ≤ 60 kg; Lodine XL 400–1000 mg 1x/day); Rheumatoid arthritis: 500 mg b.i.d.
fenoprofen calcium	Nalfon®	PO	Rheumatoid arthritis and osteoarthritis: 300–600 mg t.i.d.-q.i.d.; Pain: 200 mg q4–8 h
flurbiprofen	Ansaid®	PO	200–300 mg/day in div. doses
ibuprofen	Advil®, Motrin®	PO	Arthritis disorders: 400–800 mg/day in div. doses (max: 3200 mg/day); Pain: 400 mg q4–6 h; Dysmenorrhea: 400 mg q4 h
indomethacin	Indocin®	PO	Anti-inflammatory and analgesic: 25–50 mg b.i.d.-t.i.d. (max: 200 mg/day); Acute painful shoulder: 75–150 mg/day in 3–4 div. doses
ketoprofen	Oruvail®	PO	Inflammatory disease: 75 mg t.i.d. or 50 mg q.i.d. (max: 300 mg/day) or 200 mg sust. release q.d.; Pain or Dysmenorrhea: 12.5–50 mg q6–8 h
ketorolac tromethamine	Toradol®	PO, IM	PO: 10 mg q4–6 h p.r.n. (max: 40 mg/day); IM: 30–60 mg initially, followed by half of initial dose q6 h p.r.n.
meclofenamate sodium	(generic)	PO	Rheumatoid arthritis: 200–400 mg/day in 3–4 doses; Pain: 50 mg q4–6 h (max: 400 mg/day); Dysmenorrhea: 100 mg t.i.d.

(continues)

TABLE 21-2   Nonsteroidal Anti-inflammatory Drugs (NSAIDs)—*continued*

Generic Name	Trade Name	Route of Administration	Average Adult Dosage
mefenamic acid	Ponstel®	PO	500 mg followed by 250 mg q6 h p.r.n. (max: 1 wk of therapy)
meloxicam	Mobic®	PO	7.5–15 mg q.d.
nabumetone	Relafen®	PO	1000–2000 mg/day
naproxen sodium	Aleve®, Anaprox®	PO	Pain, primary dysmenorrhea: 500 mg initially then 250 mg q6–8 h; Arthritic disorders: 250–500 mg b.i.d.
oxaprozin	Daypro®	PO	600–1200 mg q.d.
piroxicam	Feldene®	PO	20 mg/day single dose or 10 mg b.i.d.
sulindac	Clinoril®	PO	150–200 mg b.i.d. for 1–2 wks, then reduce dose (max: 400 mg/day)
tolmetin sodium	Tolectin®	PO	400 mg b.i.d.-t.i.d. (max: 2 g / day)

Mechanism of Action

The mechanism of action of NSAIDs is unknown. It may be due to irreversible inhibition of prostaglandin (an enzyme) formation, which converts archidonic acid to prostaglandin. This action is involved in the processes of pain and inflammation. Some experts believe that NSAIDs relieve fever by central action in the hypothalamus of the brain. In low doses, baby aspirin appears to affect blood clotting by inhibiting prostaglandin formation, which prevents synthesis of platelet-aggregating substances. This can help to prevent heart attacks and strokes. NSAIDs inhibit, in varying amounts, both the COX-1 and COX-2 enzymes.

Indications

NSAIDs are used for mild to moderate pain when opioids are not indicated. Most NSAIDs are used for inflammatory conditions such as arthritis, osteoarthritis, dysmenorrhea, and dental pain. NSAIDs are available OTC in lower dosages and by prescription in larger dosages. Aspirin and ibuprofen are available as OTC drugs that are inexpensive. Ibuprofen is available in many different formulations including those designed for children.

Adverse Effects

Many NSAIDs are safe and produce adverse effects only at high doses. The most common adverse effects (at high doses) of NSAIDs are primarily GI

distress, gastric ulcers, and GI bleeding. Other NSAIDs, such as the COX-2 inhibitors, are being investigated for possible adverse effects.

Contraindications and Precautions

Nonsteroidal anti-inflammatory drugs are contraindicated in patients with known hypersensitivity to any NSAIDs. These drugs are also contraindicated in patients with nasal polyps, asthma, and angioedema. NSAIDs should be avoided during pregnancy and in patients with history of peptic ulcer, or renal or hepatic impairment.

Drug Interactions

NSAIDs should not be taken with any other OTC analgesics such as acetaminophen, aspirin, or other NSAIDs. NSAIDs may result in harmful drug interactions if taken with alcohol and a wide variety of other medications. Use of NSAIDs with phenobarbital, antacids, and glucocorticoids may decrease their effects. Insulin, methotrexate, phenytoin, sulfonamides, and penicillin may increase the effects of NSAIDs.

Cyclooxygenase Inhibitors

The two main types of **cyclooxygenase inhibitors** (COX-1 and COX-2) have been found to have an essential role in the inflammation process. Both are present in the synovial fluid of patients with arthritis. COX-2 is more specific for prostaglandin synthesis in response to an inflammatory event. It is thought to be primarily responsible for the desired anti-inflammatory, analgesic, and antipyretic effects, whereas COX-1 has a more extensive role in the body, including protection of the GI lining.

As of May 2000, the U.S. Food and Drug Administration (FDA) has approved the COX-2 inhibitors celecoxib (Celebrex) and rofecoxib (Vioxx). Recently, rofecoxib was removed from the United States market due to problems that resulted in certain patients. A third COX-2 selective inhibitor, meloxicam (Mobic), has recently been introduced. The daily role of COX appears to be the synthesis of prostaglandins that contribute to normal homeostasis.

Mechanism of Action

These agents inhibit prostaglandin synthesis by selectively targeting only the COX-2 enzymes, but they do not inhibit COX-1. The COX-2 inhibitors have similar anti-inflammatory effects without the adverse GI effects that accompany COX-1 inhibitors.

Indications

The FDA has approved celecoxib for the treatment of osteoarthritis, rheumatoid arthritis, primary dysmenorrhea, and acute pain. Rofecoxib is off the market. Meloxicam, the newest COX-2 inhibitor, has been approved by the FDA for the treatment of osteoarthritis.

Adverse Effects

The common adverse effects of COX-2 inhibitors include fatigue, flu-like symptoms, lower extremity swelling, and back pain. Dizziness, headache, hypertension, edema, heartburn, and nausea are also seen with the use of COX-2 inhibitors.

Contraindications and Precautions

COX-2 inhibitors are contraindicated in patients with known hypersensitivity to these agents, urticaria, asthma, or history of anaphylactic reaction after taking NSAIDs or aspirin. COX-2 inhibitors are also contraindicated in elderly patients, during pregnancy (third trimester), and in lactating women. These drugs should be avoided in patients with renal disease or hepatic dysfunction.

COX-2 inhibitors should be used cautiously in patients with congestive heart failure, fluid retention, or hypertension.

Drug Interactions

COX-2 inhibitors diminish the effectiveness of ACE inhibitors. Fluconazole increases concentrations of celecoxib. COX-2 inhibitors may increase lithium concentrations.

Narcotic Analgesics

Narcotic analgesics are agents that are derived from opium or opium-like compounds with potent analgesic effects associated with both significant alteration of mood and behavior and potential for dependence and tolerance. The analgesic compounds of opium have been known for hundreds of years. Morphine is extracted from raw opium and may be altered chemically to produce the semisynthetic narcotics, such as hydromorphone, oxymorphone, oxycodone, and heroin. Synthetic narcotics are produced in laboratories, with analgesic properties. Methadone, levorphanol, and meperidine are amongst the various narcotics listed in Table 21-3.

Key Concept

Narcotic analgesics are classified as Schedule II drugs, except for heroin, which is classified as a Schedule I drug.

Mechanism of Action

The effects of natural opium alkaloids occur by binding to opioid receptors. These receptors are located in the central nervous system (brain and spinal cord). Narcotic agonist effects are identified with three types of opioid receptors: the mu, kappa, and delta receptors. Most of the currently used opioid analgesics act primarily at mu receptors. Some other opioid analgesics act at the other types of receptors.

Indications

Narcotic analgesics are used to manage moderate to severe acute and chronic pain after non-narcotic analgesics have failed. They are also used as preanesthetic medications. Narcotic analgesics are indicated to relieve dyspnea

TABLE 21-3 Opioids

Generic Name	Trade Name	Route of Administration	Average Adult Dosage
Opioid Agonists with Moderate Effects			
codeine	(generic)	PO, SC, IM	15–60 mg q.i.d.
hydrocodone	Hycodan®, Robidone®	PO	5–10 mg q4–6 h prn (max: 15 mg/dose)
oxycodone	OxyContin®, Percolone®	PO	5–10 mg q.i.d. prn
propoxyphene	Darvon®, Darvon-N®	PO	65 mg (HCl form) or 100 mg (napsylate form) q4 h prn (max: 390 HCl/day; max: 600 mg napsylate/day)
Opioid Agonists with High Effects			
hydromorphone	Dilaudid®	PO, SC, IM, IV	PO:2–4 mg q4–6 h prn; SC/IM/IV: 0.75–2 mg q4–6 h
levorphanol	Levo-Dromoran®	PO	2–3 mg t.i.d.-q.i.d. prn
meperidine	Demerol®	PO, SC, IM, IV	50–150 mg q3–4 h prn
methadone	Dolophine®, Methadose®	PO, SC, IM, IV	PO/SC/IM: 2.5–10 mg q3–4 h prn; IV: 2.5–10 mg q8–12 h prn
morphine	Astramorph PF®, Duramorph®	PO	10–30 mg q4 h prn
oxymorphone	Numorphan®	PO, SC, IM	PO: 10–20 mg q4–6 h prn; SC/IM: 1–1.5 mg q4–6 h prn

of acute left ventricular failure and pulmonary edema and pain of myocardial infarction. These agents may be given to treat severe diarrhea, intestinal cramping (camphorated tincture of opium), and persistent cough (codeine).

Adverse Effects

The major adverse effect of opioid analgesics is respiratory depression, in which the respiratory rate and depth decrease. The most common adverse effects include sedation, anorexia, nausea, vomiting, constipation, dizziness, light-headedness, and sweating. Other adverse effects of agonist narcotic analgesics on different systems are as follows:

- Gastrointestinal: dry mouth and biliary tract spasms

- Central nervous system: euphoria, pinpoint pupils, insomnia, tremor, agitation, and impairment of mental and physical tasks

- Cardiovascular: tachycardia, bradycardia, palpitations, and peripheral circulatory collapse

- Genitourinary: spasms of the ureters and bladder sphincter, urinary retention or hesitancy

Contraindications and Precautions

Narcotic analgesics are contraindicated in patients with known hypersensitivity, acute bronchial asthma, emphysema, or upper airway obstruction. Narcotic analgesics are also contraindicated in patients with head injury, increased intracranial pressure, convulsive disorders, and severe hepatic or renal dysfunction. Narcotic analgesics should be avoided during pregnancy or labor (they are ranked as category C drugs), except oxycodone (which is ranked as a category B drug), because they prolong labor or produce respiratory depression in the neonate.

Narcotic analgesics should be used cautiously in patients with cardiac arrhythmias, toxic psychosis, emphysema, kyphoscoliosis (deformity of the vertebral column), and severe obesity, and in very elderly patients.

Drug Interactions

Narcotic analgesics interact with several drugs. These drugs include CNS depressants such as alcohol, other opioids, general anesthetics, sedatives, and antidepressants such as MAOIs and tricyclics. The action of opiates is increased if used with narcotic analgesics, and the risk of severe respiratory depression (and death) is also increased.

Opioid Antagonists

Opioid antagonists are agents that prevent the effects of **opioid agonists**. The opioid antagonist drugs have an affinity for a cell receptor and compete with opioid agonists for reaching the opioid receptor site (see Table 21-4).

Mechanism of Action

Pure opioid antagonists such as naloxone are able to block both mu and kappa receptors. The mechanism of action is not clearly delineated, but it appears that its competitive binding at opioid receptor sites reduces euphoria and drug cravings without supporting addiction.

Key Concept

The use of narcotic analgesics is recommended during pregnancy only if the benefit to the mother outweighs the potential harm to the fetus.

Medical Terminology Review

kyphoscoliosis
kypho = hunchback
scoliosis = lateral and rotational spinal deformity
a deformity of the spinal column causing a hunchback appearance

---

Key Concept

Yohimbe (herbal supplements) may increase the effects of morphine.

TABLE 21-4 Opioid Antagonists

Generic Name	Trade Name	Route of Administration	Average Adult Dosage
nalmefene	Revex®	SC, IM, IV	1 mg/mL concentration; nonopioid dependent: 0.5 mg/70 kg; opioid dependent: 0.1 mg/70 kg
naloxone	Narcan®	IV	0.4–2 mg, may be repeated q2–3 min up to 10 mg prn
naltrexone	ReVia®, Vivitrol®	PO	25 mg followed by another 25 mg in 1 h if no withdrawal response (max: 800 mg/day)

Indications

Opioid antagonists are used for complete or partial reversal of opioid effects in emergency conditions when acute opioid overdose is suspected. Administered intravenously, they begin to reverse opioid-initiated CNS and respiratory depression within minutes. Naloxone is the drug of choice when the nature of a depressant drug is not known and for the diagnosis of suspected acute opioid overdosage.

Adverse Effects

Opioid antagonists themselves have minimal toxicity. However, they reverse the effects of opioids and the patient may experience rapid loss of analgesia, increased blood pressure, nausea, vomiting, drowsiness, hyperventilation, and tremors.

Contraindications and Precautions

Opioid antagonists are contraindicated in respiratory depression due to nonopioid drugs. Safety during pregnancy (other than labor) (category B) or lactation is not established.

Opioid antagonist drugs should be used with caution in neonates and children, and patients with cardiac irritability and known or suspected narcotic dependence.

Drug Interactions

Opioid antagonist drug interactions include a reversal of the analgesic effects of narcotic (opiate) agonists and **agonist-antagonists**.

MIGRAINE HEADACHES

Headache is a very common type of pain. There are many categories of headache associated with different causes, and some have specific locations and characteristics. The types of headache include:

- Headaches associated with congested sinuses.

- Headaches associated with muscle spasm and tension resulting from emotional stress that causes the neck muscles to contract to a greater degree, pulling on the scalp.

- **Intracranial** headaches resulting from increased pressure inside the skull.

- Migraine headaches, which are related to abnormal changes in blood flow and metabolism in the brain. There are many precipitating factors, including atmospheric changes, stress, menstruation, hunger, and heredity. The pain of a migraine headache is usually throbbing, quite severe, and sometimes incapacitating. Characteristically, these types of headaches begin unilaterally (on one side) in the temple area, but often spread to involve the entire head. The pain is often

accompanied by dizziness, nausea, abdominal pain, fatigue, and visual disturbances. These headaches may last up to 24 hours, and there is often a prolonged recovery period.

Treatment of Migraine Headaches

Treatment is difficult, although ergotamine may be effective if administered immediately after the onset of the headache. New forms of ergotamine are available as sublingual tablets, which provide a more readily available and rapid-acting treatment. Other drugs used for migraines, and a newer group of medications, are listed in Table 21-5.

TABLE 21-5 Drugs Used to Treat Migraine Headaches

Generic Name	Trade Name	Route of Administration	Average Adult Dosage
Ergot Alkaloids			
dihydroergotamine	D.H.E. 45®, Migranal®	SC, IM, IV	1 mg repeated at 1 h intervals to a total of 3 mg IM; or 2 mg SC/IV
ergotamine	Ergomar®, Ergostat®	Sublingual	1–2 mg repeated q30 m until headache stops
ergotamine with caffeine	Cafergot®, Ercaf®	PO	1–2 mg repeated q30 m until headache stops
Triptans			
almotriptan	Axert®	PO	6.25–12.5 mg repeated in 2 h prn
electriptan	Relpax®	PO	20–40 mg repeated in 2 h prn
frovatriptan	Frova®	PO	2.5 mg repeated in 2 h prn
naratriptan	Amerge®	PO	1–2.5 mg repeated in 4 h prn
rizatriptan	Maxalt®	PO	5–10 mg repeated in 2 h prn or 5 mg with concurrent propranolol
sumatriptan	Imitrex®	PO	25 mg for 1 dose
zolmitriptan	Zomig®	PO	2.5–5 mg repeated in 2 h prn
Beta-adrenergic Blockers			
atenolol	Tenormin®	PO	25–50 mg/day
metoprolol	Lopressor®	PO	50–100 mg 1–2 times/day
propranolol	Inderal®	PO	80–240 mg/day in div. doses
timolol	Blocadren®	PO	10 mg b.i.d. up to 60 mg/day in 2 div. doses
Calcium Channel Blockers			
nifedipine	Procardia®	PO	10–20 mg t.i.d.
nimodipine	Nimotop®	PO	60 mg q4 h for 21 days, start therapy within 96 hrs of subarachnoid hemorrhage
verapamil	Isoptin®	PO	40–80 mg t.i.d.

Mechanism of Action

Anti-migraine drugs include the ergot alkaloids and the triptans, which are both serotonin agonists. Serotonergic receptors (those that are related to the neurotransmitter serotonin) are found through the CNS, GI tract, and in the cardiovascular system. These agents act by causing vasoconstriction of the cranial arteries. This vasoconstriction is moderately selective, and does not usually affect overall blood pressure.

Indications

The drugs of choice for treatment of migraine are often the triptans. Ergot alkaloids may be used to stop migraines. Prophylaxis includes various classes of drugs (such as beta blockers and calcium channel blockers) that are discussed in other chapters of this textbook.

Adverse Effects

Common adverse effects of ergot alkaloids include nausea, vomiting, abnormal pulse, weakness, and convulsive seizures. The adverse effects of triptans include warming sensations, dizziness, weakness, and tickling or prickling. The major adverse effects of triptans include: coronary artery vasospasm, heart attack, and cardiac arrest.

Contraindications and Precautions

These agents are contraindicated in patients with recent myocardial infarction, a history of angina pectoris, diabetes, and high blood pressure. Because ergot alkaloids and triptans cause vasoconstriction of blood vessels, they should be used cautiously.

Drug Interactions

Ergot alkaloids and triptans may interact with several drugs. For example, an increased effect may occur when taken with monoamine oxidase inhibitors (MAOIs) and selective serotonin reuptake inhibitors (SSRIs). Further vasoconstriction may occur.

Summary

Non-narcotic analgesics are used to relieve pain without the possibility of resulting physical dependency. Non-narcotic analgesics include the salicylates, non-salicylates (acetaminophen), and nonsteroidal anti-inflammatory drugs (NSAIDs).

Salicylates are the oldest of the nonopioid analgesics and NSAIDs. They are still commonly used as analgesics. Aspirin is the most commonly used of these agents. Some of these analgesics are also used as anti-inflammatory and antipyretic drugs.

Adverse effects of salicylate drugs are common and include heartburn, nausea, vomiting, and gastrointestinal bleeding. Acetaminophen may cause adverse reactions with chronic use or when the recommended dosage is exceeded.

New NSAIDs are available as analgesic, antipyretic, and anti-inflammatory agents. COX-2 inhibitors are more specific for prostaglandin synthesis in response to an inflammatory event. The FDA has approved the COX-2 inhibitors such as celecoxib and meloxicam.

Narcotic analgesics are controlled substances used to treat moderate to severe pain. Narcotic analgesics are classified as agonists and antagonists. One of the major adverse effects of agonist narcotic administration is respiratory depression.

Morphine is the most widely used drug in the management of chronic severe pain, and opioid antagonists are agents that prevent the effects of opioid agonists. These drugs have an affinity for a cell receptor and compete with opioid agonists for reaching the opioid receptor site.

A migraine headache is a very common type of pain. There are various agents used as anti-migraine medications. The two major drug classes used for treating migraine headaches include ergot alkaloids and triptans. Other drugs used for this purpose include beta-adrenergic blockers, calcium channel blockers, and tricyclic antidepressants.

Exploring the Web

Visit www.fda.gov

- Search for the types of drugs discussed in this chapter. Look for safety information, advisories, patient education, etc.

Visit www.healthopedia.com

- Click on "drugs and medications," and search for additional information on the drugs discussed within the chapter. You

can also find drug information at www.medicinenet.com (click "medications") or www.nlm.nih.gov/medlineplus (click on "drugs and supplements").

REVIEW QUESTIONS

Multiple Choice

1. Aspirin may be useful in the prevention of coronary thrombosis because of which of the following properties?

    A. thrombolytic
    B. antiarthritic
    C. anti-inflammatory
    D. antiplatelet

2. Celecoxib (Celebrex®) is classified as:

    A. a COX-1 and COX-2 inhibitor
    B. a COX-1 inhibitor
    C. a COX-2 inhibitor
    D. a nonselective NSAID

3. Which of the following is a main contraindication of NSAIDs?

    A. rheumatoid arthritis
    B. corticosteroid sensitivity
    C. osteoarthritis
    D. allergy to aspirin

4. Which of the following terms is used for pain-relieving drugs?

    A. antitoxins
    B. antiemetics
    C. analgesics
    D. anaphylactics

5. Examples of nonsalicylate nonsteroidal anti-inflammatory drugs include:

    A. ibuprofen and indomethacin
    B. mefenamic acid and magnesium sulfate
    C. naproxen and neomycin
    D. piroxicam and lysergic acid

6. COX-2 is more specific for synthesis of which of the following in response to an inflammatory event?

    A. histamine
    B. prostaglandin
    C. heparin
    D. epinephrine

7. Which of the following classes of drugs are *preferred* for treating migraine headaches?

    A. tricyclic antidepressants
    B. NSAIDs
    C. beta-adrenergic blockers
    D. triptans

8. Which of the following drugs is used to treat opioid dependence?

    A. hydromorphone
    B. methadone
    C. oxycodone
    D. propoxyphene

9. The main adverse effect of morphine is:

    A. diarrhea
    B. respiratory depression
    C. depression
    D. intestinal cramping

10. Narcotic analgesics are contraindicated in which of the following situations?

    A. moderate pain
    B. pulmonary edema
    C. persistent cough
    D. bronchial asthma

11. The trade name of ibuprofen is:

    A. Nalfon
    B. Advil
    C. Aleve
    D. Actron

12. Which of the following is considered an aspirin substitute?

    A. Indocin (indomethacin)
    B. Celebrex (celecoxib)
    C. Tylenol (acetaminophen)
    D. Aleve (naproxen)

13. If a patient has an allergy to aspirin, which of the following drugs may be used?

    A. sodium thiosalicylate injectable
    B. etolac
    C. acetaminophen
    D. allopurinol

14. Narcotic analgesia at the spinal level may cause which of the following?

    A. miosis and sedation
    B. physical dependence and psychosis
    C. euphoria and respiratory depression
    D. hyperventilation and tremors

15. Which of the following is an example of pure opioid antagonists?

    A. methadone
    B. oxycodone
    C. naloxone
    D. meperidine

Matching

    A. morphine

    B. methadone

    C. oxycodone

    D. hydrocodone

    E. naloxone

    _____ **1.** Often used with aspirin or acetaminophen.

    _____ **2.** Competes with opioid agonists for reaching the opioid receptor site.

    _____ **3.** More addicting than codeine.

    _____ **4.** Extracted from raw opium.

    _____ **5.** Used for detoxification of opioid addiction.

Critical Thinking

A 58-year-old patient with a history of a recent myocardial infarction is on beta-blocker and anticoagulant therapy. The patient has a history of peptic ulcer (which is not bothering him currently). During a recent flare-up, he began taking aspirin because it helped control the pain in his chest that he experienced.

    1. What recommendation would the pharmacist have for this patient?

    2. If the patient takes aspirin, what major adverse effects could occur?

    3. Name a drug that the pharmacist could advise the patient to take instead of aspirin.

Anti-infectives and Systemic Antibacterial Agents

OUTLINE

OBJECTIVES

After completing this chapter, the reader should be able to:

1. Describe the various forms of microorganisms.
2. Compare the terms *bactericidal* and *bacteriostatic*.
3. Describe various mechanisms of action of antibacterial therapy.
4. Explain the indication and contraindication of antibiotics.
5. Describe the major side effects of antibacterial agents.
6. Understand the importance of drug interactions.
7. Explain the mechanisms of action for penicillins, cephalosporins, aminoglycosides, tetracyclines, macrolides, and quinolones.
8. Compare the effectiveness of penicillins with cephalosporins.
9. Explain the first line of antituberculosis drugs.
10. Describe the significant contraindications of rifampin and ethambutol.

GLOSSARY

Antibiotics – substances that have the ability to destroy or interfere with the development of a living organism

Antimicrobial – an anti-infective drug produced from synthetic substances

Bacteria – small, one-celled microorganisms that lack a true nucleus or mechanism to provide metabolism

Bactericidal – killing bacterial growth

Bacteriostatic – suppress bacterial growth by triggering a mechanism that blocks folic acid synthesis, thereby forcing bacteria to synthesize their own folic acid

Broad-spectrum antibiotics – agent that is effective against a wide variety of

both Grampositive and Gram-negative pathogenic microorganisms

Fungi – microorganisms that grow in single cells or in colonies

Gram stains – sequential procedures involving crystal violet and iodine solutions followed by alcohol that allow rapid identification of organisms as Gram-positive or Gram-negative types

Gram-negative – microorganisms that stain red or pink with Gram stain

Gram-positive – microorganisms that stain blue or purple with Gram stain

Infection – the invasion of pathogenic microorganisms that produce tissue damage within the body

Localized infection – involve a specific area of the body such as the skin or internal organs

Mycoplasms – ultramicroscopic organisms that lack rigid cell walls and are considered to be the smallest free-living organisms

Narrow-spectrum antibiotics – antibiotics that are effective against only a few organisms

Porphyria – a group of enzyme disorders that cause skin problems (such as purple discolorations) and/or neurological complications

Protozoa – single-celled parasitic organisms with the ability to move

Rickettsia – intercellular parasites that need to be in living cells to reproduce

Red man syndrome – a rash on the upper body caused by vancomycin

Spores – bacteria in a resistant stage that can withstand an unfavorable environment

Systemic infection – impacts the whole body rather than a specific area of the body

Viruses – organisms that can live only inside cells

OVERVIEW

Pathogenic microorganisms may cause a wide spectrum of illnesses. They produce infection of different organs or systems of the body, such as upper respiratory tract infections, meningitis, pneumonia, tuberculosis, and urinary tract infections. This chapter focuses on the drugs used to treat a variety of infections.

INFECTIONS

An **infection** is described as the invasion of pathogenic microorganisms that produce tissue damage within the body. Infections may be classified primarily as either local or systemic. A **localized infection** may involve a specific area of the body such as the skin or internal organs. A localized infection can progress to a systemic infection. A **systemic infection** impacts the whole body rather than a specific area of the body. Infections are also classified as acute or chronic.

Chain of Infection

The chain of infection describes the elements of an infectious process. It is an interactive process that involves the agent, host, and environment. This process must include several essential elements or "links in the chain" for the transmission of microorganisms to occur. Figure 22-1 identifies the

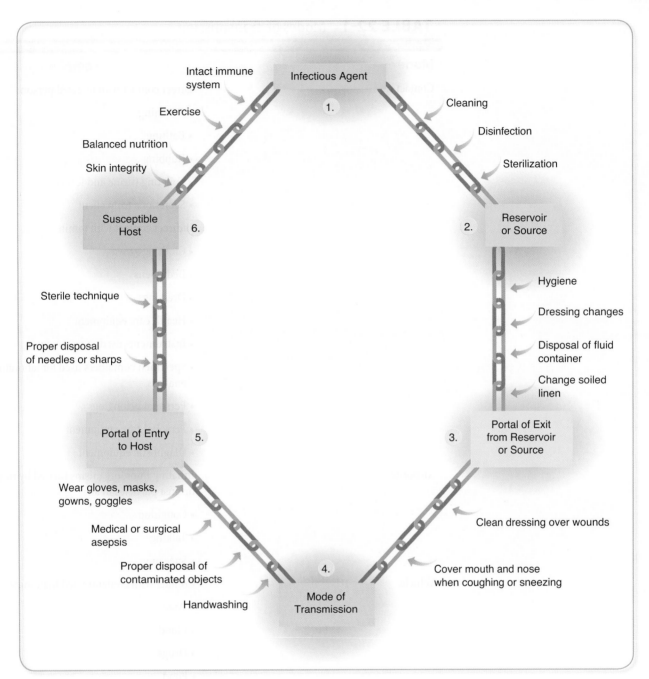

Figure 22-1 Chain of infection.

six essential links in the chain of infection. Table 22-1 summarizes modes of transmission.

Without the transmission of microorganisms, the infectious process cannot occur. Knowledge about the chain of infection facilitates control or prevention of disease by breaking the links in the chain. This is achieved by altering one or more of the interactive processes of agent, host, or environment.

TABLE 22-1   Modes of Transmission

Mode	Examples
Contact	Direct contact with infected person:
	• Touching
	• Bathing
	• Rubbing
	• Toileting (urine and feces)
	• Secretions from client
	Indirect contact with fomites:
	• Clothing
	• Bed linens
	• Dressings
	• Health care equipment
	• Instruments used in treatments
	• Specimen containers used for laboratory analysis
	• Personal belongings
	• Personal care equipment
	• Diagnostic equipment
Airborne	Inhaling microorganisms carried by moisture or dust particles in air:
	• Coughing
	• Talking
	• Sneezing
Vehicle	Contact with contaminated inanimate objects:
	• Water
	• Blood
	• Drugs
	• Food
	• Urine
Vector borne	Contact with contaminated animate hosts:
	• Animals
	• Insects

MICROORGANISMS

Microorganisms are divided into several groups: bacteria, mycoplasms, viruses, fungi, protozoa, and rickettsia. Bacteria are classified according to their shape, such as cocci, bacilli, and spirilla. They are also classified into two groups that depend upon their capacity to be stained. This staining process is

called **Gram staining**. It involves sequential procedures using crystal violet and iodine solutions followed by alcohol that allow rapid identification of organisms as Gram-positive or Gram-negative types. Gram stains can identify specific types of bacteria. **Gram-negative** microorganisms stain red or rose-pink (Figure 22-2). **Gram-positive** microorganisms stain blue or purple (Figure 22-3). Fungi may also be identified by Gram staining. The culture and sensitivity tests can determine which antibiotics should be prescribed.

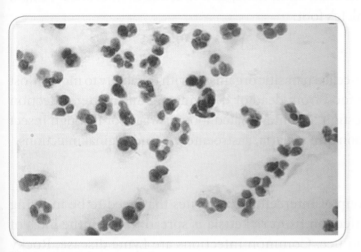

Figure 22-2 Gram-negative.

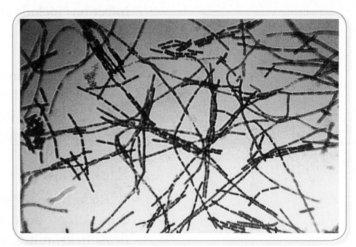

Figure 22-3 Gram-positive.

Bacteria

Bacteria are small, one-celled microorganisms that lack a true nucleus or mechanism to provide metabolism. Some forms of bacteria produce **spores**, a resistant stage that withstands an unfavorable environment. When proper environmental conditions return, spores germinate and form new cells. Spores are resistant to heat, drying, and disinfectants. Pathogenic bacteria cause a wide range of illnesses including diarrhea, pneumonia, sinusitis, urinary tract infections, and gonorrhea.

Mycoplasms

Mycoplasms are ultramicroscopic organisms that lack rigid cell walls and are considered to be the smallest free-living organisms. Some are saprophytes (a plant that lives on dead or decaying matter), some are parasites, and many are pathogens. One species is a cause of mycoplasma pneumonia, tracheobronchitis, and pharyngitis.

Viruses

Viruses are organisms that can live only inside cells. They cannot get nourishment or reproduce outside the cell. Viruses contain a core of DNA or RNA surrounded by a protein coating. Viruses damage the cell they inhabit by blocking the normal protein synthesis and by using the cell's mechanism for metabolism to reproduce themselves. Viral infections include the

common cold, influenza, measles, hepatitis, genital herpes, HIV, and the West Nile virus. Treatment of viruses will be discussed in Chapter 23.

Fungi

Fungi grow in single cells as in yeast or in colonies as in molds. Fungi obtain food from living organisms or organic matter. Disease from fungi is found mainly in individuals who are immunologically impaired. Fungi can cause infections of the hair, skin, nails, and mucous membranes. Fungal infections include athlete's foot.

Protozoa

Protozoa are single-celled parasitic organisms with the ability to move. Most protozoa obtain their food from dead or decaying organic matter. Infection is spread through ingestion of contaminated food or water, or through insect bites. Common infections are malaria, gastroenteritis, and vaginal infections.

Rickettsia

Rickettsia is a group of intercellular parasites that need to be in living cells to reproduce. Infection from rickettsia is spread through the bites of fleas, ticks, mites, and lice. Common infections are Lyme disease, Rocky Mountain spotted fever, and typhus.

PRINCIPLES OF ANTI-INFECTIVE THERAPY

Anti-infective agents are used to treat infection by destroying or suppressing the causative microorganisms. The goal is to suppress the causative agent sufficiently so that the body's own defenses can eliminate it. Anti-infective drugs derived from natural substances are called **antibiotics**. Those produced from synthetic substances are called **antimicrobials**. In past years, strong efforts have been made to change antibiotic usage policy rendering prescribing practices clinically stronger, but less costly. There is an emphasis on rapid conversion from parenteral to oral therapy for a variety of infectious processes. Major efforts are being taken to understand the underlying principles associated with the interaction of the antibiotics, host, and pathogens.

Medical Terminology Review

antibiotic

anti = against; opposite; opposing; contrary
biotic = a mode of living
suppressing the mechanism by which a microorganism lives

Selection of Agents

An anti-infective agent should be chosen on the basis of its pharmacologic properties and spectrum of activity as well as on various patient factors.

1. *Pharmacologic properties*: The drug's ability to reach the infection site and to attain a desired level of concentration in the target tissue.

2. *Spectrum of activity*: To treat an infectious disease effectively, an anti-infective agent must be effective against the causative pathogen. The effectiveness of an anti-infective drug can be confirmed by a

sensitivity test. Resistance to an anti-infective can arise by mutation in the gene that determines sensitivity/resistance to the agent.

3. *Patient factors*: There are various patient factors that determine what type of anti-infectives should be administered. These factors include: immunity of patients, age, presence of a foreign body, adverse drug reactions, pregnancy and lactation, and underlying disease. Choosing an anti-infective that doesn't offer enough protection is a common problem. Some commonly used drugs such as aminoglycosides and vancomycin are poorly absorbed and can be used to treat G.I. infections without systemic effects. Antimicrobials can be used as prophylactics for people in contact with patients with meningitis or tuberculosis; surgery to the GI, urinary tract, or dental regions; or those with rheumatoid fever. Other patient considerations in the use of anti-infective agents include:

- diminished renal function in the elderly
- partially developed hepatic function in neonates
- circulation problems such as with diabetes

Duration of Anti-infective Therapy

The most important goal of anti-infective therapy is to continue it for a sufficient duration. All antibiotics should be completed through the prescribed amount of time. Treatment for chronic infection such as osteomyelitis or endocarditis may require a longer duration, for example, 4 to 6 weeks.

Antibiotic Spectrum

Effectiveness of antibiotics against different microorganisms may be divided into two groups: broad-spectrum and narrow-spectrum. **Broad-spectrum antibiotics** are effective against a wide variety of both Gram-positive and Gram-negative pathogenic microorganisms. **Narrow-spectrum antibiotics** can be effective on a few Gram-positive or Gram-negative pathogens.

Superinfections

The normal flora (nonpathogenic microorganisms within the body) may be disrupted by administration of oral antibiotics, which causes superinfection. This process of destruction of large numbers of normal flora by antibiotics can alter the chemical environment. Therefore, uncontrolled growth of bacteria or fungal microorganisms may occur. Any antibiotic that is administered for a long time, or a repeated course of therapy, may result in superinfections. A superinfection may develop suddenly and may be serious or life-threatening. Bacterial superinfections can be seen frequently with the use of oral penicillins and involve the large intestine. Pseudomembranous colitis is a common bacterial superinfection, and moniliasis is a common type of fungal superinfection.

ANTIBACTERIAL AGENTS

Antibacterial agents are used to treat infections caused by bacteria. The major categories for antibacterial agents include: sulfonamides, penicillins, cephalosporins, aminoglycosides, macrolides, tetracyclines, fluoroquinolones, and miscellaneous antibacterial agents.

Sulfonamides

Sulfonamides are the synthetic derivatives of sulfanilamide (Table 22-2). These agents were the first drugs to prevent and cure human bacterial infection successfully. They are well-absorbed from the gastrointestinal tract. Sulfonamides readily penetrate the cerebrospinal fluid. These agents are metabolized to various degrees in the liver, and are eliminated by the kidneys. Sulfonamides were originally active against a wide range of Gram-positive and Gram-negative bacteria; however, the increasing incidence of resistance in bacteria formerly susceptible to sulfonamides has decreased the clinical usefulness of the drug. However, sulfonamides remain the drug of choice for certain infections. The major sulfonamides are generally classified as short-acting, intermediate-acting, or long-acting. Their rate of action depends on how quickly they are absorbed and eliminated.

Key Concept

Sulfonamides were the first antimicrobial agents, but their clinical use has been greatly restricted as a result of the development of resistant bacteria.

Mechanism of Action

Sulfonamides are **bacteriostatic**; they suppress bacterial growth by triggering a mechanism that blocks folic acid synthesis, thereby forcing bacteria to synthesize their own folic acid.

Medical Terminology Review

bacteriostatic

bacterio = bacteria; bacterial
static = slowing; stoppage
slowing or stopping the growth of bacteria

TABLE 22-2   Classification of Sulfonamides

Generic Name	Trade Name	Route of Administration	Common Dosage Range
Short-acting (4–8 hours)			
sulfamethizole	Thiosulfil Forte®	PO	7.5 mg–1 g
sulfasalazine	Azulfidine®	PO	1–2 g/day in 4 div. doses; may increase up to 8 g/day
sulfisoxazole	Gantrisin®	PO	2–4 g initially, followed by 1–2 g q.i.d.
Intermediate-acting (7–17 hours)			
sulfadizine	Microsulfon®	PO	2–4 g
sulfamethoxazole	Gantanol®	PO	2 g initially, followed by 1 g b.i.d.
trimethoprim-sulfamethoxazole	Bactrim®, Septra®	PO	160 mg TMP/800 mg b.i.d.
Long-acting (17+ hours)			
sulfadoxine-pyrimethamine	Fansidar®	PO	1 tablet/wk

Indications

Sulfonamides most often are used to treat urinary tract infections by *E. coli*, including acute and chronic cystitis, and chronic upper urinary tract infections. Prophylactic sulfonamide therapy has been used successfully to prevent streptococcal infections and rheumatic fever recurrences.

Adverse Effects

Key Concept

Elderly patients and patients with impairment of the kidney who are given sulfonamides have a risk for more renal damage. An increase of fluid intake up to 2,000 mL decreases the risk of crystals and stones forming in the urinary tract.

Sulfonamides may cause blood dyscrasias such as hemolytic anemia, aplastic anemia, thrombocytopenia, and agranulocytosis. Hypersensitivity reactions may occur with sulfonamide therapy. Hematuria and crystalluria are two of the major adverse effects of sulfonamide agents. Sulfonamides should be used with caution in patients with renal impairment. Life-threatening hepatitis caused by drugs is a rare adverse effect. Patients who take sulfonamides have increased susceptibility to adverse effects from sun exposure.

Contraindications and Precautions

Sulfonamides must be avoided in patients with a history of hypersensitivity to these drugs. They are contraindicated in the treatment of group A beta-hemolytic streptococcal infections or in infants less than two months of age (except in the treatment of congenital toxoplasmosis). Sulfonamides must not be used in patients with **porphyria**, advanced kidney or liver disease, intestinal obstruction, or urinary obstruction. They are contraindicated during pregnancy (if near term) and in lactating women. Sulfonamides must be used cautiously in patients with impaired kidney or liver function, severe allergy, bronchial asthma, and blood dyscrasias.

Drug Interactions

Sulfonamides may increase the effects of phenytoin, oral anticoagulants, and sulfonylureas.

Penicillins

Sir Arthur Fleming discovered the antibacterial properties of natural penicillins in 1928 while he was performing research on influenza. In 1938, British scientists realized the effects of natural penicillins on disease-causing microorganisms. In 1941, natural penicillins were used for the treatment of infections.

Natural or semisynthetic antibiotics are produced by or derived from certain species of the fungus *Penicillium*. Penicillins are the most widely used anti-infective agents; however, cephalosporin usage has increased in the last decade. Among the most important antibiotics, natural penicillins are the

preferred drugs in the treatment of many infectious diseases. The major cause of resistance to penicillin is due to production of beta-lactamases (penicillinases). Common organisms that are capable of producing penicillinase include *Staphylococcus aureus*, *Escherichia coli*, *Pseudomonas aeruginosa*, and species of *Bacillus*, *Proteus*, and *Bactericides*. Penicillins are available as penicillin G, penicillin V, penicillin G procaine, and penicillin G benzathine. Table 22-3 shows common types of penicillins and the route of administration.

Mechanism of Action

Penicillins are **bactericidal**. They inhibit bacterial cell wall synthesis in similar ways to the cephalosporins. Natural penicillins are highly active against Gram-positive and against some Gram-negative cocci. Penicillin G is ten times more active than penicillin V against Gram-negative organisms.

TABLE 22-3 Common Penicillins and Routes of Administration

Generic Name	Trade Name	Route of Administration	Common Dosage Range
Natural Penicillins			
penicillin G potassium	Pentids®	PO	400,000–800,000 units/day
penicillin V potassium	Pen Vee K®, Veetids®	PO	125–250 mg q.i.d.
penicillin G procaine	Crysticillin®	IM	600,000–1.2 million units/day
penicillin G benzathine	Bicillin®	IM	1.2 million units as a single dose
Penicillinase-Resistant Penicillins			
cloxacillin sodium	Cloxapen®	PO	250–500 mg q.i.d.
dicloxacillin sodium	Dycill®, Dynapen®	PO	125–500 mg q.i.d.
nafcillin sodium	Nafcil®, Unipen®	PO, IM, IV	500 mg–1 g q.i.d.
oxacillin sodium	Bactocill®	PO, IM, IV	500 mg–1 g q.i.d., IM/IV: 250 mg–1 g q4–6 h
Semisynthetic Penicillins			
amoxicillin	Amoxil®, Trimox®	PO	250–500 mg t.i.d.
amoxicillin and clavulanate potassium	Augmentin®	PO	250–500 mg q8–12 h
ampicillin	Polycillin®, Omnipen®	PO, IM, IV	250–500 mg q.i.d.
bacampicillin hydrochloride	Spectrobid®	PO	400–800 mg b.i.d.

Indications

Penicillin G is the drug of choice for all *Streptococcus pneumoniae* organisms. Penicillins G and V are highly effective against other streptococcal infections such as bacteremia, pharyngitis, otitis media, and sinusitis. Penicillin G is also the drug of choice against many gonococcal infections, post-exposure inhalational anthrax, syphilis, and gas gangrene. Penicillin G procaine is effective against syphilis and uncomplicated gonorrhea. Penicillin G benzathine is very effective against group A beta-hemolytic streptococcal infections. Penicillins G and V may be indicated for prophylactic treatment to prevent streptococcal infection, rheumatic fever, and neonatal gonorrhea ophthalmia.

Adverse Effects

Hypersensitivity occurs in nearly ten percent of cases. Reactions from simple rash to anaphylaxis can be observed from within two minutes and up to three days following administration. Anaphylaxis is a life-threatening reaction that most commonly occurs with parenteral administration. Signs and symptoms include severe hypotension, bronchoconstriction, nausea, vomiting, and abdominal pain. Before penicillin therapy begins, the patient's history should be evaluated for allergy to penicillin.

Key Concept

Injection of penicillin to a patient may cause anaphylactic reactions within 30 minutes after administration. Therefore, the patient must be monitored for 30 minutes.

Contraindications and Precautions

Penicillins must be avoided in patients with a history of hypersensitivity to penicillin or cephalosporins. Penicillins should be used cautiously in patients with kidney disease and during pregnancy (category C) and lactation. These drugs are to be used with caution in patients with bleeding disorders, gastrointestinal diseases, and asthma.

Drug Interactions

The most significant drugs that may increase or decrease the effects of penicillin include: probenecid, erythromycins, tetracyclines, and chloramphenicol. Probenecid increases blood levels of natural penicillin. On the other hand, chloramphenicol, erythromycins, and tetracyclines are antagonists with penicillin.

Penicillinase-resistant Penicillins

The penicillin resistance of many Gram-positive and Gram-negative bacteria is because of penicillin-destroying enzymes called beta-lactamases. The enzymes from *staphylococci, enterococci, meningococci, gonococci,* and various other bacteria were the first-known beta-lactamases and were called penicillinases.

Resistance of bacteria to penicillin cannot be explained entirely on penicillinase production because many resistant organisms produce little or no penicillinase. Nonpenicillinase-mediated resistance is called methicillin resistance.

Resistant penicillins are used predominantly for penicillinase-producing staphylococcal infections. Most staphylococci are now resistant to benzylpenillin because they produce a penicillinase. As their name suggests, penicillinase-resistant penicillins are resistant to the action of this enzyme and are therefore indicated in infections caused by penicillin-resistant *staphylococcus*. Oxacillin, cloxacillin, dicloxacillin, and nafcillin can be given orally. Methicillin is administered parenterally. Nafcillin is used parenterally for more serious infections. Penicillinase-resistant penicillins are used solely in staphylococcal infections resulting from organisms that resist natural penicillins. These agents are less potent than natural penicillins against organisms susceptible to natural penicillins. Penicillinase-resistant penicillins are the preferred choice for skin and soft tissue infections due to staphylococci. Higher doses should be used for severe infections or for infections of the lower respiratory tract. In suspension form, these agents should be taken on an empty stomach, are stable for 14 days after mixing (but refrigeration is required), and are known for having a bitter aftertaste.

Mechanism of Action

Penicillinase-resistant penicillins prevent cell wall synthesis by binding to enzymes called penicillin-binding proteins (PBPs). These enzymes are essential for the synthesis of the bacterial cell wall.

Indications

Indications of penicillinase-resistant penicillins include prevention and treatment of bacterial infections, including *streptococcus*, *enterococcus*, and *staphylococcus* strains.

Adverse Effects

The penicillinase-resistant group can also cause hypersensitivity reactions like natural penicillins. Methicillin may cause nephrotoxicity. Oxacillin can produce hepatotoxicity. They may cause nausea, vomiting, diarrhea, or skin rash.

Contraindications and Precautions

These agents are contraindicated in patients with hypersensitivity to penicillins or cephalosporins. Safe use during pregnancy (category B) is not established.

Penicillinase-resistant penicillins should be used cautiously in patients with a history of, or suspected, allergy (hives, eczema, hay fever, asthma); in premature infants and neonates; and during lactation (which may cause infant diarrhea). They also should be used with great caution in patients with renal or hepatic function impairment.

Medical Terminology Review

hypersensitivity

hyper = over; above; beyond
sensitivity = the quality or condition of being responsive or reactive
overly reactive to a particular agent

nephrotoxicity

nephro = kidney
toxicity = the quality or condition of being poisonous
poisoning of the kidney

hepatotoxicity

hepato = liver
toxicity = the quality or condition of being poisonous
poisoning of the liver

Drug Interactions

Penicillinase-resistant penicillins can inactivate aminoglycoside serum samples from patients receiving both drugs.

Semi-synthetic Penicillins (Amoxicillin/ Clavulanate Potassium)

Streptococcus pneumoniae is the most common cause of acute bacterial sinusitis (ABS) and community-acquired pneumonia (CAP). Amoxicillin/ clavulanate potassium is the first FDA-approved antibiotic for both of these infections.

Mechanism of Action

The amoxicillin component of the formulation exerts a bactericidal action against many Gram-negative and Gram-positive strains. The clavulanate potassium component protects the amoxicillin from degradation by inactivating harmful beta-lactamase enzymes.

Indications

This combination is used for the treatment of infections caused by susceptible beta-lactamase-producing organisms of upper respiratory infections such as otitis media, tonsillitis, and sinusitis. It is also used to treat lower respiratory infections such as bronchitis and pneumonia. Urinary tract, skin, and soft tissue infections are also treatable with this combination agent.

Adverse Effects

Amoxicillin/clavulanate potassium should not be used in patients with hepatic dysfunction because of the danger of transient hepatitis and cholestatic jaundice. Serious and occasionally fatal hypersensitivity reactions have been reported in patients on penicillin therapy. Diarrhea, nausea, vomiting, urticaria, and candidal vaginitis may occur.

Contraindications and Precautions

This combination should not be used in patients with hypersensitivity to penicillins, infectious mononucleosis, and during pregnancy (category B) and lactation. The combination of amoxicillin and clavulanate potassium shares the toxic potential of ampicillin.

Drug Interactions

Concurrent use of this agent with probenecid may result in increased and prolonged blood levels of amoxicillin. This agent interacts with coumarin or indandione-derivative anticoagulants, heparin, NSAIDs (especially aspirin), other platelet aggregation inhibitors or thrombolytic agents, and estrogen-containing oral contraceptives.

TABLE 22-4 Extended-spectrum Penicillins

Generic Name	Trade Name	Route of	Common Dosage Range
Carboxypenicillins			
carbenicillin	Geocillin®	PO	382–764 mg q.i.d.
ticarcillin disodium and clavulanate potassium	Timentin®	IV	>60 kg, 3.1 g q4–6 h
Ureidopenicillins			
mezlocillin	Mezlin®	IM, IV	25–50 mg/kg/day
piperacillin	Pipracil®	IM, IV	8–16 g/day

Extended-spectrum Penicillins

This group of penicillins has the widest antibacterial spectrum. Included are the carboxypenicillins and the ureidopenicillins (Table 22-4).

Mechanism of Action

Extended-spectrum penicillins are also bactericidal and inhibit bacterial cell wall synthesis.

Indications

Extended-spectrum penicillins are prescribed mainly to treat serious infections caused by Gram-negative organisms such as sepsis, pneumonia, peritonitis, osteomyelitis, and soft tissue infections.

Adverse Effects

As with other penicillins, hypersensitivity reactions may occur. Carbenicillin and ticarcillin may cause hypokalemia. The use of these two drugs may be a danger to patients with congestive heart failure because of the high sodium content of carbenicillin and ticarcillin.

Contraindications and Precautions

These agents are contraindicated in patients with hypersensitivity to penicillins and during pregnancy (category B). Safe use in children is not established.

Extended spectrum penicillins should be used cautiously in patients with a history of, or suspected, atopy or allergies, or history of allergy to cephalosporins; during lactation; in patients with impaired renal and hepatic function; and in patients on sodium restricted diets.

Drug Interactions

Extended spectrum penicillins agents may increase the risk of bleeding if used with anticoagulants. Elimination of ticarcillin is decreased by the use of probenecid.

Cephalosporins

These agents are known as beta-lactam antibiotics. Cephalosporins are semisynthetic antibiotics structurally and pharmacologically related to penicillins. Cephalosporins are usually bactericidal in action. The antibacterial activity of the cephalosporin results from inhibition of mucopeptide synthesis in the bacterial cell wall. The cephalosporins are classified into four different "generations." Particular cephalosporins may be differentiated within each group according to the bacteria that are sensitive to them (see Table 22-5).

First-generation cephalosporins are effective against most Gram-positive organisms and some Gram-negative organisms. They are used mainly for *Klebsiella* infections, and for those who have penicillin- and sulfonamide-resistant urinary tract infections. Cephapirin and cefazolin are used parenterally; others can be administered orally. Cephalosporins do not penetrate the cerebrospinal fluid (CSF).

Second-generation cephalosporins extend the spectrum of the first generation to include *Haemophilus influenzae* and some *Proteus*. Second-generation cephalosporins are used primarily in the treatment of urinary tract, bone, and soft tissue infections, and prophylactically in various surgical procedures. All are administered parenterally except for cefaclor and cefuroxime, which may be given orally.

Third-generation cephalosporins have even broader Gram-negative activity and less Gram-positive activity than do second-generation agents. High third-generation cephalosporins include cefotaxime, which is potent against *Haemophilus influenza*, *Neisseria gonorrhea*, and *Enterobacteria*. All are administered parenterally. Third-generation agents are used primarily for serious Gram-negative infections, alone or in combination with aminoglycosides. Cefixime is given orally.

Fourth-generation cephalosporins have the greatest action against Gram-negative organisms among the four generations and minimal action against Gram-positive organisms.

Mechanism of Action

The mechanism of action of cephalosporins lies in preventing cell wall synthesis as they bind to enzymes called penicillin-binding proteins (PBPs). These enzymes are essential for the synthesis of the bacterial cell wall.

Indications

Cephalosporins are used to treat community-acquired and hospital-acquired infections of the skin, soft tissue, urinary tract, and respiratory tract. Parenteral first-generation agents are used for surgical wound prophylaxis. The cephamycin group is useful for mixed aerobic/anaerobic infections of the skin and soft tissues, intra-abdominal, and gynecologic infections, as well as for surgical prophylaxis.

TABLE 22-5 Classification of Cephalosporins

Generic Name	Trade Name	Route of Administration	Common Dosage Range
First-generation			
cephradine	Velosef®	PO	250–500 mg q6 h
cephapirin	Cefadyl®	IM, IV	500 mg–1 g q4–6 h
cephalexin	Keflex®	PO	250–500 mg q.i.d.
cefadroxil	Duricef®	PO	1–2 g/day in 1–2 div. doses
cefazolin sodium	Ancef®, Zolicef®, Kefzol®	IM, IV	250 mg–2 g t.i.d.
Second-generation			
cefoxitin sodium	Mefoxin®	IM, IV	1–2 g q6–8 h
cefaclor	Ceclor®	PO	250–500 mg t.i.d.
cefuroxime sodium	Zinacef®	PO	250–500 mg b.i.d.
cefonicid	Monocid®	IM	1–2 g/day
cefprozil	Cefzil®	PO	250–500 mg, 1–2 times/day
cefmetazole	Zefazone®	IV	1–2 g q6–12 h
cefotetan	Cefotan®	IM, IV	1–2 g q12 h
Third-generation			
cefdinir	Omnicef®	PO	300 mg b.i.d.
cefditoren pivoxil	Spectracef®	PO	200 mg b.i.d.
cefpodoxime proxetil	Vantin®	PO	200 mg b.i.d.
ceftazidime	Fortaz®	IM, IV	1–2 g b.i.d.
ceftibuten	Cedax®	PO	400 mg/day
ceftizoxime sodium	Cefizox®	IM, IV	1–2 g b.i.d. or t.i.d.
cefotaxime sodium	Claforan®	IM, IV	1–2 g, 12–24 h
cefixime	Suprax®	PO	400 mg/day in 1–2 div. doses
ceftriaxone sodium	Rocephin®	IM, IV	1–2 g, 12–24 h
cefoperazone sodium	Cefobid®	IM, IV	1–2 g, q12 h
Fourth-generation			
cefepime hydrochloride	Maxipime®	IM, IV	0.5–1 g, q12 h

Adverse Effects

The kidneys eliminate all cephalosporins except cefoperazone. Doses must be adjusted for patients with renal impairment. They can cause hypersensitivity reactions similar to penicillin. The most common adverse

Key Concept

Nephrotoxicity may occur with the use of cephalosporins. A decrease in urine output is an early sign of the adverse effect on patients with kidney impairments.

effects include nausea, vomiting, diarrhea, and nephrotoxicity. Adverse effects of cephalosporins include hypoprothrombinemia and bleeding, alcohol intolerance, hypersensitivity reactions, and thrombophlebitis.

Contraindications and Precautions

Cephalosporins are contraindicated if the patient has a history of allergies to these agents or penicillins. Cephalosporins should be avoided in pregnant and lactating women. Cephalosporins are to be used cautiously in patients with renal or hepatic impairment, and in patients with bleeding disorders.

Drug Interactions

Cephalosporins have drug interactions with alcohol, diarrhea medications, birth control pills, anticoagulants, blood viscosity reducing medicines, and antiseizure medicines. Cephalosporins are contraindicated for use with alcohol, alcohol-containing medications, aminoglycosides, anticoagulants, carbenicillin by injection, dipyridamole, divalproex, heparin, pentoxifylline, plicamycin, sulfinpyrazone, ticarcillin, thrombolytic agents, valproic acid, potent diuretics, iron-iron supplements, and probenecid.

Aminoglycosides

Aminoglycosides are broad-spectrum antibiotics. The toxic potential of these drugs limits their use. Since their introduction into clinical use 50 years ago, aminoglycosides continue to play an important role in the treatment of severe infections. Major aminoglycosides include amikacin, gentamicin, kanamycin, neomycin, netilmicin, streptomycin, and tobramycin. These agents are shown in Table 22-6.

Mechanism of Action

Aminoglycosides are bactericidal; they inhibit bacterial protein synthesis, causing cell death. Their mechanism of action is not fully known.

Indications

Aminoglycosides are prescribed for a variety of disorders and infectious diseases.

- Streptomycin: This can be used to treat tularemia, acute brucellosis, bacterial endocarditis, tuberculosis, and plague.

- Amikacin, gentamycin, netilmicin, and tobramycin: These are prescribed for serious Gram-negative bacillary infections such as *Enterobacter*, *klebsiella*, bacteremia, meningitis, and peritonitis.

- Neomycin: This is used for pre-operative bowel sterilization, hepatic coma, and in topical form for burns.

TABLE 22-6 Major Aminoglycosides

Generic Name	Trade Name	Route of Administration	Common Dosage Range
amikacin sulfate	Amikin®	IM, IV	5–7.5 mg/kg/day in 2–3 divided doses
gentamicin sulfate	Garamycin®	IM, IV	1.5–2.0 mg/kg/day (standard dose)
kanamycin	Kantrex®	IM, IV	15 mg/kg each 8–12 hours for serious infections
neomycin sulfate	Mycifradin®	PO, IM, Topical	PO: 50 mg/kg in 4 div. doses for 2–3 days; IM: 1.3–2.6 mg/kg q.i.d.; Topical: apply 1–3 times/ day
netilmicin	Netromycin®	IM	4 mg/kg in 2 div. doses
paromomycin sulfate	Humatin®	PO	25–35 mg/kg t.i.d.
streptomycin	generic only	IM	15 mg/kg up to 1 g/d as a single dose
tobramycin sulfate	Tobrex®	IM, IV	3 mg/kg t.i.d.

Adverse Effects

Aminoglycosides can cause serious adverse effects such as ototoxicity (including hearing loss) and nephrotoxicity. Neomycin is the most nephrotoxic aminoglycoside, and streptomycin is the least nephrotoxic. Gentamycin and tobramycin are nephrotoxic to the same degree. Aminoglycosides are also potentially neurotoxic, and these adverse effects may cause permanent damage to the organs.

Contraindications and Precautions

History of hypersensitivity or toxic reaction to an aminoglycoside antibiotic is contraindicated. Safety during pregnancy (category C) and lactation, in neonates and infants, or use for a period exceeding 14 days is not established. Aminoglycosides should be used cautiously in patients with impaired renal function, eighth cranial (auditory) nerve impairment, or in older adults. Other cautions include use in premature infants, neonates, and infants.

Drug Interactions

The risks of nephrotoxicity may increase by using an aminoglycoside with cephalosporins. If an aminoglycoside is used with loop diuretics (furosemide, ethacrynic acid, etc.), there is an increased risk of ototoxicity.

TABLE 22-7 Most Commonly Used Macrolides

Generic Name	Trade Name	Route of Administration	Common Dosage Range
erythromycin base	Eryc®, E-mycin®	PO	250–500 mg q.i.d.
erythromycin estolate	Ilosone®	PO, IM, IV	250–500 mg
erythromycin stearate	SK-Erythromycin®	PO	250–500 mg
clarithromycin	Biaxin®	PO	250–500 mg b.i.d.
azithromycin	Zithromax®, Zmax®	PO	500 mg on day 1, then 250 mg/d
dirithromycin	Dynabac®	PO	500 mg once/day

Macrolides

The macrolides include erythromycin, azithromycin, and clarithromycin. Erythromycin is produced by *Streptomyces erythreus*. They are also used as alternative agents when the patient is allergic to penicillin. Table 22-7 shows common macrolides.

Mechanism of Action

Macrolides may be bactericidal (bringing death to bacteria) or bacteriostatic (tending to restrain the development or reproduction of bacteria). They inhibit bacterial protein synthesis by binding to cell membranes. Erythromycins generally penetrate the cell wall of Gram-positive bacteria more readily than those of Gram-negative bacteria.

Indications

Macrolides are effective in the treatment of infections caused by a wide range of Gram-negative and Gram-positive microorganisms. They are the drug of choice for the treatment of *Mycoplasma pneumoniae*, campylobacteria infections, Legionnaires' disease, chlamydial infections, and pertussis. In patients with penicillin allergy, erythromycins are the best alternatives in the treatment of gonorrhea, syphilis, and pneumococcal pneumonia. Erythromycins may be given prophylactically before dental procedures to prevent bacterial endocarditis.

Adverse Effects

Macrolides rarely cause serious adverse effects. Nausea, vomiting, and diarrhea may occur with all forms of macrolides.

Contraindications and Precautions

Macrolides are contraindicated in patients with hypersensitivity, and in patients with liver diseases. These drugs should be used cautiously during

pregnancy and lactation. Erythromycin and azithromycin are contraindicated in pregnancy (category B); and clarithromycin and troleandomycin are pregnancy category C drugs. Macrolides must be used with great caution in patients with liver diseases.

Drug Interactions

Macrolides inhibit the hepatic metabolism of theophylline. They may interfere with the metabolism of digoxin, corticosteroids, and cyclosporin. Use of antacids decreases the absorption of most macrolides. Chloramphenicol, clindamycin, and lincomycin are able to decrease the therapeutic activity of the macrolides if they are used concurrently.

Tetracyclines

Tetracyclines are broad-spectrum agents that are effective against certain bacterial strains that resist other antibiotics. The major tetracyclines and the administration routes are shown in Table 22-8.

Mechanism of Action

Tetracyclines are bacteriostatic (capable of slowing the multiplication of bacteria). They inhibit bacterial protein synthesis, which is a process necessary for reproduction of the microorganism.

TABLE 22-8 Major Tetracyclines and Administration Routes

Generic Name	Trade Name	Route of Administration	Common Dosage Range
demeclocycline hydrochloride	Declomycin®	PO	150 mg q.i.d. or 300 mg b.i.d.
doxycycline hyclate	Vibramycin®	PO, IV	100 mg b.i.d. on day 1, then 100 mg/day
methacycline hydrochloride	Rondomycin®	PO	600 mg/day in 2–4 div. doses
minocycline hydrochloride	Minocin®	PO	4 mg/kg/day–200 mg/day; 200 mg followed by 100 mg b.i.d.
oxytetracycline	Terramycin®	PO, IM, IV	PO: 250–500 mg b.i.d.-q.i.d.; IM: 100 mg t.i.d.; IV: 250–500 mg b.i.d.
tetracycline hydrochloride	Achromycin®, Sumycin®	PO	250–500 mg b.i.d.
tigecycline	Tygacil®	IV	100 mg followed by 50 mg q12 h

Indications

Tetracyclines are active against Gram-negative and Gram-positive organisms, spirochetes, mycoplasmal and chlamydial organisms, rickettsial species, and certain protozoa. They are the drugs of choice in rickettsial infections (such as Rocky Mountain spotted fever), chlamydial infections, amebiasis, cholera, brucellosis, and tularemia. Tetracyclines are prescribed as an alternative to penicillin in the treatment of anthrax, syphilis, gonorrhea, Lyme disease, and *Haemophilus influenzae* respiratory infections. Oral or topical tetracycline may be used as a treatment for acne. Doxycycline is highly effective in the prophylaxis of "traveler's diarrhea."

Adverse Effects

Abdominal discomfort, nausea, diarrhea, and anorexia are common adverse effects of tetracyclines. Cross-sensitivity within the tetracyclines are also common. Use of the drugs in infants has resulted in retardation of bone growth. Because tetracyclines localize in the dentin and enamel of developing teeth, use of the drugs during tooth development may cause enamel hypoplasia and permanent yellow-gray to brown discoloration of the teeth. Tetracycline can cause fetal toxicity when administered to pregnant women (e.g., retardation of skeletal development). Liver toxicity has occurred following IV administration of tetracyclines to pregnant women. Oxytetracycline is the least hepatotoxic. Phototoxicity may occur in patients when they are exposed to strong sunlight (ultraviolet), especially with demeclocycline (Declomycin). Minocycline can cause vestibular toxicity. IV administration of tetracyclines is irritating and may cause phlebitis.

Contraindications and Precautions

Tetracyclines are contraindicated in patients who are allergic to them, or to any ingredient used in their formulations. Tetracyclines should not be used in children younger than eight years of age unless other appropriate drugs are ineffective or are contraindicated. Tetracyclines should be avoided in patients with severe renal or hepatic impairment. They are also contraindicated in those individuals with common bile duct obstruction.

Tetracyclines should be used cautiously in patients with renal function impairment or a history of liver dysfunction. History of allergy, asthma, and undernourished patients are other factors that cause tetracyclines to be used with caution.

Drug Interactions

There are certain foods (dairy products) and agents such as iron preparations, laxatives, and antacids that contain aluminum and calcium, which may effect a reduction of tetracycline absorption. Therefore, they are

Key Concept

Tetracyclines should not be used during pregnancy, infancy, and childhood (up to eight years of age), or during lactation, because they cause permanent discoloration of teeth in children.

recommended to be taken on an empty stomach. Barbiturates and phenytoin can decrease the effectiveness of tetracyclines.

Fluoroquinolones

Fluoroquinolones (also known as quinolones) are related to nalidixic acid and are bactericidal for growing bacteria. The most commonly used quinolones are shown in Table 22-9.

Mechanism of Action

Fluoroquinolones exert their bactericidal (bacteria-destroying) effects by interfering with an enzyme (DNA gyrase) that is required by bacteria for the synthesis of DNA. This action results in the prevention of cell reproduction and in bacterial death.

Indications

Fluoroquinolones are used in the treatment of infections caused by Gram-positive and Gram-negative microorganisms. The indications of

TABLE 22-9　Fluoroquinolones

Generic Name	Trade Name	Route of Administration	Common Dosage Range
First-generation			
nalidixic acid	NegGram®	PO	500 mg–1 g q.i.d.
Second-generation			
ciprofloxacin hydrochloride	Cipro®, Cipro XR®	PO, IV	PO: 250 mg q12h or 500 mg (Cipro XR) q.d. × 3 days; IV: 200 mg q12h, infused over 60 min
lomefloxacin hydrochloride	Maxaquin®	PO	400 mg q.d. × 10 days
norfloxacin	Noroxin®	PO	400 mg b.i.d.
ofloxacin	Floxin®	PO	400 mg for 1 dose
Third-generation			
gatifloxacin	Zymer®	PO	400 mg/day
levofloxacin	Levaquin®	PO, IV	500 mg/day
Fourth-generation			
gemifloxacin	Factive®	PO	320 mg/day
moxifloxacin hydrochloride	Avelox®, Vigamox®	PO, IV	400 mg/day
trovafloxacin	Trovan®	PO	100–300 mg/day

fluoroquinolones are primarily in the treatment of urinary tract and lower respiratory infections, skin and skin structure infections, and sexually transmitted diseases. Ciprofloxacin, norfloxacin, and ofloxacin are used in ophthalmic forms for eye infections.

Adverse Effects

Fluoroquinolone agents may produce nausea, headache, dizziness, dyspepsia, insomnia, photosensitivity, and hypoglycemia. Crystalluria can occur with high doses at alkaline pH. Therefore, fluoroquinolones should be taken with water and the patient should stay well-hydrated. These drugs may cause pain, inflammation, or rupture of a tendon (the most common tendon to be ruptured is the Achilles tendon).

Contraindications and Precautions

Fluoroquinolones are contraindicated in patients with a history of hypersensitivity, during pregnancy (category C) and lactation, and in children younger than 18 years. These agents are also contraindicated in patients who have syphilis, viral infections, tendon inflammation, and tendon pain. Fluoroquinolones should be used cautiously in patients with a history of seizures, in patients with renal dysfunction, in patients on dialysis, or in elderly adults.

Drug Interactions

Ciprofloxacin may increase theophylline levels in blood. Antacids and iron can decrease the absorption of fluoroquinolones. They may increase prothrombin times in patients receiving warfarin.

Miscellaneous Antibacterial Agents

Some antibiotics are classified as miscellaneous antibacterial agents, such as chloramphenicol, clindamycin, dapsone, spectinomycin, and vancomycin (Table 22-10). A few examples of these drugs are detailed below.

Chloramphenicol

This antibiotic is highly effective against rickettsia as well as many Gram-positive and Gram-negative organisms.

Mechanism of Action.   Chloramphenicol is principally bacteriostatic but may be bactericidal against a few bacterial strains (e.g., Haemophilus influenzae) or when given in higher concentrations. Chloramphenicol inhibits protein synthesis.

Indications.   Chloramphenicol is used only for specific infections that cannot be treated effectively with other antibiotics. It is particularly effective against typhoid fever, rickettsial infections in pregnant women, and meningococcal infections in cephalosporin-allergic patients. Chloramphenicol is also used for infections in patients who have a history of allergies to tetracycline.

TABLE 22-10 Miscellaneous Antibacterial Agents

Generic Name	Trade Name	Route of Administration	Average Adult Dosage
chloramphenicol	Chloromycetin®	PO, IV	50 mg/kg q.i.d.
clindamycin hydrochloride	Cleocin®	PO, IM, IV	PO: 150–450 mg q.i.d.; IM/IV: 600–1200 mg/day in div. doses
dapsone	Aczone®	PO	100 mg/day (with 6 months of rifampin at 600 mg/day for a minimum of 3 years)
ertapenem sodium	Invanz®	IM, IV	1 g/day
lincomycin hydrochloride	Lincocin®	IM, IV	IM: 600 mg every 12–24 h; IV: 600 mg–1 g b.i.d. or t.i.d.
methenamine	Mandelamine®, Hiprex®	PO	1 g b.i.d. (Hiprex) or q.i.d. (Mandelamine)
nitrofurantoin	Furadantin®, Macrobid®	PO	50–100 mg q.i.d.
spectinomycin hydrochloride	Trobicin®	IM	2 g as single dose or q12 h for 7 days until switched to an oral medication
telithromycin	Ketek®	PO	800 mg/day
vancomycin hydrochloride	Vancocin®	IV	500 mg q.i.d. or 1 g b.i.d.

Adverse Effects.   Chloramphenicol can cause suppression of bone marrow (in high doses) with resulting pancytopenia. This agent can lead to aplastic anemia in rare, non–dose-related cases. Chloramphenicol therapy can also lead to gray baby syndrome in neonates.

Contraindications and Precautions.   Chloramphenicol is contraindicated in patients with a history of hypersensitivity or toxic reaction to chloramphenicol. This agent should be avoided in the treatment of minor infections, for prophylactic use, in typhoid carrier state, in patients with a history or family history of drug-induced bone marrow depression, and during pregnancy (category C) and lactation.

Chloramphenicol should be given cautiously to patients with impaired hepatic or renal function. This drug may be used cautiously in premature and full-term infants and children.

Drug Interactions.   Chloramphenicol may inhibit the metabolism of phenytoin, dicumarol, and tolbutamide, leading to prolonged action and increased effects of these drugs. Phenobarbital can reduce the effect of chloramphenicol therapy. Acetaminophen elevates chloramphenicol levels and may cause toxicity. Penicillins can cause antibiotic antagonism.

Key Concept

Chloramphenicol may cause non–dose-related and irreversible aplastic anemia and pancytopenia (abnormal reduction in the number of all circulating blood cells).

Clindamycin

Clindamycin is an anti-infective and antibiotic that has marked toxicity. Clindamycin should be prescribed for special infections when it has been determined to be the most effective drug to treat them.

Mechanism of Action.   Clindamycin is bacteriostatic and inhibits bacterial protein synthesis. This agent is active against most Gram-positive and many anaerobic organisms.

Indications.   Clindamycin is used in serious infections when less toxic alternatives are inappropriate. Clindamycin is used for joint, bone, and abdominal infections. Topical applications are used in the treatment of acne vulgaris. Vaginal applications are used in the treatment of bacterial vaginosis in non-pregnant women.

Adverse Effects.   Clindamycin may cause rash, nausea, vomiting, diarrhea, and pseudomembranous colitis. Leukopenia, agranulocytosis, and thrombocytopenia may also occur.

Contraindications and Precautions.   Clindamycin is contraindicated in patients with a history of hypersensitivity to clindamycin or lincomycin. This agent also should not be used in patients with a history of regional enteritis, ulcerative colitis, or antibiotic-associated colitis. Clindamycin is contraindicated in pregnancy (category B) and lactation. It must be used cautiously in patients with history of GI disease, renal or hepatic disease, eczema, asthma, and hay fever.

Drug Interactions.   Clindamycin may potentiate the effects of neuromuscular blocking agents, atracurium, tubocurarine, and pancuronium. It is antagonistic to chloramphenicol and erythromycin.

Dapsone

Dapsone is the primary agent in the treatment of all forms of leprosy.

Mechanism of Action.   Dapsone is bacteriostatic and bactericidal for Mycobacterium leprae by blocking folic acid synthesis, thereby forcing microorganisms to synthesize their own folic acid.

Indications.   Dapsone is the drug of choice for treating leprosy. It is also used prophylactically in contacts of patients with all forms of leprosy except tuberculoid and indeterminate leprosy. Dapsone may be indicated for treatment of dermatitis herpetiformis. The topical (gel) form of dapsone is used for acne vulgaris.

Adverse Effects.   Nausea, vomiting, and anorexia are common adverse effects of dapsone. This agent may cause skin rash, peripheral neuropathy, blurred vision, hepatitis, hemolysis (destruction of red blood cells), and cholestatic jaundice.

Contraindications and Precautions.   Dapsone is contraindicated in patients with history of hypersensitivity to sulfones or their derivatives,

advanced renal dysfunction, and anemia. Safe use of dapsone during pregnancy (category C) or lactation is not established. Dapsone may be used with caution in patients with hepatic dysfunction, anemia, severe cardiopulmonary disease, and during pregnancy.

Drug Interactions. Probenecid can elevate blood levels of dapsone that may result in toxicity. Otherwise, there are no significant drug-drug interactions associated with the use of dapsone.

Spectinomycin

Spectinomycin is a wide-spectrum antibiotic with moderate activity against both Gram-positive and Gram-negative bacteria.

Mechanism of Action. Its action is usually bacteriostatic, but it has variable activity against a wide variety of Gram-negative and Gram-positive organisms.

Indications. Spectinomycin is used clinically for only one purpose, namely, to treat or prevent acute gonorrhea when the organism is resistant to penicillin, or when the patient is allergic to penicillin. It is not as effective as ceftriaxone.

Adverse Effects. Untoward effects include frequent pain at the injection site, an infrequent headache, nausea, vomiting, insomnia, chills, fever, mild pruritus, and urticaria.

Contraindications and Precautions. Safety during pregnancy (category B) or lactation, and in infants and children age eight years or under, is not established. Spectinomycin should be used with caution in those with a history of allergies.

Drug Interactions. No clinically significant interactions with spectinomycin have been established.

Vancomycin

Vancomycin can destroy most Gram-positive organisms.

Mechanism of Action. Vancomycin is bactericidal and bacteriostatic. It inhibits bacterial cell wall synthesis. Vancomycin acts against susceptible Gram-positive bacteria.

Indications. Vancomycin usually is reserved for serious infections, especially those caused by methicillin-resistant staphylococci, or other serious Gram-positive infections that do not respond to treatment with other anti-infective agents. It is useful in patients who are allergic to penicillin or cephalosporins. Typical uses include treatment of osteomyelitis, endocarditis, and staphylococcal pneumonia.

Adverse Effects. Vancomycin (in higher doses) may cause ototoxicity and nephrotoxicity, which can lead to uremia. It may cause rash on the upper

Key Concept

IV administration of vancomycin should be over a minimum of 60 minutes for a 1 gm dose.

body, sometimes called "**Red man syndrome**." This condition can produce facial flushing and hypotension due to very rapid infusion of the drug.

Contraindications and Precautions.   Vancomycin is contraindicated in patients with known hypersensitivity. This medication is used cautiously in patients with hearing impairment or renal dysfunction and during pregnancy (category C) and lactation.

Key Concept

Vancomycin may be used orally only in Clostridium difficile colitis.

Drug Interactions.   Vancomycin may have added toxicity if used with aminoglycosides, cisplatin, polymyxin B, cyclosporine, and amphotericin B. These drugs (with vancomycin) will result in additive effects of ototoxicity and nephrotoxicity.

ANTITUBERCULAR DRUGS

Tuberculosis is a highly contagious infection caused by *Mycobacterium tuberculosis*. While tuberculosis most commonly affects the lungs, it can also invade any part of the body, including bone, the gastrointestinal tract, and the kidneys. Tuberculosis lesions are characterized by the death of affected tissue with sloughing of tissue and formation of cavities.

Antitubercular drugs are used to treat tuberculosis by suppressing or killing the slow-growing mycobacteria that causes this disease. Antitubercular agents fall into two main categories: primary and re-treatment agents. Because the causative organisms tend to develop resistance to any single drug, combination drug therapy has become standard in the treatment of tuberculosis. Agents chosen for therapy must eradicate mycobacterium. Drugs available include isoniazid, streptomycin, ethambutol, rifampin, pyrazinamide, and rifabutin. Combination drug therapy is essential. Agents showing the lowest incidence of resistance such as isoniazid, rifampin, and streptomycin are usually used in combination with ethambutol or pyrazinamide. Most patients are started on isoniazid, rifampin, and pyrazinamide. A fourth drug (ethambutol or streptomycin) is added with suspected resistance (see Table 22-11 for a list of antitubercular drugs). Some antitubercular drugs are discussed in detail below.

Key Concept

General treatment for any bacterial infection is the administration of a single antibiotic. For tuberculosis, as many as four different drug combinations may be required. These combinations are divided into the first- and second-line antituberculotics on the basis of their efficacy.

Primary Antitubercular Drugs

These include isoniazid, ethambutol, rifampin, pyrazinamide, and streptomycin. These drugs usually offer the greatest effectiveness with the least toxicity. In most cases, the combination of isoniazid, rifampin, and pyrazinamide is most effective. These antibiotics must be administered concurrently during the 6- to 24-month treatment period.

Isoniazid

This agent is the mainstay of antitubercular therapy and is used in all therapeutic regimens.

TABLE 22-11 Antituberculotics

Generic Name	Trade Name	Route of Administration	Average Adult Dosage
First-line agents			
ethambutol hydrochloride	Myambutol®	PO	15–25 mg/kg/day
isoniazid	INH®, Laninzid	PO, IM	5 mg/kg/day
pyrazinamide	PZA®	PO	15–35 mg/kg t.i.d.-q.i.d. (max: 2 g/day)
rifampin	Rifadin®, Rimactane®	PO, IV	600 mg/day as a single dose
rifapentine	Priftin®	PO	600 mg 2x/wk for 2 mo; then 1x/wk for 4 mo
streptomycin sulfate	Streptomycin®	IM	15 mg/kg up to 1 g/day as a single dose
Second-line agents			
amikacin sulfate	Amikin®	IM, IV	5–7.5 mg/kg loading dose; then 7.5 mg/kg b.i.d.
capreomycin	Capastat Sulfate®	IM, IV	1 g/day (not to exceed 20 mg/kg/day) for 60–120 days, then 1 g 2–3 times/wk
ciprofloxacin hydrochloride	Cipro®	PO	250–750 mg b.i.d.
cycloserine	Seromycin®	PO	250 mg q12h for 2 wk; may increase to 500 mg q12 h (max: 1 g/day)
ethionamide	Trecator ®	PO	0.5–1.0 g/day div. q8–12 h
kanamycin	Kantrex®	IM, IV	15 mg/kg b.i.d.-t.i.d.
ofloxacin	Floxin®	PO	400 mg in 1 dose
rifabutin	Mycobutin®	PO	300 mg q.i.d., may give 150 mg b.i.d. if nausea is a problem

Mechanism of Action.   Isoniazid is bacteriostatic and bactericidal, but bacteriostatic for dormant mycobacteria. It is postulated to act by interfering with biosynthesis of bacterial proteins, nucleic acid, and lipids. The mechanism of action is not completely known.

Indications.   Isoniazid is the most widely prescribed antitubercular drug. It should be used in combination with another antitubercular agent to prevent drug resistance in tuberculosis. In the majority of cases of tuberculosis, isoniazid should be recommended at least for six months. Its agent, though, may last from six months to two years depending on the severity of the disease. During isoniazid therapy, the patient should be given

Key Concept

Prophylactic isoniazid may be given alone for up to one year in adults or children who have a positive tuberculin test result, but lack active lesions.

pyridoxine (vitamin B6) supplements to prevent neuritis (inflammation of a nerve).

Adverse Effects. The most common adverse effects of isoniazid are fever, jaundice, peripheral neuritis, and skin rash. Hepatitis can be severe and fatal. Aplastic or hemolytic anemia and thrombocytopenia may occur. Isoniazid may increase the excretion of pyridoxine, which can lead to peripheral neuritis, particularly in poorly nourished patients.

Contraindications and Precautions. Isoniazid is contraindicated in patients with history of isoniazid-associated hypersensitivity reactions, including hepatic injury or acute liver damage (from any cause). Isoniazid should be avoided during pregnancy (category C) unless the risk is warranted.

Isoniazid should be used cautiously in chronic liver disease, renal dysfunction, and chronic alcoholism. This drug must be used cautiously in people over 35 years of age, and during lactation.

Drug Interactions. Food and antacids that contain aluminum decrease the absorption of isoniazid. Disulfiram may cause coordination difficulties or psychotic reactions. Drinking alcohol with isoniazid may increase the risk of liver damage.

Ethambutol

Ethambutol is a synthetic water-based compound. It is an anti-tuberculosis and anti-infective drug.

Mechanism of Action. Ethambutol is bacteriostatic. The actual mechanism of action is unknown, but it appears to inhibit RNA synthesis and thus arrest multiplication of tubercle bacilli. The emergence of resistant strains is delayed by administering ethambutol in combination with other antituberculosis drugs.

Indications. Ethambutol is prescribed in the treatment of pulmonary tuberculosis in conjunction with at least one other antituberculosis drug.

Adverse Effects. Ethambutol may cause optic neuritis (a decrease in visual acuity and changes in color perception), drug fever, dizziness, confusion, hallucinations, and joint pains.

Contraindications and Precautions. Ethambutol is contraindicated in patients with a history of hypersensitivity. The drug should be avoided for children under the age of six years, or in patients with optic neuritis. Ethambutol should be used with caution in patients with renal and hepatic impairment, during lactation, or pregnancy (category B). Ethambutol is given to patients with diabetic retinopathy because of the danger of optic neuritis.

Drug Interactions. Aluminum-containing antacids can decrease absorption of ethambutol.

Rifampin

Rifampin is a complex macrocyclic agent.

Mechanism of Action. Rifampin has both bacteriostatic and bactericidal actions. This agent inhibits DNA-dependent RNA polymerase activity in susceptible bacterial cells, thereby suppressing RNA synthesis.

Indications. The combination of rifampin and isoniazid is the most effective drug for treatment of tuberculosis. It should not be given alone because it may cause drug-resistance for organisms. Rifampin may be prescribed in combination with dapsone for the treatment of leprosy. Rifampin is also effective against prevention of Neisseria meningitides, and a wide range of Gram-negative and Gram-positive organisms.

Adverse Effects. Liver damage can result from rifampin therapy. Liver function tests should be routinely checked. Headache, dizziness, fatigue, confusion, skin rash, nausea, and vomiting may occur.

Contraindications and Precautions. Rifampin is contraindicated in patients with a history of hypersensitivity, hepatic and renal impairment, meningococcal disease, and lactation. Safe use during pregnancy (category C) or in children less than five years of age is not established. Rifampin should be used cautiously in patients with hepatic disease or history of alcoholism.

Drug Interactions. Rifampin may decrease the effect of many drugs, such as warfarin, oral contraceptives, oral hypoglycemics, digitoxin, and corticosteroids. There is also a decrease in the effects of phenytoin, verapamil, and chloramphenicol. Probenecid may increase blood levels of rifampin.

Streptomycin

Streptomycin is one of the aminoglycosides that is given in combination with other antitubercular agents (see discussion of aminoglycosides).

Key Concept

Rifampin may change the colors of urine, tears, saliva, sweat, and feces to orange-red.

Key Concept

Patients who wear soft contact lenses should be instructed that rifampin therapy may permanently stain these lenses.

Summary

The invasion of pathogenic microorganisms may cause either local or systemic infection. The pathogen can be present in the blood circulation causing bacteremia. Anti-infective drugs, generally called antibiotics, are used to treat infection. Selection of antibiotics depends on various factors such as pharmacologic properties and spectrum activity of the drugs, and patient factors such as immunity, age, adverse drugs reactions, and underlying diseases. Pregnancy and lactation also play a major role. There are broad classifications of anti-infective drugs that may affect specific pathogens such as bacteria viruses, fungi, protozoa, and mycoplasms. Penicillins are the most widely used anti-infective agents. However, cephalosporin usage has increased in the last decade. There are specific antibiotics that are used predominantly for penicillinase-resistant penicillins. The first drugs used successfully to prevent and treat human bacterial infections were sulfonamides.

Exploring the Web

Visit any of the following Web sites to search for information on various types of diseases caused by infectious agents or the drugs used to treat them that were discussed in this chapter.

- *http://healthresources.caremark.com*
- *www.cdc.gov*
- *www.mayoclinic.com*
- *www.nfid.org*
- To learn more about the concerns and adverse affects of using antibiotics, review the information found at *www.tufts.edu/med/apua.*

Review Questions

Multiple Choice

1. Third-generation cephalosporins are potent against all of the following, except:

   A. Neisseria gonorrhea
   B. mycobacterium tuberculosis
   C. Haemophilus influenzae
   D. enterobacteria

2. Which of the antibiotics should not be used in children under age 18 years?

   A. chloramphenicol
   B. penicillins
   C. isoniazid
   D. ciprofloxacin

3. All of the following agents are in the class of macrolides, antibiotics, except:

    A. sulfonamide
    B. erythromycin
    C. troleandomycin
    D. clarithromycin

4. Penicillinase may be produced by:

    A. Streptococci
    B. Necesseria gonorrhea
    C. Staphylococci
    D. Haemophilus influenzae

5. Streptomycin is an aminoglycoside-like antibiotic indicated for the treatment of which of the following:

    A. tuberculosis
    B. Gram-negative bacillary septicemia
    C. penicillin-resistant gonococcal infection
    D. syphilis

6. Which of the following antibiotics may cause enamel hypoplasia and permanent yellow-gray color of the teeth in young children?

    A. isoniazid
    B. streptomycin
    C. rifampin
    D. tetracyclines

7. Which of the following antibiotics may lead to gray baby syndrome?

    A. tetracyclines
    B. chloramphenicol
    C. streptomycin
    D. metronidazole

8. A person who lacks resistance to an agent and is vulnerable to a disease is called a:

    A. compromised host
    B. susceptible host
    C. virulent host
    D. parasitic host

9. Viable bacteria which is present in the circulatory system is called:

    A. bacteremia
    B. virimia
    C. anemia
    D. hyperemia

10. The reservoir is a place where:

    A. an infectious agent leaves the body
    B. an organism invades the host
    C. an agent can be spread to others
    D. the agent can survive, colonize, and reproduce

11. Anti-infective drugs derived from natural substances are called:

    A. antivirals
    B. Gram stains
    C. antibiotics
    D. antifungals

12. A 42-year-old man has an upper respiratory infection. Four years ago, he experienced an episode of bronchospasm following penicillin V therapy. The culture now reveals a Gram-positive *Streptococcus pneumoniae* that is sensitive to all of the following drugs. Which of the following drugs would be the best choice for this patient?

    A. cefaclor
    B. ampicillin
    C. amoxicillin/clavulanate
    D. erythromycin

13. Isoniazid is a primary antitubercular agent that:

    A. may be nephrotoxic and ototoxic
    B. requires vitamin B_6 (pyridoxine supplementation)
    C. should never be used due to hepatotoxic potential
    D. causes ocular complications that are reversible if the drug is discontinued.

14. All of the following drugs are suitable oral therapy for a lower urinary tract infection due to Gram-negative bacteria, except:

    A. ciprofloxacin
    B. norfloxacin
    C. sulfadiazine
    D. cefoxitin

15. Which of the following is the drug of choice for Chlamydial organisms and rickettsial species?

    A. tetracycline
    B. isoniazid
    C. rephampin
    D. penicillin

Matching

_____ 1. Contraindicated in children younger than eight years of age

A. isoniazid

_____ 2. Causes aplastic anemia in infants

B. erythromycin

_____ 3. Changes the color of urine or saliva to orange-red

C. sulfonamide

_____ 4. This agent is used for preoperative bowel sterilization and hepatic coma

D. neomycin

_____ 5. The drug of choice for the treatment Legionnaires' disease, and pertussis

E. rifampin

_____ 6. The first drug discovered to prevent and cure human bacterial infections

F. chloramphenicol

_____ 7. The most widely prescribed antitubercular drug

G. tetracyclines

Critical Thinking

Christian is a 16-year-old who goes to a private school. He wanted to work at a local hospital as a volunteer. Therefore, they required that he had to have a tuberculin test. His physician diagnosed that his TB test was positive with a reading of 16 mm, and ordered a chest x-ray. The result of the chest x-ray was negative, so the physician recommended that Christian go to the local Health Department for tuberculosis evaluation. They determined that he had been exposed to tuberculosis, but did not have the primary form of tuberculosis himself.

1. What drug or drugs would the Health Department recommend for this patient?

2. How long do you think he will need to take the drug or drugs that he is prescribed?

3. Since Christian had been exposed to tuberculosis, will his entire family also need to receive preventative medications?

Antiviral, Antifungal, and Antiprotozoal Agents

OBJECTIVES

After completing this chapter, the reader should be able to:

1. Describe why antiviral drug treatments are limited compared with other antibacterial agents.

2. Identify viral diseases that may benefit from drug therapy.

3. Describe the expected outcomes of HIV drug therapy.

4. Define HAART and explain why it is commonly used in the drug therapy of HIV infection.

5. Explain the mechanisms of action of antiviral, antifungal, and antiprotozoal agents.

6. Explain the four commonly used antifungal agents.

7. Compare the drug therapy of superficial and systemic fungal infections.

8. Name common drugs used for malarial parasites.

9. Explain the important adverse effects of systemic antifungal and antiprotozoal drugs.

10. Name three important amebicides and their mechanisms of action.

GLOSSARY

Acquired Immunodeficiency Syndrome (AIDS) – a severe immunological disorder caused by the retrovirus HIV, resulting in a defect in cell-mediated immune response

Amebicides and trichomonacides – drugs use to treat amebic and trichomonal infections

Antimalarial agents – drugs used to treat malaria infections

Epidemic – an outbreak of a disease or infection that spreads widely and rapidly

Fungi – a distinct group of organisms that are neither plant nor animal

Human immunodeficiency virus (HIV) – a retrovirus that infects helper T cells of the immune system, leading to AIDS

Malaria – a severe generalized infection caused by the bite of an *anopheles* mosquito that is infected with a *Plasmodium* protozoon

Mycoses – fungal diseases

Pro-drug – inactive or partially active drug that is metabolically changed in the body to an active drug

Protozoa – single-celled parasitic organisms, many of which are motile (able to move spontaneously)

Replication – the process of reproduction or copying of genetic material

Superficial mycoses – involving a surface or a shallow depth of tissue

Systemic mycoses – relating to or affecting an entire body or an entire organism

Viruses – intracellular parasites that take over the metabolic machinery of host cells and use it for their own survival and replication

OVERVIEW

Many infections may be caused by viruses, fungi, and protozoa. Some of these infections may result in no permanent damage, and usually disappear within seven to ten days if the patient is otherwise healthy. Many of these infections may cause serious viral infections that may be fatal, such as HIV, and may require aggressive drug therapy. Fungal infections are seen commonly in patients with immune deficiency diseases. Fungi and protozoans are more complex than bacteria and there are fewer medications to treat these types of infections.

VIRUSES

Viruses are intracellular parasites that take over the metabolic machinery of host cells and use it for their own survival and replication, often resulting in the destruction of the infected cells. Viral diseases are the most common causes of disease in humans. Viruses result in a wide variety of diseases ranging from the common cold and the "cold sore" of herpes immune simplex to several types of cancers and AIDS.

Key Concept

Ebola virus, Dengue virus, and human immunodeficiency virus are examples of emerging viruses that threaten the public health and kill thousands of people each year.

Viruses are extremely small, and contain their genetic information in either deoxyribonucleic acid (DNA) or ribonucleic acid (RNA), which are surrounded by a protein coat (capsid). After infection, viruses usually make multiple copies of their genetic material and produce the necessary viral proteins for replication. Some animal viruses are responsible for diseases such as hemorrhagic fever (Ebola virus), influenza virus, and measles (rubeola virus).

Antiviral Drugs

Antiviral drugs are used to treat viral infections by influencing viral **replication**. Viruses are not able to independently provide their metabolic activity, and can replicate only within living host cells. Therefore, antiviral agents tend to damage the host as well as viral cells. The majority of antivirals are active against only one virus, either DNA or RNA types. These viruses may include herpes simplex virus (HSV) 1 and 2, varicella-zoster virus (VZV), cytomegalovirus (CMV), and influenza A. Table 23-1 shows

TABLE 23-1   Antiviral Drugs and Their Therapeutic Uses

Generic Name	Trade Name	Route of Administration	Common Adult Dosage
Non-HIV Antivirals			
acyclovir	Zovirax®	Topical, PO, IV	Topical: Apply 5 times/day for 4 days; PO: 400 mg t.i.d.; IV: 5 mg/kg t.i.d.
amantadine	Symmetrel®	PO	200 mg once/day
cidofovir	Vistide®	IV	5 mg/kg once weekly for 2 weeks
famciclovir	Famvir®	PO	500 mg t.i.d.
ganciclovir	Cytovene®	IV	5 mg/kg b.i.d.
rimantadine	Flumadine®	PO	100 mg b.i.d.
ribavirin	Rebetrol®, Virazole®	PO	600 mg b.i.d. for 24–48 weeks
valacyclovir	Valtrex®	PO	1 g t.i.d.
HIV Antivirals			
abacavir sulfate	Ziagen®	PO	300 mg b.i.d.
didanosine (DDI)	Videx®	PO	250 mg q.d.
indinavir sulfate	Crixivan®	PO	800 mg t.i.d.
nevirapine	Viramune®	PO	200 mg once daily
stavudine (D4T)	Zerit®	PO	40 mg b.i.d.
zidovudine (formerly azidothymidine, AZT)	Retrovir®	PO, IV	PO: 300 mg b.i.d.; IV: 1–2 mg/kg q4 h

antiviral agents that are currently approved for treatment of some viruses. The following antiviral drugs are a few examples.

Acyclovir

Acyclovir is a synthetic acyclic analog of guanosine with activity against various herpes viruses. Herpes viruses can infect neonates, children, and adults, causing a wide spectrum of diseases. Herpes simplex type 1 virus is responsible for systemic infections involving the liver and other organs, including the central nervous system, and localized infections that may involve the skin, eyes, and mouth. Other medically important herpes viruses include cytomegalovirus (CMV), varicella (Chicken Pox), and varicella-zoster (shingles). Acyclovir is available in capsules ranging from 200 to 800 mg.

Mechanism of Action.   Acyclovir is taken up selectively by cells that are infected with herpes viruses. Its activity depends upon conversion to the

triphosphate where it becomes incorporated into viral DNA and inhibits viral replication.

Indications.   Acyclovir is most effective against HSV-1 and HSV-2. IV acyclovir is used for HSV encephalitis, neonatal HSV, and life-threatening HSV and VZV infections in immunocompromised patients. Oral acyclovir is indicated for the treatment of primary and recurrent genital herpes. Acyclovir ophthalmic ointment is effective for herpes simplex keratitis.

Adverse Effects.   Acyclovir may cause nausea, vomiting, and diarrhea. The drug can precipitate in the renal tubules with excessive dosages or when it is given by rapid infusion, which may cause acute renal failure. Other adverse effects of acyclovir include headache, drowsiness, fatigue, uncontrollable rhythmic shaking, confusion, and seizures.

Contraindications and Precautions.   Acyclovir is contraindicated in patients with hypersensitivity to this agent. Acyclovir should be used with caution in lactation, pregnancy (category B), dehydration, and renal insufficiency.

Drug Interactions.   Amphotericin B may raise the plasma and renal concentrations of acyclovir. Probenecid decreases acyclovir elimination. Zidovudine may cause increased drowsiness and lethargy.

Famciclovir

Famciclovir is a **pro-drug** (inactive or partially active drug that is metabolically changed in the body to an active drug) of the antiviral agent penciclovir.

Mechanism of Action.   Famciclovir prevents viral replication by inhibition of DNA formation.

Indications.   Famciclovir is used for the management of acute herpes zoster (shingles) and recurrent genital herpes in immunocompetent patients. It is effective against HSV-1, HSV-2, and VZV.

Adverse Effects.   Common adverse effects resulting from famciclovir use include fatigue, nausea, diarrhea, vomiting, constipation, and anorexia. Headache is also frequently reported.

Contraindications and Precautions.   Famciclovir is contraindicated in patients with known hypersensitivity to this agent and lactation. This drug should be used cautiously in patients with renal or hepatic impairment, or carcinoma, in older adults, and during pregnancy (category B). Safety of this drug in children less than 18 years is not established.

Drug Interactions.   Probenecid can increase plasma concentration of penciclovir. Famciclovir may increase digoxin levels.

Amantadine

Amantadine is an antiviral and anticholinergic agent effective for viral respiratory infections such as influenza A virus (it is not effective against influenza B infections), and Parkinson's disease.

Mechanism of Action.   The mechanism of the antiviral activity of amantadine is unknown. Its action appears to occur early in the course of viral infection.

Indications.   Amantadine is indicated for the prophylaxis and treatment of influenza A virus infections, as well as for Parkinson's disease. Individuals who have not received vaccine prophylaxis can benefit from amantadine prophylaxis given for at least ten days after a known exposure to influenza A.

Adverse Effects.   Amantadine causes mild adverse effects, including blurred vision, anxiety, insomnia, and dizziness. Urinary retention is another potential adverse effect. Serious adverse effects in patients treated for Parkinson's disease have included congestive heart failure, hypotension, peripheral edema, depression, seizures, psychosis, and leukopenia.

Contraindications and Precautions.   Amantadine is contraindicated in pregnancy (category C), lactation, and in children less than one year. Amantadine should be used cautiously in patients with history of epilepsy, congestive heart failure, peripheral edema, drops in blood pressure when the patient stands up from a lying or sitting position, psychoses, and hepatic disease.

Drug Interactions.   Amantadine interacts with anticholinergic drugs to produce atropine-like effects unless the dosage of the anticholinergic drug is reduced. Amantadine prophylaxis or treatment does not interfere with the immune response to influenza vaccination given concurrently.

Ganciclovir

Ganciclovir is an antiviral agent and synthetic purine nucleoside analog that is approved for the treatment of cytomegalovirus (CMV) infection.

Mechanism of Action.   After conversion to ganciclovir triphosphate, ganciclovir is incorporated into viral DNA, and inhibits the replication of the DNA virus. By this mechanism, it can terminate viral replication.

Indications.   Ganciclovir is prescribed for CMV retinitis, prophylaxis and treatment of systemic CMV infections in immunocompromised patients, including HIV-positive and transplant patients.

Adverse Effects.   Ganciclovir has black box warnings concerning increased potential for dose-limited neutropenia, thrombocytopenia, and anemia. The FDA issues black box warnings when a serious problem concerning the use of a drug has been discovered, so that medical practitioners are aware of the problem and its resulting adverse effects. Inflammation of a vein and pain may occur at the site of infusion.

Contraindications and Precautions.   Ganciclovir is contraindicated in patients with known hypersensitivity, and during lactation. This drug should be used cautiously in patients with renal impairment, older adults, and during pregnancy (category C). Safety and efficacy in children are not established.

Drug Interactions.   Probenecid may increase ganciclovir levels and possibly toxicity.

Antiretroviral Drugs for HIV-AIDS

In 1981, an **epidemic** of fatal infections first appeared in homosexual men. The spread of this illness to these groups suggested that an infectious agent, transmissible through blood and semen, caused the immunodeficiency that was common to all the patients. The term **Acquired Immunodeficiency Syndrome**, or **AIDS**, was coined to describe this illness. At the outset of the epidemic, most people with AIDS died within a year of this diagnosis. In 1983, researchers isolated the virus that causes AIDS. Today, we have learned much about AIDS since the first case reports. We now know that AIDS is caused by **human immunodeficiency virus (HIV)**, its modes of transmission, and who is at risk for HIV infection. We know that HIV kills lymphocytes (cells in the blood stream necessary to respond to bacteria, fungi, protozoa, and viruses). Antiviral medications for HIV-AIDS slow the growth of HIV in several different ways.

None of the available medications can cure the disease and, due to the rapid mutation of HIV and its resistant strains, new HIV antiviral agents are constantly being developed. The decision of exactly when to begin pharmacotherapy must be made early enough after the diagnosis is established in order to give each patient the best chance of receiving effective treatment. HIV may remain dormant for either months or years after initial exposure. It is important to begin treatment during the latent stage in order to delay acute symptoms and the onset of full-blown AIDS.

HAART Therapy

Highly Active Anti-Retroviral Therapy (HAART) has been shown to reduce viral load and increase CD4 lymphocytes in persons infected with HIV, delay onset of AIDS, and prolong survival with AIDS. The incidence and mortality of AIDS has declined substantially since 1996 due to HAART. The benefits of HAART, which involves the combination of three to four drug combinations against HIV, have been widely publicized. However, HAART presents formidable challenges, including adverse effects and the potential for the rapid spread of drug resistance. Protease inhibitors do not work as well with HIV drugs such as non-nucleoside analogues, and they should not be taken alone. If one of the drugs involved in multiple drug therapy is not well tolerated, or if a patient's HIV infection becomes resistant to it, a

whole new set of drugs must be prescribed for the regimen to be effective. Currently, due to the limited number of HAART medications available in the U.S. market, only a few different drug combinations are possible. HAART regimens can also fail because of the lack of viral load response, or poor treatment adherence. Missing a single dose of HAART medication even twice a week can cause the development of drug-resistant HIV—a real danger, because adherence to the drug regimens is difficult. For each group of antiretroviral drugs for HIV-AIDS, only one selected drug will be discussed here. Table 23-2 shows antiretroviral drugs used for HIV-AIDS.

TABLE 23-2 Antiretroviral Drugs used for HIV-AIDS

Generic Name	Trade Name	Route of Administration	Common Adult Dosage
Non-Nucleoside Reverse Transcriptase Inhibitors (NNRTIs)			
delavirdine mesylate	Rescriptor®	PO	400 mg t.i.d.
efavirenz	Sustiva®	PO	600 mg/day
nevirapine	Viramune®	PO	200 mg/day x 14 days, then increase to b.i.d.
Nucleoside Reverse Transcriptase Inhibitors (NRTIs)			
abacavir sulfate	Ziagen®	PO	300 mg b.i.d.
didanosine (DDI)	Videx®	PO	400 mg q.d.
emtricitabine	Emtriva®	PO	200 mg/day
lamivudine	Epivir®	PO	300 mg/day
stavudine (D4T)	Zerit®	PO	40 mg b.i.d.
zalcitabine (DDC)	Hivid®	PO	0.75 mg t.i.d.
zidovudine (formerly AZT)	Retrovir®	PO, IV	PO: 300 mg b.i.d.; IV: 1–2 mg/kg q4 h
Protease Inhibitors (PIs)			
amprenavir	Agenerase®	PO	1200 mg b.i.d.
atazanavir	Reyataz®	PO	400 mg/day
indinavir sulfate	Crixivan®	PO	800 mg t.i.d.
nelfinavir mesylate	Viracept®	PO	750 mg t.i.d.
ritonavir	Norvir®	PO	600 mg t.i.d. w/meals
saquinavir mesylate	Invirase	PO	600 mg t.i.d.
Miscellaneous Drugs			
enfuvirtide	Fuzeon®	SC	90 mg b.i.d.
tenofovir disoproxil fumarate	Viread®	PO	300 mg once/day

Delavirdine

Delavirdine is a nonnucleoside reverse transcriptase inhibitor that prevents the replication of HIV-1 virus.

Mechanism of Actions. Delavirdine binds directly to reverse transcriptase of HIV-1 and blocks RNA- and DNA- dependent DNA polymerase activities.

Indications. Delavirdine is used in the treatment of HIV infection in combination with other antiretroviral agents.

Adverse Effects. Delavirdine may cause headache, fatigue, allergic reaction, chills, edema, and joint pain. Administration of delavirdine may also cause abnormal coordination, amnesia, anxiety, confusion, and dizziness. Common adverse effects of delavirdine include nausea, vomiting, diarrhea, abdominal cramps, and anorexia.

Contraindications and Precautions. Delavirdine is contraindicated in patients with hypersensitivity to this agent, and during lactation. Delavirdine must be used cautiously in patients with impaired liver function, pregnancy (category C). Safety and efficacy in children younger than 16 years have not been established.

Drug Interactions. Antacids and H2-receptor antagonists decrease the absorption of delavirdine. Didanosine and delavirdine should be taken one hour apart to avoid decreased delavirdine levels.

Lamivudine

Lamivudine is one example of a nucleoside reverse transcriptase inhibitor (NRTI). This agent is used in combination with other medications to treat HIV infection in patients with AIDS. It is not a cure, and may not decrease the number of HIV-related illnesses. Lamivudine does not prevent the spread of HIV to other people. It is also used to treat hepatitis B infection. It is often used in combination with zidovudine.

Mechanism of Action. Lamivudine is in a class of medications called nucleoside reverse transcriptase inhibitors (NRTIs), which work by interfering with viral reproduction by preventing the creation of new viral RNA. It should never be used alone due to resistance, which can occur very rapidly.

Indications. Lamivudine is used to treat HIV infection in combination with zidovudine. It is also used in the treatment of chronic hepatitis B. The combination of these two drugs may stop the spread of both viruses.

Adverse Effects. The most serious adverse effects of lamivudine include rash, stomach pain, vomiting or upset stomach (in children), fever, muscle pain, and a numbness, tingling, or burning sensation in the fingers or toes.

Contraindications and Precautions.   Lamivudine is contraindicated in patients with hypersensitivity to this agent. Lamivudine should be avoided during lactation. This drug is used with caution in patients with renal impairment, during pregnancy (category C), and in children.

Drug Interactions.   The use of lamivudine with trimethoprim/sulfamethoxazole can increase the amount of lamivudine in the body. However, it is not necessary to change the dosages of either of these agents. Lamivudine increases the risk of lactic acidosis in combination with other reverse transcriptase inhibitors and antiretroviral agents.

Ritonavir

Ritonavir is an anti-HIV drug that is a protease inhibitor. It is used to treat HIV infection when therapy is warranted.

Mechanism of Action.   By interfering with the formation of essential proteins and enzymes, ritonavir blocks the maturation of the HIV virus and causes the formation of nonfunctional, immature, noninfectious virions.

Indications.   Ritonavir is used to treat HIV in adults and children, in combination with other antiretroviral agents. Because it inhibits the metabolism of other protease inhibitors, it is increasingly used for boosting and maintaining plasma concentrations of protease inhibitors.

Adverse Effects.   One of the more serious effects of ritonavir is potentially fatal pancreatitis. Other serious adverse effects include body fat redistribution and accumulation, increased bleeding in patients with hemophilia type A and B, hyperglycemia, hyperlipidemia, new-onset diabetes mellitus, and the exacerbation of existing diabetes mellitus.

Contraindications and Precautions.   Ritonavir is contraindicated in patients with hypersensitivity to this drug. Ritonavir should not be given in patients with antimicrobial resistance to protease inhibitors, or those suffering from pancreatitis. Safety and efficacy in children less than two years are not established.

Ritonavir is used with caution in pregnancy (category B), hepatic diseases, advanced HIV disease, diabetes mellitus, hyperlipidemia, and renal insufficiency.

Drug Interactions.   When ritonavir is given in combination with other protease inhibitors, the dosage of the other protease inhibitors may be reduced. Drug interactions may occur when ritonavir is administered with a wide variety of other drugs, mostly due to pharmacokinetic interactions. Concomitant use of ritonavir with lovastatin or simvastatin is not recommended. Caution should also be taken when ritonavir is used with atorvastatin, cerivastatin, St. John's wort, sildenafil, astemizole, or cisapride.

Tenofovir

Tenofovir is one of the miscellaneous agents for treatment of HIV-AIDS. This agent is an antiviral drug that is approved for the treatment of HIV infection. It is able to reduce the amount of HIV in the blood and, when used in combination with other antiviral drugs, it can help prevent or reverse damage to the immune system and reduce the risk of AIDS-related illnesses. It is also an experimental treatment for hepatitis B.

Mechanism of Action.   Tenofovir is a potent inhibitor of retroviruses, including HIV-1. It may be active against nucleoside-resistant HIV strains. The active form of tenofovir persists in HIV-infected cells for prolonged periods; thus, it results in sustained inhibition of HIV replication. It reduces the viral load and CD4 counts.

Indications.   Tenofovir is used in combination with other antiretrovirals for the treatment of HIV.

Adverse Effects.   Tenofovir may cause asthenia, anorexia, neutropenia, increased creatine kinase, AST, ALT, serum amylase, triglycerides, or serum glucose. Nausea, vomiting, diarrhea, flatulence, abdominal pain, and anorexia are common adverse effects of tenofovir.

Contraindications and Precautions.   Tenofovir is contraindicated in patients with hypersensitivity to tenofovir, hepatitis, and lactic acidosis. Tenofovir should be avoided with concurrent administration of nephrotoxic agents, in patients with renal failure, and during lactation. Tenofovir must be used cautiously in patients with hepatic dysfunction, alcoholism, renal impairment, and obesity, during pregnancy (category B), and in children.

Drug Interactions.   Tenofovir may increase didanosine toxicity. Use of this agent with acyclovir, amphotericin B, cidofovir, foscarnet, ganciclovir, probenecid, valacyclovir, or valganciclovir may increase tenofovir toxicity by decreasing its renal elimination.

FUNGI

Fungi are a distinct group of organisms that are neither plant nor animal. Fungi grow in single cells, as in yeast, or in colonies, as in molds. Fungi obtain food from living organisms or organic matter. Disease from fungi is found mainly in individuals who are immunologically impaired, but is also seen (less commonly) in other patients. Fungi can cause infections of the hair, skin, nails, and mucous membranes. Fungi infections include athlete's foot, histoplasmosis, cryptococcosis, *Candida* infections, and tinea.

Antifungal Drugs

Antifungal agents are used to treat systemic, local, and topical fungal infections. As fungi are single-celled or multicellular organisms that are

more complex than bacteria, most antibacterial agents are ineffective against fungi. The human body is generally resistant to infection by fungi, but patients infected with HIV may frequently exhibit fungal infections, some of which may need intensive drug therapy. Fungal diseases are called **mycoses**.

Fungal infections may be classified into two groups: **superficial mycoses** (of the skin) and **systemic mycoses**, which affect internal organs such as the lungs, digestive organs, and brain. Antifungals are used to treat systemic, local fungal, and topical fungal infections. A table of antifungal drugs can be found in Table 23-3. A selective few agents will be discussed here in detail.

TABLE 23-3 Antifungal Agents

Generic Name	Trade Name	Route of Administration	Common Dosage Range
amphotericin B	Fungizone®, Amphocin®	IV	0.25–0.3 mg/kg/day
butoconazole nitrate	Femstat 3®, Gynazole 1®	Vaginal	One full applicator h.s.
caspofungin	Cancidas®	IV	70 mg on day one; then 50 mg q.d. thereafter
clotrimazole	Mycelex®, Lotrimin®	Topical, Vaginal	Topical: 10 mg b.i.d. prn; Vaginal: 5–100 mg in applicator h.s.
econazole nitrate	Spectazole®	Topical	15–85 g prn
fluconazole	Diflucan®	PO, IV	PO: 100–200 mg/day; IV: 200 mg for 14–21 (max: 400 mg q.i.d.)
griseofulvin	Grifulvin®, Fulvicin®	PO	500 mg–1 g/day
itraconazole	Sporanox®	PO	100–400 mg/day
ketoconazole	Nizoral®	PO , Topical	200–400 mg single dose/day
miconazole nitrate	Monistat®	Topical, Vaginal	Apply cream or insert suppository into vagina h.s.
nystatin	Mycostatin®	PO, Vaginal , Topical	PO: 500,000–1,000,000 units q.i.d.; Vaginal: 1–2 times/day for 2 weeks
terbinafine hydrochloride	Lamisil®	Topical	Apply thin layer to affected area
tioconazole	Vagistat-1®	Vaginal	5 mg (one applicator) once/day
tolnaftate	Tinactin®	Topical	2 oz prn

Amphotericin B

Amphotericin B is the most effective agent available for the treatment of most systemic fungal infections.

Mechanism of Action. Amphotericin B is fungistatic, antibiotic, and may be fungicidal at higher concentrations, depending on the sensitivity of the fungus. It has a wide spectrum of activity on most of the fungi pathogenic to humans. Amphotericin B acts by binding to fungal cell membranes, causing them to become permeable.

Indications. Amphotericin B is used intravenously for a wide spectrum of potentially fatal systemic fungal (mycotic) infections, including aspergillosis, blastomycosis, coccidiomycosis, cryptococcosis, disseminated candidiasis, and histoplasmosis. Treatment may continue for several months. Unlike antibiotics, resistance to amphotericin B is not common. Topical preparations are used to treat cutaneous and mucocutaneous infections caused by *Candida (monilia)*.

Adverse Effects. Amphotericin B can cause many serious adverse effects. Therefore, it should be administered in a hospital. Adverse effects include fever, chills, nausea, vomiting, headache, hypotension, muscle pain, dyspnea, and tachypnea. Nephrotoxicity, anaphylactoid reactions, phlebitis, and liver damage may occur. Amphotericin B for parenteral use should only be mixed in D5W and should be protected from light. Sometimes patients may be pre-medicated with diphenhydramine IV or acetaminophen prior to administration.

Contraindications and Precautions. Amphotericin B is contraindicated in patients with a known hypersensitivity and during lactation. This agent is used cautiously in patients with severe bone marrow depression or renal function impairment. Amphotericin B should be used during pregnancy (category B) only when there is a life-threatening situation.

Drug Interactions. When amphotericin B is given with corticosteroids, severe hypokalemia may occur, and the hypokalemia increases the risk of digitalis toxicity. Aminoglycosides, colistin, furosemide, and vancomycin may interact with amphotericin B and cause the possibility of nephrotoxicity.

Griseofulvin

Griseofulvin is a drug that is deposited in the skin, and bound to keratin. It is an antifungal, antibiotic, and anti-infective agent.

Mechanism of Action. Griseofulvin is fungistatic. It inhibits fungal cell activity. This agent is active against various strains of Microsporum, Trichophyton, and Epidermophyton. Griseofulvin has no effect on other fungi, including Candida, bacteria, and yeast.

Key Concept

Topical administration of amphotericin B is also possible, and includes the application of creams, lotions, ointment, tinctures, sprays, and powders to the surface of skin and mucous membranes.

Key Concept

Kidney damage is the most serious adverse effect of amphotericin B. Reduction of dosage or increasing time between dosages is essential. Serum creatinine levels and blood urea nitrogen levels are checked frequently during the course of therapy to monitor kidney function.

Indications.   Griseofulvin is effective in mycotic infections of the nails, hair, and skin. It is available only in oral form.

Adverse Effects.   Griseofulvin may produce fatigue, headache, confusion, syncope, and lethargy. It also occasionally causes leukopenia and, in rare cases, serum sickness and hepatotoxicity. Heartburn, nausea, vomiting, diarrhea, flatulence, dry mouth, and unpleasant taste are common adverse effects of griseofulvin.

Contraindications and Precautions.   Griseofulvin must be avoided in patients with known hypersensitivity and severe liver disease. Griseofulvin is used cautiously during pregnancy (category C) and lactation.

Drug Interactions.   Griseofulvin may increase the metabolism of anticoagulants and decrease the effects of these agents. Barbiturates can reduce absorption of griseofulvin. A decrease in the effects of an oral contraceptive may occur with the administration of griseofulvin, causing breakthrough bleeding, amenorrhea, or pregnancy. Alcohol consumption can cause flushing and tachycardia when griseofulvin is used.

Nystatin

The chemical structure of nystatin is similar to amphotericin B, and is the common topical treatment for thrush, which can show up in the mouth or on the tongue, gums, or skin. It is not considered a systemic antifungal, but acts locally. It is available in tablets or a liquid suspension, as well as a cream, ointment, and topical powder; and therapy is usually continued for two weeks to be effective.

Mechanism of Action.   Nystatin is fungicidal and fungistatic. It is effective against a variety of yeasts and fungi (Candida infections).

Indications.   Nystatin is prescribed primarily as a local infection of skin and mucous membranes caused by Candida albicans (e.g. vulvovaginal, orpharyngeal, and intestinal candidiasis). It is also used for candidal diaper rashes. It is often used prophylactically on the diaper area when an oral Candida infection is present.

Adverse Effects.   Nystatin can temporarily affect the sense of taste, and thus decrease appetite. Other adverse effects include nausea, vomiting, diarrhea, and stomach pain. If used to treat vaginal infections, the patient should avoid using sanitary napkins and refrain from sexual contact until the infection subsides.

Contraindications and Precautions.   Vaginal tablets of nystatin are contraindicated during pregnancy (category C), and with vaginal infections caused by Trichomonas species. Nystatin should be used cautiously during lactation.

Drug Interactions.   There are no listed drug interactions with Nystatin.

Itraconazole

Itraconazole is an antifungal indicated in the treatment of histoplasmosis, aspergillosis, and blastomycosis. Liver function should be monitored during treatment with itraconazole.

Mechanism of Action.   Itraconazole is fungistatic, and may also be fungicidal depending on the concentration. Itraconazole interferes with the formation of ergosterol, the principal sterol in the fungal cell membrane that, when depleted, interrupts membrane functions.

Indications.   Itraconazole is used in the treatment of systemic fungal infections caused by blastomycosis, histoplasmosis, and aspergillosis due to dermatophytes of the toenail with or without fingernail involvement, or mouth and throat candidiasis.

Adverse Effects.   Itraconazole may cause heart failure. With high doses, hypertension may occur. Other adverse effects include headache, dizziness, fatigue, euphoria, drowsiness, gynecomastia, hypokalemia (low potassium level), hypertriglyceridemia, impotence, rash, pruritus, and adrenal insufficiency.

Contraindications and Precautions.   Itraconazole is contraindicated in patients with a known hypersensitivity or renal failure, and during pregnancy (category C) and lactation.

Itraconazole should be used cautiously in patients with hypochlorhydria, hepatitis, and HIV. Itraconazole also must be used with great caution in patients with pulmonary, renal, and valvular heart diseases.

Drug Interactions.   Itraconazole may increase levels and toxicity of oral hypoglycemic agents. Combination with oral midazolam, pimozide, levomethadyl, or quinidine may cause severe cardiac events including cardiac arrest or sudden death. Itraconazole levels are decreased by carbamazepine, phenytoin, phenobarbital, isoniazid, and rifampin.

Fluconazole

Fluconazole is an antifungal for both systemic and superficial mycoses.

Mechanism of Action.   Fluconazole interferes with the formation of ergosterol, resulting in decreased cell wall integrity and leakage of essential cellular components. Fluconazole is fungistatic and it may also be fungicidal, depending on the concentration used.

Indications.   Fluconazole has been shown to be effective against meningitis, as well as oropharyngeal and systemic candidiasis, both of which are commonly seen in AIDS patients. Fluconazole is also used for vaginal candidiasis.

Adverse Effects.   The most common adverse effects of fluconazole include elevated liver enzymes, gastrointestinal complaints, headache, and skin rash.

Key Concept

Herbal supplements such as St. John's wort and garlic may affect itraconazole levels.

Key Concept

In the use of fluconazole in elderly patients or those who have renal impairments, a creatinine clearance test should be provided before administration of the drug.

Contraindications and Precautions.   Fluconazole is contraindicated in patients with known hypersensitivity and during pregnancy (category C) and lactation. Fluconazole is used cautiously in patients with renal impairment. This agent may be given during pregnancy if the benefit of the drug outweighs any possible risk to the fetus.

Drug Interactions.   Fluconazole administration may increase the effect of oral hypoglycemics and decreases the metabolism of phenytoin and warfarin.

Ketoconazole

Ketoconazole is an antifungal agent effective for the treatment of candidiasis, histoplasmosis, blastomycosis, and aspergillosis.

Mechanism of Action.   Ketoconazole is fungistatic and may also be fungicidal depending on the concentration used. Ketoconazole interferes with the formation of ergosterol, the principal sterol in the fungal cell wall, interrupting membrane function.

Indications.   Ketoconazole is used for severe systemic fungal infections, including candidiasis (e.g., oral thrush, candiduria), chronic mucocutaneous and pulmonary candidiasis. Topical forms are available for superficial mycoses.

Adverse Effects.   Ketoconazole is usually well-tolerated. In some cases, nausea, vomiting, dizziness, headache, abdominal pain, and pruritus have been reported. Most adverse effects are mild and transient. In rare cases, fatal hepatic necrosis may occur. Periodic hepatic function tests should be used to monitor for hepatic toxicity.

Contraindications and Precautions.   Ketoconazole is contraindicated in patients with known hypersensitivity to ketoconazole or to any component in its formulation, as well as chronic alcoholism. Safe administration of ketoconazole during pregnancy (category C) and lactation, or in children less than two years of age is not established.

Drug Interactions.   Ketoconazole increases the anticoagulant effects of warfarin and causes hepatotoxicity when administered with alcohol. The absorption of ketoconazole is decreased when this agent is given with histamine antagonists and antacids.

PROTOZOA

Protozoa are single-celled parasitic organisms, many of which are motile. Most protozoa obtain their food from dead or decaying organic matter. Infection is spread through the ingestion of contaminated food or water, or through insect bites. Some protozoa are agents of disease, and some cause infections among the most serious known to humanity. Common

TABLE 23-4   Protozoa That Cause Major Diseases and Preferred Site of Infection

Protozoan Group	Genus	Preferred Site of Infection	Disease
Amoebae	Entamoeba	Intestine	Amebiasis
Sporozoa	Plasmodium	Bloodstream, liver	Malaria
	Toxoplasma	Intestine	Toxoplasmosis
Flagellates	Trypanosoma	Blood	Trypanosomiasis
	Trichomonas	Genital tract	Trichomoniasis
	Giardia	Intestine	Giardiasis

infections caused by protozoa include amebiasis, malaria, toxoplasmosis, trypanosomiasis, trichomoniasis, and giardiasis. Although many of these diseases are rare in the United States, travelers to Africa, South America, and Asia may acquire them overseas and return home with the infection. Table 23-4 shows the characteristics of each group.

Antiprotozoal Drugs

Antiprotozoal drugs fall into two main categories: **antimalarial agents** used to treat malaria infection; and **amebicides** and **trichomonacides**, which are prescribed to treat amebic and trichomonal infections.

Amebicides and Trichomonacides

These drugs are very important in the treatment of amebiasis, giardiasis, and trichomoniasis. These drugs include metronidazole, iodoquinol, and paromomycin (Table 23-5).

Metronidazole.   Metronidazole is an antitrichomonal, amebicide, and antibiotic.

Mechanism of Action.   Metronidazole is a synthetic compound with direct trichomonacidal and amebicidal activity as well as antibacterial activity against anaerobic bacteria and some Gram-negative bacteria.

Indications.   Metronidazole is the drug of choice in amebic dysentery, giardiasis, and trichomoniasis. It is used in asymptomatic and symptomatic dysentery, which is a gastrointestinal disorder resulting from ulcerative inflammation of the colon caused chiefly by infection with Entamoeba histolytica. Entamoeba, Giardia, toxoplasma, and trypanosomia are commonly found in Africa, Asia, and Latin America. These infections are rare in the U.S. Trichomona Vaginalis is usually transmitted through sexual contact, which is frequently seen in the United States in females and males. Metronidazole is also used in an acute intestinal amebiasis and amebic liver abscess. This agent

TABLE 23-5   Drug Effects on Protozoal Infections

Generic Name	Trade Name	Route of Administration	Common Adult Dosage
Antiprotozoals (nonmalarial)			
metronidazole	Flagyl®	PO, IV	PO: 250–500 mg t.i.d.; IV: loading dose 15 mg/kg, maintenance dose 7.5 mg/kg q6 h
pentamidine isoethionate	Nebupent®	IM, IV	4 mg/kg daily × 14–21 days: infuse over 60 min
trimetrexate	Neutrexin®	IV	45 mg/m² daily
Antimalarials			
atovaquone	Mepron®	PO	750 mg b.i.d. × 21 days
chloroquine phosphate	Aralen®	PO	600 mg initial dose, then 300 mg weekly
hydroxychloroquine	Plaquenil®	PO	620 mg initial dose, then 310 mg weekly
mefloquine hydrochloride	Lariam®	PO	Prevention: begin with 250 mg once a week × 4 weeks, then 250 mg every other week; Treatment: 1250 mg as a single dose
primaquine phosphate	Primaquine®	PO	30 mg/day
pyrimethamine	Daraprim®	PO	25 mg once per week × 10 weeks
quinine	Quinamm®	PO	260–650 mg t.i.d. for 3 days
Amebicides			
doxycycline	Vibramycin®	PO	100 mg/day
iodoquinol	Yodoxin®	PO	650 mg t.i.d. × 20 days (max: 2 g/day)
paromomycin sulfate	Humatin®	PO	25–35 mg/kg divided in 3 doses for 5–10 days

Key Concept

Alcohol must be avoided while a patient is taking metronidazole to prevent profound vomiting.

commonly indicates for preoperative prophylaxis in colorectal surgery, elective hysterectomy, or vaginal repair. IV metronidazole is used for the treatment of serious infections caused by susceptible anaerobic bacteria in intra-abdominal infections, skin infections, and septicemia.

Adverse Effects.   Metronidazole causes nausea, vomiting, diarrhea, metallic taste or bitter taste, and, occasionally, neurologic reactions. This agent may also cause polyuria, dysuria, pyuria, incontinence, cystitis, decreased libido, and vaginal dryness.

Contraindications and Precautions.   Metronidazole is contraindicated in patients with known hypersensitivity, blood dyscrasias, and active CNS disease. Metronidazole cannot be used in the first trimester of pregnancy (category B), or during lactation. This drug should be cautiously used in patients with coexistent candidiasis, alcoholism, and liver disease, and during the second and third trimesters of pregnancy.

Drug Interactions.   Alcohol may elicit disulfiram reaction, which consists of flushing, a throbbing headache, nausea, vomiting, arrhythmias, and many other unpleasant effects. Metronidazole interacts with many drugs, including oral solutions of citalopram ritonavir and IV formulations of sulfamethoxazole. Trimethoprim and nitroglycerin, if used with metronidazole, may elicit disulfiram reaction due to the alcohol content of the dosage form. Phenobarbital increases metronidazole metabolism.

Antimalarial Agents

Malaria is a severe generalized infection caused by the bite of an *anopheles* mosquito that is infected with *Plasmodium* protozoa. The most important human parasite among the sporozoa is *Plasmodium*, which causes malaria. There are four different types of *Plasmodium*: *P. falciparum*, *P. malariae*, *P. vivax*, and *P. ovale*. According to Integrated Regional Information Networks (www.irinnews.org), it has been estimated that more than 100 million people are infected, and about one million die annually of malaria in Africa alone. Antimalarial drugs are selectively active during different phases of the protozoan life cycle. Antimalarial drugs include chloroquine, primaquine, quinine, and hydroxychloroquine. Agents that are employed in the prevention of malaria include mefloquine, quinacrine, and folic acid antagonists. Mefloquine is chemically related to quinine. It is used both in the prevention of malaria and in the treatment of acute malarial infections. Quinacrine was once the most popular drug for malaria prophylaxis, but the use of quinacrine has declined sharply with the development of safer and more effective agents. Folic acid antagonists such as pyrimethamine and sulfa drugs interfere with the synthesis of folic acid. They may be used alone or in combination to suppress and prevent malaria caused by susceptible strains of *Plasmodium*.

Mechanism of Action.   Chloroquine and hydroxychloroquine bind to and alter the properties of *Plasmodium*. The mechanism of action of primaquine and quinine is unknown.

Indications.   Chloroquine is the drug of choice to suppress malaria symptoms and treat acute malaria attacks resulting from *P. falciparum* and

P. malariae infections. Chloroquine is the most useful antimalarial agent. Hydroxychloroquine is prescribed as an alternative to chloroquine in patients that cannot tolerate chloroquine or when chloroquine is unavailable. Primaquine is used to cure relapses of *P. vivax* and *P. ovale* malaria, to prevent malaria in exposed persons, and in the prevention and treatment of chloroquine-resistant strains of *P. falciparum*. Quinine is prescribed for acute malaria caused by chloroquine-resistant strains. Quinine is always given in combination with another antimalarial agent.

Adverse Effects. Chloroquine and hydroxychloroquine can concentrate in the liver and must be used carefully in patients with liver diseases. They may cause visual disturbances, headache, and skin rash.

Primaquine may cause anemia, granulocytopenia, nausea, vomiting, and abdominal cramps.

Quinine overdose or hypersensitivity reactions may be fatal. Toxicity of quinine produces visual and hearing disturbances, headache, fever, syncope, and cardiovascular collapse.

Contraindications and Precautions. Chloroquine is contraindicated with patients with hypersensitivity to this agent and renal disease, or who are suffering from psoriasis. Chloraquine should be avoided for long-term therapy in children and during pregnancy (category C) and lactation. Safe use in women of childbearing potential has not been established.

Chloroquine should be used with caution in patients with impaired hepatic function, alcoholism, and eczema, and in infants and children.

Primaquine is contraindicated in patients with rheumatoid arthritis and lupus erythematosus. Primaquine is also contraindicated in patients with recent or concomitant use of agents capable of bone marrow depression (e.g., quinacrine). This drug is not used during pregnancy (category C) or lactation.

Quinine is contraindicated in patients with myasthenia gravis, tinnitus, and optic neuritis, and during pregnancy (category X). This drug should be avoided during lactation. Quinine is used cautiously in patients with cardiac arrhythmias.

Drug Interactions. Antacids containing aluminum and magnesium decrease chloroquine absorption. Toxicity of both primaquine and quinacrine are increased. Quinine may increase digoxin levels. Anticonvulsants, barbiturates, and rifampin increase the metabolism of quinine.

Key Concept

Chloroquine may cause irreversible retinal damage in patients who are on this drug for a long-term therapy.

Key Concept

If patients experience itching, rash, fever, difficulty breathing, or vision problems, they must stop taking quinine.

SUMMARY

Antiretroviral drugs are undergoing constant changes as new products are added to the market. It is an area of intense research interest, and new information is being discovered every day that will help patients with immune deficiency problems. Most antiviral drugs act by inhibiting viral DNA or RNA replication in the virus, causing viral death. These agents have limited use because they are effective against only a small number of specific viral infections.

Superficial mycotic (fungal) infections occur on the surface of, or just below, the skin or nails. Deep mycotic infections develop inside the body, such as the lungs. Treatment for deep mycotic infections is often difficult and prolonged. Antiprotozoal drugs include antimalarial, antiamebia, antitrichomoniasis, and others. Diseases caused by protozoa are rare in the U.S. They are seen commonly in Africa, Asia, and Latin America.

EXPLORING THE WEB

Look for additional information on HIV and AIDS and the treatments used to combat the diseases on the following sites:

- ***www.aegis.com***
- ***www.thebodypro.com***
- ***www.unicef.com***

REVIEW QUESTIONS

Multiple Choice

1. Amantadine is prescribed for the prophylaxis and treatment of:

   A. malaria
   B. *Candida* infections
   C. HIV
   D. influenza A

2. Which of the following antimicrobial agents is similar to amphotericin B (in its chemical structure)?

   A. ribavirin
   B. streptomycin
   C. amantadin
   D. nystatin

3. Which of the following are parasitic, minute organisms that may invade normal cells, and cause disease?

   A. fungi
   B. protozoa
   C. viruses
   D. bacteria

4. Herpes simplex virus type 2 (HSV-2) causes which of the following conditions or diseases?

   A. cold sores
   B. AIDS
   C. fever blisters
   D. genital herpes

5. Ketoconazole is contraindicated in children less than how old?

   A. 2 years
   B. 6 years
   C. 12 years
   D. 18 years

6. All of the following parasitic organisms include the classification of protozoa, except:

   A. flagellates
   B. spriochetes
   C. sporozoa
   D. amoebae

7. IV metronidazole is used for the treatment of which of the following serious infections?

   A. susceptible anaerobic bacteria
   B. trichomoniasis
   C. giardiasis
   D. amebic dysentery

8. Which of the following is the reason to decline sharply the use of quinacrine in the treatment of malaria?

   A. less safe and less effective
   B. price is higher than others
   C. discontinuation of the products
   D. none of the above

9. Which of the following agents is indicated to treat cytomegalovirus?

   A. zidovudine
   B. abacavir
   C. ganciclovir
   D. nelfinavir

10. The trade names of enfuvirtide (miscellaneous drug for treatment of HIV-AIDS) include which of the following?

    A. Fuzeon
    B. Viread
    C. Hivid
    D. Norvir

11. Which of the following antiviral drugs may be indicated for treatment of Parkinson's disease?

    A. famciclovir
    B. ritonavir
    C. acyclovir
    D. amantadine

12. All of the following diseases may be caused by protozoa, except:

    A. giardiasis
    B. aspergillosis
    C. trichomoniasis
    D. malaria

13. HAART therapy in HIV-AIDS patients has been shown to reduce viral load, resulting in which of the following?

    A. increased CD4 lymphocytes
    B. decreased length of survival with AIDS
    C. decreased CD4 lymphocytes
    D. increased risk of mortality of AIDS patients

14. The first cases of AIDS were seen in which of the following years?

    A. 1969
    B. 1975
    C. 1981
    D. 1996

Matching

Generic Name	Trade Name
_____ 1. tioconazole	A. Fulvicin
_____ 2. fluconazole	B. Monistat
_____ 3. nystatin	C. Nizoral
_____ 4. ketoconazole	D. Sporanox
_____ 5. miconazole	E. Fungizone
_____ 6. griseofulvin	F. Diflucan
_____ 7. amphotericin B	G. Mycostatin
_____ 8. itraconazole	H. Vagistat

Critical Thinking

A young female client who was recently diagnosed with insulin-dependent diabetes has been given a prescription for metronidazole (Flagyl) for a vaginal infection.

1. What would be the most important recommendations by her physician regarding this vaginal infection?

2. What foods or beverages must be avoided with this medication?

PHARMACOLOGY FOR SPECIFIC POPULATIONS

Drug Therapy During Pregnancy and Lactation

OBJECTIVES

After completing this chapter, the reader should be able to:

1. Identify how normal physiologic changes with pregnancy alter the pharmacokinetics of drug therapy.
2. Define "teratogenic effect" and its relevance in managing drug therapy in pregnant patients.
3. Differentiate the classifications of drugs for use in pregnancy.
4. Describe why adverse effects of drug therapy may be overlooked in pregnant patients.
5. Identify how drug therapy in pregnant or breast-feeding patients may vary from drugs in other groups.
6. Discuss FDA pregnancy categories.
7. Identify potential drugs that cause problems during breast-feeding.
8. Explain pharmacodynamics of drugs during pregnancy.
9. Describe the common conditions affecting pregnant patients.
10. Define *preeclampsia* and *eclampsia*.

GLOSSARY

Affinity – the force that impels certain atoms to unite with certain others

Eclampsia – the occurrence of seizures (convulsions) in a pregnant woman, usually occurring after the twentieth week of pregnancy

Floppy infant syndrome – also called "infantile hypotonia", this is a condition of abnormally low muscle tone, often with reduced muscle strength

Hemodynamic – related to blood circulation or blood flow

Hyperemesis gravidarum – pernicious vomiting during pregnancy

Lipophilic – fat-soluble

Organogenesis – from implantation to about 60 days after, the time when major fetal organs form

Preeclampsia – the development of elevated blood pressure and protein in the urine after the twentieth week of pregnancy; it may also cause swelling of the face and hands

Teratogenic – causing developmental malformations

OVERVIEW

A developing fetus must always be carefully considered when drugs are administered to a pregnant woman. Each drug prescribed for a woman during pregnancy must be evaluated for its utmost effectiveness while weighing this against its potential adverse effects. Practitioners must always consider the dangers these drugs may present to the fetus. There are many conditions that occur which are secondary to pregnancy, including **preeclampsia** (high blood pressure, weight gain, and protein in the urine), **eclampsia** (a seizure disorder that may follow preeclampsia), or gestational diabetes. Sometimes, fetal conditions are treated by administering drugs to the mother, who passes them to the fetus through the placenta. An example of this is digoxin, used to treat fetal congestive heart failure or tachycardia.

> **Medical Terminology Review**
>
> **preeclampsia**
> *pre = before*
> *eclampsia = a serious complication of pregnancy involving convulsions*
> a condition that exists prior to a more serious condition of pregnancy

PHARMACOKINETICS DURING PREGNANCY

During pregnancy, physiologic and anatomic changes occur that can alter drug pharmacokinetics. These changes involve the endocrine, cardiovascular, circulatory, gastrointestinal (GI), and renal systems.

Absorption

The function of the gastrointestinal tract may be greatly altered by hormonal action during pregnancy. Peristalsis and gastric emptying may be slowed to such a degree as to affect the amount of drug absorbed from the gut. Gastric acid secretion is also more erratic, which can affect the degree of absorption of acidic agents. However, because of individual differences in the effects of pregnancy, the observed effects on absorption can vary greatly, and are difficult to predict. Nevertheless, an awareness of the kinds of pharmacokinetic effects that can be expected during pregnancy is valuable, even if these effects don't occur every time.

> **Medical Terminology Review**
>
> **pharmacokinetic**
> *pharmaco = related to drugs*
> *kinetic = putting into motion; activity*
> the movement of drugs within the body

Distribution

Because of **hemodynamic** changes (those that relate to the mechanics of blood circulation), many alterations occur in a pregnant woman's body. The heart rate increases by about 10 to 15 beats per minute. The blood volume increases by 40 percent. Plasma volume increases by 50 percent throughout pregnancy. These changes alter drug transportation and distribution. Other factors that determine distribution during pregnancy include plasma protein concentration and **affinity** for the drug, body fluid levels, drug solubility, body fat content, and the tissue blood flow. Therefore, distribution of drugs in pregnant women can be altered.

The fetus receives drugs from the mother's circulatory system, which passes them through the placenta. Drugs are affected by pregnancy

Medical Terminology Review

hemodynamic

hemo = blood
dynamic = properties; actions
the actions of blood in the body

Medical Terminology Review

lipophilic

lipo = fat
philic = soluble
ability to dissolve in fatty substances

hormones, which can result in a larger than normal amount of free drugs in circulation, which can cross the placental membrane easily. Fat-soluble drugs especially pass through the placenta's lipid membrane with ease.

Drugs can be distributed in a mother's breast milk, usually in low concentrations. It is important to note that drugs with increased lipid solubility and low protein binding (such as CNS agents), may be present in high concentrations in breast milk. Since breast milk contains a high percentage of fats, **lipophilic** (fat-soluble) drugs pass easily through breast milk. Other drugs that easily diffuse in breast milk include those with lower molecular weights or organic bases.

Drug levels in breast milk are not the same as drug levels in the mother's blood. This is because of the influence of factors that was discussed above. Those with poor bioavailability don't usually achieve high concentrations in a neonate's circulation. Less than 2 percent of the mother's total dose of these drugs is usually ingested by a nursing infant.

Metabolism

Drug metabolism may be altered in patients with liver disease, hepatic blood flow, conditions that affect hepatic enzyme levels, or diet in general, but drug metabolism is not altered by breast-feeding or pregnancy.

Excretion

Changes in renal plasma flow (usually 40 to 50 percent), glomerular filtration rates, and tubular reabsorption cause changes in renal function during pregnancy. Increased renal plasma flow causes greater capillary pressure and increased glomerular filtration (by approximately 50 percent). Drug excretion rates are therefore increased during pregnancy.

PHARMACODYNAMICS

Medical Terminology Review

pharmacodynamics

pharmaco = related to drugs
dynamic = properties; actions
the actions and properties of drugs

By the 32nd week of pregnancy, a woman's cardiac output has increased by 50 percent. Her arterial blood pressure increases, beginning in the second trimester. Because of these changes, a drug's pharmacodynamics must be carefully evaluated before administration. Therefore, the mechanism of action of any drug that is used in pregnant women has important clinical applications. Knowledge of therapeutic indexes, dose-response relationships, and drug receptor interactions will help pharmacy technicians provide cautious, safe, and effective treatment during pregnancy.

PREGNANCY DRUG CATEGORIES

Pregnancy drug categories were developed in 1980 by the Food and Drug Administration to help classify drugs by the risks they pose to a developing fetus. See Table 24-1 for a listing of these categories.

TABLE 24-1 Pregnancy Drug Categories

Category	Explanation
A	Controlled studies in pregnant women show no risk to the fetus
B	Animal studies fail to show fetal risk, but no controlled human studies were conducted; or animal studies show fetal risk that is not confirmed in human studies
C	Animal studies show fetal risk, but no controlled human studies were conducted; or there are no animal or human studies—these drugs are given if their benefit justifies their risks
D	Controlled human studies show fetal risk; the benefit of these drugs may be acceptable, despite risks, in life-threatening situations
X	Controlled human studies show fetal risk that outweighs any possible benefit; these drugs are contraindicated for use in pregnant or potentially pregnant women

Drug manufacturers are required to state these pregnancy categories in all printed drug reference materials and package inserts. There are many stated concerns about these categories and how accurate they are in describing the dangers of various drugs. Category C in particular is being revised because it contains drugs that have undergone no human studies, but animal studies have indicated fetal harm. Animal studies do not always accurately predict human responses to the studied drug. The FDA is working to clarify the categorization of drugs with more focus on their actual fetal risks.

Adverse Effects

There are two major considerations that need to be remembered when evaluating the adverse effects of drug therapy in pregnant women. They are as follows:

- Common side effects of pregnancy
- The adverse effect that maternal drug therapy can have upon the fetus

Many of the side effects of pregnancy can mask the adverse effects of drug therapy in pregnant patients. These signs and symptoms include:

- Light-headedness or hypotension
- Constipation
- Heartburn
- Nausea and vomiting
- Heart palpitations
- Fatigue
- Frequent urination

The dose and duration of drug therapy, the type of adverse effects that may occur, and the stage of pregnancy must all be considered in determining

TABLE 24-2 Common Non-teratogenic Drugs with Adverse Fetal Effects

Non-teratogenic Drug	Adverse Fetal Effects
Acetaminophen	Renal failure
Adrenocortical hormones	Adrenocortical suppression, electrolyte imbalance
Amphetamines	Withdrawal
Cocaine	Vascular disruption, withdrawal, intrauterine growth retardation
Meperidine	Neonatal depression
Phenobarbital (if excessively used)	Neonatal bleeding, death
Cigarette smoking	Premature births, intrauterine growth retardation
Thiazide diuretics	Thrombocytopenia, salt and water depletion, possible neonatal death

Key Concept

The timing of drug exposure is critical because of the vulnerability of the fetus during constant changes in development.

Key Concept

The effects of most approved drugs on a developing human fetus are unknown.

drug administration and potential fetal risks. Before a fertilized ovum is implanted in the uterus, certain drugs such as alcohol can produce a hostile environment capable of preventing implantation or causing a spontaneous abortion.

Some drugs that are not normally **teratogenic** (causing developmental malformations) can cause a situation wherein a neonate cannot correctly adapt to life outside the uterus (see Table 24-2). Benzodiazepines can cause **floppy infant syndrome**, while nonsteroidal anti-inflammatory drugs such as aspirin or indomethacin can cause premature closing of the neonate's ductus arteriosus.

Contraindications and Precautions

Some drugs are contraindicated for use during the first trimester of pregnancy. Caution is advised for using others because certain drugs may pass through the placenta to the fetus and cause teratogenic effects. Some others should not be used at all during pregnancy and lactation. As the above categories of drugs show, the prescribing or administration of medications during pregnancy must be done cautiously.

During the period of **organogenesis** (from implantation to about 60 days after, the time when major fetal organs form), teratogenic drugs may cause serious malformations, or even spontaneous abortion, to occur (see Table 24-3). Drug therapy should be delayed until after this time if possible. The embryonic phase is completed at about 60 days, when the fetal phase begins. Effects that may occur during this phase include:

- Damage to structures or organs that were normally formed during organogenesis
- Damage to systems currently undergoing tissue development

Medical Terminology Review

organogenesis

organo = related to organs
genesis = development
development of organs

TABLE 24-3   Common Teratogenic Drugs

Drug or Drug Class	Indications
Aminopterin, methylaminopter, busulfan, cyclophosphamide, thalidomide	Antineoplastic
Androgenic hormones, diethylstilbestrol	Hormone replacement
Coumarin	Anticoagulant
Etretinate	Psoriasis
Isotretinoin	Recalcitrant cystic acne
Lithium	Antimanic
Methimazole	Antithyroid
Penicillamine	Cystinuria and rheumatoid arthritis
Phenytoin, trimethadione, valproic acid	Anticonvulsant
Tetracycline	Antibiotic

Key Concept

The minimum therapeutic dose should be used for as short a time as possible during pregnancy. If possible, drug therapy should be delayed until after the first trimester of pregnancy.

- Retardation of growth
- Fetal death or stillbirth

Combinations of drug effects may occur, with growth retardation being the most common fetal effect. For example, coumarin derivatives that are used as anticoagulants can produce eye and brain defects due to hemorrhagic accidents in the developing fetus.

LACTATION DRUG CATEGORIES

The American Academy of Pediatrics published a report in 2001 that identified several categories of drugs that may cause problems during breast-feeding. These categories are listed below:

- Cytotoxic drugs that can interfere with a nursing infant's cellular metabolism
- Abused drugs with reported adverse effects on nursing infants
- Radioactive agents that require the stopping of breast-feeding
- Drugs that have unknown but possibly dangerous effects on nursing infants
- Drugs that have caused harm to some nursing infants and should be given to nursing mothers only with caution
- Maternal medications that are usually compatible with breast-feeding
- Food and environmental agents that affect nursing infants

It is recommended that all drugs of abuse be avoided by lactating women, regardless of documented effects on nursing infants. Women should not breast-feed while they are taking active radioactive agents. Drugs that have unknown neonatal effects include antianxiety drugs, antidepressants, and neuroleptics and must be used with caution. Nursing mothers should be informed that these drugs may be passed to their infant, and can affect the development of the central nervous system with long-term effects. Other drugs that may have adverse effects on neonates include anti-infectives, aspirin, phenobarbital, and sulfasalazine. While most drugs that are administered to nursing mothers are safe for use, with only minimal effects, many drugs are not part of large research studies and realistically need to be further tested in order to ensure safety.

Key Concept

Drugs may be excreted into breast milk, although the total amount received by the infant is a small percentage of the maternal dose.

COMMON CONDITIONS AFFECTING THE PREGNANT PATIENT

Pregnant patients who have pre-existing conditions requiring drug therapy have special needs. Physicians must consider how drug therapy will affect the developing fetus. Also, any adverse effects caused by pregnancy must be identified so that drug therapy may be changed if needed. If the pregnancy causes health changes that require new drug therapy, adverse effects of these new drugs upon the fetus must also be considered.

During pregnancy, special attention should be given to cardiovascular problems that may develop. The cardiovascular system changes and experiences more stress during pregnancy, possibly requiring changes in drug selection or dosage. The use of over-the-counter drugs, which can pose additional risks to the fetus, must also be assessed.

Seizure Disorders

Seizure disorders are important to consider during pregnancy. A woman with a seizure disorder who is planning to become pregnant must first discuss her condition with her physician, and seriously consider how anticonvulsant drug therapy might affect her fetus. Anticonvulsant drug therapy may adversely affect a developing fetus. Physicians must carefully assess how pregnant women with seizure disorders should be treated to avoid possible teratogenic effects to the fetus. It is believed by many experts that seizures in a pregnant woman can cause fetal hypoxia, which leads to central nervous system damage. The anticonvulsants known as trimethadione and valproic acid should be avoided in pregnant women. However, only drugs of pregnancy category X are strictly contraindicated. The decision whether to maintain therapy with category D or even category C drugs must be made based on the ratio of risks to benefits.

Depression

Though little accurate information exists, the use of antidepressants by pregnant women must be carefully controlled. Drugs such as selective serotonin reuptake inhibitors (SSRIs) do not appear to cause increased risk for fetal complications. However, high doses of fluoxetine (Prozac) have been shown to cause low birth weight.

Diabetes

According to the Food and Drug Administration approximately 9 percent of all women in the U.S. have diabetes and about one-third of these women don't know they have the disorder. Also, gestational diabetes may develop in 2 to 5 percent of all pregnancies and resolves after birth. During pregnancy, production of hormones increases thus insulin demands also increase. This can cause insulin resistance in the pregnant patient. Insulin therapy may be required to prevent hyperglycemia, which can cause congenital anomalies that can harm the fetus. Insulin is preferred over oral hypoglycemic drugs because it does not cross the placenta. After the baby is delivered, insulin therapy is usually no longer required for women who have developed gestational diabetes, because their blood sugar levels return to normal.

Women with diabetes or who acquire diabetes during their pregnancies are at risk for having babies with higher birth weights resulting in an increase in cesarean sections. These women are also at an increased risk of developing toxemia.

Hyperemesis During Pregnancy

Hyperemesis gravidarum (pernicious vomiting during pregnancy) may require antiemetic drug therapy. This currently consists of piperazines and phenothiazines. Of these classes of antiemetic drugs, piperazines are not known to be teratogenic, while the phenothiazines are generally considered safe in low, infrequent doses.

Key Concept

When using antiemetics, especially during the first trimester, the risk for adverse fetal effects must be considered.

Preeclampsia

Preeclampsia is a hypertensive condition developing usually after the twentieth gestational week. It is characterized by hypertension, cerebral edema, and proteinuria. Preeclampsia may lead to eclampsia, and the primary goal of preeclampsia treatment is to prevent this condition from developing. Treatment is aimed at decreasing central nervous system irritability and reducing maternal blood pressure. The drugs of choice for preeclampsia are magnesium sulfate (to prevent convulsions) and hydralazine (to treat hypertension). Other medications used in the treatment of hypertension in preeclampsia include diazoxide, nifedipine, and labetalol (see Chapter 12).

Eclampsia

Eclampsia is a more serious condition in which the blood pressure is higher, and kidney dysfunction is indicated by proteinuria, weight gain, and generalized edema (of the face, hands, feet, and legs). In some patients, preeclampsia may progress to eclampsia, in which the blood pressure becomes extremely high, and generalized seizures (*grand mal*) or coma develops. Immediate hospitalization is required for adequate treatment of eclampsia.

SUMMARY

Drug therapy may be required to manage preexisting or newly developed conditions in pregnant or lactating women. However, drug therapy can adversely affect the fetus or infant. Since physiologic changes related to pregnancy can alter drug absorption, distribution, and elimination, potential risks must always be considered before administering any drug. Also, potential fetal risks must be compared with maternal benefits when drug therapy is needed. Drugs may be excreted into breast milk in varying amounts. Limiting drug use during pregnancy and lactation decreases adverse effects to both the mother and infant.

EXPLORING THE WEB

Visit *www.aafp.org*

- Search for and read the article "Medications in the Breastfeeding Mother."

Visit the following Web sites and search by "pregnancy"; read additional articles relevant to the discussion presented in this chapter.

- *www.drugtopics.com*
- *www.emedicine.com*
- *www.fda.gov*
- *www.perinatology.com*
- *www.uspharmacist.com*

REVIEW QUESTIONS

Multiple Choice

1. Which of the following is a result of pharmacokinetics of orally administered drugs that may be altered by progesterone during pregnancy?
   A. increased opening of the center of the iris of each eye
   B. decreased volume of the respiratory system to absorb more inhaled medications
   C. decreased gastric tone and motility
   D. increased the time it takes the urinary bladder to empty

2. Which of the following is a true statement?

   A. Drug levels in breast milk are more than the drug levels in the mother's blood.
   B. Drug levels in breast milk are not the same as the drug levels in the mother's blood.

C. Drugs with increased lipid solubility and low protein binding may be present in low concentrations in breast milk.

D. Fat-soluble drugs are not able to pass easily through breast milk.

3. By the eighth month of pregnancy, a female's cardiac output has:

A. increased by 50 percent
B. increased by 80 percent
C. decreased by 50 percent
D. decreased by 80 percent

4. Which of the following pregnancy drug categories are absolutely contraindicated for use in pregnant women?

A. category B
B. category C
C. category D
D. category X

5. Women should *not* breast-feed while they are taking:

A. tetracycline
B. aspirin
C. acetaminophen
D. radioactive agents

6. Which of the following drugs is non-teratogenic and may be used during pregnancy?

A. cocaine
B. coumarin
C. meperidine
D. thiazide diuretics

7. Methimazole is a teratogenic drug that is indicated for:

A. congestive heart failure
B. hypertension
C. thyroid conditions
D. diabetes mellitus

8. Which of the following conditions during pregnancy may be accompanied by convulsions?

A. depression
B. diabetes
C. preeclampsia
D. eclampsia

9. Seizures in pregnant women can cause fetal:

A. hypertension
B. hypoxia
C. pernicious vomiting
D. all of the above

10. Administration of high doses of fluoxetine (Prozac) during pregnancy may cause which of the following in newborns?

A. low birth weight
B. high birth weight

C. low blood sugar
D. high blood sugar

11. Which of the following drugs may be required to prevent hyperglycemia during pregnancy?

   A. oral hypoglycemics
   B. insulin
   C. vitamin B_6
   D. none of the above

12. Which of the following medications may be used for pernicious vomiting during pregnancy?

   A. vitamin C
   B. vitamin B_{12}
   C. piperazine
   D. minocycline

13. Drug excretion rates during pregnancy are:

   A. increased
   B. decreased
   C. not changed
   D. changed only in depressed women

14. Which of the following classes of drugs are safer during pregnancy in women with severe depression?

   A. monoamine oxidase inhibitors
   B. tricyclic antidepressants
   C. selective serotonin reuptake inhibitors
   D. A and B

15. Which of the following is an adverse fetal effect of acetaminophen during pregnancy?

   A. renal failure
   B. heart failure
   C. liver failure
   D. low birth weight

16. Common teratogenic drugs include which of the following?

   A. methimazole
   B. coumarin
   C. tetracycline
   D. all of the above

17. Lithium is classified as:

   A. a hormone replacement
   B. an antithyroid agent
   C. an antimanic agent
   D. an anticonvulsant

18. Which of the following antibiotics is contraindicated during pregnancy?

   A. penicillin
   B. erythromycin
   C. tetracycline
   D. none of the above

19. Which of the following is a consequence of cigarette smoking during pregnancy?

    A. premature birth
    B. intracranial pressure in the newborn
    C. intrauterine growth retardation
    D. A and C

20. Which of the following is an appropriate treatment in women with gestational diabetes after delivery?

    A. insulin injections
    B. oral hypoglycemic drugs
    C. tranquilizers
    D. observation only

Critical Thinking

A 37-year-old woman had a root canal procedure at her local dentist's office. The dentist ordered ibuprofen to be taken every four hours for pain. This woman also had a painkiller at home, so she did not get her dentist's prescription filled. Every four hours, she took this painkiller, which was Tylenol III. Unknowingly, she continued to breast-feed her 4-month-old baby while taking Tylenol III. After several sessions of breast-feeding, the baby went into deep sleep, could not be awoken, and was rushed to the emergency unit, where the baby died.

1. What was the likely cause of the baby's death?

2. What drugs are combined in Tylenol III?

3. If she had filled her dentist's prescription and used it as instructed, would there have been any danger to her baby?

Drug Therapy for Pediatric Patients

OBJECTIVES

After completing this chapter, the reader should be able to:

1. Recognize common childhood respiratory diseases.
2. Identify treatment of asthma in children.
3. Describe otitis media in children.
4. Understand the factors affecting pharmacokinetics and pharmacodynamics in children.
5. Identify cardiovascular and blood disorders.
6. Define sickle cell anemia.
7. List five common examples of infectious diseases in pediatrics.
8. Explain acute bacterial meningitis.
9. Describe diabetes mellitus in pediatrics.
10. Explain international classification of seizures.

GLOSSARY

Apnea – the cessation of respiration for more than 20 seconds with or without cyanosis, hypotonia, or bradycardia

Asthma – a chronic, reversible, obstruction of the bronchial airways

Bacteremia – a condition in which bacteria are recovered from blood cultures of a patient and may or may not be associated with the disease

Congestive heart failure – a disorder in which the heart cannot pump the blood returning to the right side of the heart or provide adequate circulation to meet the needs of organs and tissues in the body

Croup – a viral infection that affects the larynx and the trachea

Epiglottitis – an acute bacterial infection of the epiglottis (an appendage which closes the glottis while food or drink is passing through the pharynx) and the surrounding areas that causes airway obstruction

Eustachian tubes – tubes within the ear by which fluids drain

Gestational age – the time measured from the first day of the mother's last menstrual cycle to the current date

Insulin-dependent diabetes mellitus – a disorder caused by complete lack of insulin secretion by the pancreas

Iron deficiency anemia – anemia characterized by low serum iron, increased serum iron-binding capacity, decreased serum ferritin, and decreased marrow iron stores

Kernicterus – yellow staining and degenerative lesions in basal ganglia associated with high levels of unconjugated bilirubin in infants; also known as "bilirubin encephalopathy"

Neonatal period – the time from birth to approximately 28 days of age

Otitis media – an inflammation of the middle ear

Patent ductus arteriosus – a condition in which the normal channel between the pulmonary artery and the aorta fails to close at birth

Pediatric period – the period from birth to approximately age 18

Pneumonia – an inflammation or infection of the pulmonary parenchyma; caused by viruses, bacteria, mycoplasmas, and aspiration of foreign substances

pneumonitis – inflammation of the lungs

Respiratory distress syndrome (RDS) – the result of the absence, deficiency, or alteration of the components of pulmonary surfactant

Respiratory syncytial virus (RSV) – the major cause of bronchiolitis and pneumonia in infants under one year of age; caused by a virus and exhibits mild cold-like symptoms

Septicemia – bacteremia associated with active disease, whether localized or systemic

Sickle cell anemia – an inherited disorder characterized by the presence of abnormal hemoglobin; hemoglobin contains hemoglobin S (HbS)

OVERVIEW

Pediatric drug therapy is a special consideration in medicine. It is problematic even for practitioners with extensive experience. To put it simply, a child's age, weight, development, and lack of information about the clinical pharmacology of specific agents for pediatric patients can all complicate drug therapy. A drug undergoes the same processes in a child as it does in an adult, but a child's body is distinctive and constantly changing, which affects how it responds to a drug. During the past few decades, drug administration, usage, and research in pediatric patients have been challenging. Children are not merely miniature adults. Therefore, knowledge about pediatric medications cannot simply be extrapolated from the adult research, literature, and clinical trials. In fact, if a label does not contain a pediatric dose, do not assume that the drug is safe for anyone less than 12 years of age. The pharmacy technician should be sure that a drug is safe for children by asking the doctor or pharmacist. Effective and safe drug therapy in newborns, infants, and children requires an understanding of maturational changes that affect drug action, metabolism, and disposition.

TABLE 25-1   Stages of Childhood Growth and Development

Age	Description
Newborn	Birth to one month
Infancy	One month to one year
Toddlerhood	One to three years
Preschool age	Three to six years
School age	Six to 12 years
Adolescence	12 to 18 years

Pediatric drug dosage must be adjusted for the characteristics of individual drugs, and for the patient's age, disease states, sex, and individual needs to prevent ineffective treatment or toxicity.

DEFINING THE NEONATAL AND PEDIATRIC POPULATION

The **neonatal period** generally covers the time from birth to approximately 28 days of age. This general category also includes premature infants of varying gestational ages. **Gestational age** (the time measured from the first day of the mother's last menstrual cycle to the current date) will factor in dosing for various medications and may even preclude the use of some. The **pediatric period** covers a wide range of ages, from birth to approximately age 18 (see Table 25-1).

UNIQUE CHARACTERISTICS IN PEDIATRIC MEDICATION ADMINISTRATION

A child's body surface area, metabolism, development, and tolerance are quite different from those of an adult. For many drugs, safe and effective use in children requires additional pharmacokinetic and pharmacodynamic data. According to the American Academy of Pediatrics, 20 percent of all medications marketed today do not have U.S. Food and Drug Administration (FDA) approved labeling for use in neonates, infants, children, and adolescents, and only 5 of the 80 drugs most often used in newborns and infants are labeled for pediatric use. The FDA has recently made regulatory changes to facilitate labeling of drugs for pediatric use.

To complicate matters even more, most drugs are not tested on children. In many instances, no one knows for sure if a given drug is safe or effective in children, or what dosage is appropriate. Only about 30 percent of FDA-approved drugs have been approved for specific pediatric indications,

Key Concept

Children younger than two years should not be given any OTC drug without a doctor's approval.

Children will respond differently to some drugs than adults. For example, certain barbiturates which make adults feel sluggish will make a child hyperactive. Amphetamines, which stimulate adults, can calm children.

and few approved drugs come in child-appropriate dosage forms, which means that health care professionals must formulate pediatric doses.

It is essential that pharmacy technicians be familiar with most common diseases and conditions of neonatal and young children, the principles of pharmacology, and the required drug therapy. The technician should also consider the four processes involved in pharmacokinetics: absorption, distribution, metabolism, and excretion.

Pharmacokinetics

Pharmacokinetics focuses on how drugs move throughout the body. This includes the processes of absorption, distribution, biotransformation, and excretion. Pharmacokinetics deals with how drugs enter the body, reach their site of action (in what concentration), and how the body eliminates them. The body's effects on drugs, or how the body handles drugs, can be described as pharmacokinetics.

Neonates, infants, and children have different pharmacokinetic processes than adults. It is important to understand the developmental differences of children in order to understand how drugs are concentrated at the site of action, how intense their effects will be, and how long their action will last.

Absorption

Absorption involves the movement of drugs from their site of administration into the bloodstream. Two factors that influence oral drug absorption are gastric emptying time and pH. In neonates and infants, gastric emptying time is slower than in adults, reaching adult values at around six months of age. Delayed gastric emptying delays drug absorption of drugs designed to be absorbed from the intestine. More complete absorption may occur for drugs that are absorbed mostly from the stomach.

In newborns, gastric pH is more alkaline, becoming more acidic at around two to three years of age. Acidic drugs are better absorbed from an acidic environment while basic (alkaline) drugs are better absorbed from an alkaline environment. During infancy, basic drugs are more easily absorbed from the stomach, while acidic drugs are less well-absorbed. This is different in comparison to older children and adults.

Topical medications are absorbed more rapidly by infants and children. This is because they have a greater ratio of body surface area (BSA) to weight. Also, their skin is thinner, and thus more permeable.

Distribution

The movement or transport of drugs throughout the body is known as distribution. In this process, drugs are made available to body tissues and fluids. Body composition, fluid distribution, blood flow to the tissues, special membrane barriers, and protein binding all influence drug distribution in the body.

Neonates, infants, and young children have more body water than adults. Premature neonates have 85 percent body water, neonates have 70 to 75 percent, and adults have only 50 to 60 percent body water. Body fat percentage is different, based on age and gender, and even differs between individual children. A neonate's body is comprised of 15 to 16 percent fat. Premature infants may have as little as 1 percent fat. Body fat percentage peaks at about nine months of age, decreasing (between one and five years) to between 8 and 12 percent, increasing again around adolescence. Girls have a higher percentage of body fat than boys.

Lipid-soluble drugs can be stored in body fat, and have a high affinity for adipose (fat) tissue. As a result, lower levels of drug may be left available in circulation and at the site of action. People with higher percentages of body fat need a higher mg/kg dose of lipid-soluble drugs than people who have a lower percentage of body fat.

Children under two years of age have an immature blood-brain barrier that allows a relatively easy access to their central nervous systems. Therefore, they are more sensitive to drugs that affect the brain, with increased risk of CNS toxicity. To protect young children from undesired drug effects, lower doses of certain drugs may be required.

Key Concept

*Sulfonamide antimicrobials compete with serum bilirubin for binding to albumin. Drugs given to a neonate with jaundice can displace bilirubin from albumin. Because of the greater permeability of the neonatal blood-brain barrier, substantial amounts of bilirubin may enter the brain and cause **kernicterus** (yellow staining and degenerative lesions in basal ganglia associated with high levels of unconjugated bilirubin in infants; also known as "bilirubin encephalopathy").*

Metabolism

Metabolism (biotransformation) involves the alteration or transformation of chemicals from their original form, aiding in the eventual excretion of the substance via the renal system. Most biotransformation of drugs happens in the liver. In infants and neonates, liver immaturity influences drug-metabolizing capacity. Hepatic enzyme activity is not mature until 1 to 2 years of age. At this stage of life, drugs metabolized by the liver have a longer half-life and there is more chance for toxicity. A drug's half-life is the time needed for 50 percent of a drug's administered dose to be eliminated.

As a result, reduction of some drug dosages and less frequent drug administration may be required. Young children have higher metabolic rates and metabolize drugs more rapidly. Between 2 and 6 years of age, this condition is more pronounced. Higher doses or more frequent administration is required, and this condition can continue until 10 to 12 years of age.

Excretion

The process involving the removal of drugs, active metabolites, and inactive metabolites from the body is known as excretion. Most drugs are excreted via the kidneys. Renal function increases rapidly during infancy, reaching adult levels by 6 to 12 months of age. During infancy, reduced renal excretion causes longer drug half-lives and the increased possibility of toxicity to drugs primarily excreted through the renal system. Especially during the neonatal period, reduced dosages are required. By three years of

age, drugs are eliminated more rapidly because the glomerular filtration rate surpasses the adult rate. In toddlers, a drug's half-life may be shorter than in older children and adults.

Pharmacodynamics

The way drugs affect the body and how they accomplish this can be explained as pharmacodynamics. This can be further described as the biochemical and physical effects of drugs (drug effects and the responses resulting from drug action) and their mechanisms of drug action. Most drugs are believed to act at the cellular level. They do this by attaching to cell receptors where they block or mimic the action of endogenous molecules that regulate cell action.

A drug's mechanism of action is the same in all individuals. However, drug effects may be different in infants and children than in adults. This is because of immaturity of target organs and the sensitivity of receptors. As a result, an infant or child may need either a lower or higher dose of a drug than may be expected, and usually has a heightened sensitivity to drugs.

FEVER

Fever is a common reason why parents seek medical attention for their children, and approximately 30 percent of visits to pediatricians are fever-related. Parents believe that fever is a disease rather than a symptom. Fever is part of the febrile response, which includes the activation of numerous physiologic, endocrinologic, and immunologic systems. Microbes, toxins, or products of microbial origin, antigen-antibody complexes, complement (a group of proteins in the blood that assist the function of antibodies in the immune system) and other chemical agents are pyrogens that cause fever.

This evidence indicates that fever is an important defense mechanism and that treating the fever may have detrimental effects. In varicella, for example, acetaminophen prolongs the time of crusting of skin lesions. Nevertheless, many clinicians and caregivers believe that fever is harmful. A small percentage of children younger than five years may develop a seizure when they have a fever.

Acetaminophen is one of the most widely used antipyretics. Like aspirin and other nonsteroidal anti-inflammatory drugs (NSAIDs), acetaminophen blocks the conversion of arachidonic acid to prostaglandin. Current evidence still suggests that acetaminophen is the drug of choice for antipyresis in children.

Ibuprofen (Motrin) is another option as an antipyretic. This agent has been shown to provide a greater temperature decrement in febrile children and a longer duration of antipyresis than noted with acetaminophen when

the two drugs were administered in equal doses (10 mg/kg). Physical methods to reduce temperature are ineffective if shivering is not prevented, and such methods do not alter the hypothalamic set point.

CHILDHOOD RESPIRATORY DISEASES

The patterns of respiratory tract diseases in childhood are modified by age, sex, race, season, geography, and environmental and socioeconomic conditions. Immediately after birth, tuberculosis can be transmitted to the newborn, presenting after several weeks of life as a severe **pneumonitis**. Lung immaturity and other events related to the perinatal period predispose to hyaline membrane disease. The incidence of respiratory tract infections also peaks during the first 2 to 3 school years. Respiratory diseases affect many children each year. Respiratory syncytial virus (RSV) and asthma are two specific problems quite often treated in the pediatric/neonatal patient population. Apnea is seen in the neonatal age group, especially in premature infants.

> **Medical Terminology Review**
>
> pneumonitis
> pneumo(n) = breathing; the lungs
> itis = inflammation; condition
> **inflammation of the lungs impairing breathing**

> **Medical Terminology Review**
>
> **cyanosis**
> cyan/o = blue
> -osis = condition of
> **condition characterized by blue coloring of skin and membranes**
>
> **hypotonia**
> hypo- = decreasing, below
> -tonia = tone, tension
> **decreased tone or tension in muscles**

Apnea

Apnea is the cessation of respiration for more than 20 seconds with or without cyanosis, hypotonia, or bradycardia. Apnea may be a symptom of another disorder that resolves upon treatment of the disorder. These disorders may include infection, gastroesophageal reflux, hypoglycemia, metabolic disorders, drug toxicity, hydrocephalus, or thermal instability in newborns. Immaturity of the central nervous system often accounts for apnea of the newborn, which occurs most commonly during active sleep.

Treatment for Apnea

The airway should be opened and cardio-respiratory resuscitation should be initiated when a child presents with apnea. The treatment of central apnea that is most commonly used for premature infants includes minimizing potential causes such as temperature variances and feeding intolerance. The use of xanthine medications such as caffeine and theophylline (see Chapter 14) provide CNS stimulation. Pulmonary function support may include the use of supplemental oxygen and continuous positive airway pressure at low pressures.

Respiratory Syncytial Virus (RSV)

Respiratory syncytial virus (RSV) is the major cause of bronchiolitis and pneumonia in infants younger than one year. It is the most important respiratory tract pathogen of early childhood. It causes mild cold-like symptoms in infants and most children. However, RSV can cause a more serious respiratory disease in premature infants that sometimes requires hospitalization. The at-risk group includes infants born at less than 36 weeks' gestation or those with chronic lung disease. The respiratory disease occurs

because of the immaturity of the infants' lungs and because these infants have not received sufficient antiviral substances from their mothers. In most parts of the U.S., RSV infection occurs seasonally, generally from fall through spring (October through March). At-risk infants are now treated before discharge from the hospital to provide some immunoprophylaxis.

Treatments for Respiratory Syncytial Virus

Palivizumab (Synagis) is used for immunoprophylaxis against severe lower respiratory tract RSV infections. In infants with uncomplicated bronchiolitis, treatment is symptomatic. Humidified oxygen is usually indicated for hospitalized infants because most have hypoxia. Fluids should be carefully administered. Often, intravenous or tube feeding is helpful when sucking is difficult. Bronchodilators should not be routinely used. However, a course of epinephrine should be used in children with wheezing who are older than one year, and bronchodilators should be administered if found to be beneficial. The use of corticosteroids is not indicated except as a last resort in patients whose condition is critical. Sedatives are rarely necessary. The antiviral drug ribavirin, delivered by small-particle aerosol and breathed along with the required concentration of oxygen for 20 to 24 hours per day for 3 to 5 days, has a beneficial effect on the course of pneumonia caused by RSV.

Asthma

Asthma is a leading cause of chronic illness in childhood, and is responsible for a significant proportion of school days missed because of chronic illness. Asthma is a chronic, reversible obstruction of the bronchial airways. The airways become over-reactive because of this inflammation and increased mucus secretion; mucosal swelling and muscle contraction then occur. This leads to airway obstruction, chest tightness, coughing, wheezing, and, if asthma is severe, shortness of breath and low blood oxygen levels. Most children experience their first symptoms by 4 to 5 years of age. Allergies, viral respiratory infections, and airborne irritants produce the inflammation that can lead to asthma. Childhood asthma is a disease with a strong allergic component and a genetic predisposition. Approximately 75 to 80 percent of children with asthma have allergies.

Treatment for Asthma

Treatment for asthma generally involves two types of medications: quick-relief medications (also called bronchodilators), and controller medications. Controller medications get their name because they help control inflammation to make breathing easier. These medications must be taken daily to be effective. Medications in the bronchodilators and controller group are listed in Table 25-2.

TABLE 25-2 Bronchodilators and Controller Groups for Asthma

Generic Name	Trade Name	Route of Administration
Bronchodilators		
albuterol	Ventolin®, Proventil®	PO, Nasal
bitolterol mesylate	Tornalate®	Nasal
epinephrine	Adrenalin®, Primatene Mist®	SC, IM, IV, Nasal
isoproterenol hydrochloride	Isuprel®	IV
metaproterenol sulfate	Alupent®, Metaprel®	PO, Nasal
pirbuterol acetate	Maxair®	Nasal
salmeterol xinafoate	Serevent®	Nasal
terbutaline sulfate	Brethaire®	Nasal, SC
Xanthine Derivatives		
aminophylline	Truphylline®	PO, IV
theophylline	Elixophyllin®	PO, IV
Leukotriene Inhibitors		
montelukast	Singulair®	PO
zafirlukast	Accolate®	PO
Corticosteroids		
dexamethasone	Decadron®	PO, IM, IV
hydrocortisone sodium	Solu-Cortef®	PO
prednisolone	Prelone®	PO
beclomethasone sodium phosphate	Beconase AQ®	Intranasal
budesonide	Rhinocort®	Nasal
fluticasone	Flovent®	Nasal, Intranasal
Mast Cell Stabilizers		
cromolyn sodium	Intal®	Nasal
nedocromil sodium	Tilade®, Alocril®	Nasal
IM, intramuscular; IV, intravenous; SC, subcutaneous		

Respiratory Distress Syndrome

Respiratory distress syndrome (RDS), or hyaline membrane disease, is the result of the absence, deficiency, or alteration of the components of pulmonary surfactant. Surfactant, a lipoprotein complex, is an ingredient of the film-like surface of each alveolus that prevents alveolar collapse. When the amount of surfactant is inadequate, alveolar collapse and hypoxia result.

Medical Terminology Review

lipoprotein
lipo = fats; triglycerides
protein = amino acid complex
amino acid complex with fatty
substance

The younger the infants are, the greater the incidence of RDS. However, the occurrence of RDS appears to be more dependent on lung maturity than actual gestational age. The severity of RDS is decreased in infants whose mothers received corticosteroids 24 to 48 hours before delivery. Corticosteroids are most effective when newborns are less than 34 weeks' gestational age, and they are administered for at least 24 hours, but no longer than seven days before delivery.

Treatment for Respiratory Distress Syndrome

Infants at risk for RDS, as well as infants with respiratory failure due to meconium aspiration syndrome, persistent pulmonary hypertension, or pneumonia, are treated with natural, animal-derived, or synthetic surfactant. Continuous positive airway pressure, via nasal prongs, is required to prevent volume loss during expiration or mechanical ventilation via endotracheal tube for severe hypoxemia and/or hypercapnia. Aerosol administration of bronchodilators is also prescribed.

Croup

Croup, or acute laryngo-tracheobronchitis, is a viral infection that affects the larynx and the trachea, resulting in subglottic edema with upper respiratory tract obstruction accompanied by thick secretions. Children are susceptible to airway obstruction because the diameter of the subglottic area is narrow. Croup is caused by any virus associated with upper respiratory tract infection. Spasmodic croup is a sudden attack of croup, which usually occurs during the night, and can be associated with an upper respiratory tract infection, fever, or allergies. The incidence of croup is higher in the late fall and early winter. The age range of occurrence is 6 months to 6 years. The peak age of onset is 2 years.

Treatment for Croup

When a child with suspected croup is seen at the hospital, supplemental humidified oxygen is given as indicated by the child's appearance, result of pulse oximetry, and vital signs. The child can be treated with bronchodilators, usually administered with epinephrine if humidification alone is ineffective. The use of corticosteroids is controversial. Children who receive corticosteroids need endotracheal intubation less often, and their stridor is more quickly resolved. Antibiotics are administered if secondary bacterial infection is suspected.

Epiglottitis

Epiglottitis is an acute bacterial infection of the epiglottis (an appendage that closes the glottis while food or drink is passing through the pharynx) and the surrounding areas that causes airway obstruction. The infection is caused by *Haemophilus influenzae* type B or, on rare occasions, streptococci

and pneumococci. The use of *H. influenzae* type B vaccine in infants has resulted in a dramatic reduction in the incidence of epiglottitis. Onset is sudden and infection progresses rapidly, causing acute respiratory difficulty. This condition requires emergency airway stabilization and medical measures because a fatal outcome can occur. Boys between ages 2 to 7 are most often affected. The incidence of epiglottitis is highest in the winter.

Medical Terminology Review
epiglottitis
epi = above
glott = the tongue
itis = inflammation; condition
inflammation of the tissue above the tongue in the airway

Treatment for Epiglottitis

Visual examination of the throat is contraindicated until a tracheostomy is performed. The child is observed in the intensive care area until swelling of the epiglottis decreases (usually by the third day). Antibiotics are given for a total of 7 to 10 days.

Pneumonia

Pneumonia is an inflammation or infection of the pulmonary parenchyma. Pneumonia is caused by viruses, bacteria, *Mycoplasma* organisms, and aspiration of foreign substances. Viral pneumonia occurs more often than bacterial pneumonia.

Treatment for Pneumonia

Medical treatment is primarily supportive and includes improving oxygenation with oxygen and respiratory treatments. Antibiotics are used to treat bacterial pneumonia based on culture and sensitivity testing. Hospitalization depends on the severity of illness, the child's age, and the suspected organism.

COMMON CHILDHOOD ILLNESSES

It is impossible to discuss all pediatric disorders and illnesses in one chapter. Therefore, some selective examples of the most common childhood illnesses will be discussed.

Otitis Media

Otitis media is an inflammation of the middle ear. Children six years of age and younger are at particular risk for otitis media because their **eustachian tubes** are shorter and more horizontal. Otitis media is the most commonly encountered diagnosis in office visits for children younger than 15 years of age in the United States. Otitis media occurs most often in children between 3 months and 3 years with peak incidences occurring between 5 to 24 months and 4 to 6 years. Boys have more ear infections than girls. Tympanic membrane rupture with discharge and short-term conductive hearing loss are common complications of otitis media.

Treatment for Otitis Media

The efficacy of steroid therapy, decongestants, and antihistamines for the resolution of otitis media has not been proven. Their use should not be encouraged. Surgical removal of tonsils or adenoids is not recommended for the treatment of otitis media with effusion in the absence of specific tonsil or adenoid pathological conditions. The first-line antibiotic medication most often prescribed is amoxicillin or ampicillin. The second-line medication regimen (to be used when an amoxicillin-resistant organism is suspected) includes amoxicillin with clavulanate, cefaclor, cotrimoxazole, erythromycin, or sulfisoxazole. In the penicillin-allergic child, erythromycin with a sulfonamide or trimethoprim-sulfamethoxazole may be used. Generic names, trades names, and routes of administration were discussed in Chapter 22. Myringotomy is the surgical procedure of inserting pressure-equalizing tubes into the tympanic membrane. This allows ventilation of the middle ear, relieves the negative pressure, and permits drainage of fluid. The tubes usually fall out after 6 to 12 months.

Diabetes Mellitus

Insulin-dependent diabetes mellitus (IDDM), or Type I (juvenile-onset) diabetes, is caused by complete lack of insulin secretion by the pancreas. Insulin is necessary for many physiological functions of the body. Insulin deficiency results in unrestricted glucose production without appropriate use, resulting in hyperglycemia and increased production of ketones in the blood. Age ranges of peak incidence are 5 to 7 years and puberty. Among children 5 to 10 years of age, the disease is more commonly diagnosed in girls. Type I diabetes usually starts with polyphagia, weight loss, polydipsia, and polyuria. Long-term effects of IDDM include failure to grow at a normal rate, neuropathy (the impairment of sensory and motor nerve functions), recurrent infection, renal microvascular disease, and ischemic heart disease.

Treatment for Insulin-dependent Diabetes Mellitus (IDDM)

As soon as hyperglycemia or glucosuria is detected, immediate medical attention is needed because of the potential for rapid deterioration of the patient's condition. The initial therapy will depend on how early the diagnosis is made, and on the state of the child. Medical management includes the regulation of serum glucose, fluid, and electrolyte levels. Once glucose levels are stabilized, the child's insulin dose is typically dictated by a sliding scale based on the serum glucose level. Regulation of nutrition and exercise is also a key factor in managing diabetes. For older children, or children who are in the midst of the adolescent growth spurt, a regimen of twice-daily injections of a mixture of preferably NPH and regular insulin before breakfast and before supper may be started immediately. Table 25-3 shows types and action of insulins (see Chapter 16).

Medical Terminology Review

polyphagia
poly = much
phagia = to eat
excessive eating

polydipsia
poly = much
dipsia = thirst
excessive thirst

polyuria
poly = much
uria = urine
excessive urine

TABLE 25-3 Types and Action of Insulin

Type and Action	Action (in hours)	
	Peak	Duration
Fast		
Regular	2–4	5–7
Semilente	2–8	8–16
Intermediate		
NPH	8–12	18–24
Lente	8–12	18–28
Slow		
Ultralente	16–18	20–36
Protamine zinc	16–20	24–36

Treatment of Diabetes in Infants

Symptomatic hyperglycemia can occur in newborn infants. These babies usually suffer from severe intrauterine malnutrition and, therefore, are small for their gestational age. They are hypoinsulinemic and their pancreas fails to release insulin in response to any of the standard body demands. They must be treated with divided doses of exogenous insulin of up to 1–2 units/kg/24 h. Insulin requirements are best established by starting a continuous intravenous insulin infusion at rates to provide at least 0.5 units/kg/24 h. Insulin treatment is simplified by using diluted insulin so that inadvertent overdoses do not occur. In most cases, pancreas function develops sometime between the age of 6 and 12 weeks. The children do well after the newborn period and do not appear to be at increased risk of developing Type I diabetes at a later age. See Chapter 16 for more information on the endocrine system, hormones, and related subjects.

Seizure Disorders

Seizure is a sudden, transient alteration in brain function as a result of abnormal neuronal activity and excessive cerebral electric discharge. The causes of seizure include perinatal factors, infectious disease (encephalitis and meningitis), febrile illness, metabolic disorders, trauma, neoplasms, toxins, circulatory disturbances, and degenerative diseases of the nervous system. Epilepsy is a disorder characterized by recurrent, unprovoked seizures, in which seizures are of primary cerebral origin, indicating underlying brain dysfunction. Epilepsy is not a disease in itself.

Medical Terminology Review

encephalitis
encephal = brain
itis = inflammation
inflammation of the brain

Treatment for Epilepsy

Antiepileptic drug therapy is the mainstay of medical management. Single-drug therapy is the most desirable, with the goal of establishing a

balance between seizure control and adverse side effects. The drug of choice is based on seizure type, epileptic syndrome, and patient variables. Drug combinations may be needed to achieve seizure control. Complete control is achieved in only 50 to 75 percent of children with epilepsy. The most commonly used anticonvulsants were discussed in Chapter 8.

CARDIOVASCULAR AND BLOOD DISORDERS

Medications to support cardiovascular functions in the pediatric/neonatal patient population differ little from those used with adults. Digoxin, diuretics, and, occasionally, antihypertensives are utilized. Their indications and dosage generally are the same in all groups. Discussion in this section will focus on a topic unique to the neonatal population, (patent ductus arteriosus), and the use of inotropic agents to support blood pressure. The pharmacy technician may need to recognize the medications used and prepare them for proper use.

Patent Ductus Arteriosus

During fetal life, most of the pulmonary arterial blood is shunted through the ductus arteriosus into the aorta. Functional closure of the ductus normally occurs soon after birth, but if the ductus remains patent when pulmonary vascular resistance falls, aortic blood is shunted into the pulmonary artery. **Patent ductus arteriosus** (PDA) is one of the most common congenital cardiovascular anomalies associated with maternal rubella (German measles) during early pregnancy. The entire phenomenon of transition is not completely understood, and the transition period of infants is a particularly important time. In uncomplicated PDA, the ductus closes spontaneously within the first weeks or months of life.

Treatment for Patent Ductus Arteriosus

When a large symptomatic PDA is present, general treatment may include fluid restriction, correction of anemia, digitalization, and diuretic therapy. Ductus arteriosus patency is mediated through the prostaglandins, and the ductus arteriosus in the pre-term infant with RDS can be constricted and closed by the administration of inhibitors of prostaglandin synthesis such as indomethacin. Early administration of indomethacin in the course of RDS associated with large ductal left-to-right shunts is approximately 80 percent effective in closing the ductus. Surgical closure is a safe and effective backup technique for management when indomethacin is contraindicated or indomethacin treatment has not been successful. Administration is by intravenous infusion over at least 30 minutes to minimize adverse effects on cerebral, renal, and gastrointestinal blood flow. Usually, three doses per course are given, with a maximum of two courses. Urine output must

be closely monitored and if anuria (no urine output) or oliguria occurs, subsequent doses should be delayed.

Congestive Heart Failure

Congestive heart failure (CHF) occurs when the heart cannot pump the blood returning to the right side of the heart or provide adequate circulation to meet the needs of organs and tissues in the body. Causes of CHF include the following:

1. High output state, usually related to congenital heart diseases in which there is increased pulmonary blood flow, returning to the right side of the heart.

2. Low output state, related to (1) congenital heart diseases in which there are left-side heart obstructions causing the heart to pump harder to bypass the restrictive area, such as with coarctation of the aorta or aortic valve stenosis, (2) a primary heart muscle disease, such as a cardiomyopathy, or (3) rhythm disturbances (tachycardia or bradycardia). Ninety percent of infants with congenital heart defects develop CHF within the first year of life. The majority of affected infants manifest symptoms within the first few months of life.

Treatment for Congestive Heart Failure

The initial management of CHF is accomplished by the use of pharmacologic agents that act to improve the function of the heart muscle and reduce the workload on the heart. Digitalis is given to increase cardiac output by slowing conduction through the atrioventricular node to make each contraction stronger. Diuretics decrease preload volume because as their actions result in decreased extracellular fluid volume. Fluids are usually restricted to two-thirds of maintenance levels, and attention is given to nutrition and rest. Medical management continues with the plan for interventional cardiac catheterization or surgical intervention if indicated. See Chapter 11 for more information about the cardiovascular system and related subjects.

Iron Deficiency Anemia

Iron deficiency anemia is the most common anemia affecting children in North America. The full-term infant born of a well-nourished, nonanemic mother has sufficient iron stores until the birth weight is doubled, generally at 4 to 6 months. Iron deficiency anemia is generally not evident until nine months of age. After that period, iron must be available from the diet to meet the child's nutritional needs. If dietary iron intake is insufficient, iron deficiency anemia results. Pre-term infants, those with significant perinatal blood loss, or infants born to a poorly nourished mother with iron deficiency, may have inadequate iron stores. This infant would have a significantly higher

risk for iron deficiency anemia before the age of six months. Iron deficiency anemia may also result from chronic blood loss. In the infant, this may be due to chronic intestinal bleeding caused by the heat-labile protein in cow's milk. Other causes of iron deficiency anemia include nutritional deficiencies such as folate (vitamin B_{12}) deficiency, sickle cell anemia, infections, and chronic inflammation.

Treatment for Iron Deficiency Anemia

Treatment efforts are focused on prevention and intervention. Prevention includes encouraging mothers to breast-feed (only until the infant is between 4 to 6 months), to eat foods that are rich in iron, and to take iron-fortified prenatal vitamins (approximately 1 mg/kg of iron supplement per day). Therapy to treat iron deficiency anemia consists of a medication regimen. Iron is administered by mouth in doses of 2 to 3 mg/kg of elemental iron. All forms of iron (ferrous sulfate, ferrous fumarate, ferrous succinate, and ferrous gluconate) are equally effective. Vitamin C must be administered simultaneously with iron (ascorbic acid increases iron absorption). Iron is best absorbed when it is taken one hour before a meal. Iron therapy should continue for a minimum of six weeks after the anemia is corrected to replenish iron stores. Injectable iron is seldom used unless small bowel malabsorption disease is present.

Sickle Cell Anemia

Sickle cell anemia is an inherited disorder. Children with sickle cell anemia have abnormal hemoglobin. Their hemoglobin contains hemoglobin S (HbS). Sickled red blood cells are crescent-shaped, have decreased oxygen-carrying capacity, and are destroyed at a higher rate than that for normal red blood cells. Sickling results in clumping of red blood cells in the vessels, decreased oxygen transport, and increased destruction of red blood cells. Ischemia and tissue death result from the obstruction of vessels and decreased blood flow. Sickle cell traits occur in 8 to 10 percent of African Americans. Most commonly, death occurs in children at 1 to 3 years of age from organ failure or thrombosis of major organs, usually the lungs and brain. With new treatments, 85 percent of affected individuals survive to the age of 20.

Treatment of Sickle Cell Anemia

Medical management focuses on pain control, oxygenation, hydration, and careful monitoring for other complications of vasoocclusion. Administration of prophylactic penicillin to prevent septicemia should be initiated at 2 to 3 months of age and continued through five years of life. Additional immunizations required are:

- pneumococcal vaccine at two years of age with a booster at 4 to 5 years
- influenza vaccine

Analgesics are used to control pain during a crisis period. The only cure is thought to be a bone marrow transplant, which also involves risks. This may be a promising treatment modality in the near future.

INFECTIOUS DISEASES

Various types of infectious agents have effects on different body systems in newborns and children, which can cause infectious diseases. Discussion of the many infectious diseases that exist is beyond the scope of this text, but the following are a few examples of symptoms or complications resulting from infectious diseases that are seen more often in children.

Diarrhea

Diarrhea is one of the most common problems encountered by pediatricians. Diarrhea is defined as an increase in frequency, fluidity, and volume of feces. During the first three years of life, it is estimated that a child will experience an acute, severe episode of diarrhea one to three times. It may be caused by a variety of infectious agents such as bacteria, viruses, protozoans, and parasites. Hospitalization is usually necessary for severe diarrhea because of the possibility of bacterial disease, which should be treated there, and because hydration often requires fluid therapy.

Treatment for Diarrhea

Treatment for diarrhea is symptomatic. Antipyretic drugs are recommended for fever. Codeine, morphine, and the phenothiazine derivatives, often used for pain and vomiting but rarely needed for children, should be avoided because they may induce misleading signs and symptoms.

Bacteremia and Septicemia

The terms *bacteremia* and *septicemia* describe the presence of bacteria in the blood. In **bacteremia**, bacteria are recovered from blood cultures of a patient and may or may not be associated with the disease. **Septicemia** is bacteremia associated with active disease, whether localized or systemic. In some patients, bacteremia or septicemia may be associated with focal infection (e.g., pneumonia, osteomyelitis, endocarditis, or meningitis). Primary bacteremia, however, also occurs in normal infants and children.

Treatment for Bacteremia and Septicemia

Treatment may be initiated with ampicillin and a semisynthetic penicillinase-resistant penicillin (methicillin, oxacillin, nafcillin) administered intravenously. In some patients, the use of chloramphenicol may also be indicated.

Medical Terminology Review

bacteremia
bacter = bacteria; bacterial
emia = blood
bacteria in the blood

septicemia
septic = presence of pathogens or toxins
emia = blood
pathogens in the blood

TABLE 25-4 Most Common Infectious Agents Causing Meningitis in Different Age Groups

Age Group	Infective Causes
Neonates	Group B streptococci, *Escherichia coli*
Infants	*Haemophilus influenzae* type B, *Streptococcus pneumoniae*
Young Children	*Streptococcus pneumoniae* or *Neisseria meningitidis*

Acute Bacterial Meningitis

The incidence of bacterial meningitis (especially that caused by *Haemophilus influenzae* type B and group B *β-hemolytic streptococci*) is increasing. Mortality and morbidity are significant, but the reported number of deaths has decreased over time. Acute bacterial meningitis may be caused by several types of bacteria, depending on the age group of the child. Table 25-4 shows the most common infectious agents that cause meningitis in different age groups.

Treatment for Meningitis

Initial therapy includes immediate administration of multiple antibiotics including a third-generation cephalosporin (such as ceftriaxone or cefotaxime) after an intravenous line has been placed and blood has been drawn for cultures. Vancomycin, with or without rifampin, is usually added, as is ampicillin or gentamycin. Heparin therapy should be considered for patients with the syndrome of disseminated intravascular coagulation. Corticosteroids have been suggested as a therapeutic adjunct that may reduce cerebral edema and inflammation.

Streptococcal Infections

Streptococci are among the most common causes of bacterial infections in infancy and childhood. Group A streptococci are the most common bacteria causing acute pharyngitis.

Treatment for Streptococcal Infections

Penicillin is the drug of choice for the treatment of streptococcal infections. The goal of therapy is to maintain, for at least ten days, blood and tissue levels of penicillin sufficient to kill streptococci. Various subjects related to antimicrobial infections and the agents used to treat them were covered in Chapter 22.

Human Immunodeficiency Virus and Acquired Immunodeficiency Syndrome

The cause of acquired immunodeficiency syndrome (AIDS) is the human immunodeficiency virus (HIV). This virus attaches to lymphocytes and

Key Concept

For an intramuscular injection, the vastus lateralis is the preferred site. Because of underdevelopment of the gluteal muscles, they are not recommended for use in children under three years of age.

other immunological cells, which results in a gradual destruction of T-helper lymphocytes. Therefore, HIV is able to reduce and damage immune functions of the body. The virus is transmitted only through direct contact with infected blood or blood products and body fluids through intravenous drug use, sexual contact, perinatal transmission from mother to infant, and breast-feeding. There is no evidence that HIV infection is acquired through casual contact. Zidovudine is given to pregnant HIV-infected women, which significantly reduces the probability of transmission from mother to child. Infants infected through perinatal transmission from infected mothers accounts for more than 85 percent of children with AIDS who are younger than 13 years. Infants who have been breast-fed (primarily in developing countries) and children who have received blood products (especially children with hemophilia) account for the remaining 15 percent of children with AIDS.

Treatment for AIDS

There is currently no cure for HIV infection and AIDS. Management begins with a staging evaluation to determine disease progression and the appropriate course of treatment. Zidovudine (AZT, ZDV), didanosine (DDI), zalcitabine (DDC), and lamivudine (3TC) slow down multiplication of the virus. Combination drug treatment is used, and many children are enrolled in research drug protocols. Trimethoprim-sulfamethoxazole (Septra, Bactrim) and pentamidine are used for treatment and prophylaxis of *Pneumocystis carinii* pneumonia. Monthly administration of intravenous immunoglobulin has been useful in preventing serious bacterial infections in children, as well as hypogammaglobulinemia. Immunizations are recommended for children with HIV infection, but instead of the oral poliovirus vaccine, the inactivated poliovirus vaccine is given. See Chapter 23 for more information about immunological agents and related subjects.

SUMMARY

The administration of drugs to a growing and developing infant or child may present a unique problem to the physician, who must be constantly aware of the changes in drug dosages that are determined by alterations in processes of disposition at different ages. Underlying this approach is the concept that there are complex changes in the anatomy, physiology, biochemistry, and behavior from one stage of development to another over the time frame of growth from conception to adulthood. Drugs are double-edged swords. Although they can save lives, they can also endanger lives. Effective and safe drug therapy in neonates, infants, and children requires an understanding of the differences in drug action, metabolism, and disposition that are apparent during growth and development. Virtually all pharmacokinetic parameters change with age. Therefore, pediatric drug dosage regimens must be adjusted for age, disease state, sex, and individual needs. Failure to make such adjustments may lead to ineffective treatment or even to toxicity. Pharmacy technicians must be educated so that they have the required knowledge about, and can pay proper attention to, this important matter. It is impossible to cover each topic or aspect of pediatric diseases, conditions, and pharmacology in this chapter. Therefore, special considerations for selected diseases and their therapies were chosen for discussion.

EXPLORING THE WEB

Visit *www.aap.org*

- Look for information on the disorders covered in this chapter. You may also find information on disorders that are not covered in this chapter. Create flashcards of the diseases and disorders and their treatments to use for preparation of exams.

Visit the following Web sites to research articles related to pediatric illnesses and treatments.

- *www.emedicine.com*

- *www.medscape.com*

- Visit *www.nichd.nih.gov* and search for the information related to the Pediatric Pharmacology Research Units (PPRU) Network. What are the goals of this network? What research is being conducted? What are the results of some of the research to date?

REVIEW QUESTIONS

Multiple Choice

1. Which of the following factors may cause slower drug excretion and increase the risk of drug toxicity in an infant?

   A. kidney stones
   B. pyelonephritis
   C. urethritis
   D. renal immaturity

2. Complications of apnea include which of the following?

   A. sudden infant death syndrome
   B. hypertension
   C. asthma
   D. congestive heart failure

3. Palivizumab (Synagis) is used for immunoprophylaxis against which of the following infections?

   A. epiglottitis
   B. pneumonia
   C. respiratory syncytial virus
   D. asthma

4. Which of the following years of age exhibits the peak onset for croup?

   A. 1
   B. 2
   C. 4
   D. 6

5. Which of the following is the most commonly encountered diagnosis of respiratory disorders in office visits for children younger than the age of 15 in the United States?

   A. pneumonia
   B. flu
   C. epiglottitis
   D. otitis media

6. Patent ductus arteriosus is one of the most common congenital cardiovascular anomalies associated with which of the following maternal infections?

   A. hepatitis b
   B. rubella
   C. AIDS
   D. pneumonia

7. Ninety percent of infants with congenital heart defects develop which of the following complications within the first year of life?

   A. iron deficiency anemia
   B. cystic fibrosis
   C. sickle cell anemia
   D. congestive heart failure

8. The most common cause of death in children between 1 to 3 years who are suffering from sickle cell anemia is:

    A. thrombosis of major organs
    B. encephalitis
    C. kidney failure
    D. meningitis

9. The first-line antibiotic medication most often prescribed for otitis media is:

    A. tetracycline
    B. gentamycin
    C. tobramycin
    D. amoxicillin

10. Which of the following infectious diseases may be related to bacteremia?

    A. hepatitis b
    B. cystitis
    C. osteomyelitis
    D. epiglottitis

11. The goal of therapy for treatment of streptococcal infections is to:

    A. maintain for at least 10 days blood and tissue levels of penicillin sufficient to kill streptococci
    B. prevent myocarditis by using corticosteroids
    C. maintain for at least 3 days blood and tissue levels of corticosteroids to deal with stress
    D. prevent nephritic syndrome by using antineoplastic agents

12. Which of the following infectious diseases probably requires monthly administration of intravenous immunoglobulin to prevent serious bacterial infections in children?

    A. epiglottitis
    B. croup
    C. asthma
    D. AIDS

13. Which of the following types of insulins is classified as intermediate action?

    A. NPH
    B. regular
    C. ultralente
    D. protamine zinc

14. The drug of choice for epilepsy is based on which of the following factors?

    A. types of seizure
    B. pregnancy
    C. maturation of patients
    D. race and age of patients

15. Treatment for patent ductus arteriosus includes which of the following agents?

    A. oxygen
    B. morphine
    C. indomethacin
    D. acetaminophen

Fill in the Blank

1. In children, bacteremia may be associated with infections such as:

    a. _____
    b. _____
    c. _____ or _____

2. The two mainstays of treatment for congestive heart failure are _____ and _____.

3. The most common congenital cardiovascular anomaly is _____, which may indicate indomethacin therapy.

4. 97 percent of all juvenile patients with newly diagnosed diabetes have insulin _____.

5. Epiglottitis infection is commonly caused by _____, type B.

6. Respiratory distress syndrome or hyaline membrane disease is the result of the absence of _____.

7. The most widely used antipyretic in children is _____.

Critical Thinking

A 15-month-old infant who has only been breast-fed without any formula or other foods is brought into the pediatrician's office. He examines her and orders blood tests, which reveal that she has severe anemia.

1. With this history of the infant, what type of anemia do you think she has?

2. What would be the way to prevent an infant from developing this type of anemia?

3. What other types of anemia can be seen in children of this age?

CHAPTER 26

Drug Therapy in Geriatrics

OBJECTIVES

After completing this chapter, the reader should be able to:

1. Identify the most popular types of drugs that elderly patients need.
2. Discuss clinical concerns of drug therapy and the way elderly patients react to certain drugs differently than younger patients.
3. Compare the way aging affects drug interaction, absorption, and distribution.
4. Understand how drug metabolism changes with age.
5. Discuss differences in renal function in elderly patients.
6. List some of the adverse effects that certain drugs have upon older patients.
7. Review some of the ways aging can be slowed with a healthy diet and exercise.
8. Identify age-related changes to the integumentary system.
9. Discuss common disorders in the elderly.
10. Describe the use of cold remedies in elderly people, and potential related consequences.

GLOSSARY

Collagen – a strong fibrous protein found in connective tissue

Dermis – a thick layer of loose connective tissue that is well-supplied with blood vessels, lymphatic vessels, nerves, and accessory organs

Elastin – an extracellular connective tissue protein

Pharmacodynamic interactions – differences in effects produced by a given plasma level of a drug

Pharmacokinetic interactions – differences in the plasma levels of a drug achieved with a given dose of that drug

Polypharmacy – the practice of prescribing multiple medicines to a single patient simultaneously

OVERVIEW

The phenomenon of aging is unavoidable because aging is a universal process. The difference between aging and disease is that the aging process is intrinsic and depends on genetic factors, whereas disease is intrinsic and extrinsic, depending on both genetic and environmental factors. Aging is always progressive, whereas disease may be discontinuous, and may progress, regress, or be arrested entirely. Aging is irreversible, whereas disease may be treatable and often has a known cause. The average life expectancy in the U.S. has increased largely because of improvements in sanitation, food, and water supplies, and the advent of antibiotics and vaccinations.

AGING PATIENTS

The impact of age on medical care is substantial, and thus a significantly altered approach to treatment is needed for the older patient. As individuals age, they are more likely to be affected by many chronic disorders and disabilities. Consequently, they use more drugs than any other age group. Combined with a decrease in physiological reserve, these added burdens (if present) make the older person more vulnerable to environmental, pathologic, or pharmacologic illnesses. Understanding these facts is essential for optimal care of older patients. Aging alters pharmacodynamics and pharmacokinetics, affecting the choice, dose, and rate of administration of many drugs. In addition, pharmacotherapy may be complicated by an elderly patient's inability to purchase or obtain drugs, or to comply with drug regimens.

Many drugs benefit elderly persons. Some can save lives, such as antibiotics and thrombolytic therapy in acute illness. Oral hypoglycemic drugs can improve independence and quality of life while controlling chronic disease. Antihypertensive drugs and influenza vaccines can help prevent or decrease morbidity. Analgesics and antidepressants can control debilitating symptoms. Therefore, the appropriateness of the potential benefits in outweighing the potential risks should guide therapy. The health problems and medical management of elderly patients differs from those of younger ones in important ways, which explains the development of training in geriatrics as a medical specialty. Prescribing medications for elderly patients is always a challenge for physicians. Body functions decline dramatically in elderly patients. Safe, effective pharmacotherapy remains one of the greatest challenges in the practice of clinical geriatrics. Therefore, the normal aging process can lead to altered drug effects and the need for altered doses.

PHYSIOLOGIC AGING

Not all functions in the human body show age-related changes. For example, the hematocrit does not change with age. However, testosterone, cortisol, thyroxine, and insulin do show age-related declines.

It is extremely difficult to differentiate among primary age changes (physiological), secondary age changes (pathophysiological), and tertiary age changes (sociogenic and behavioral). Age-related changes may be responsible for the atypical presentation of diseases in elderly persons, which can be observed in hyperthyroidism, depression, uncontrolled diabetes mellitus, and rheumatoid arthritis. Although aging changes may lessen the severity of some diseases, they may also be responsible for more severe presentations. For example, normal human aging is associated with a progressive reduction in dopamine concentrations in the brain, which may influence the onset or severity of Parkinson's disease. Menopause clearly is related to an increase in osteoporosis and atherosclerosis. Arteriosclerosis accounts for the age-related increase in diastolic blood pressure, a major risk factor for cerebrovascular disease (stroke).

The Blood and Lymphatic Systems

The effect of the aging process on the blood results mainly from a reduced capacity to make new blood cells quickly when disease has occurred. After age 70 (approximately), the amount of bone marrow space that is occupied by tissue that produces blood cells declines progressively. This decrease in the ability to produce new blood cells when disease has occurred is a serious problem for elderly patients.

In the lymphatic system, age-related changes affect immune responses. Specific antibody responses to foreign antigens are impaired by the aging process. Elderly individuals may be more susceptible to infections and malignancies due to decreased immunity. In the elderly, infections are a leading cause of morbidity and mortality (see Table 26-1).

The Cardiovascular System

With advancing age, the heart weight increases significantly. In the myocardium (the heart muscle) fat, **collagen** (a strong fibrous protein found in connective tissue), and **elastin** (an extracellular connective tissue protein) increase. Arterial compliance in the internal and external carotid pathways significantly decrease. Fibrous plaques are present in many individuals' arteries at ages 15 to 24 years. Within another decade of life, 85 percent of blood vessels have these plaques. More than 60 percent of hearts at ages 55 to 64 years show vascular calcification. Narrowing heart vessels are also more prevalent with age, and occlusion may occur in at least one of the three major coronary arteries. See Chapter 12 for more information on the cardiovascular system.

TABLE 26-1 Common Infections in the Elderly

Disorder	Causes	Prevention or Treatment
Pneumonia	Bacterial	Vaccine and Antibiotics
Influenza	Viral	Vaccine
Urinary Tract	Bacterial	Antibiotics
Herpes zoster (shingles)	Viral	Vaccine

The Urinary System

Age-associated kidney changes can be categorized as anatomic or functional. Anatomic changes include loss of glomeruli, decreased kidney size, renal tubular changes, and renal vascular changes. Anatomic changes involving the lower urinary tract make men more susceptible to prostatic hypertrophy. Women become prone to pelvic relaxation, urinary incontinence, urinary tract infections, and the development of uterine and cervical cancers. Renal function declines progressively starting in the fifth decade, so that by age 70 normal renal function greatly declines in comparison to people at age 30. Glomerular filtration rate declines by about 1 mL/min/year. Even in the absence of cardiovascular, renal, or acute illness, the decline is more rapid in men than in women. Renal blood flow and plasma flow also decrease with age. Drug metabolism is often impaired in the elderly because of a decrease in the glomerular filtration rate, as well as reduced hepatic clearance. See Chapter 18 for more information on the urinary system.

The Endocrine System

Specific age-related disturbances in extrahepatic hormonal regulatory mechanisms have been proposed. The reduced availability of hormones results in diminished endocrine regulatory mechanisms, deficiencies in hormonal feedback mechanisms, and decreased binding affinities and receptors. Altered pancreatic and adrenal hormone concentrations decrease glucose tolerance with age. Insulin release is impaired in some older individuals, whereas others have fewer insulin receptors or exhibit postreceptor abnormalities. The peripheral glucose disposal rate is significantly lower in older than in younger persons. Production of sex hormones also decreases with age. In postmenopausal women, reduced estrogen concentrations have been linked to increased incidences of osteoporosis and cardiovascular disease. See Chapter 17 for more information on the endocrine system.

The Skeletal System

Normal age-related changes of the musculoskeletal system affect mobility in most cases. The musculoskeletal system gradually loses bone mass after age 50 because bone formation and resorption becomes unstable. The skeletal systems of elderly people are affected by a decrease in total body mass. Bone mass,

density, and strength all decrease, and at the same time, bone fragility increases. Elderly skeletal system diseases and disorders are influenced by these factors. See Chapter 10 for more information on the musculoskeletal system.

The Respiratory System

Changes in the respiratory system with age have been reviewed. The diameters of the trachea and central airways increase, enlarging anatomic dead space. The volume of the alveolar ducts increases, whereas the membranous bronchioles narrow. Lung weight decreases dramatically, and chest wall compliance also decreases. These and other changes result in less elastic recoil in the lung, increased closing volume, and decreased maximal expiratory flow.

Thus, elderly persons have an increased risk for respiratory failure. Aspiration or inhalation of foreign material into the tracheobronchial tree can produce major respiratory illness, which is more likely to occur in older than younger people. Finally, asthma in elderly persons must be differentiated from other causes of airflow obstruction, such as acute bronchitis or congestive heart failure. See Chapter 14 for more information on the respiratory system.

The Gastrointestinal System

Age-associated changes in the gastrointestinal system have been reviewed. The gastrointestinal system starts with the oral cavity, where age-related changes reflect perturbation in oral health resulting from poor hygiene, disease, or disease treatment, rather than from dysfunction directly related to age. Nevertheless, oral disorders are common among elderly persons. As many as 50 percent of older people experience traumatic lesions of the oral cavity, which may be ulcerative, atrophic, or hyperplastic. These changes make the oral mucosa more susceptible to disease, a problem that can be exacerbated by corticosteroids, antibiotics, cytotoxic agents, and immunosuppressive therapy. Elderly persons may have an increased risk of local adverse drug reactions such as fixed eruptions (round or oval patches of reddened blisters on the skin), swelling, glossitis (inflammation of the tongue), and stomatitis (inflammation of the mouth).

Gastric secretion declines with age. Gastric cell function decreases and gastric pH rises. Gastric emptying is about 2.5 times faster in younger than in older persons, perhaps because it is under the control of the CNS, which may lose efficiency with advancing age. Slowing of gastric emptying also follows a reduction in gastric acid secretion. Gastric emptying is reduced by stress, lack of ambulation, gastric ulcer, intestinal obstruction, myocardial infarction, and diabetes mellitus. Emptying is delayed by fatty meals in the elderly more so than in younger people. Bleeding is a fairly common complication of ulcers in elderly persons. The normal aging process leads to a reduction in vitamin D absorption and a profound decline in the intestinal absorption of calcium. There is little existing evidence that the motility of the small intestine is altered by the aging process. Constipation is common because of alteration of motility in the large intestine.

The liver is the organ least affected by primary age changes. It continues to function in those persons not affected by disease. In general, just a small part can perform the tasks of the entire liver. Liver weight correlates with body weight, and both decrease starting in the fifth or sixth decade.

Primary aging may be responsible for decreased hepatic blood flow. Hepatic blood flow decrease probably affects the metabolic clearance of certain drugs. These functional changes are thought to be most relevant with drugs that have a high first-pass extraction ratio. Clearance is limited by the capacity of the organ, and hepatic clearance cannot exceed hepatic blood flow, which is approximately 1.5 L/min. Thus, reduced blood flow can alter drug action in the elderly. For at least some drugs, hepatic metabolism in the elderly apparently is altered.

The reduction in hepatic clearance is due to the decreased activity of microsomal enzymes and reduced hepatic perfusion with aging. The distribution of drugs is also affected. In addition, serum albumin levels decrease, especially in sick patients, so that protein binding of some drugs (such as warfarin and phenytoin) is reduced. This leaves more free (active) drugs available. Also, older individuals often have altered responses to a given serum drug level. See Chapter 15 for more information on the gastrointestinal system.

The Nervous System

With age, cellular brain mass and cerebral blood flow decrease. Sensory conduction takes longer, and the blood-brain barrier may become more permeable. These changes may decrease coordination, prolong reaction time, and impair short-term memory. Manifestations include more falls (particularly among elderly women), urinary incontinence, and confusion. Homeostatic response (the balance of the internal body systems) also declines.

In short, the brain shrinks with advancing age and loses nerve cells. The brain weighs less at 70 years of age than it weighs at age 30. Various areas of the brain lose substantial amounts of their nerve cells, although the nerve cells that control eye movement are not affected. The greatest loss of cells appears to take place in the temporal area, but the functional effect is surprisingly small. Cerebral blood flow is controlled by autoregulation, metabolic regulation, and chemical factors. Its regulation is influenced by the disease processes prevailing in old age, such as dementia, atherosclerosis, diabetes mellitus, stroke, and hypertension.

Short-term memory is significantly affected by aging, a loss that can be minimized by teaching methods of memorization to older adults. The declines in both learning facility and information retrieval, and perhaps also the loss in processing speed, appear to contribute to failing short-term memory.

Serotonin (a neurotransmitter) is widely distributed throughout the CNS. It is implicated in a variety of neural functions, such as pain, feeding, sleep, sexual behavior, cardiac regulation, and cognition. Changes in the serotonin system occur in association with healthy aging. See Chapter 4 for more information on the nervous system.

The Special Senses (Eye and Ear)

Vision impairment is one of the three most common medical problems among the elderly. Significant visual difficulties are caused by the aging process, resulting in difficulty reading or conducting daily activities independently. With aging, the size of the pupil decreases, necessitating brighter lighting in order to see. Sensitivity to glares also increases because of age-related changes in the eyes' lens opacity. As we age, color discrimination decreases and depth perception becomes altered.

Hearing impairment is the second-most common health problem seen in elderly patients. High frequencies often become inaudible by the age of 50, with a marked decline occurring after age 65. The term "hard of hearing" may relate more to high-frequency hearing loss than an overall decline in hearing perception. Therefore, it is usually easier for an elderly adult to hear voices, telephones, doorbells, and horns since they have lower tones and are of high intensity.

The Integumentary System

Cells in the epidermis, which contain melanocytes (that produce the melanin pigment), must be continuously replaced with new cells that divide, by mitosis, in the lower layers. The rate of production of these new cells decreases between ages 20 and 70. It is clear that during long periods of time, individual epidermal cells are exposed to carcinogens (cancer-causing agents), such as ultraviolet light from the sun. Furthermore, the number of melanocytes and the amount of protective melanin pigment decreases with age, making ultraviolet light more dangerous.

The **dermis** is a thick layer of loose connective tissue that is well-supplied with blood vessels, lymphatic vessels, nerves, and accessory organs. The predominant cells found in the dermis are fibroblasts, mast cells, and macrophages. Fibroblasts produce and release collagen and elastin into the extracellular matrix, which give skin its strength and elasticity, respectively.

The amount of collagen and elastin in the dermis decreases as people age, accounting for the thinning and wrinkling of the skin in elderly persons. Loss of collagen makes the skin more susceptible to wear and tear, whereas loss of elastin causes skin to lose its resiliency over time.

Perhaps the most striking age-related changes in the integumentary system are the graying, thinning, and loss of the hair. Hair color depends on varying amounts of melanin pigment within the specialized cells.

The Reproductive System

As men age, testosterone levels decrease, sperm production slows, the scrotum loses muscle tone, and the testicles lose size and firmness. With age,

the prostate gland enlarges considerably. Sexual activity is still normal and possible in elderly patients if they have no major health problems.

In women, physical changes occur after menopause. The ovaries cease producing ova (eggs), and lowered estrogen levels may cause physiological symptoms. Women experience a general atrophy of the genitalia that is related to hormonal changes, including less fat, the loss of external hair, and flattening of the labia. An elderly female's uterus is about one-half the size of the uterus of a young adult female. With age, the vagina also becomes drier and narrower.

After menopause, women experience changes in breast tissue resulting in less glandular tissue, reduced elasticity, more connective tissue, and more fat. As a result, the breasts experience sagging, though the size of the breasts may not change. Many of the physiological changes in body systems are summarized in Table 26-2.

TABLE 26-2 Physiological Changes Due to Aging

System or Process	Changes
Muscular system	Strength and flexibility decline.
Metabolism	Slows down, generally causing weight gain.
Nervous system	Motor nerves deteriorate, slowing reaction time.
Skeletal system	Bones lose calcium, weakening them.
Body temperature	Ability to maintain normal temperature declines.
Bloodstream	Ability to use glucose in the bloodstream declines, increasing risk for diabetes. Good (HDL) cholesterol level lowers while bad (LDL) cholesterol level raises.
Cardiovascular system	The heart becomes less efficient, working harder to pump blood.
Digestive system	Motions of this system decrease, altering digestion. Secretions decrease, altering defecation. Mouth secretions decrease, causing greater tooth decay; speaking, swallowing, and tasting may be affected.
Urinary system	Kidney function declines. Muscles of the bladder weaken, causing loss of urine control. In men, the prostate enlarges, also causing loss of urine control.
Brain processes	Memory becomes less efficient. Reflexes become slower; coordination decreases.
Special senses	Degeneration of eye structures causes poor vision; tear production declines. Hearing ability decreases.
Integumentary system	Skin thins and dries, becoming wrinkled. Nail growth slows.
Reproductive system	The vagina narrows and becomes drier. The penis becomes less able to achieve or maintain erections.

PRINCIPLES OF DRUG THERAPY IN ELDERLY PATIENTS

The principal clinical concerns of drug therapy include efficacy and safety, dosage, complexity of regimen, number of drugs, cost, and patient compliance. There are several reasons for the greater incidence of adverse reactions of drugs in the elderly population.

Thus, the elderly are more sensitive to some drugs, (e.g., opioids), and less sensitive to others (e.g., β-blocking agents). Finally, the older patient with multiple chronic conditions is likely to be receiving many drugs, including non-prescribed agents. Drug doses in elderly patients must often be reduced, although dose requirements may vary considerably from person to person. In general, starting doses of about one-third to one-half the usual adult dose are indicated for drugs with a low therapeutic index.

THE PHYSIOPATHOLOGY OF AGING

Many of the physiological changes associated with aging can be slowed to some extent with a healthy diet and consistent regimen of moderate exercise. Many of the chronic diseases prevalent in elderly persons are either preventable or modifiable with healthy lifestyle habits. Reduction of dietary fat (especially saturated fats and cholesterol) lowers the risk of coronary artery disease and stroke, as well as breast and colon cancer. It is clear that our health and well-being depend on the degree to which our organ systems can successfully work together to maintain homeostasis (internal stability) in the body. Diminished function in one organ system is lessened by appropriate compensatory mechanisms in other systems. The aging process affects all body systems physiologically.

COMMON DISORDERS IN THE ELDERLY

Some disorders occur almost exclusively in elderly persons, and some occur in persons of all ages but are far more common in elderly persons than in other age groups. For example, multiple disorders, accidental hypothermia, and urinary incontinence are almost exclusively found in elderly persons. Some other examples include lymphoma, chronic lymphocytic leukemia, prostate cancer, degenerative osteoarthritis, dementia, falls, hip fracture, osteoporosis, Parkinsonism, hypertension, heart failure, stroke, and herpes zoster. These disorders are available for study and review in many medical textbooks. In this chapter, the most common disorders in elderly persons will be discussed selectively.

Multiple Disorders

Normal and abnormal effects of the aging process on different systems of the body in elderly persons may cause multiple disorders after middle age. A patient may suffer from several disorders, such as peptic ulcer, hypertension,

and diabetes mellitus. Therefore, some patients are receiving several different medications that may cause drug interactions and side effects.

Cardiovascular Disorders

The incidence and prevalence of most cardiovascular disorders increases markedly with advancing age. Significant fat accumulations and calcifications in blood vessels of the heart (coronary arteries), brain, or peripheral arterial system are found in the majority of men and women older than 70 years of age. The combined effects of the pathological and physiological changes contribute to a high prevalence of problems, such as heart failure and cardiac arrhythmias in the elderly. There is good evidence that risk factors such as hypertension and hyperlipidemia can be successfully modified in older people, reducing the risk of ischemic vascular events. Multiple disorders are common in old age and coexistent diseases often can influence the choice of drugs for a cardiovascular condition. In addition, both pharmacokinetic and pharmacodynamic drug profiles may be altered in older subjects. These can influence both choice of drug and dosing regimen.

Ischemic Heart Disease

Aging is associated with a progressive rise in morbidity and mortality due to ischemic heart disease, which is the most common cause of death in elderly people in the United States. The three main groups of drugs used to treat angina pectoris are β-adrenergic receptor blocking agents, calcium channel blockers, and nitrates, which are discussed in Chapter 11.

Acute Myocardial Infarction

Acute myocardial infarction (AMI) is painless in many persons older than 70 years of age. The mortality from AMI is greater in older subjects than in young and middle-aged subjects. This is due to a number of factors, including increased severity of underlying coronary artery disease, a greater prevalence of previous myocardial infarction, and an associated increase in the incidence of cardiac failure. The aims of treatment are to relieve symptoms, reduce mortality, and prevent late cardiovascular disability. Pain relief is usually attempted by the use of intravenous opiates such as diamorphine. Intravenous nitrates are sometimes used to reduce opiate requirements, and may also be helpful in the treatment of associated cardiac failure; however, adverse effects, including hypotension and bradycardia, are more common in elderly subjects. When used in elderly persons, the dosage should be reduced.

Aspirin has been shown to significantly reduce mortality, reinfarction, and stroke rate after AMI in older patients. Treatment with the combination of thrombolytic agents and oral aspirin confers additional benefit.

Cardiac Failure

The incidence and prevalence of cardiac failure increase sharply with increasing age. In postmortem examinations of elderly persons, the most common underlying pathologic conditions are ischemia and hypertensive heart disease. The appropriate treatment of cardiac failure depends on accurate diagnosis including the underlying cardiac pathological conditions. Treatments for cardiac failure are discussed in Chapter 11.

Hypertension

The major causes of death and morbidity associated with hypertension are myocardial infarction and stroke. In addition, congestive heart failure is more common in elderly hypertensive patients than in their younger counterparts. Blood pressure rises with age up to about 75 years. Hypertension is perhaps best defined as the blood pressure level at which treatment is likely to be beneficial.

The best choice of antihypertensive treatment for elderly patients remains highly controversial. Drugs that are effective in younger patients also will lower blood pressure in the elderly patients. In the absence of specific contraindications, different agents seem to be tolerated equally well in elderly patients, though some patients may develop adverse reactions requiring a change of drug. Treatment of hypertension is discussed in Chapter 12.

Cerebrovascular Disease

Stroke continues to be a significant public health problem in the United States. It is estimated that every minute, one person in the United States suffers a stroke, making it the third leading cause of death and the major cause of long-term disability in adults. Because two-thirds of all patients affected by stroke are older than 65 years, this disease mostly affects the elderly population.

The most significant unmodifiable risk factor for stroke is advanced age. The risk for stroke in African Americans is much higher than in Caucasians, even after controlling for the effects of age, hypertension, and diabetes. Cigarette smoking and excessive alcohol consumption are important independent risk factors for stroke. Hypertension is by far the most important modifiable risk factor. It is a contributing factor in more than two-thirds of strokes, and lowering diastolic blood pressure significantly reduces stroke risk by 40 percent.

General therapeutic measures for stroke patients include maintaining an open airway, hydration with intravenous fluids, and judicious treatment of hypertension and hypoglycemia.

Cancer

The management of cancer with aging is an increasingly common problem as the number of elderly patients with cancer grows. Elderly persons comprise approximately 12 percent of the U.S. population. According to the

Journal of Allied Health, the number of elderly people (those aged 65 years or older) is projected to reach almost 40 million by 2010. After heart disease, cancer is the second leading cause of death in the U.S.

Malignant tumor incidence increases progressively with age, although the increase is not uniform for each type of cancer. The reason for the increased incidence of cancer with age is not fully understood. The duration of carcinogenesis (agents that cause cancers), and the prolonged exposure to chemical, physical, or biologic carcinogens may explain the association.

Cancer in older persons should be considered differently because of the physiological effects of aging. There are two important pharmacokinetic factors that occur with aging: a change in the volume of distribution, and a decrease in the concentration of serum albumin. The treatment of different cancers was discussed in Chapter 20.

Arthritis

Arthritis is the most common chronic ailment in elderly persons. Most people aged 70 years or older report having arthritis, occasionally resulting in physical limitations. After age 65, the prevalence is approximately 50 percent, and it increases every decade thereafter. The two most common forms of arthritis in elderly persons are rheumatoid arthritis (RA), and osteoarthritis (OA).

Rheumatoid Arthritis

The clinical manifestations of RA in elderly people may differ from those of the typical younger adult patient with this disease. The abrupt appearance of symptoms is more common in elderly-onset disease, whereas bone erosions and nodules are less common. A multidisciplinary treatment approach is required for elderly patients with RA. It includes physical therapy, occupational therapy, pharmacotherapy, and, occasionally, surgical intervention. The goals of therapy for elderly patients are the same as those for younger patients: to relieve symptoms, reduce inflammation, avoid joint destruction, prevent deformities, maintain functional capacity, and preserve quality of life. The pharmacotherapy of RA is similar in young and old patients. Age alone does not contraindicate the use of the first- or second-line antirheumatic drugs. The adverse effects of some drugs are more pronounced in elderly patients. Nonsteroidal anti-inflammatory drugs (NSAIDs), including aspirin and nonacetylated salicylates, are useful in treating arthritic symptoms in elderly subjects. Drug therapy must be monitored vigilantly in elderly patients because of the increased risk of complications. Anti-inflammatory complications of NSAIDs in elderly patients include cardiovascular (congestive heart failure and hypertension), CNS (confusion, dizziness, headaches, and hearing loss), gastrointestinal (gastritis, ulcers, and epigastric pain), and renal (electrolyte imbalances, fluid retention, and renal insufficiency) complications.

Osteoarthritis (OA)

The other common type of arthritis is osteoarthritis (OA), which is characterized by degeneration of cartilage, bone remodeling, and overgrowth of bone. This form of arthritis, also referred to as degenerative joint disease, is the most common form in elderly people. Radiographic evidence of OA is present in the majority of those older than age 65, yet many are asymptomatic. Pain is the primary complaint of patients with OA. Pain can be absent despite severe joint damage. Joint stiffness, pain at night, pain at rest, and crepitus (a feeling of crackling as the joint is moved) also are common symptoms. Commonly affected joints include the interphalangeal joints of the hands, knees, hips, first metatarsophalangeal joint, and the lumbar and cervical spine.

The primary goals in treating OA are to minimize joint pain, maintain functional mobility, and allow use of the affected joints. A combination of pharmacotherapy and nonpharmacological therapeutic interventions is often necessary. Resting the joints sometimes relieves pain. Joint replacement may be the treatment of choice in patients with severe OA that cannot be adequately managed with other modalities. For more information for pharmacotherapy, refer to Chapter 10.

Osteoporosis

Osteoporosis is a metabolic bone disorder in which the rate of bone reabsorption accelerates while the rate of bone formation slows down, causing a loss of bone mass. Bones affected by this disease lose calcium and phosphate salts, and thus become porous, brittle, and abnormally vulnerable to fractures. Osteoporosis may be primary or secondary to an underlying disease. Primary osteoporosis is often called postmenopausal osteoporosis because it develops more commonly in postmenopausal women. Osteoporosis is usually discovered when an elderly person bends to lift something, hears a snapping sound, then feels a sudden pain in the lower back. Osteoporosis can develop insidiously with increasing deformity, kyphosis, and loss of height. As bones weaken, spontaneous wedge fractures, pathological fractures of the neck or femur and hip, become increasingly common. Osteoporosis, often affecting older people, is a major risk factor in vertebral compression fractures and hip fractures.

The aims of treatment are to prevent additional fractures and control pain. A physical therapy program, emphasizing gentle exercise and activity, is an important part of the treatment. Hormone replacement therapy (HRT) with estrogen and progesterone may retard bone loss and prevent the occurrence of fractures. HRT decreases bone reabsorption and increases bone mass. Other medications may include alendronate (Fosamax) and calcitonin; however, adequate calcium and vitamin D intakes are needed for maximum effect. Drug therapy merely arrests osteoporosis; it does not cure it. Surgery can correct pathologic fractures. For information on pharmacotherapy, refer to Chapter 17.

Ophthalmic Disorders

One of the consequences of aging is a gradual impairment of vision. Like other tissues and organs in the body, the eye is constantly undergoing changes, both physical and functional. Changes may be a consequence of the aging process, diet, environment, or disease. Conditions that are commonly associated with age-related deterioration of ocular function include reduction in precorneal tear production; changes affecting the clarity and flexibility of the crystalline lens; an elevation in intraocular pressure, and changes in vessels supplying blood to regions in the eye.

Dry Eye Syndrome

Dry eye syndrome (xerosis) in elderly persons may be caused by a number of conditions, including trachoma, vitamin A deficiency, chemical burn, radiation, and chemotherapy. Dry eye is a common disorder affecting the elderly population, especially individuals older than 40 years. In elderly persons, a thinned conjunctiva and diminished corneal sensation add to the problem of dry eyes.

The primary treatment for dry eyes is replacement of deficient tear production with artificial tear preparations. Sterile isotonic saline preparations have been used to replace aqueous tear deficiencies, but the duration of relief is extremely short, requiring frequent dosing. Relief can be prolonged by the addition of water-soluble polymers, which increase the viscosity of the solution and provide an aqueous film over the corneal surface for an extended period.

Presbyopia

In the normal resting state, the eye can focus on an image of a distant object. However, to focus on a near object, the refractive power of the lens must increase. This is accomplished by contraction of the ciliary muscles, which causes the lens to become more spherical. This process is referred to as accommodation. The closest distance that the eye is able to accommodate (near point) is extremely short in infancy, and it progressively increases with age. When a person reaches the mid-40s, presbyopia, a condition in which the near point of accommodation moves beyond a comfortable reading distance, gradually develops. Presbyopia is presently treated using corrective eyeglasses. Bifocal or trifocal contact lenses are also available, but they have had limited acceptance.

Cataract

A cataract is defined as any opacity or loss in transparency in the crystalline lens of the eye. When a cataract interferes with transmission of light to the retina, some loss in visual acuity, and possibly complete loss of vision, may result. Cataracts are a leading cause of blindness and visual impairment worldwide.

Cataracts may be congenital or acquired (secondary). Most cataracts have no known etiology, and they usually occur in individuals older than 50 years of age. There is significant correlation between age and the occurrence of lens opacities, which are found to some degree in most people older than 60.

At present, no medical treatment will restore an opaque lens to its transparent state. Surgery remains the only effective method of treatment.

Glaucoma

Glaucoma includes a group of ocular diseases that are characterized by increased intraocular pressure, which may produce compression of the optic disk, resulting in damage to the optic nerve that leads to loss of the peripheral visual field and visual acuity.

Glaucoma is the second leading cause of blindness in the world. According to the Glaucoma Foundation, it is estimated that 67 million people worldwide have primary glaucoma. It is also a common cause of blindness in the United States.

The treatment of glaucoma centers on the reduction of the elevated intraocular pressure. Currently, this is accomplished with medical, laser, or surgical treatment.

DRUG INTERACTIONS

A drug interaction occurs whenever the pharmacological action of a drug is altered by a second substance. This change may be related to **pharmacokinetic interactions** (differences in the plasma levels of a drug achieved with a given dose of that drug), and **pharmacodynamic interactions** (differences in effects produced by a given plasma level of a drug). The duration and intensity of the action of a drug are a function of the plasma level of the drug, which is related directly to the absorption, distribution, metabolism, and excretion of that drug. These rates may be altered by previous drug therapy, dietary factors, and exposure to environmental chemicals (chemicals not used for therapeutic purposes). Physical factors such as ambient temperature and effects of disease (e.g., fever) may also have an impact.

Pharmacokinetics

Pharmacokinetics is the study of the activities of drugs occurring within the body after a drug is administered, including absorption, distribution, excretion, and metabolism. It also involves the amount of time that each of these processes requires. Pharmacokinetics is also the study of the onset of action, duration of effect, biotransformation, and routes of excretion of the metabolites of the drug. It is difficult to determine the amount of drug reaching its site of action as a function of time after administration. In most cases, this is not feasible; therefore, it is the plasma concentration of the drug

that is measured. This provides useful information, since the amount of drug in the tissues is related to plasma concentration. Pharmacokinetics are also greatly affected by the aging process.

Drug Absorption

Physiological changes with aging, such as changes of gastric pH, slowed gastric emptying rate, reduced cardiac output (blood flow), reductions of absorptive surfaces, and slowed gastrointestinal (GI) track motility, are factors that affect not only drug absorption but also drug distribution and metabolism. Different diseases and conditions of the GI tract are also obvious factors that affect drug absorption. Examples are peptic ulcer, diarrhea, and constipation.

Drug Distribution

Alterations in drug distribution in elderly patients depend on many factors, such as a reduction of total body water content, decreased plasma albumin concentration, reduced lean body mass, and increased body fat. Many drugs, especially acidic ones, bind to plasma proteins. Drugs can compete for plasma protein-binding sites. Plasma protein-binding sites are especially significant when a high percentage of the drug (more than 90 percent) is normally protein-bound, as with coumarin anticoagulants, sulfonamides, salicylates, indomethacin, and most other nonsteroidal anti-inflammatory agents. Lipid-soluble drugs such as lidocaine and diazepam have a large volume of distribution in elderly persons, whereas water-soluble drugs such as ethanol and acetaminophen have a smaller volume of distribution. Digoxin also has a lower volume of distribution in elderly persons, and therefore, doses must be reduced.

Drug Metabolism

The most common and most important cause for differences in the plasma levels of a drug is a change in the rate of biotransformation of the drug. Variations in a person's plasma drug levels are more common with drugs that undergo extensive GI metabolism or first-pass hepatic metabolism. The total liver blood flow declines significantly with aging because of a reduction of cardiac output. Therefore, if severe and progressive liver damage is present in an elderly person, drug metabolism would be affected. Otherwise, the decline in the ability of elderly persons to metabolize most drugs is relatively small and difficult to predict. In older persons, presystemic (first-pass) metabolism of some drugs given orally is decreased and their serum concentration and bioavailability are increased. Examples of these drugs include labetalol, propranolol, and verapamil. Consequently, initial doses of these drugs should be reduced as required. However, presystemic metabolism of other metabolized drugs such as imipramine, amitriptyline, morphine, and meperidine is not decreased. The effects of cigarette smoking, diet, and alcohol consumption may be more important than the physiological changes in the liver.

Key Concept

The differences in pharmacokinetics can lead to stronger or weaker drug effects in the elderly compared with those in young adults.

Drug Elimination

Drugs may be eliminated from the body by many routes, including urine, feces (e.g., unabsorbed drugs or those secreted in bile), saliva, sweat, tears, breast milk, and lungs (e.g., alcohols and anesthetics). Any route may be important for a given drug, but the kidney is the most important route for the elimination of the majority of drugs. Some drugs are excreted unchanged in the urine, whereas other drugs are so extensively metabolized that only a small fraction of the original chemical substance is excreted unchanged. Different responses to drug therapy may be seen in elderly individuals because of a decline in hepatic and renal function, which is often accompanied by a concurrent disease process. The rate of elimination of any drug by the kidney is reduced in elderly persons. Renal blood flow, mainly in the renal cortex, decreases significantly with aging. This physiological change causes a decrease in renal drug elimination.

Because renal function is dynamic, maintenance doses of drugs should be adjusted when a patient becomes acutely ill or dehydrated or has recently recovered from dehydration. In addition, because renal function continues to decline, the dose of drugs given long-term should be reviewed periodically. Examples of these drugs are the aminoglycosides, chlorpropamide, digoxin, and lithium carbonate. To prevent drug toxicity, renal function must be estimated, and the dosage of the drug should be adjusted. Most elderly patients do not have normal renal function, and the majority require adjustments in the dosages of drugs that are eliminated primarily by the kidneys. See Chapter 3 for more information on drug elimination and the renal system.

Pharmacodynamics

Drug action is defined as physiological changes in the body caused by a drug, or responses to the pharmacological effects of a drug. Pharmacodynamics refers to the chemical reaction of drugs in the body. This can be different in elderly persons because of physiological changes that occur with aging. Drugs can modify the way the body acts, but they do not give body organs and tissues new functions. They usually either slow down or speed up ordinary cell processes.

The most common way in which drugs display their action is by forming a chemical bond with specific receptors within the body. This binding may occur if the drug and its receptors have a compatible chemical shape. Figure 26-1 illustrates a drug-receptor interaction.

The effects of similar concentrations of drugs at the site of action may be greater or lesser in elderly persons than they are in younger persons. The difference may be due to changes in drug-receptor interactions. The increased sensitivity that occurs with aging must be considered when drugs that can have serious adverse effects are used. These drugs include morphine, pentazocine, warfarin, angiotensin-converting enzyme inhibitors, diazepam (especially when it is given parenterally), and levodopa. Some drugs whose

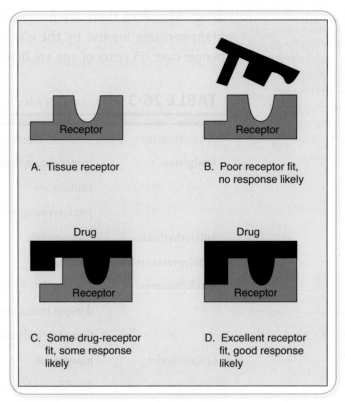

Figure 26-1 Drug-receptor interaction.

effects are reduced in elderly persons include tolbutamide, glyburide, and β-blockers, which should also be used with caution because serious dose-related toxicity can still occur, and signs of toxicity may be delayed.

POLYPHARMACY

Polypharmacy is the practice of prescribing multiple medicines simultaneously to a single patient. It increases costs for treatment as well as the chances for drug interactions and multiple adverse effects. Polypharmacy is more common in elderly patients because they often need several medical specialists and also may be using OTC drugs and herbal supplements. Herbal supplements must be considered to be drugs because of their potential to interact adversely with prescribed and OTC drugs.

Liver dysfunction, confusion, falls, and malnutrition may all be caused by polypharmacy. Liver dysfunction contributes to confused mental states and delirium, with perception disturbances and misinterpretations of information commonly seen.

SPECIFIC DRUG CONSIDERATIONS FOR THE ELDERLY

Several classes of drugs that are commonly prescribed for elderly persons will be selectively discussed here. They include cardiovascular drugs, central nervous system drugs, anti-inflammatory drugs, and gastrointestinal

drugs. However, there are many different types of drugs that are potentially inappropriate for use by the elderly. Drugs that are dangerous if used by people over 65 years of age are listed in Table 26-3.

TABLE 26-3 Dangerous Medications for Adults over 65 Years of Age

Classification	Generic Name	Trade Name
Analgesics	meperidine hydrochloride	Demerol®
	pentazocine	Talwin®
	propoxyphene hydrochloride	Darvon, Darvocet N®
Antiarrhythmics	disopyramide	Norpace®
Antidepressants and Antipsychotics		
Antidepressants	amitriptyline hydrochloride	Enovil®
	doxepin hydrochloride	Sinequan®
	fluoxetine hydrochloride	Prozac®
Antipsychotics	haloperidol	Haldol®
	thioridazine hydrochloride	Mellaril®
Antiemetics	trimethobenzamide hydrochloride	Tigan®
Antihypertensives	clonidine hydrochloride	Catapres®
	hydrochlorothiazide	Esidrix®, HydroDIURIL®
	methyldopa	Aldomet®
	propranolol	Inderal®
	reserpine	Serpasil®
Anti-infectives and Antihistamines		
Anti-infectives	nitrofurantoin	Macrodantin®
Antihistamines	chlorpheniramine maleate	Chlor-Trimeton®
	diphenhydramine hydrochloride	Benadryl®, Tylenol PM®
	hydroxyzine pamoate	Vistaril®, Atarax®
	promethazine hydrochloride	Phenergan®
Antispasmodics	belladonna alkaloids	Donnatal® and others
	dicyclomine hydrochloride	Bentyl®
	hyoscyamine sulfate	Levsin®
	oxybutynin chloride	Ditropan®
	tolterodine tartrate	Detrol®
Decongestants	oxymetazoline	Afrin®, Dristan®, others
	phenylephrine hydrochloride	Neo-Synephrine®
	pseudoephedrine hydrochloride	Sudafed®

(continues)

TABLE 26-3 Dangerous Medications for Adults over 65 Years of Age—*continued*

Classification	Generic Name	Trade Name
Histamine-2 Blockers	cimetidine	Tagamet®
Iron	ferrous sulfate	Feosol® and others
Muscle Relaxants	carisoprodol	Soma®
	cyclobenzaprine hydrochloride	Flexeril®
	methocarbamol	Robaxin®
	orphenadrine	Norflex®
NSAIDs	indomethacin	Indocin®
	ketorolac tromethamine	Toradol®
	phenylbutazone	Butazolidin®
Oral Hypoglycemics	chlorpropamide	Diabinese®
Platelet Inhibitors	dipyridamole	Persantine®
Sedative-Hypnotics	alprazolam	Xanax®
	chlordiazepoxide	Librium®, Limbitrol®
	diazepam	Valium®
	flurazepam	Dalmane®
	lorazepam	Ativan®
	meprobamate	Miltown®
	oxazepam	Serax®
	temazepam	Restoril®
	triazolam	Halcion®

Cardiovascular Drugs

Almost one-third of all deaths in Western countries can be attributed to heart disease. Many cardiovascular drugs must be used cautiously in the elderly for the treatment of hypertension, congestive heart failure, myocardial infarction, and stroke, amongst other disorders and conditions.

Blood pressure increases with age, leading to serious health problems. Treatment of hypertension is effective in older patients. Antihypertensive drugs include thiazides, which are the most commonly prescribed class of diuretics. In the elderly, because of potential adverse effects, these agents should be used in lowered doses. Unfortunately, thiazides can increase the risk of worsening gout, which is a common elderly condition. Beta blockers and ACE inhibitors are prescribed less than thiazides because they may

conflict with certain elderly disorders. Alpha$_1$ blockers are infrequently used for elderly patients because of their adverse effects.

The toxic effects of cardiac glycosides are particularly dangerous in elderly patients because of their increased susceptibility to arrhythmias. Renal function should be considered when dosing regimens are being contemplated. Digoxin is considered safe for older adults if there is close monitoring of serum digoxin levels, creatinine clearance tests, and monitoring of vital signs.

Because older people exhibit changes in hemodynamic reserve, treating patients in this age group who have arrhythmias (dysrhythmias) is challenging. Disopyramide should be avoided due to its major toxicities. Patients with arrhythmias should receive therapy that is designed to control their ventricular rate without conversion to normal sinus rhythm. The prevention of possible thromboembolism in chronic atrial fibrillation is an important goal.

Anticoagulants

Many elderly patients with atrial fibrillation are not given anticoagulants because physicians fear injuries and secondary bleeding due to falls. Head injuries from falling are usually of greatest concern. Given that anticoagulation can result in an annual absolute reduction in the risk of stroke, the benefits of anticoagulation outweigh the risks of falling in most instances (see Chapter 13).

Central Nervous System Drugs

Central nervous system drugs may act by blocking receptors and preventing transmitters from binding them. CNS drugs for geriatric patients include sedative-hypnotics, narcotic analgesics, antidepressants, antipsychotics, and drugs used for Alzheimer's disease.

The second most common group of drugs prescribed for (or taken OTC) by the elderly are sedatives and hypnotics. The half-lives of many of these drugs show a greatest age-related increase in people who are 60 to 70 years of age. Reduced renal function or liver disease affects the rate at which these drugs can be eliminated. Ataxia and other motor impairments should be closely watched for in older patients when they are taking these drugs, which include barbiturates and benzodiazepines.

Narcotic analgesics may cause dose-related adverse effects in the elderly. Because of the way respiratory function changes as we age, geriatric patients are often more sensitive to the respiratory effects of these drugs. Use of narcotics may cause hypotension in the elderly. Opioids are often underutilized in the elderly, though good pain management plans are easily obtained for this age group.

Antidepressants and antipsychotics have sometimes been overused in the elderly for the treatment of such disorders as schizophrenia, dementia, aggressiveness, delirium, and paranoia. Older drugs of this type, such as chlorpromazine, should be avoided in the elderly because they induce orthostatic hypotension. According to the patient's tolerance, drug doses should be gradually increased to achieve the desired therapeutic effect, with close monitoring for adverse effects.

Some phenothiazines should be started at just a fraction of the amounts used for young adults when they are being used for the elderly. Due to its clearance by the kidneys, lithium must be dosage-adjusted, and it should never be used concurrently with thiazide diuretics. Antidepressants often cause more toxicity in older adults, and those with reduced antimuscarinic effects (such as nortriptyline and desipramine) should be used. It is important to remember that major depression and senile dementia must be carefully diagnosed due to the possibility of them resembling each other.

Alzheimer's disease is characterized by progressive memory and cognitive function impairment. Cholinomimetic drugs are usually used for this condition, to decrease the release of gamma-aminobutyric acid (GABA), and increase the release of norepinephrine, dopamine, and serotonin from nerve endings. Some agents, such as donepezil, rivastigmine, and galantamine have been shown to improve cognitive activity in some Alzheimer's patients, and may even reduce morbidity from other diseases. This is important in prolonging the life of the patient. However, these agents should be used with caution in patients receiving other cytochrome P450 enzyme inhibitors.

Anti-inflammatory Drugs

About one-half of patients with cancer who are dying have severe pain. Patients perceive pain differently, depending on factors such as fatigue, insomnia, anxiety, depression, and nausea. Addressing these factors together with a supportive environment can help control pain.

Key Concept

For the administration of drugs in elderly patients, neurological status and parameters relating to renal, liver, cardiac, and respiratory function should be noted.

The choice of analgesic depends largely on pain intensity, which can be determined only by talking with and observing the patient. All pain can be relieved by an appropriately potent drug at the right dosage, which may also produce sedation or confusion. Commonly used drugs are aspirin, acetaminophen, or NSAIDs for mild pain; codeine or oxycodone for moderate pain; and hydromorphone or morphine for severe pain. For a detailed discussion of analgesic use, see Chapter 21.

Cold Remedies

Over-the-counter cold remedies often cause adverse effects in elderly people. The anticholinergic properties of many create confusion, impair bladder emptying, or cause constipation and decongestants may cause urinary hesitance or retention in men.

Gastrointestinal Drugs

Many seriously ill patients experience nausea, often without vomiting. Contributors to nausea include GI problems such as constipation and gastritis, metabolic abnormalities such as hypercalcemia and uremia (elevation of urea in blood), drug side effects, and increased intracranial pressure due to brain cancer. Treatment should be guided by the probable etiology, such as discontinuation of NSAIDs and administration of H_2-receptor blockers such as ranitidine (Zantac), famotidine (Pepcid), and cimetidine (Tagamet) in a patient with gastritis. In contrast, a patient with known or suspected brain metastasis may have nausea due to increased intracranial pressure and would best be treated with a course of corticosteroids. Metoclopramide, orally or by injection, is useful for nausea caused by gastric distension. If a reason for mild nausea is not identifiable, nonspecific treatment with phenothiazines such as promethazine or prochlorperazine before meals may be given. Anticholinergic drugs such as scopolamine and the antihistamine meclizine prevent recurrent nausea in many patients. Second-line drugs for intractable nausea include haloperidol and granisetron. Constipation is common in elderly people because of inactivity, use of opioid and anticholinergic drugs, and decreased fluid and dietary fiber intake. Laxatives help prevent fecal impaction, especially for those receiving opioids. Laxative drugs are discussed in Chapter 15.

Antimicrobial Drugs

Due to alterations in their T-lymphocyte function, many elderly patients appear to have reduced host defenses, and are more susceptible to serious infections and diseases such as cancer. It is important to remember that decreased renal function greatly affects the use of certain antimicrobial drugs, such as aminoglycosides, in the elderly. Antimicrobial drugs that are considered safe for the elderly include penicillins, cephalosporins, sulfonamides, and tetracyclines. Drug doses should be decreased if the patient has decreased renal drug clearance or the drug has a prolonged half-life.

SUMMARY

Throughout the aging process, individuals are more likely to be affected by many chronic disorders and disabilities. Consequently, elderly persons use more drugs than any other age group. The normal function of each system and organ of the body changes during the aging process. However, some functions in the human body do not show age-related changes. There are three factors that are associated with the aging process: physiological, pathophysiological, and sociogenic or behavioral. The principles of drug therapy in elderly patients are based on efficacy and safety, dosage, complexity of regimen, number of drugs, cost, and patient compliance. Many disorders and conditions are more common in elderly men, women, or both. The most common diseases seen in elderly persons in the United States have been selectively discussed. Several classes of drugs that are commonly prescribed for elderly patients should be given special consideration because of their side effects, drug interactions, and dosages. They include anticoagulants, glaucoma medications, analgesics, antihypertensives, cold remedies, antiemetics, and benzodiazepines.

EXPLORING THE WEB

Visit the following Web sites and search for articles and information related to the body as it ages and the effects of pharmacotherapy in the elderly:

- *www.nlm.nih.gov/medlineplus*
- *www.postgradmed.com*
- *http://healthlibrary.stanford.edu*
- *www.4therapy.com/consumer/medications/ item.php?uniqueid=4712&categoryid=163&*
- *www.adaa.org/aboutADAA/newsletter/AnxietyandAging.htm*
- *Visit www.ageworks.com*
- Look at the various online courses and continuing education courses. Choose a course you feel would enhance your understanding of the factors affecting aging and health.

REVIEW QUESTIONS

Multiple Choice

1. Which of the following disorders is the most common cause of death in the United States?

    A. cancer

    B. AIDS

C. rheumatoid arthritis

D. myocardial infarction

2. The goal of treatment for osteoporosis includes:

A. stopping the aging process

B. preventing additional fractures and controlling pain

C. preventing surgery for pathologic fractures and controlling pain

D. stopping the use of hormone replacement

3. In postmenopausal women, reduced estrogen blood levels have been linked to increased incidence of which of the following conditions or diseases?

A. upper respiratory tract infections

B. rheumatoid arthritis

C. breast cancer

D. cardiovascular disease

4. Which of the following drugs requires a lower dosage in elderly persons because of reduction of renal function?

A. warfarin

B. gentamicin

C. digoxin

D. ranitidine

5. Which of the following medications in elderly patients may cause falls and hip fractures?

A. thiazides

B. diazepam

C. vitamin B_{12}

D. cimetidine

6. Physiological changes with aging may alter all of the following, except:

A. reduction of cardiac output

B. reduction of absorptive surfaces

C. increased gastric emptying rate

D. changes in gastric pH

7. All of the following are reasons for the greater incidence of adverse reactions of drugs in elderly individuals, except:

A. increased total body fluid

B. impaired drug metabolism

C. decreased serum albumin levels

D. medication errors are more likely to occur

8. Which of the following drugs has a large volume of distribution?

A. diazepam

B. acetaminophen

C. digoxin

D. ethanol

9. Which of the following body systems is the most important for elimination of the majority of drugs?
   A. digestive
   B. respiratory
   C. reproductive
   D. urinary

10. Which of the following agents can cause systemic side effects such as bradycardia, asthma, and heart failure?
    A. diazepam
    B. diphenhydramine
    C. warfarin
    D. bethanechol

11. The number of melanocytes and the amount of protective melanin _____ in elderly people.
    A. increases
    B. decreases
    C. does not change
    D. depends on what types of medications are being taken

12. The most important route for the elimination of the majority of drugs includes which of the following?
    A. sweat
    B. saliva
    C. lungs
    D. kidneys

13. The effects of similar drug concentrations at the site of action are called:
    A. pharmacology
    B. pharmacokinetic
    C. pharmacodynamic
    D. pharmacogenetic

14. In the United States, about _____ of persons older than 65 years take prescription and nonprescription (over-the-counter) drugs.
    A. one-half
    B. one-fourth
    C. two-thirds
    D. three-fifths

15. Primary age changes are also known as _____ age changes.
    A. physiological
    B. pathophysiological
    C. sociogenic
    D. tertiary

Fill in the Blank

1. Anticholinergic properties of many over-the-counter cold remedies often cause adverse effects in elderly people, such as:

   a. _____

   b. _____

   c. _____

   d. _____

2. Scopolamine and the antihistamine meclizine prevent recurrent _____ in many elderly patients.

3. Longer-acting benzodiazepines should be avoided in elderly people because _____.

4. Many elderly patients with atrial fibrillation are not given anticoagulants because physicians fear _____ and secondary bleeding due to _____.

5. The most significant unmodifiable risk factor for stroke is _____.

6. Digoxin has a lower volume of distribution in elderly patients; therefore, doses _____.

7. Topical β-blockers can cause systemic side effects in elderly patients, such as _____, _____, and _____.

Critical Thinking

A 65-year-old man has had a history of alcoholism for the past 20 years. He has been taking warfarin for the past ten days. It is known that with cirrhosis of the liver, serum albumin decreases, as does hepatic blood flow.

1. What would be the consequences of taking warfarin in his condition?

2. Explain the hepatic clearance in elderly people who are suffering from liver diseases.

3. If this patient also takes phenytoin, what would be the potential outcome?

1. A 4-year-old boy presents with the following symptoms. He is experiencing a fever of 101.9° F, chills, sore throat, and rash. The best recommendation for treating this child's fever is:

   A. choline salicylate, because it is in the liquid form, and therefore more easily swallowed
   B. acetaminophen, since the specific disease condition is not known
   C. pediatric aspirin, because it is flavored and will ensure patient compliance
   D. any of the above recommendations are acceptable

Questions 2–4

A 60-year-old hypertensive woman brings three prescriptions to your pharmacy. They include furosemide, enalapril, and irbesartan.

2. Which of the following is an example of an ACE inhibitor?

   A. furosemide
   B. enalapril
   C. digoxin
   D. irbesartan

3. Which of the following is the trade name of furosemide?

   A. Midamor
   B. Hygroton
   C. Aldactone
   D. Lasix

4. Irbesartan is classified as which of the following antihypertensive drugs?

   A. peripheral vasodilator
   B. angiotensin II receptor antagonist
   C. adrenergic blocker
   D. angiotensin-converting enzyme inhibitor

5. A 31-year-old woman presents with a 2-month history of depressed mood, absence of pleasure from the performance of any act, increased appetite, weight gain, and suicidal ideation. This is the patient's first episode of major depression. Which of the following agents would be most appropriate in the treatment of this patient?

   A. sertraline (Zoloft)
   B. chlorpromazine (Thorazine)
   C. thioridazine (Mellaril)
   D. ritodrine (Yutopar)

Questions 6–7

A 56-year-old man has been diagnosed with acute gouty arthritis of the right large toe.

6. Which of the following is the drug of choice for relieving pain and inflammation, and for ending the acute gout attack?

   A. mivacurium
   B. gold sodium thiomalate
   C. aspirin
   D. colchicine

7. If the traditional drug of choice is not an analgesic, which of the following agents may be used in combination in the management of pain for acute gout?

   A. succinylcholine
   B. allopurinol
   C. acetaminophen
   D. oxycodone

Questions 8–9

A 72-year-old man with advanced inoperable throat cancer is hospitalized for pain management. He is given a morphine solution (40 mg orally) every 3 hours for pain. He complains of difficulty swallowing and about the frequency with which he must take the morphine.

8. An appropriate analgesic alternative for this patient would be:

   A. intramuscular methadone
   B. controlled-release oral morphine
   C. transdermal fentanyl
   D. not another medication; simply increase the dose of the oral morphine solution

9. If there is no other analgesic alternative and the attending physician increases the oral dosage of morphine, which of the following might be the consequence?

   A. excellent pain relief
   B. worsening renal function
   C. excessive appetite
   D. overdose

Questions 10–12

A 21-year-old, previously healthy man is brought to the emergency room with a 2-week history of excessive elimination of urine, excessive thirst, and an unintentional weight loss of 25 pounds. No retinopathy is present. Laboratory values reveal high blood glucose and high glucose in the urine.

10. What is the most likely diagnosis for this patient?

    A. Type I diabetes mellitus
    B. Type II diabetes mellitus
    C. Type III diabetes mellitus
    D. diabetes insipidus

11. Which of the following is the appropriate initial therapy?

    A. intravenous fluids and a sulfonylurea agent
    B. intravenous fluids and intravenous regular insulin
    C. intravenous fluids and 10 units of subcutaneous regular insulin
    D. intravenous fluids alone

12. The patient is at risk for developing which of the following complications?

    A. coronary artery disease
    B. retinopathy
    C. hypoglycemia
    D. all of the above

Questions 13–15

A 75-year-old man with a history of cigarette smoking for 50 years is brought to the emergency room with a fever of 103°F (which he has had for 4 days), cough, chills, and chest pain. Chest x-ray reveals pneumonia with confirmation via blood tests.

13. If this patient was diagnosed with bacterial pneumonia, which of the following antibiotics is the most appropriate to administer intravenously?

    A. chloramphenicol
    B. cephradine
    C. amphotericin B
    D. rifampin

14. If the patient has an allergy to the drug of choice (which is one of the four choices in Question 13), which of the following would be the best drug of choice?

    A. chloramphenicol
    B. cephradine
    C. amphotericin B
    D. rifampin

15. The physician orders chloramphenicol 50 mg/kg/day in divided doses (every 6 hours). Which of the following is the most serious adverse effect of this drug?

    A. ototoxicity
    B. nephrotoxicity
    C. phlebitis at injection site
    D. bone marrow depression

Questions 16–17

A 25-year-old man has burns on over 75% of his body. He has been admitted for two weeks at a local hospital, where he developed Zollinger-Ellison syndrome (a hypersecretion condition of the stomach with gastric ulcers).

16. Which of the following prototypes of H_2-receptor antagonists is used in the treatment of this condition?

    A. cimetidine
    B. famotidine
    C. nizatidine
    D. ranitidine

17. Which of the following prototype H_2-receptor antagonists is the most potent?

   A. ranitidine
   B. cimetidine
   C. famotidine
   D. nizatidine

18. Erythromycin 500 mg bid × 8 days is prescribed. The pharmacy technician has only the 250 mg dose in stock. How many capsules will the technician dispense for this patient?

   A. 16
   B. 24
   C. 32
   D. 48

Questions 19–21

A 62-year-old female has been diagnosed with congestive heart failure and pulmonary edema. Her physician orders digitalis, a diuretic, ACE inhibitors, and beta-blockers.

19. Which of the following diuretics are preferred?

   A. loop diuretics
   B. thiazide and thiazide-like diuretics
   C. potassium-sparing diuretics
   D. carbonic anhydrase inhibitors

20. If the order is for thiazide or loop diuretics, which of the following is the most dangerous adverse effect?

   A. hypertension
   B. hyperkalemia
   C. hypokalemia
   D. loss of appetite

21. If the physician orders spironolactone, which of the following adverse effects may occur?

   A. hyperkalemia
   B. gynecomastia
   C. hyponatremia
   D. all of the above

22. A pediatrician orders penicillin for an 11-year-old patient without closely checking the patient's chart. While the pharmacy technician is dispensing the prescription, he notices that the computer chart indicates that the patient has an allergy to penicillin.

Which of the following would be the best drug of choice in this case?

   A. ciprofloxacin
   B. clarithromycin
   C. amikacin
   D. vancomycin

23. A 75-year-old patient with advanced metastatic prostate cancer and a long history of renal failure presents with severe bone pain. He is given meperidine. Two days later, he develops a generalized seizure condition. What is the likely mechanism of this complication?

   A. worsening renal failure
   B. buildup of meperidine metabolite levels
   C. hypercalcemia
   D. brain metastasis

24. A 55-year-old patient with a history of hypertension and recent edema in her legs is treated with a thiazide diuretic. She should be monitored regularly for altered plasma levels of:

   A. uric acid
   B. calcium
   C. glucose
   D. potassium

25. A 27-year-old woman who breast-feeds her 7-month-old infant presents with chronic panic disorder. Her physician prescribes a benzodiazepine for her. All of the following properties of this drug are desirable for breastfeeding, except:

   A. hepatic metabolism to inactive metabolites
   B. a tendency to bind to milk proteins
   C. a rapid onset of action
   D. a short half-life

Answer Key

1. B	2. B	3. D	4. B	5. A	6. D
7. B	8. C	9. D	10. A	11. B	12. D
13. B	14. A	15. D	16. A	17. C	18. C
19. A	20. C	21. D	22. B	23. B	24. D
25. B					

APPENDIX
B Top 200 Drugs by Prescription

Number	Generic Name	Trade Name
1	hydrocodone w/APAP	Hydrocodone w/APAP®
2	atorvastatin	Lipitor®
3	amoxicillin	Trimox®
4	lisinopril	Prinivil®, Zestril®
5	hydrochlorothiazide	Diaqua®, Esidrix®
6	atenolol	Tenormin®
7	azithromycin	Zithromax®
8	furosemide	Lasix®
9	alprazolam	Xanax®
10	metoprolol	Toprol XL®
11	albuterol	Proventil®
12	amlodipine	Norvasc®
13	levothyroxine	Synthroid®
14	metformin	Glucophage®, Glucophage XR®
15	sertraline	Zoloft®
16	escitalopram	Lexapro®
17	ibuprofen	Motrin®
18	cephalexin	Keflex®
19	zolpidem	Ambien®
20	prednisone	Deltasone®
21	esomeprazole magnesium	Nexium®
22	triamterene	Dyrenium®
23	propoxyphene napsylate	Darvon-N®
24	simvastatin	Zocor®
25	montelukast	Singulair®
26	lansoprazole	Prevacid®
27	metoprolol tartrate	Lopressor®
28	fluoxetine	Prozac®
29	lorazepam	Ativan®
30	clopidogrel	Plavix®

Number	Generic Name	Trade Name
31	oxycodone w/APAP	Oxycodone w/APAP®
32	salmeterol	Serevent®
33	alendronate	Fosamax®
34	venlafaxine	Effexor®, Effexor XR®
35	warfarin	Coumadin®
36	paroxetine hydrochloride	Paxil®
37	clonazepam	Klonopin®
38	cetirizine	Zyrtec®
39	pantoprazole	Protonix®
40	potassium chloride	Potassium Chloride®
41	acetaminophen/codeine	Tylenol-Codeine®
42	trimethoprim/ sulfamethoxazole	TMP-SMZ®
43	gabapentin	Neurontin®
44	conjugated estrogens	Premarin®
45	fluticasone	Flonase®
46	trazodone	Desyrel®
47	cyclobenzaprine	Flexeril®
48	amitriptyline	Elavil®, Enovil®
49	levofloxacin	Levaquin®
50	tramadol	Ultram®
51	ciprofloxacin	Cipro®
52	amlodipine/benazepril	Lotrel®
53	ranitidine	Zantac®
54	fexofenadine	Allegra®
55	levothyroxine	Levoxyl®
56	valsartan	Diovan®
57	enalapril	Vasotec®
58	diazepam	Valium®
59	naproxen	Anaprox®, Naprosyn®
60	fluconazole	Diflucan®

Number	Generic Name	Trade Name
61	lisinopril/HCTZ	Zestoretic®
62	potassium chloride	Klor-Con®
63	ramipril	Altace®
64	bupropion	Wellbutrin®, Wellbutrin XL®
65	celecoxib	Celebrex®
66	sildenafil citrate	Viagra®
67	doxycycline hyclate	Vibra-Tabs®
68	ezetimibe	Zetia®
69	rosiglitazone maleate	Avandia®
70	lovastatin	Mevacor®
71	valsartan/ hydrochlorothiazide	Diovan HCT®
72	carisoprodol	Soma®, Rela®
73	drospirenone/ ethinyl estradiol	Yasmin 28®
74	allopurinol	Alloprin®
75	clonidine	Catapres®
76	methylprednisolone	Medrol®
77	pioglitazone hydrochloride	Actos®
78	pravastatin	Pravachol®
79	risedronate sodium	Actonel®
80	norelgestromin/ ethinyl estradiol	Ortho Evra®
81	citalopram hydrobromide	Celexa®
82	verapamil	Calan®
83	isosorbide mononitrate	Ismotic®
84	penicillin V	Penicillin VK®
85	glyburide	Micronase®
86	amphetamine sulfate	Adderall®
87	mometasone furoate	Nasonex®
88	folic acid	Folacin®

Number	Generic Name	Trade Name
89	quetiapine fumarate	Seroquel®
90	losartan potassium	Cozaar®
91	fenofibrate	Tricor®
92	carvedilol	Coreg®
93	methylphenidate hydrochloride	Concerta®
94	ezetimibe	Vytorin®
95	insulin glargine	Lantus®
96	promethazine hydrochloride	Phenergan®
97	meloxicam	Mobic®
98	tamsulosin hydrochloride	Flomax®
99	rosuvastatin	Crestor®
100	glipizide	Glucotrol XL®
101	norgestimate/ ethinyl estradiol	Ortho Tri-Cyclen Lo®
102	temazepam	Restoril®
103	omeprazole	Prilosec®
104	cefdinivir	Omnicef®
105	albuterol	Ventolin®
106	risperidone	Risperdal®
107	rabeprazole sodium	AcipHex®
108	digoxin	Digitek®
109	spironolactone	Aldactone®
110	valacyclovir hydrochloride	Valtrex®
111	latanoprost	Xalatan®
112	metformin	Fortamet®
113	losartan potassium/ hydrochlorothiazide	Hyzaar®
114	quinapril	Accupril®
115	clindamycin	Cleocin®
116	metronidazole	Flagyl®
117	triamcinolone	Atolone®
118	topiramate	Topamax®

Number	Generic Name	Trade Name
119	ipratropium bromide/ albuterol sulfate	Combivent®
120	benazepril	Lotensin®
121	gemfibrozil	Lopid®
122	irbesartan	Avapro®
123	glimepiride	Amaryl®
124	norgestimate/ethinyl estradiol	Trinessa®
125	estradiol	Alora®, Climara®
126	hydroxyzine	Atarax®
127	metoclopramide	Maxolon®, Reglan®
128	fexofenadine/ pseudoephedrine	Allegra-D 12 Hour®
129	doxazosin mesylate	Cardura®
130	warfarin	Jantoven®
131	glipizide	Glucotrol®
132	diclofenac sodium	Voltaren®
133	raloxifene hydrochloride	Evista®
134	diltiazem	Cardizem®, Tiazac®
135	tolterodine tartrate	Detrol®, Detrol LA®
136	meclizine	Antivert®, Bonamine®
137	glyburide/metformin	Glucovance®
138	atomoxetine	Strattera®
139	duloxetine hydrochloride	Cymbalta®
140	nitrofurantoin	Furadantin®
141	promethazine/codeine	Phenergan with Codeine®
142	olmesartan medoxomil	Benicar®
143	mirtazapine	Remeron®
144	bisoprolol/HCTZ	Ziac®
145	desloratadine	Clarinex®
146	oxycodone	OxyContin®
147	minocycline	Arestin®, Minocin®
148	sumatriptan	Imitrex®

Number	Generic Name	Trade Name
149	nabumetone	Relafen®
150	olanzapine	Zyprexa®
151	lamotrigine	Lamictal®
152	cetirizine/ pseudoephedrine	Zyrtec-D®
153	polyethylene glycol	Glycolax®
154	acyclovir	Zovirax®
155	propranolol	Inderal®
156	triamcinolone acetonide	Nasacort AQ®
157	donepezil hydrochloride	Aricept®
158	butalbital/ acetaminophen/caffeine	Fioricet®
159	niacin	Niaspan®
160	azithromycin	Zmax®
161	divalproex sodium	Depakote®
162	buspirone	Buspar®
163	norgestimate/ethinyl estradiol	Tri-Sprintec®
164	methotrexate	Amethopterin®, MTX®
165	oxycodone	Roxicodone®
166	budesonide	Rhinocort Aqua®
167	olmesartan medoxomil hydrochlorothiazide	Benicar HCT®
168	terazosin	Hytrin®
169	metaxalone	Skelaxin®
170	clotrimazole/ betamethasone	Lotrisone®
171	tadalafil	Cialis®
172	irbesartan/ hydrochlorothiazide	Avalide®
173	fexofenadine	Telfast®
174	norgestimate/ethinyl estradiol	Ortho Tri-Cyclen®
175	bupropion hydrochloride	Wellbutrin®, Zyban®
176	benzonatate	Tessalon®

Number	Generic Name	Trade Name
177	olopatadine hydrochloride	Patanol®
178	quinine	Quinamm®, Quiphile®
179	diltiazem hydrochloride	Cartia XT®
180	insulin lispro, rDNA origin	Humalog®
181	paroxetine	Paxil CR®
182	levonorgestrel and ethinyl estradiol	Aviane®
183	digoxin	Lanoxin®
184	amphetamine	Adderall XR®
185	famotidine	Pepcid®, Pepcid AC®
186	digoxin	Lanoxicaps®
187	levothyroxine	Levothroid®
188	nifedipine	Adalat®, Procardia®

Number	Generic Name	Trade Name
189	nortriptyline	Aventyl®
190	hydrocodone polistirex/ chlorpheniramine polistirex	Tussionex®
191	nitroglycerin	NitroQuick®
192	phenytoin	Dilantin®
193	budesonide	Endocet®
194	etodolac	Lodine®, Lodine XL®
195	atenolol/chlorthalidone	Tenoretic®
196	phentermine	Fastin®
197	tramadol/ acetaminophen	Ultracet®
198	tizanidine	Zanaflex®
199	cetirizine hydrochloride/ pseudoephedrine	Virlix-D®
200	divalproex sodium	Depakote ER®

Generic Names	Brand Names	Possible Dangers
celecoxib citalopram hydrobromide fosphenytoin	Celebrex® Celexa® Cerebyx®	Mix-ups may cause decreased mental ability, lack of pain or seizure control, and other serious adverse events.
cisplatin carboplatin	Platinol® Paraplatin®	Though the generic names are similar, safe doses of carboplatin usually exceed the maximum safe dose of cisplatin, potentially causing toxicity and death.
clonidine clonazepam	Catapres® Klonopin®	Easily confused generic or trade names.
concentrated liquid morphines versus conventional liquid morphine concentrations	Concentrated: Roxanol®, MSIR® Conventional: morphine oral liquid	Concentrated forms can be confused with standard concentrations can lead to fatal errors due to differences in labeling or prescribing by volume versus milligrams, e.g., 10 mg versus 10 mL.
ephedrine epinephrine	Ephedrine® Adrenalin®	Similar names and clinical uses can cause these drugs to be stored close to each other; also, they are packaged in similar amber-colored vials and ampules.
fentanyl sufentanil	Sublimaze® Sufenta®	These non-interchangeable drugs have very different potencies, and can cause respiratory arrest if misused.
hydromorphone injection morphine injection	Dilaudid® Astramorph®, Duramorph®, Infumorph®	Hydromorphone is not the generic equivalent of morphine and they are not interchangeable. Due to close storage and similar concentrations, they may be easily misused, causing death because of potency differences influencing respiratory arrest.
insulin glargine insulin zinc suspension human insulin insulin lispro human insulin aspart 70% isophane insulin NPH/ 30% insulin regular 70% insulin aspart protamine suspension and 30% insulin aspart	Lantus® Lente® Humulin®, Novolin® Humalog® Novolog® Novolin 70/30® Novolog Mix 70/30®	Similar names, strengths, and concentrations can cause medication errors; also mix-ups between 100 units/mL and 500 units/mL can occur.

lipid-based:
  doxorubicin liposomal
  daunorubicin citrate liposomal
conventional:
  daunorubicin
  doxorubicin
	Doxil®
	Daunoxome®
	
	Cerubidine®
	Adriamycin®, Rubex®
		Confusion between liposomal and conventional formulations can occur easily, but these products are not interchangeable; accidental use of liposomal forms instead of conventional forms has resulted in severe side effects and death.

nefazodone quetiapine	Serzone® Seroquel®	Similar names and available dosages, as well as use in similar clinical settings, can cause many adverse events and potentially dangerous drug interactions with other agents that may be used concurrently.

Generic Names	Brand Names	Possible Dangers
paclitaxel docetaxel	Taxol® Taxotere®	These cancer agents have different dosing recommendations and can cause serious adverse outcomes.
vinblastine vincristine	Velban® Oncovin®	Fatal errors can occur due to name similarity and wide variances in safe recommended dosages of each.
olanzapine cetirizine	Zyprexa® Zyrtec®	Name similarity can easily cause mix-ups; Zyrtec is an antihistamine, while Zyprexa is an antipsychotic; serious physical or mental injury or impairment can occur.

Drug	U.S. Drug Schedule	Canadian Drug Schedule
alfentanil	II	I
alprazolam	IV	IV
amobarbital	II	IV
amphetamine	II	III
aprobarbital	III	IV
benzophetamine	III	III
buprenorphine	III	I
butabarbital	III	IV
butorphanol	IV	IV
chloral hydrate	IV	Not controlled
chlordiazepoxide	IV	IV
clonazepam	IV	IV
clorazepate	IV	IV
cocaine	II	I
codeine	II	I
dexmethylphenidate	II	Not available
dextroamphetamine	II	III
dextropropoxyphene (bulk)	II	I
dextropropoxyphene (dosage forms)	IV	I
diazepam	IV	IV
diethylpropion	IV	IV
difenoxin products	V	I
diphenoxylate products	V	I
dronabinol	III	Not controlled
estazolam	IV	IV
ethchlorvynol	IV	IV
fentanyl	II	I
fluoxymesterone	III	IV
flurazepam	IV	IV

Drug	U.S. Drug Schedule	Canadian Drug Schedule
glutethimide	II	IV
halazepam	IV	IV
hydrocodone	Only available in C-III combination drugs	I
hydromorphone	II	I
ketamine	III	Not controlled
levorphanol	II	I
lorazepam	IV	IV
mazindol	IV	IV
meperidine	II	I
mephobarbital	IV	IV
meprobamate	IV	IV
methadone	II	I
methamphetamine	II	III
methandrostenalone	III	IV
methylphenidate	II	III
methyltestosterone	III	IV
midazolam	IV	IV
modafinil	IV	Not controlled
morphine	II	I
nandrolone	III	IV
opium opium products	II V	I I
oxandrolone	III	IV
oxazepam	IV	IV
oxycodone	II	I
oxymetholone	III	IV
oxymorphone	II	I
paraldehyde	IV	Not controlled
paregoric	III	I

Drug	U.S. Drug Schedule	Canadian Drug Schedule
pemoline	IV	Not controlled
pentazocine	IV	I
pentobarbital sodium		
PO	II	IV
rectal	III	IV
phencyclidine	II	I
phendimetrazine	III	IV
phenobarbital	IV	IV
phentermine	IV	IV
prazepam	Not available	IV
quazepam	IV	IV
remifentanil	II	Not available
secobarbital	II	IV
sibutramine	IV	Not available
stanolone	III	IV
stanozolol	III	IV
sufentanil	II	I
temazepam	IV	IV
testosterone	III	IV
thiopental	III	IV
triazolam	IV	IV
zaleplon	IV	Not available
zolpidem	IV	Not available

Drug Dosage Calculations

Using Ratios and Proportions to Calculate Dosages

1. Ratios may be written as follows: 3 : 4, which means 3 parts of drug #1 to 4 parts of solution or solvent. *Ratios* are used to express the relationship between two or more quantities. Ratios are usually expressed as fractions in drug calculations, as follows:

$$\frac{3 \text{ parts of drug \#1}}{4 \text{ parts of a solution}} = \frac{3}{4}$$

Proportions show the relationship between two ratios, as follows:

$$\frac{\text{Dose on hand}}{\text{Quantity on hand}} = \frac{\text{Desired dose}}{\text{Desired quantity (X)}}$$

The same formula can be written as follows by using cross multiplication:

$$\text{Desired quantity (X)} = \frac{\text{Desired dose}}{\text{Dose on hand} \times \text{Quantity on hand}}$$

If the dose on hand is 200 mg, the desired dose is 400 mg, and the quantity on hand is 10 mL, what is the desired quantity (X)?

$$\frac{\text{Dose on hand (200 mg)}}{\text{Quantity on hand (10 mL)}} = \frac{\text{Desired dose (400 mg)}}{\text{Desired quantity (X)}}$$

When cross-multiplying, we find:

$$200 \times X = 10 \text{ mL} \times 400$$

$$200X = 4{,}000 \text{ mL}$$

$$X = 20 \text{ mL}$$

The dose to be administered is 20 mL.

2. The same proportion method can solve solid dosage calculations, as follows:

If the dose on hand is available as 5 mg tablets, and the desired dose is 25 mg/day, how many tablets should be administered each day?

$$\frac{\text{Dose on hand (5 mg)}}{1 \text{ tablet}} = \frac{\text{Desired dose (25 mg)}}{\text{Desired quantity (X)}}$$

By cross-multiplying, it is found that:

$$5 \text{ mg} \times X = 25 \text{ mg} \times 1 \text{ tablet}$$

$$5X = 25 \text{ mg}$$

$$X = 5 \text{ tablets/day}$$

Therefore, 5 tablets should be administered daily.

Dosage Calculations by Weight

Drug dosages are often expressed as milligrams per unit of body weight (usually kilograms rather than pounds), and are commonly used in depicting pediatric doses. An example recommended dose of a drug might be 1 mg/kg/24 hours. This information can be used to calculate the dose for a specific patient, or to check that prescribed doses are correct and not significantly under or over the required doses for that patient.

Caution must always be used in converting between pounds and kilograms.
The formula that should be understood is as follows:

Body weight $\times$ (dose in mg/kg) $=$ X mg of drug

Example: Chewable tablets for a 110-pound child are to be administered at the rate of 20 mg/kg/dose. How many tablets, if they are 500 mg each, should be administered to this patient for each dose?

First, convert the patient's weight to kilograms as follows:

$$1 \text{ kg} = 2.2 \text{ lbs}$$

$$\frac{1 \text{ kg}}{2.2 \text{ lbs}} = \frac{X \text{ kg}}{110 \text{ lbs}}$$

$$X = 50 \text{ kg}$$

Next, calculate the total daily dose as follows. For each kg of body weight, you should give 20 mg of the drug.

$$\frac{20 \text{ mg}}{1 \text{ kg}} = \frac{X \text{ mg}}{50 \text{ kg}}$$

$$X = 1,000 \text{ mg}$$

Finally, calculate the number of tablets needed to supply 1,000 mg per dose.

Remember that the concentration of the tablets on hand is 500 mg per tablet.

$$\frac{500 \text{ mg}}{1 \text{ tablet}} = \frac{1,000 \text{ mg}}{X \text{ tablets}}$$

$$X = 2 \text{ tablets per dose}$$

Calculating Dosage by Body Surface Area

Using body surface area to calculate pediatric dosages is a very accurate method. Nomograms are charts that use patient weight and height to determine body surface area in square meters (m^2). This body surface area (BSA) is then placed into a ratio with the average adult's body surface area (1.73 m^2). The following formula is then used:

$$\text{Child's dose} = \frac{\text{Child's BSA in m}^2}{1.73 \text{ m}^2} \times \text{Adult dose}$$

Nomogram scales contain metric and avoirdupois values for height and weight, enabling body surface area to be determined in pounds and inches or kilograms and centimeters without needing to make conversions. See the figure of the nomogram scale at the end of this Appendix.

WEST NOMOGRAM

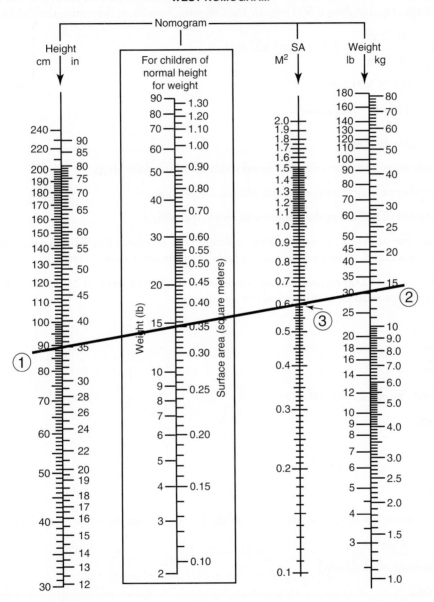

To determine BSA, a ruler or straightedge is recommended. After determining the patient's height and weight, place the ruler or straightedge on the nomogram and connect the two points on the height and weight scales that represent the patient's values. Where the ruler or straightedge crosses the center column (BSA), the corresponding reading is the value of the BSA in

square meters. Substitute the BSA value in the formula to calculate the dosage for this patient. If this child's BSA is 0.52 m², and the adult dosage of the required drug is 500 mg, use the following formula to determine the child's dose:

$$\text{Child's dose} = \frac{0.52 \text{ m}^2}{1.73 \text{ m}^2} \times \text{Adult dose (500 mg)}$$

$$= 0.3 \times 500 \text{ mg}$$

$$= 150 \text{ mg (child's dose)}$$

Calculating IV Infusion Rates

To calculate the flow rate using the ratio and proportion method, follow these steps:

1. Determine the number of milliliters the patient will receive per hour.

2. Determine the number of milliliters the patient will receive per minute.

3. Determine the number of drops per minute that will equal the number of milliliters calculated above. The IV set's drop rate must be considered. This is expressed as a ratio of drops per milliliter (gtt/mL).

Example: The prescriber orders 3,000 mL of dextrose 5% in water (D_5W) IV over 24 hours. If the IV set delivers 15 drops per milliliter, how many drops must be administered per minute?

First, calculate mL/hr.

$$\frac{3,000 \text{ mL}}{24 \text{ hrs}} = \frac{X \text{ mL}}{1 \text{ hr}}$$

$$X = 125 \text{ mL/hr or } 125 \text{ mL/60 min}$$

Next, calculate mL/min.

$$\frac{125 \text{ mL}}{60 \text{ min}} = \frac{X \text{ mL}}{1 \text{ min}}$$

$$X = 2 \text{ mL/min}$$

Finally, calculate gtt/min using the drop rate per minute of the IV set. (IV set drop rate = 15 drops/mL)

$$\frac{15 \text{ gtt}}{1 \text{ mL}} = \frac{X \text{ gtt}}{2 \text{ mL (amount needed/min)}}$$

$$X = 30 \text{ gtt/min}$$

DEPARTMENT OF HEALTH AND HUMAN SERVICES • CENTERS FOR DISEASE CONTROL AND PREVENTION

Recommended Immunization Schedule for Persons Aged 0–6 Years—UNITED STATES • 2007

Vaccine▼ Age ▶	Birth	1 month	2 months	4 months	6 months	12 months	15 months	18 months	19–23 months	2–3 years	4–6 years	
Hepatitis B[1]	HepB	HepB		see footnote 1		HepB				HepB Series		Range of recommended ages
Rotavirus[2]			Rota	Rota	Rota							
Diphtheria, Tetanus, Pertussis[3]			DTaP	DTaP	DTaP		DTaP				DTaP	
Haemophilus influenzae type b[4]			Hib	Hib	*Hib[4]*	Hib			Hib			
Pneumococcal[5]			PCV	PCV	PCV	PCV				PCV / PPV		Catch-up immunization
Inactivated Poliovirus			IPV	IPV		IPV					IPV	
Influenza[6]						Influenza (Yearly)						
Measles, Mumps, Rubella[7]						MMR					MMR	Certain high-risk groups
Varicella[8]						Varicella					Varicella	
Hepatitis A[9]						HepA (2 doses)				HepA Series		
Meningococcal[10]										MPSV4		

This schedule indicates the recommended ages for routine administration of currently licensed childhood vaccines, as of December 1, 2006, for children aged 0–6 years. Additional information is available at http://www.cdc.gov/nip/recs/child-schedule.htm. Any dose not administered at the recommended age should be administered at any subsequent visit, when indicated and feasible. Additional vaccines may be licensed and recommended during the year. Licensed combination vaccines may be used whenever any components of the combination are indicated and other components of the vaccine are not contraindicated and if approved by the Food and Drug Administration for that dose of the series. Providers should consult the respective Advisory Committee on Immunization Practices statement for detailed recommendations. Clinically significant adverse events that follow immunization should be reported to the Vaccine Adverse Event Reporting System (VAERS). Guidance about how to obtain and complete a VAERS form is available at http://www.vaers.hhs.gov or by telephone, 800-822-7967.

1. Hepatitis B vaccine (HepB). *(Minimum age: birth)*
At birth:
- Administer monovalent HepB to all newborns before hospital discharge.
- If mother is hepatitis surface antigen (HBsAg)-positive, administer HepB and 0.5 mL of hepatitis B immune globulin (HBIG) within 12 hours of birth.
- If mother's HBsAg status is unknown, administer HepB within 12 hours of birth. Determine the HBsAg status as soon as possible and if HBsAg-positive, administer HBIG (no later than age 1 week).
- If mother is HBsAg-negative, the birth dose can only be delayed with physician's order and mother's negative HBsAg laboratory report documented in the infant's medical record.

After the birth dose:
- The HepB series should be completed with either monovalent HepB or a combination vaccine containing HepB. The second dose should be administered at age 1–2 months. The final dose should be administered at age ≥24 weeks. Infants born to HBsAg-positive mothers should be tested for HBsAg and antibody to HBsAg after completion of ≥3 doses of a licensed HepB series, at age 9–18 months (generally at the next well-child visit).

4-month dose:
- It is permissible to administer 4 doses of HepB when combination vaccines are administered after the birth dose. If monovalent HepB is used for doses after the birth dose, a dose at age 4 months is not needed.

2. Rotavirus vaccine (Rota). *(Minimum age: 6 weeks)*
- Administer the first dose at age 6–12 weeks. Do not start the series later than age 12 weeks.
- Administer the final dose in the series by age 32 weeks. Do not administer a dose later than age 32 weeks.
- Data on safety and efficacy outside of these age ranges are insufficient.

3. Diphtheria and tetanus toxoids and acellular pertussis vaccine (DTaP). *(Minimum age: 6 weeks)*
- The fourth dose of DTaP may be administered as early as age 12 months, provided 6 months have elapsed since the third dose.
- Administer the final dose in the series at age 4–6 years.

4. *Haemophilus influenzae* type b conjugate vaccine (Hib). *(Minimum age: 6 weeks)*
- If PRP-OMP (PedvaxHIB® or ComVax® [Merck]) is administered at ages 2 and 4 months, a dose at age 6 months is not required.
- TriHiBit® (DTaP/Hib) combination products should not be used for primary immunization but can be used as boosters following any Hib vaccine in children aged ≥12 months.

5. Pneumococcal vaccine. *(Minimum age: 6 weeks for pneumococcal conjugate vaccine [PCV]; 2 years for pneumococcal polysaccharide vaccine [PPV])*
- Administer PCV at ages 24–59 months in certain high-risk groups. Administer PPV to children aged ≥2 years in certain high-risk groups. See *MMWR* 2000;49(No. RR-9):1–35.

6. Influenza vaccine. *(Minimum age: 6 months for trivalent inactivated influenza vaccine [TIV]; 5 years for live, attenuated influenza vaccine [LAIV])*
- All children aged 6–59 months and close contacts of all children aged 0–59 months are recommended to receive influenza vaccine.
- Influenza vaccine is recommended annually for children aged ≥59 months with certain risk factors, health-care workers, and other persons (including household members) in close contact with persons in groups at high risk. See *MMWR* 2006;55(No. RR-10):1–41.
- For healthy persons aged 5–49 years, LAIV may be used as an alternative to TIV.
- Children receiving TIV should receive 0.25 mL if aged 6–35 months or 0.5 mL if aged ≥3 years.
- Children aged <9 years who are receiving influenza vaccine for the first time should receive 2 doses (separated by ≥4 weeks for TIV and ≥6 weeks for LAIV).

7. Measles, mumps, and rubella vaccine (MMR). *(Minimum age: 12 months)*
- Administer the second dose of MMR at age 4–6 years. MMR may be administered before age 4–6 years, provided ≥4 weeks have elapsed since the first dose and both doses are administered at age ≥12 months.

8. Varicella vaccine. *(Minimum age: 12 months)*
- Administer the second dose of varicella vaccine at age 4–6 years. Varicella vaccine may be administered before age 4–6 years, provided that ≥3 months have elapsed since the first dose and both doses are administered at age ≥12 months. If second dose was administered ≥28 days following the first dose, the second dose does not need to be repeated.

9. Hepatitis A vaccine (HepA). *(Minimum age: 12 months)*
- HepA is recommended for all children aged 1 year (i.e., aged 12–23 months). The 2 doses in the series should be administered at least 6 months apart.
- Children not fully vaccinated by age 2 years can be vaccinated at subsequent visits.
- HepA is recommended for certain other groups of children, including in areas where vaccination programs target older children. See *MMWR* 2006;55(No. RR-7):1–23.

10. Meningococcal polysaccharide vaccine (MPSV4). *(Minimum age: 2 years)*
- Administer MPSV4 to children aged 2–10 years with terminal complement deficiencies or anatomic or functional asplenia and certain other high-risk groups. See *MMWR* 2005;54(No. RR-7):1–21.

The Recommended Immunization Schedules for Persons Aged 0–18 Years are approved by the Advisory Committee on Immunization Practices (http://www.cdc.gov/nip/acip), the American Academy of Pediatrics (http://www.aap.org), and the American Academy of Family Physicians (http://www.aafp.org).

SAFER • HEALTHIER • PEOPLE™

CS103164

DEPARTMENT OF HEALTH AND HUMAN SERVICES • CENTERS FOR DISEASE CONTROL AND PREVENTION

Recommended Immunization Schedule for Persons Aged 7–18 Years—UNITED STATES • 2007

Vaccine ▼ Age ►	7–10 years	11–12 YEARS	13–14 years	15 years	16–18 years
Tetanus, Diphtheria, Pertussis[1]	see footnote 1	Tdap	Tdap		
Human Papillomavirus[2]	see footnote 2	HPV (3 doses)	HPV Series		
Meningococcal[3]	MPSV4	MCV4		MCV4[3] / MCV4	
Pneumococcal[4]		PPV			
Influenza[5]		Influenza (Yearly)			
Hepatitis A[6]		HepA Series			
Hepatitis B[7]		HepB Series			
Inactivated Poliovirus[8]		IPV Series			
Measles, Mumps, Rubella[9]		MMR Series			
Varicella[10]		Varicella Series			

Range of recommended ages

Catch-up immunization

Certain high-risk groups

This schedule indicates the recommended ages for routine administration of currently licensed childhood vaccines, as of December 1, 2006, for children aged 7–18 years. Additional information is available at http://www.cdc.gov/nip/recs/child-schedule.htm. Any dose not administered at the recommended age should be administered at any subsequent visit, when indicated and feasible. Additional vaccines may be licensed and recommended during the year. Licensed combination vaccines may be used whenever any components of the combination are indicated and other components of the vaccine are not contraindicated and if approved by the Food and Drug Administration for that dose of the series. Providers should consult the respective Advisory Committee on Immunization Practices statement for detailed recommendations. Clinically significant adverse events that follow immunization should be reported to the Vaccine Adverse Event Reporting System (VAERS). Guidance about how to obtain and complete a VAERS form is available at http://www.vaers.hhs.gov or by telephone, 800-822-7967.

1. Tetanus and diphtheria toxoids and acellular pertussis vaccine (Tdap).
(Minimum age: 10 years for BOOSTRIX® and 11 years for ADACEL™)
- Administer at age 11–12 years for those who have completed the recommended childhood DTP/DTaP vaccination series and have not received a tetanus and diphtheria toxoids vaccine (Td) booster dose.
- Adolescents aged 13–18 years who missed the 11–12 year Td/Tdap booster dose should also receive a single dose of Tdap if they have completed the recommended childhood DTP/DTaP vaccination series.

2. Human papillomavirus vaccine (HPV). *(Minimum age: 9 years)*
- Administer the first dose of the HPV vaccine series to females at age 11–12 years.
- Administer the second dose 2 months after the first dose and the third dose 6 months after the first dose.
- Administer the HPV vaccine series to females at age 13–18 years if not previously vaccinated.

3. Meningococcal vaccine. *(Minimum age: 11 years for meningococcal conjugate vaccine [MCV4]; 2 years for meningococcal polysaccharide vaccine [MPSV4])*
- Administer MCV4 at age 11–12 years and to previously unvaccinated adolescents at high school entry (at approximately age 15 years).
- Administer MCV4 to previously unvaccinated college freshmen living in dormitories; MPSV4 is an acceptable alternative.
- Vaccination against invasive meningococcal disease is recommended for children and adolescents aged ≥2 years with terminal complement deficiencies or anatomic or functional asplenia and certain other high-risk groups. See *MMWR* 2005;54(No. RR-7):1–21. Use MPSV4 for children aged 2–10 years and MCV4 or MPSV4 for older children.

4. Pneumococcal polysaccharide vaccine (PPV). *(Minimum age: 2 years)*
- Administer for certain high-risk groups. See *MMWR* 1997;46(No. RR-8):1–24, and *MMWR* 2000;49(No. RR-9):1–35.

5. Influenza vaccine. *(Minimum age: 6 months for trivalent inactivated influenza vaccine [TIV]; 5 years for live, attenuated influenza vaccine [LAIV])*
- Influenza vaccine is recommended annually for persons with certain risk factors, health-care workers, and other persons (including household members) in close contact with persons in groups at high risk. See *MMWR* 2006;55 (No. RR-10):1–41.
- For healthy persons aged 5–49 years, LAIV may be used as an alternative to TIV.
- Children aged <9 years who are receiving influenza vaccine for the first time should receive 2 doses (separated by ≥4 weeks for TIV and ≥6 weeks for LAIV).

6. Hepatitis A vaccine (HepA). *(Minimum age: 12 months)*
- The 2 doses in the series should be administered at least 6 months apart.
- HepA is recommended for certain other groups of children, including in areas where vaccination programs target older children. See *MMWR* 2006;55 (No. RR-7):1–23.

7. Hepatitis B vaccine (HepB). *(Minimum age: birth)*
- Administer the 3-dose series to those who were not previously vaccinated.
- A 2-dose series of Recombivax HB® is licensed for children aged 11–15 years.

8. Inactivated poliovirus vaccine (IPV). *(Minimum age: 6 weeks)*
- For children who received an all-IPV or all-oral poliovirus (OPV) series, a fourth dose is not necessary if the third dose was administered at age ≥4 years.
- If both OPV and IPV were administered as part of a series, a total of 4 doses should be administered, regardless of the child's current age.

9. Measles, mumps, and rubella vaccine (MMR). *(Minimum age: 12 months)*
- If not previously vaccinated, administer 2 doses of MMR during any visit, with ≥4 weeks between the doses.

10. Varicella vaccine. *(Minimum age: 12 months)*
- Administer 2 doses of varicella vaccine to persons without evidence of immunity.
- Administer 2 doses of varicella vaccine to persons aged <13 years at least 3 months apart. Do not repeat the second dose, if administered ≥28 days after the first dose.
- Administer 2 doses of varicella vaccine to persons aged ≥13 years at least 4 weeks apart.

The Recommended Immunization Schedules for Persons Aged 0–18 Years are approved by the Advisory Committee on Immunization Practices (http://www.cdc.gov/nip/acip), the American Academy of Pediatrics (http://www.aap.org), and the American Academy of Family Physicians (http://www.aafp.org).
SAFER • HEALTHIER • PEOPLE™

CS100131

Catch-up Immunization Schedule

for Persons Aged 4 Months–18 Years Who Start Late or Who Are More Than 1 Month Behind

The table below provides catch-up schedules and minimum intervals between doses for children whose vaccinations have been delayed. A vaccine series does not need to be restarted, regardless of the time that has elapsed between doses. Use the section appropriate for the child's age.

CATCH-UP SCHEDULE FOR PERSONS AGED 4 MONTHS–6 YEARS

Vaccine	Minimum Age for Dose 1	Minimum Interval Between Doses			
		Dose 1 to Dose 2	Dose 2 to Dose 3	Dose 3 to Dose 4	Dose 4 to Dose 5
Hepatitis B[1]	Birth	4 weeks	8 weeks (and 16 weeks after first dose)		
Rotavirus[2]	6 wks	4 weeks	4 weeks		
Diphtheria, Tetanus, Pertussis[3]	6 wks	4 weeks	4 weeks	6 months	6 months[3]
Haemophilus influenzae type b[4]	6 wks	4 weeks if first dose administered at age <12 months **8 weeks (as final dose)** if first dose administered at age 12-14 months **No further doses needed** if first dose administered at age ≥15 months	4 weeks[4] if current age <12 months **8 weeks (as final dose)[4]** if current age ≥12 months and second dose administered at age <15 months **No further doses needed** if previous dose administered at age ≥15 months	8 weeks (as final dose) This dose only necessary for children aged 12 months–5 years who received 3 doses before age 12 months	
Pneumococcal[5]	6 wks	4 weeks if first dose administered at age <12 months and current age <24 months **8 weeks (as final dose)** if first dose administered at age ≥12 months or current age 24–59 months **No further doses needed** for healthy children if first dose administered at age ≥24 months	4 weeks if current age <12 months **8 weeks (as final dose)** if current age ≥12 months **No further doses needed** for healthy children if previous dose administered at age ≥24 months	8 weeks (as final dose) This dose only necessary for children aged 12 months–5 years who received 3 doses before age 12 months	
Inactivated Poliovirus[6]	6 wks	4 weeks	4 weeks	4 weeks[6]	
Measles, Mumps, Rubella[7]	12 mos	4 weeks			
Varicella[8]	12 mos	3 months			
Hepatitis A[9]	12 mos	6 months			

CATCH-UP SCHEDULE FOR PERSONS AGED 7–18 YEARS

Vaccine	Minimum Age for Dose 1	Dose 1 to Dose 2	Dose 2 to Dose 3	Dose 3 to Dose 4	
Tetanus, Diphtheria/ Tetanus, Diphtheria, Pertussis[10]	7 yrs[10]	4 weeks	8 weeks if first dose administered at age <12 months **6 months** if first dose administered at age ≥12 months	6 months if first dose administered at age <12 months	
Human Papillomavirus[11]	9 yrs	4 weeks	12 weeks		
Hepatitis A[9]	12 mos	6 months			
Hepatitis B[1]	Birth	4 weeks	8 weeks (and 16 weeks after first dose)		
Inactivated Poliovirus[6]	6 wks	4 weeks	4 weeks	4 weeks[6]	
Measles, Mumps, Rubella[7]	12 mos	4 weeks			
Varicella[8]	12 mos	4 weeks if first dose administered at age ≥13 years **3 months** if first dose administered at age <13 years			

1. Hepatitis B vaccine (HepB). *(Minimum age: birth)*
- Administer the 3-dose series to those who were not previously vaccinated.
- A 2-dose series of Recombivax HB® is licensed for children aged 11–15 years.

2. Rotavirus vaccine (Rota). *(Minimum age: 6 weeks)*
- Do not start the series later than age 12 weeks.
- Administer the final dose in the series by age 32 weeks. Do not administer a dose later than age 32 weeks.
- Data on safety and efficacy outside of these age ranges are insufficient.

3. Diphtheria and tetanus toxoids and acellular pertussis vaccine (DTaP). *(Minimum age: 6 weeks)*
- The fifth dose is not necessary if the fourth dose was administered at age ≥4 years.
- DTaP is not indicated for persons aged ≥7 years.

4. *Haemophilus influenzae* type b conjugate vaccine (Hib). *(Minimum age: 6 weeks)*
- Vaccine is not generally recommended for children aged ≥5 years.
- If current age <12 months and the first 2 doses were PRP-OMP (PedvaxHIB® or ComVax® [Merck]), the third (and final) dose should be administered at age 12–15 months and at least 8 weeks after the second dose.
- If first dose was administered at age 7–11 months, administer 2 doses separated by 4 weeks plus a booster at age 12–15 months.

5. Pneumococcal conjugate vaccine (PCV). *(Minimum age: 6 weeks)*
- Vaccine is not generally recommended for children aged ≥5 years.

6. Inactivated poliovirus vaccine (IPV). *(Minimum age: 6 weeks)*
- For children who received an all-IPV or all-oral poliovirus (OPV) series, a fourth dose is not necessary if third dose was administered at age ≥4 years.
- If both OPV and IPV were administered as part of a series, a total of 4 doses should be administered, regardless of the child's current age.

7. Measles, mumps, and rubella vaccine (MMR). *(Minimum age: 12 months)*
- The second dose of MMR is recommended routinely at age 4–6 years but may be administered earlier if desired.
- If not previously vaccinated, administer 2 doses of MMR during any visit with ≥4 weeks between the doses.

8. Varicella vaccine. *(Minimum age: 12 months)*
- The second dose of varicella vaccine is recommended routinely at age 4–6 years but may be administered earlier if desired.
- Do not repeat the second dose in persons aged <13 years if administered ≥28 days after the first dose.

9. Hepatitis A vaccine (HepA). *(Minimum age: 12 months)*
- HepA is recommended for certain groups of children, including in areas where vaccination programs target older children. See *MMWR* 2006;55(No. RR-7):1–23.

10. Tetanus and diphtheria toxoids vaccine (Td) and tetanus and diphtheria toxoids and acellular pertussis vaccine (Tdap). *(Minimum ages: 7 years for Td, 10 years for BOOSTRIX®, and 11 years for ADACEL™)*
- Tdap should be substituted for a single dose of Td in the primary catch-up series or as a booster if age appropriate; use Td for other doses.
- A 5-year interval from the last Td dose is encouraged when Tdap is used as a booster dose. A booster (fourth) dose is needed if any of the previous doses were administered at age <12 months. Refer to ACIP recommendations for further information. See *MMWR* 2006;55(No. RR-3).

11. Human papillomavirus vaccine (HPV). *(Minimum age: 9 years)*
- Administer the HPV vaccine series to females at age 13–18 years if not previously vaccinated.

Information about reporting reactions after immunization is available online at http://www.vaers.hhs.gov or by telephone via the 24-hour national toll-free information line 800-822-7967. Suspected cases of vaccine-preventable diseases should be reported to the state or local health department. Additional information, including precautions and contraindications for immunization, is available from the National Center for Immunization and Respiratory Diseases at http://www.cdc.gov/nip/default.htm or telephone, 800-CDC-INFO (800-232-4636).

DEPARTMENT OF HEALTH AND HUMAN SERVICES • CENTERS FOR DISEASE CONTROL AND PREVENTION • SAFER • HEALTHIER • PEOPLE

CS103164

Poisonings account for approximately 5 million injuries per year in the United States. Of these, 5,000 people die annually. Poisonings are responsible for 9 percent of all ambulance transports, 10 percent of all hospital emergency visits, and 5 percent of all hospital inpatient admissions. In children, many poisonings result from failure to store hazardous household substances and medications in a safe place. Poisons are often classified according to the body organ they primarily affect. The following table lists the specific antidotes for toxic substances.

Toxin	Antidote (s)
Acetaminophen	acetylcysteine (Mucomyst)
Anticholinergic agents (such as tricyclic antidepressants)	physostigmine salicylate (Antilirium)
Anticholinesterase agents (such as organophosphate insecticides)	pralidoxime chloride, PAM (Protopam Chloride)
Arsenic	dimercaprol (BAL in Oil)
Benzodiazepines	flumazenil (Romazicon)
Calcium and digitalis	edentate disodium (Endrate, Sodium Versenate)
Cholinergic agents	atropine
Cyanide	amyl nitrite, sodium thiosulfate
Digoxin	digoxin immune FAB (Digibind)
Folic acid antagonists (such as methotrexate)	leucovorin calcium
Gold	dimercaprol
Heparin	protamine sulfate
Ifosfamide	mesna (Mesnex)
Insulin	glucagon
Iron	deferoxamine mesylate (Desferal Mesylate)
Lead	edentate calcium disodium (Calcium Disodium Versenate), succimer (Chemet), dimercaprol, cuprimine
Mercury	dimercaprol
Narcotics (opiates)	naloxone HCl (Narcan), nalmefene HCl (Revex)
Warfarin	vitamin K

Reporting of Medical Errors

Medical errors can potentially cause great harm to patients. Hundreds of thousands of people die each year as a result of medical errors or accidents. Some studies have shown that medication errors account for 10 to 25 percent of all medical errors. The following form is used by the FDA to document adverse events related to medications, medical devices, and other medical products.

U.S. Department of Health and Human Services

MEDWATCH

The FDA Safety Information and
Adverse Event Reporting Program

For VOLUNTARY reporting of
adverse events, product problems and
product use errors

Page ____ of ____

Form Approved: OMB No. 0910-0291, Expires: 10/31/08
See OMB statement on reverse.

FDA USE ONLY

Triage unit
sequence #

A. PATIENT INFORMATION

1. Patient Identifier

In confidence

2. Age at Time of Event, or
Date of Birth:

3. Sex
☐ Female
☐ Male

4. Weight
____ lb
or
____ kg

B. ADVERSE EVENT, PRODUCT PROBLEM OR ERROR

Check all that apply:

1. ☐ Adverse Event   ☐ Product Problem *(e.g., defects/malfunctions)*
☐ Product Use Error   ☐ Problem with Different Manufacturer of Same Medicine

2. Outcomes Attributed to Adverse Event
(Check all that apply)

☐ Death: _____
(mm/dd/yyyy)
☐ Life-threatening
☐ Hospitalization - initial or prolonged
☐ Required Intervention to Prevent Permanent Impairment/Damage (Devices)

☐ Disability or Permanent Damage
☐ Congenital Anomaly/Birth Defect
☐ Other Serious (Important Medical Events)

3. Date of Event *(mm/dd/yyyy)*   4. Date of this Report *(mm/dd/yyyy)*

5. Describe Event, Problem or Product Use Error

6. Relevant Tests/Laboratory Data, Including Dates

7. Other Relevant History, Including Preexisting Medical Conditions *(e.g., allergies, race, pregnancy, smoking and alcohol use, liver/kidney problems, etc.)*

PLEASE TYPE OR USE BLACK INK

C. PRODUCT AVAILABILITY

Product Available for Evaluation? *(Do not send product to FDA)*

☐ Yes   ☐ No   ☐ Returned to Manufacturer on: _____
(mm/dd/yyyy)

D. SUSPECT PRODUCT(S)

1. Name, Strength, Manufacturer *(from product label)*
#1
#2

2. Dose or Amount   Frequency   Route
#1
#2

3. Dates of Use *(If unknown, give duration) from/to (or best estimate)*
#1
#2

5. Event Abated After Use
Stopped or Dose Reduced?
#1 ☐ Yes ☐ No ☐ Doesn't Apply
#2 ☐ Yes ☐ No ☐ Doesn't Apply

4. Diagnosis or Reason for Use *(Indication)*
#1
#2

8. Event Reappeared After
Reintroduction?
#1 ☐ Yes ☐ No ☐ Doesn't Apply
#2 ☐ Yes ☐ No ☐ Doesn't Apply

6. Lot #   7. Expiration Date
#1   #1
#2   #2

9. NDC # or Unique ID

E. SUSPECT MEDICAL DEVICE

1. Brand Name

2. Common Device Name

3. Manufacturer Name, City and State

4. Model #   Lot #   5. Operator of Device
☐ Health Professional
Catalog #   Expiration Date *(mm/dd/yyyy)*   ☐ Lay User/Patient
Serial #   Other #   ☐ Other: _____

6. If Implanted, Give Date *(mm/dd/yyyy)*   7. If Explanted, Give Date *(mm/dd/yyyy)*

8. Is this a Single-use Device that was Reprocessed and Reused on a Patient?
☐ Yes   ☐ No

9. If Yes to Item No. 8, Enter Name and Address of Reprocessor

F. OTHER (CONCOMITANT) MEDICAL PRODUCTS

Product names and therapy dates *(exclude treatment of event)*

G. REPORTER *(See confidentiality section on back)*

1. Name and Address

Phone #   E-mail

2. Health Professional?   3. Occupation   4. Also Reported to:
☐ Yes ☐ No   ☐ Manufacturer
☐ User Facility
5. If you do NOT want your identity disclosed
to the manufacturer, place an "X" in this box: ☐   ☐ Distributor/Importer

FORM FDA 3500 (10/05)   Submission of a report does not constitute an admission that medical personnel or the product caused or contributed to the event.

ADVICE ABOUT VOLUNTARY REPORTING

Detailed instructions available at: http://www.fda.gov/medwatch/report/consumer/instruct.htm

Report adverse events, product problems or product use errors with:

- Medications *(drugs or biologics)*
- Medical devices *(including in-vitro diagnostics)*
- Combination products *(medication & medical devices)*
- Human cells, tissues, and cellular and tissue-based products
- Special nutritional products *(dietary supplements, medical foods, infant formulas)*
- Cosmetics

Report product problems - quality, performance or safety concerns such as:

- Suspected counterfeit product
- Suspected contamination
- Questionable stability
- Defective components
- Poor packaging or labeling
- Therapeutic failures (product didn't work)

Report SERIOUS adverse events. An event is serious when the patient outcome is:

- Death
- Life-threatening
- Hospitalization - initial or prolonged
- Disability or permanent damage
- Congenital anomaly/birth defect
- Required intervention to prevent permanent impairment or damage
- Other serious (important medical events)

Report even if:

- You're not certain the product caused the event
- You don't have all the details

How to report:

- Just fill in the sections that apply to your report
- Use section D for all products except medical devices
- Attach additional pages if needed
- Use a separate form for each patient
- Report either to FDA or the manufacturer *(or both)*

Other methods of reporting:

- 1-800-FDA-0178 -- To FAX report
- 1-800-FDA-1088 -- To report by phone
- www.fda.gov/medwatch/report.htm -- To report online

If your report involves a serious adverse event with a device and it occurred in a facility outside a doctor's office, that facility may be legally required to report to FDA and/or the manufacturer. Please notify the person in that facility who would handle such reporting.

If your report involves a serious adverse event with a vaccine call 1-800-822-7967 to report.

Confidentiality: The patient's identity is held in strict confidence by FDA and protected to the fullest extent of the law. FDA will not disclose the reporter's identity in response to a request from the public, pursuant to the Freedom of Information Act. The reporter's identity, including the identity of a self-reporter, may be shared with the manufacturer unless requested otherwise.

-Fold Here-   -Fold Here-

FORM FDA 3500 (10/05) (Back)   Please Use Address Provided Below -- Fold in Thirds, Tape and Mail

---

DEPARTMENT OF
HEALTH & HUMAN SERVICES

Public Health Service
Food and Drug Administration
Rockville, MD 20857

Official Business
Penalty for Private Use $300

NO POSTAGE
NECESSARY
IF MAILED
IN THE
UNITED STATES
OR APO/FPO

BUSINESS REPLY MAIL
FIRST CLASS MAIL   PERMIT NO. 946   ROCKVILLE MD

MEDWATCH
The FDA Safety Information and Adverse Event Reporting Program
Food and Drug Administration
5600 Fishers Lane
Rockville, MD 20852-9787

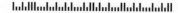

Drug/Food Interactions

A. DRUGS THAT SHOULD BE TAKEN WHILE FASTING

Alendronate
Ampicillin
AzoGantanol/Gantrisin
Bacampicillin
Bethanechol (may experience N&V)
Bisacodyl
Calcium carbonate
Captopril
Carbenicillin
Castor oil
Chloramphenicol
Claritin
Cyclosporine gel caps only
  (avoid fatty meals)
Demeclocycline (avoid high
  calcium foods/dairy products)
Dicloxacillin
Digoxin (avoid high fiber
  cereals and oatmeal)
Disopyramide
Digitalis preparations (not
  with high fiber foods)
Erythromycin base/estolate
Etidronate
Ferrous salts (not with tea,
  coffee, egg, cereals,
  fiber, or milk)
Fexofenadine
Flavoxate
Furosemide
Isoniazid
Isosorbide dinitrate
Ketoprofen (if GI distress
  occurs, may take with food)
Lansoprazole
  Levodopa (not with high protein
  foods; meals delay absorption and
  peak plasma concentration;
  avoid caffeine)
Lisinopril
Lomustine (empty stomach will
  reduce nausea)
Methotrexate (milk, cream, or yogurt
  may decrease absorption)
Methyldopa (not with high protein
foods; meals delay absorption and
peak plasma concentration;
avoid caffeine)
Nafcillin (inactivated by
  stomach acid; absorption variable
  with/without food)
Nalidixic acid
Naltrexone
Norfloxacin (milk, cream,
  or yogurt may decrease
  absorption)
Oxytetracycline (avoid dairy products
  and foods high in calcium)
Penicillamine (antacids, iron,
  and food decreases absorption)
Penicillin
Phenytoin (if GI distress occurs,
  may take with food; food effect
  depends on preparation)
Propantheline
Rifampicin
Sotalol
Sulfamethoxazole
Tetracycline (avoid dairy
  products and foods
  high in calcium)
Theophylline (absorption
  of controlled release varies
  by preparation)
Thyroid hormone preparations
  (limit foods containing goitrogens)
Terbutaline sulfate
Trientine (antacids, iron,
  and food reduces absorption)
Trimethoprim
Zyrtec

B. DRUGS THAT SHOULD BE TAKEN WITH FOOD

Allopurinol (after meal)
Atovaquone
Augmentin
Aspirin
Amiodarone
Baclofen
Bromocriptine
Buspirone
Carbamazepine (erratic absorption)
Carvedilol
Cefpodoxime
Chloroquine
Chlorothiazide
Cimetidine
Clofazimine
Diclofenac
Divalproex
Doxycyline
Felbamate
Fenofibrate (TriCor)
Fiorinal
Fludrocortisone
Fenoprofen
Gemfibrozil
Glyburide
Griseofulvin (high fat meals)
Hydrocortisone
Hydroxychloroquine (Plaquenil)
Indomethacin
Iron products
Isotretinoin
Itraconazole capsules
Ketorolac
Labetalol
Lithium
Lovastatin
Mebendazole
Methenamine
Methylprednisolone
Metoprolol
Metronidazole
Misoprostol
Metoprolol
Naltrexone
Naproxen
Nelfinavir (Viracept)
Niacin
Nifedipine (grapefruit juice
  increases bioavailability)
Nitrofurantoin
Olsalazine
Oxcarbazepine
Pentoxifylline
Pergolide
Piroxicam
Potassium salts
Prednisone
Probucol (high fat meals)

Procainamide
Propranolol
Ritonavir
Salsalate
Saquinavir
Sevelamer
Spironolactone
Sulfasalazine
Sulfinpyrazone
Sulindac
Ticlopidine
Tolmetin
Trazodone
Verapamil SR (absorption varies by
  manufacturer; too rapid absorption
  may cause heart block)

C. CONSTIPATING AGENTS

Antacids
Anticholinergic drugs
Anticonvulsants
Antihistamines
Antiparkinsonian drugs
BP meds (calcium channel blockers)
Clonidine
Corticosteroids
Diuretics
Ganglionic blocking agents
Iron supplements
Laxatives (when abused)
Lithium
MAO Inhibitors
Muscle relaxants
NSAIDs
Octreotide
Opioids
Phenothiazines
Prostaglandin synthesis inhibitors
Tranquilizers
Tricyclic antidepressants

D. DIARRHEAL AGENTS

Adrenergic neuron blockers:
  reserpine, guanethidine
Antacids (Mg containing)
  H_2 receptor antagonists
  (i.e., ranitidine) PPIs

(i.e, Omeprazole)
Antiarrhythmics (i.e., quinidine)
Antibiotics (especially
  broad spectrum agents)
Antihypertensives (beta blockers,
  ACE Inhibitors)
Anti-inflammatory drugs
  (NSAIDs, colchicine)
Chemotherapy agents
Cholinergic agonists and
  cholinesterase inhibitors
Glucophage
Metoclopramide
Misoprostol
Osmotic and stimulant laxatives
Theophylline

E. TYRAMINE CONTAINING FOODS

Moderate amounts of tyramine:
Banana peel
Broad beans
Cheese (all except cream
  cheese and cottage cheese)
Chianti, vermouth
Concentrated yeast extracts/
  Brewer's yeast
Fermented cabbage products:
  sauerkraut, kimchee
Fermented soy products:
  fermented bean curd,
  soya bean paste, miso soup
Hydrolyzed protein extracts for
  sauces, soups, gravies
Imitation cheese
Liquid and powdered protein
  supplements
Meat extracts
Nonalcoholic beers
Prepared meats (sausage, chopped
  liver, pate, salami, mortadella)
Raspberries
Some non-United States
  brands of beer
Yeast products

Significant amounts of tyramine:
Avocado
Chocolate

Cream from fresh pasteurized milk
Distilled spirits
Peanuts
Red and white wines, port wines
Soy sauce
Yogurt

F. FOODS CONTAINING GOITROGENS

Asparagus
Brocolli
Brussels sprouts
Cabbage
Cauliflower
Kale
Lettuce
Millet
Mustard
Other leafy green vegetables
Peaches
Peanuts
Peas
Radishes
Rutabaga
Soy beans
Spinach
Strawberries
Turnip greens
Watercress

G. COUMARIN ANTICOAGULANTS AND DIETARY EFFECTS

Consumption of vitamin K-enriched foods may counteract the effects of anticoagulants since the drugs act through antagonism of vitamin K. Advise client on anticoagulants to maintain a steady, consistent intake of vitamin K-containing foods. The drug monograph for warfarin clearly lists these foods. Additionally, certain herbal teas (green tea, buckeye, horse chestnut, Woodruff, tonka beans, melitot) contain natural coumarins that can potentiate the effects of coumadin and should be

avoided. Large amounts of avocado also potentiate the drug's effects. Brussels sprouts, broccoli, spinach, kale, turnip greens, and other cruciferous vegetables increase the catabolism of warfarin thereby decreasing its anticoagulant activities. Caffeinated beverages (i.e., cola, coffee, tea, hot chocolate, chocolate milk) can affect therapy. Alcohol intake of more than three drinks per day can affect clotting times. Herbal supplements can also affect bleeding time: Coenzyme Q10 is structurally similar to vitamin K, feverfew, garlic, and ginseng. Avoid herbal medications while on warfarin therapy.

H. GENERAL DRUG CLASS RECOMMENDATIONS

ACE inhibitors: Take captopril and moexipril 1 h before or 2 h after meals; food decreases absorption. Avoid high potassium foods as ACE increases K^+.

Analgesic/Antipyretic: Take on an empty stomach as food may slow the absorption.

Antacids: Take 1 h after or between meals. Avoid dairy foods as the protein in them can increase stomach acid.

Anti-anxiety agents: Caffeine may cause excitability, nervousness, and hyperactivity lessening the anti-anxiety drug effects.

Antibiotics: Penicillin generally should be taken on an empty stomach; may take with food if GI upset occurs. Do not mix with acidic foods: coffee, citrus fruits, and tomatoes; the acid interferes with absorption of penicillin, ampicillin, erythromycin and cloxacillin.

Anticoagulants: High vitamin K produces blood-clotting substance and may reduce drug effectiveness. Vitamin E >400 IU may prolong clotting time and increase bleeding risk.

Antidepressant drugs: May be taken with or without food.

Antifungals: Avoid taking with dairy products; avoid alcohol.

Antihistamines: Take on an empty stomach to increase effectiveness.

Bronchodilators with theophylline: High-fat meals may increase bio-availability while high-carbohydrate meals may decrease it. Food increases absorption of Theo-24 and Uniphyl which may cause increased N&V, headache, and irritability.

Cephalosporins: Take on an empty stomach 1 h before or 2 h after meals. May take with food if GI upset occurs.

Diuretics: Vary in interactions; some cause loss of potassium, calcium, and magnesium. Avoid salty food and natural black licorice as these increase K and Mg losses. Large doses of vitamin D can elevate blood pressure.

H_2 blockers: May take with or without regard to food.

HMG-CoA reductase inhibitors: Take lovastatin with the evening meal to enhance absorption.

Laxatives: Avoid dairy foods as calcium can decrease absorption.

Macrolides: Take on an empty stomach 1 h before or 2 h after meals. May take with food for GI upset.

MAO inhibitors: Have many dietary restrictions, so follow dietary guidelines as prescribed. Foods or alcoholic beverages containing tyramine may cause a fatal increase in BP.

Narcotic analgesics: Avoid alcohol as it may increase sedative effects.

Nitroimadazole (metronidazole): Avoid alcohol or food prepared with alcohol for at least three days after finishing the medicine. Alcohol may cause nausea, abdominal cramps, vomiting, headaches, and flushing.

NSAIDs: Take with food or milk to prevent irritation of the stomach.

Quinolones: Take on an empty stomach 1 h before or 2 h after meals. May take with food for GI upset but avoid calcium containing foods such as milk, yogurt, vitamins/minerals containing iron and antacids because they decrease drug concentrations. Caffeine containing products may lead to excitability and nervousness.

Sulfonamides: Take on an empty stomach 1 h before or 2 h after meals. May take with food if GI upset occurs.

Tetracyclines: Take on an empty stomach 1 h before or 2 h after meals. May take with food but avoid dairy products, antacids, and vitamins containing iron with tetracycline.

Reprinted from Spratto, G. and Woods, A. (2009) Delmar Nurse's Drug Handbook. Delmar, Cengage Learning: Clifton Park, NY.

Drugs That Should not Be Crushed

As a rule of thumb, any sustained-release or extended-release formulation should never be crushed. Instead, attempt to get a liquid formulation of the product so that it can be administered in that form. Coated products also should not be crushed. They were coated for a specific purpose, e.g., to prevent stomach irritation by the product, to prevent destruction of the product by stomach acid, to prevent an unwanted reaction, or to produce a prolonged or an extended effect.

These are some of the drugs that should not be crushed:

Accutane®
Aciphex®
Adalat cc SR®
Advicor ER®
Afrinol Repetab®
Allerest® capsule
Allegra D®
Aminodur Duratab®
Artane Sequel®
Arthrotec®
ASA E.C.®
ASA Enseal®
Augmentin XR®
Azulfadine Entab®
Betaphen-VK®
Biaxin XL®
Biscodyl EC®
Calan SR®
Cardizem LA, SR®
Ceclor CD®
Ceftin®
Chlortrimeton SR®
Choledyl SR®
Cipro XR®
Claritin-D®
Colace®
Colestid®
Compazine Spansule®
Concerta SR®
Creon EC®
Depakote ER®
Desyrel®
Dexedrine SR®
Diamox Sequel®
Dilacor XR®
Dimetapp SR®

Ditropan XL®
Donnatal Extentab®
Drixoral® tablet
Ecotrin® tablet
Effexor XR®
E-Mycin® tablet
Entex LA®
Erythromycin EC®
Feldene®
Feosol Spansule®
Feosol® tablet
Ferro Grad-500® tablet
Flomax®
Glucophage XR®
Glucatrol XL®
Humibid DM, LA®
Imdur SR, LA®
Indocin SR®
Isoptin SR®
Isordil® sublingual
Isordil Tembids®, Dinitrate
Kaon® tablet
K-Dur®, K-tab®
Klor-Con®
Levbid SR®
Lithobid SR®
Macrobid SR®
Mestinon Timespans®
Metadate CD, SR®
MS Contin®
Mucinex®
Nexium®
Niaspan®
Nitroglycerin® tablet
Nitrospan® capsule
Norpace CR®

Ornade Spansule®
OxyContin®
Pancrease EC, MT®
Paxil CR®
Pentosa®
Phazyme®
Plendil SR®
Prevacid®
Prilosec SR®
Procardia XL®
Protonix®
Proventil Repetabs®
Prozac weekly®
Quinaglute Duratab®
Quinidex Extenutab®
Slow K® tablet; Slow Mag®, Slow Fe®
Sorbitrate
Sudafed SA® capsule
Tegretol XR®
Teldrin® capsule
Tenuate Dospan®
Tessalon Perles®
Theobid Duracaps®
Theolair SR®
Thorazine Spansules®
Tiazac SR®
Toprol XL®
Trental SR®
Tylenol ER®
Uniphyl SR®
Verelan PM®
Volmax SR®
Voltaren EC®
Voltaren SR®
Wellbutrin SR®

Xanax SR®
Zerit XR®
Zomig ZMT®
Zyban®
Zyrtec-D®

Reprinted from Spratto, G. and Woods, A. (2009) Delmar Nurse's Drug Handbook. Delmar, Cengage Learning: Clifton Park, NY.

ACARBOSE
Precose
BAYER
*Antidiabetic, oral;
alpha-glucosidase inhibitor*

25 mg 50 mg 100 mg

ACETAMINOPHEN AND HYDROCODONE BITARTRATE
Vicodin
ABBOTT
Analgesic

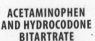
500 mg / 5 mg

Vicodin ES
ABBOTT

7.5 / 750 mg

Vicodin HP
ABBOTT

10 mg / 660 mg

ACETAMINOPHEN AND OXYCODONE HCl
Percocet
ENDO
Analgesic

325 mg / 2.5 mg

325 mg / 5 mg

325 mg / 7.5 mg

325 mg / 10 mg

500 mg / 7.5 mg

650 mg / 10 mg

ALENDRONATE SODIUM
Fosamax
MERCK
*Bone growth regulator,
biphosphonate*

5 mg

10 mg 35 mg

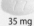 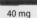
40 mg 70 mg

AMLODIPINE AND BENAZEPRIL
Lotrel
NOVARTIS
Calcium channel blocker

2.5 mg

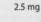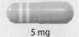
5 mg

10 mg

AMPHETAMINE MIXTURES
Adderall XR
SHIRE
CNS stimulant

5 mg

ATENOLOL
Tenormin
ASTRAZENECA
Beta-adrenergic blocking agent

ATOMOXETINE HCl
Strattera
ELI LILLY
*Antidepressant, selective
serotonin reuptake inhibitor*

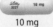
10 mg

18 mg

 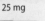
25 mg

40 mg

60 mg

BENAZEPRIL HCl
Lotensin
NOVARTIS
Antihypertensive, ACE inhibitor

5 mg 10 mg

20 mg 40 mg

Lotensin HCT
NOVARTIS

5 mg

Lotensin HCT
NOVARTIS

10 mg

Lotensin HCT
NOVARTIS

20 mg

BUDESONIDE
Pulmicort Respules
ASTRAZENECA
Glucocorticoid

CANDESARTAN CILEXETIL
Atacand
ASTRAZENECA LP
*Antihypertensive, angiotensin II
receptor blocker*

CAPECITABINE
Xeloda
LA ROCHE
Antineoplastic, antimetabolite

150 mg

500 mg

CARBAMAZEPINE
Tegretol
NOVARTIS
Anticonvulsant

 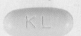
100 mg 200 mg

CEPHALEXIN HCl MONOHYDRATE
Keflex
ADVANCIS
Cephalosporin, first generation

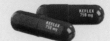
750 mg

CIPROFLOXACIN HCl
Cipro
BAYER
Antibiotic, fluoroquinolone

100 mg 250 mg

500 mg

750 mg

Cipro XR
BAYER

500 mg

Cipro XR
BAYER

1000 mg

CLARITHROMYCIN
Biaxin
ABBOTT
Antibiotic, macrolide

250 mg

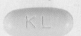
500 mg

Biaxin XL
ABBOTT

500 mg

CLONAZEPAM
Klonopin
LA ROCHE
Anticonvulsant

  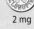
0.5 mg 1 mg 2 mg

CYCLOBENZAPRINE HCI

Flexeril
MERCK

Skeletal muscle relaxant, centrally acting

DEXMETHYLPHENIDATE HCI

Focalin
NOVARTIS

CNS stimulant

2.5 mg

5 mg

10 mg

DIAZEPAM

Valium
LA ROCHE

Antianxiety, benzodiazepine

2 mg

5 mg

10 mg

DICLOFENAC SODIUM

Voltaren
NOVARTIS

Non steroidal anti-inflammatory

25 mg   50 mg   75 mg

ESOMEPRAZOLE MG

Nexium
ASTRAZENECA

Proton pump inhibitor

20 mg

EZETIMIBE

Zetia
MERCK

Antihyperlipidemic, HMG-CoA reductase inhibitor

FELODIPINE

Plendil
ASTRAZENECA

Calcium channel blocker

FENOFIBRATE

Tricor
ABBOTT

Antihyperlipidemic

48 mg

145 mg

FINASTERIDE

Proscar
ABBOTT

Androgen hormone inhibitor

5 mg

FLUOXETINE HCI

Prozac
ELI- LILLY

Antidepressant, selective serotonin reuptake inhibitor

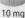
10 mg

20 mg

FLUVASTATIN SODIUM

Lescol
NOVARTIS

Antihyperlipidemic, HMG-CoA reductase inhibitor

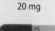
20 mg

40 mg

GRANISETRON HCI

Kytril
LA ROCHE

Antiemetic, 5-HT3 receptor antagonist

1 mg

HYDROCODONE BITARTRATE/ HOMATROPINE METHYBROMIDE

Hycodan
ENDO

Analgesic

KETOROLAC

Toradol oral
LA ROCHE

Nonsteroidal anti-inflammatory

10 mg

LEVOTHYROXINE SODIUM (T4)

Levoxyl
KING

Thyroid product

23 mg   50 mg

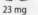
75 mg   88 mg

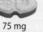
100 mg   112 mg

125 mg   137 mg

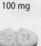
150 mg   175 mg

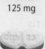
200 mg   300 mg

LEVOTHYROXINE SODIUM (T4)

Synthroid
ABBOTT

Thyroid product

LISINOPRIL

Prinivil
MERCK

Antihypertensive, ACE inhibitor

2.5 mg

---

5 mg

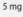
10 mg

20 mg

40 mg

LISINOPRIL

Zestril
ASTRAZENECA

Antihypertensive, ACE inhibitor

LOPINAVIR/RITONAVIR

Kaletra
ABBOTT

HIV protease inhibitor

LOSARTAN HCTZ

Hyzaar
MERCK

Angiotensin II receptor antagonist and diuretic

LOSARTAN POTASSIUM

Cozaar
MERCK

Antihypertensive, angiotensin II receptor blocker

25 mg

50 mg

100 mg

LOVASTATIN

Mevacor
MERCK

Antihyperlipidemic, HMG-CoA reductase inhibitor

10 mg

---

20 mg

40 mg

METAXALONE

Skelaxin
KING

Muscle relaxant

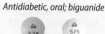

METFORMIN

Fortamet
FIRST HORIZON

Antidiabetic, oral; biguanide

METHYLPHENIDATE HCI

Ritalin
NOVARTIS

CNS stimulant

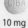
5 mg

10 mg

20 mg

METOPROLOL SUCCINATE

Toprol
ASTRAZENECA

Beta-adrenergic blocking agent

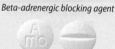

METOPROLOL TARTRATE

Lopressor
NOVARTIS

Beta-adrenergic blocking agent

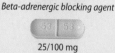
25/100 mg

50/100 mg

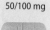
50 mg

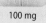
100 mg

MONTELUKAST SODIUM

Singulair
MERCK

*Antiasthmatic, leukotriene
receptor antagonist*

MOXIFLOXACIN HCl

Avelox
BAYER

Antibiotic, fluoroquinolone

NAPROXEN

Naprosyn
LA ROCHE

Nonsteroidal anti-inflammatory

NAPROXEN SODIUM

Anaprox
LA ROCHE

Nonsteroidal anti-inflammatory

NITROFURANTOIN

Macrobid
PROCTOR AND GAMBLE

Antibiotic

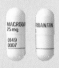

NITROFURANTOIN

Macrodantin
PROCTOR AND GAMBLE

Antibiotic

OLANZAPINE

Zyprexa
ELI LILLY

Antipsychotic

2.5 mg

5 mg

7.5 mg

10 mg

15 mg

20 mg

Zyprexa Zydia
ELI LILLY

15 mg

Zyprexa Zydia
ELI LILLY

20 mg

OSELTAMIVIR PHOSPHATE

Tamiflu
LA ROCHE

Antiviral

75 mg

QUETIAPINE FUMARATE

Seroquel
ASTRAZENECA

Antipsychotic

OXYCODONE AND
ACETAMINOPHEN

Endocet
ENDO

Analgesic

5 mg / 325 mg

7.5 mg / 325 mg

10 mg / 325 mg

7.5 mg / 500 mg

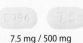
10 mg / 650 mg

POTASSIUM SALTS

Klor-con and Klor-con M20
UPSHER SMITH

Electrolyte

RALOXIFENE HCl

Evista
ELI LILLY

Estrogen receptor modulator

RISEDRONATE SODIUM

Actonel
PROCTOR AND GAMBLE

*Bone growth regulator,
biphosphonate*

5 mg

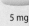
5 mg

30 mg

RIVASTIGMINE TARTRATE

Exelon
NOVARTIS

Treatment of Alzheimer's Disease

1 mg

3 mg

4.5 mg

6 mg

RIZATRIPTAN BENZOATE

Maxalt
MERCK

5 mg

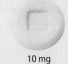
10 mg

Maxalt MLT
MERCK

5 mg

Maxalt MLT
MERCK

Antimigraine

10 mg

ROFECOXIB

Vioxx
MERCK

*Nonsteroidal anti-inflammatory;
COX-2 inhibitor*

ROSUVASTATIN

Crestor
ASTRAZENECA

*Antihyperlipidemic, HMG-CoA
reductase inhibitor*

SIMVASTATIN

Zocor
MERCK

*Antihyperlipidemic, HMG-CoA
reductase inhibitor*

5 mg

10 mg

20 mg

40 mg

80 mg

SPIRONOLACTONE

Aldactone
MYLAN

Diuretic, potassium-sparing

TAMOXIFEN CITRATE

Nolvadex
ASTRAZENECA

Antiestrogen

TEGASEROD MALEATE

Zelnorm
NOVARTIS

*Drug for irritable bowel
syndrome in women*

5 mg   **6 mg**

TEMAZEPAM

Restoril
MALLINCKRODT
*Sedative-hypnotic,
benzodiazepine*

7.5 mg

15 mg

22.5 mg

30 mg

TRIAMTERENE AND HYDROCHLOROTHIAZIDE

Maxide
MYLAN

*Antihypertensive,
combination drug*

VALGANCICLOVIR HCl

Valcyte
LA ROCHE
Antiviral

20 mg

ZAFIRLUKAST

Accolate
ASTRAZENECA
Antiasthmatic

ZOLMITRIPTAN

Zomig
ASTRAZENECA
Antimigraine

Used under license from Bayer: Precose , Cipro, Avelox.

Abbott Laboratories: Vicodin, Biaxin, Tricor, Synthroid, Kaletra.

Endo Pharmaceuticals: Percocet, Hycodan, Endocet.

Used with permission of Merck & Co. Inc.: Fosamax, Flexeril, Proscar, Prinvil, Hyzaar, Cozaar, Mevacor, Maxalt, Vioxx, Zocor.

Used with permission of Merck/Schering-Plough Pharmaceuticals: Zetia.

Novartis Pharmaceuticals: Lotrel, Lotensin, Tegretol, Focalin, Voltaren, Lescol, Ritalin, Lopressor, Singulair, Exelon, Zelnorm.

Shire Pharmaceuticals: Adderall XR.

AstraZeneca: Atenolol, Pulmicort, Atacand, Nexium, Plendil, Zestril, Toprol XL, Seroquel, Crestor, Nolvadex, Accolate, Zomig.

© Copyright Eli Lilly and Company. All rights reserved. Used with permission. ® Evista, Prozac, Strattera, and Zyprexa are registered trademarks of Eli Lilly and Company.

Reprinted with Permission of Roche Laboratories Inc. All rights reserved: Xeloda, Klonopin, Valium, Kytril, Toradol, Naprosyn, Anaprox, Anaprox DS, Tamiflu, Valcyte.

Advancis: Keflex.

King Pharmaceuticals: Levaxyl.

First Horizon: Fortamet.

Proctor and Gamble: Macrobid, Macrodantin, Actonel.

Upsher Smith: Klor-Con, Klor-Con MZO.

Mallinckrodt Inc.: Restoril.

A

Absence seizure – generalized seizure that does not involve motor convulsions; also referred to as "petit mal"

Absorption – the movement of a drug from its site of administration into the bloodstream

Acetylcholine – a neurotransmitter that plays a major role in cognitive function and memory formation as well as motor control

Acquired Immunodeficiency Syndrome (AIDS) – a severe immunological disorder caused by the retrovirus HIV, resulting in a defect in cell-mediated immune response

Acromegaly – overdevelopment of the bones of the head, face, and feet

Active transport – a process that moves particles in fluid through membranes from a region of lower concentration to a region of high concentration

Acute pain – pain that is of sudden onset and brief course; can also mean "severe"

Adrenergic blocker agents – drugs that antagonize the secretion of epinephrine and norepinephrine from sympathetic terminal neurons; also known as sympatholytics

Adrenergic receptor – receptors that mediate responses to epinephrine (adrenaline) and norepinephrine

Adrenocorticotropic hormone (ACTH) – another hormone from the anterior pituitary gland that stimulates the growth of the adrenal gland cortex and the secretion of corticosteroids

Adrenogenital syndrome – congenital adrenal hyperplasia; a group of disorders involving steroid hormone production in the adrenal glands, leading to a deficiency of cortisol

Adsorbent agents – drugs with the ability to adsorb gases, toxins, and bacteria

Affinity – the force that impels certain atoms to unite with certain others

Aggregation – the clumping together of platelets to form a clot

Agonist – the drug that produces a functional change in a cell

Agonist-antagonists – agents that can initiate or resist actions

Allergic rhinitis – inflammation of the nasal mucosa that is due to the sensitivity of the nasal tissue to an allergen

Allergy – a state of hypersensitivity induced by exposure to a particular antigen

Alopecia – loss of hair from anywhere on the body, sometimes until complete baldness is reached

Alpha-receptors – an adrenergic receptor; there are two types: alpha$_1$ and alpha$_2$

Alzheimer's disease – a disorder causing severe cognitive dysfunction in older persons in which the brain experiences atrophy (shrinkage) and exhibits senile plaques

Amebicides and trichomonacides – drugs use to treat amebic and trichomonal infections

Amenorrhea – the absence of a menstrual period in a woman of reproductive age

Analgesic – a compound that relieves pain by altering perception without producing anesthesia or loss of consciousness

Anaphylactic reaction – a severe, life-threatening allergic reaction to a drug

Anaphylactic shock – a severe and sometimes fatal allergic reaction

Androgen – the generic term for any natural or synthetic compound, usually a steroid hormone, that stimulates or controls the development of masculine characteristics by binding to androgen receptors

Anesthesia – a loss of feeling or sensation

Anesthetic – an agent that partially or completely numbs or eliminates sensitivity with or without loss of consciousness

Angina pectoris – an episodic, reversible oxygen insufficiency

Angiotensin II receptor antagonists – drugs that block the binding of angiotensin II to the angiotensin II type 1 receptor

Angiotensin-converting enzyme inhibitors – drugs that competitively inhibit conversion of angiotensin I to angiotensin II, a potent vasoconstrictor, through the angiotensin-converting enzyme activity, with resultant lower levels of angiotensin II

Anorexia nervosa – an eating disorder characterized by a psychological fear of being overweight; view of body image is distorted

Antacids – neutralize hydrochloric acid and raise gastric pH, thus inhibiting pepsin (a gastric enzyme)

Antagonist – the drug blocks a functional change in the cell

Antianxiety agents – drugs that relieve anxiety; also known as anxiolytics

Antibiotics – substances that have the ability to destroy or interfere with the development of a living organism

Anticoagulants – agents used to prevent the formation of a blood clot

Anticonvulsant – a drug that prevents or stops a convulsive seizure

Antidepressants – drugs used to treat depression

Antidiuretic hormone (ADH) – released when the body is low on water, and causes the kidneys to conserve water, but not salt, by concentrating the urine and reducing urine volume

Antiemetic – a drug that stops vomiting

Antigen – a substance that is introduced into the body and induces the formation of antibodies

Antihistamines – drugs that counteract the action of histamine

Antimalarial agents – drugs used to treat malaria infections

Antimetabolite – a substance that is produced to alter the actions of liver enzymes

Antimetabolites – prevent cancer cell growth by affecting its DNA production

Antimicrobial – an anti-infective drug produced from synthetic substances

Antineoplastic agents – used to treat cancers or malignant neoplasms

Antiplatelet agents – drugs that inhibit normal platelet function, usually by reducing their ability to aggregate and inappropriately form blood clots

Antipsychotic drugs – the major therapeutic modality for psychotic disorders; also known as neuroleptic drugs

Antithyroid drug – a chemical agent that lowers the basal metabolic rate by interfering with the formation, release, or action of thyroid hormones

Antitussives – agents that relieve or prevent coughing

Anuria – inability to produce urine

Anxiety – state of apprehension and autonomic nervous system activation resulting from exposure to a nonspecific or unknown cause

Anxiolytics – drugs that relieve anxiety; also known as antianxiety agents

Apnea – the cessation of respiration for more than 20 seconds with or without cyanosis, hypotonia, or bradycardia

Aromatic water – a mixture of distilled water with an aromatic volatile oil

Arrhythmias – deviations from the normal pattern of the heartbeat; also called dysrhythmias

Arteriosclerosis – degenerative changes in small arteries, commonly occurring in older individuals and diabetics; walls of arteries lose elasticity and become thick and hard

Articular – related to the joints of the body

Ascorbic acid – a water-soluble vitamin that is essential for the formation of collagen and fibroid tissue for teeth, bones, cartilage, connective tissue, and skin; also known as vitamin C

Asthma – a chronic inflammatory disorder of the airways of the respiratory system

Ataxia – loss of the ability to coordinate muscular movement

Atheromas – plaques consisting of lipids, cells, and cell debris, often with attached thrombi, which form inside the walls of large arteries

Atherosclerosis – disease of the arteries characterized by the presence of atheromas (plaques consisting of lipids, cells, and cell debris, often with attached thrombi, which form inside the walls of large arteries)

Atrophy – wasting away or "without development"

B

Bacteremia – a condition in which bacteria are recovered from blood cultures of a patient and may or may not be associated with the disease

Bacteria – small, one-celled microorganisms that lack a true nucleus or mechanism to provide metabolism

Bactericidal – killing bacterial growth

Bacteriostatic – suppress bacterial growth by triggering a mechanism that blocks folic acid synthesis, thereby forcing bacteria to synthesize their own folic acid

Barbiturates – drugs that depress multiple aspects of central nervous system function and can be used for sleep, seizures, and general anesthesia

Basal nuclei – clusters of nerve cells at the base of the brain; responsible for body movement and coordination

Benign – cellular growth that is nonprogressive, and non–life-threatening

Benzodiazepines – drugs of first choice for treating anxiety and insomnia

Beriberi – a deficiency caused by deficiency of thiamine, characterized by neurological symptoms, cardiovascular abnormalities, and edema

Beta-adrenergic blockers – drugs used to reverse sympathetic heart action caused by exercise, stress, or physical exertion

Beta-receptors – an adrenergic receptor; there are two types: $beta_1$ and $beta_2$

Bioavailability – measurement of the rate of absorption and total amount of drug that reaches the systemic circulation

Biotin – a water-soluble B complex vitamin that aids in fatty acid production, and in the oxidation of fatty acids and carbohydrates; also known as vitamin B_7

Biotransformation – the conversion of a drug within the body; also known as metabolism

Bipolar disorder – a type of mental illness characterized by periods of extreme excitation, or mania, and deep depression

Blood coagulation – the process by which blood clots

Bradykinesia – a decrease in spontaneity and movement, as seen in Parkinson's disease

Bradykinin – a polypeptide that mediates inflammation, increases vasodilation, and contracts smooth muscle

Broad-spectrum antibiotics – antibiotics that are used for the treatment of diseases caused by multiple organisms

Bronchiectasis – a destruction and widening of the large airways

Bronchodilators – agents that relax the smooth muscle of the bronchial tubes

Buffered tablet – a type of tablet manufactured to prevent irritation of the stomach

Bulimia nervosa – an eating disorder characterized by recurrent (at least twice a week) episodes of binge eating, during which the patient consumes large amounts of food and feels unable to stop eating

Bulk-forming laxatives – natural or synthetic polysaccharide derivatives that absorb water to soften the stool and increase bulk to stimulate peristalsis

Buspirone – an anxiolytic drug that differs significantly from the benzodiazepines

C

Cachexia – weight loss, wasting of muscle, loss of appetite, and general debility that can occur during a chronic disease

Calciferol – a fat-soluble vitamin chemically related to steroids; calciferol is essential for the normal formation of bones and teeth and important for the absorption of calcium and phosphorus from the GI tract; also known as vitamin D

Calcitonin (CT) – produced primarily by the parafollicular cells of the thyroid gland

Calcium (Ca) – the fifth-most abundant element in the human body, present mainly in the bones

Calcium carbonate – a substance that causes acid rebound, which may delay ulcer-related pain relief and ulcer healing

Calcium channel blockers – drugs used to treat stable angina

Caplet – a tablet shaped like a capsule

Capsule – a solid dosage form in which the drug is enclosed in either a hard or soft shell of soluble material

Carcinogens – any agent directly involved in or related to the promotion of cancer

Cardiac output – the amount of blood the heart pumps to the body in one minute

Carotenoids – any of a class of yellow to red pigments, including the carotenes and xanthophylls

Catecholamines – a group of chemically related compounds having a sympathomimetic action

Cheilosis – fissures on the lips caused by deficiency of riboflavin

Chemical digestion – the alteration of food into different forms through chemicals and enzymes

Chemical mediators – substances released by mast cells and platelets into interstitial fluid and blood; these substances include histamines, leukotrienes, serotonin, and prostaglandins

Chemical name – a drug's full name, that refers to its complete chemical makeup

Chloride (Cl) – involved in the maintenance of fluid and the body's acid-base balance

Cholinergic receptor – receptors that mediate responses to acetylcholine

Chronic obstructive pulmonary disease (COPD) – a group of common chronic respiratory disorders that are characterized by progressive tissue damage and obstruction in the airways of the lungs

Chronic pain – pain that is persistent or long-term; can also mean "low-intensity"

Clinical pharmacology – an area of medicine devoted to the evaluation of drugs used for human benefit

Collagen – a strong fibrous protein found in connective tissue

Compulsion – a ritualized behavior or mental act that a patient is driven to perform in response to his or her obsessions

Congenital megacolon – congenital dilation and hypertrophy of the colon due to reduction in motor neurons of the parasympathetic nervous system, resulting in extreme constipation, and if untreated,

growth retardation; also known as Hirschsprung's disease

Congestive heart failure – a disorder in which the heart cannot pump the blood returning to the right side of the heart or provide adequate circulation to meet the needs of organs and tissues in the body

Congestive heart failure (CHF) – condition in which the heart is not able to pump enough blood to meet the body's metabolic demands

Conn's syndrome – a disease of the adrenal glands involving excess production of the hormone *aldosterone*

Controlled substances – drugs recognized by the Drug Enforcement Agency (DEA) as having abuse potential

Contusion – an injury to body part or tissue without a break in the skin

Convulsions – abnormal motor movements

Copper (Cu) – important for the synthesis of hemoglobin because it is part of a co-enzyme involved in its synthesis; also a component of several important enzymes in the body, and essential to good health

Coronary arterial bypass graft (CABG) – a procedure wherein a vein graft is surgically implanted to bypass the part of the occlusion in the coronary artery

Coronary artery disease (CAD) – a condition in which there is an insufficient supply of oxygen to the myocardium (cardiac muscle); also referred to as "coronary heart disease" and "ischemic heart disease"

Corpus striatum – a layer of nervous tissue within the brain

Cream – a semisolid emulsion of either the oil-in-water or the water-in-oil type, ordinarily intended for topical use

Cretinism – arrested physical and mental development with dystrophy of bones and soft tissues due to congenital lack of thyroid secretion

Croup – a viral infection that affects the larynx and the trachea

Cushing's syndrome – a disease caused by the excessive body production of cortisol; it can also be caused by excessive use of cortisol or other steroid hormones

Cyanocobalamin – a water-soluble substance that is the common pharmaceutic form of vitamin B_{12}; involved in the metabolism of protein, fats, and carbohydrates, and also in normal blood formation and neural function

Cyclooxygenase inhibitors – drugs that prevent the action of one of two enzymes that have an essential role in the inflammation process

Cycloplegia – paralysis of the ciliary muscles of the eye, resulting in loss of visual accommodation

Cystic fibrosis – a genetic disorder affecting the exocrine glands, causing thick mucus to obstruct the bronchioles in the lungs

D

Dementia – a chronic deterioration of intellectual function and other cognitive skills severe enough to interfere with the ability to perform activities of daily living

Depot-medroxyprogesterone acetate (Depo-Provera®) – a long-acting progestin

Depression – a mood disorder

Dermis – a thick layer of loose connective tissue that is well-supplied with blood vessels, lymphatic vessels, nerves, and accessory organs

Diabetes mellitus – a complex disorder of carbohydrate, fat, and protein metabolism caused by lack of or inefficient use of insulin in the body; classified as type I (insulin-dependent diabetes mellitus [IDDM]), or type II (non-insulin-dependent diabetes mellitus [NIDDM])

Diastolic blood pressure – the pressure measured at the moment the ventricles relax

Diffusion – the process of particles in a fluid moving from an area of higher concentration to an area of lower concentration, resulting in an even distribution of the particles in the fluid

Diuretics – a drug that promotes urine formation and elimination. Sodium passing through the kidneys attract water from the circulatory system and increases the volume of urine

Dopamine – a neurotransmitter that is naturally produced in the brain, affecting motor control, memory, attention span, the ability to problem solve, motivation, pleasure, and creative thought

Dopamine receptors – an adrenergic receptor

Dose-effect relationship – the relationship between drug dose and blood, or other biological fluid concentrations

Drug clearance – elimination rate over time divided by the drug's concentration

Drug Enforcement Agency (DEA) – the government agency concerned with controlled substances that enforces laws against drug activities, including illegal drug use, dealing, and manufacturing

Dry powder inhaler (DPI) – a device used to deliver medication in the form of micronized powder into the lungs

Dwarfism – a condition of lack of growth of the arms and legs in proportion to the head and trunk; it may be caused by over 200 different other conditions, including achondroplasia, kidney disease, genetic conditions, and problems with hormones or metabolism

E

Eclampsia – the occurrence of seizures (convulsions) in a pregnant woman, usually occurring after the twentieth week of pregnancy

Elastin – an extracellular connective tissue protein

Electrical threshold – an individual's balance between excitatory and inhibitory forces in the brain; also known as seizure threshold

Electrolytes – compounds, particularly salts, that when dissolved in water or another solvent, dissociate into ions and are able to conduct an electric current

Elixir – a clear, sweetened, flavored, hydroalcoholic liquid medication intended for oral use

Embolism – obstruction or occlusion of a vessel

Emetic – a drug that induces vomiting

Emollient laxatives – substances that act as surfactants by allowing absorption of water into the stool

Emphysema – the destruction of the alveolar walls and septae, which leads to large, permanently inflated alveolar air space

Emulsion – a system containing two liquids that cannot be mixed together in which one is dispersed in the form of very small globules throughout the other

Encephalitis – inflammation of the brain's connective tissue framework

Enteral nutrition (EN) – feeding by tube directly into the patient's digestive tract

Enteric-coated tablet – a tablet covered in a special coating to protect it from stomach acid, allowing the drug to dissolve in the intestines

Epidemic – an outbreak of a disease or infection that spreads widely and rapidly

Epidural anesthesia – injection of an anesthetic into the space immediately outside of the dura mater that contains a supporting cushion of fat and other connective tissues

Epiglottitis – an acute bacterial infection of the epiglottis (an appendage which closes the glottis while food or drink is passing through the pharynx) and the surrounding areas that causes airway obstruction

Epilepsy – condition characterized by periodic or recurrent seizures or convulsions

Epinephrine – a major transmitter released by the adrenal medulla

Epinephrine (adrenaline) – produced by the medulla of adrenal glands, and is a "fight or flight" hormone that is released when danger threatens

Epiphyses – the ends of long bones that are originally separated from the main bone by a layer of cartilage, becoming unified through ossification

Essential hypertension – idiopathic (occurring spontaneously from an unknown cause); also known as primary hypertension

Estrogen – substances capable of producing sexual receptivity in female individuals

Eustachian tubes – tubes within the ear by which fluids drain

Excretion – the process whereby the undigested residue of food and waste products of metabolism are eliminated, material is removed to regulate composition of body fluids and tissues, or substances are expelled to perform functions on an exterior surface

Exfoliative dermatitis – a skin disorder characterized by reddening and scaling of 100% of the skin; erythroderma

Expectorants – agents that promote the removal of mucus secretions from the lung, bronchi, and trachea, usually by coughing

Extrapyramidal – nerves in the brain that control movement

F

Fibrin – gel-like threads

Fibrinogen – a plasma protein

Fibrinolysis – the breakdown of fibrin

Filtration – the movement of water and dissolved substances from the glomerulus to the Bowman's capsule

First-pass effect – drugs reaching the liver where they are partially metabolized before being sent to the body

Floppy infant syndrome – also called "infantile hypotonia," this is a condition of abnormally low muscle tone, often with reduced muscle strength

Fluidextract – a pharmacopoeial liquid preparation of vegetable drugs, made by filtration, containing alcohol as a solvent or as a preservative, or both

Fluorine – a chemical element that is used as a diagnostic aid in various tissue scans

Folic acid – essential for cell growth and the reproduction of red blood cells; also known as vitamin B_9

Follicle-stimulating hormone (FSH) – a gonadotropin that stimulates the growth and maturation of follicles in the ovary in females and promotes spermatogenesis (the process by which male gametes develop into mature spermatozoa) in males

Food additive – any substance that becomes part of a food product

Food and Drug Administration (FDA) – the branch of the U.S. Department of Health and Human Services that is responsible for the regulation of foods, drugs, cosmetics, and medical devices

Fungi – a distinct group of organisms that are neither plant nor animal. Fungi grow in single cells or in colonies

G

Gamma-aminobutyric acid (GABA) – a neurotransmitter distributed throughout the brain and spinal cord; now considered to be the major inhibitory neurotransmitter

in the CNS, acting to modulate the activity of excitatory pathways

Gel – a jelly or the solid or semisolid phase of a colloidal solution

Gelcap – an oil-based medication that is enclosed in a soft gelatin capsule

General anesthesia – provision of a pain-free state for the entire body

Generalized anxiety disorder – difficult-to-control, excessive anxiety that lasts six months or more

Generalized seizure – seizure originating and involving both cerebral hemispheres

Generic name – a drug not protected by a trademark, but regulated by the FDA. Also called the *official name*

Genetic engineering – techniques wherein genes from one organism are spliced into the chromosomes of another organism; also known as recombinant DNA technology

Gestational age – the time measured from the first day of the mother's last menstrual cycle to the current date

Gigantism – condition produces excessive growth (a "giant") if the hypersecretion of GH occurs before puberty

Glomerular filtration rate (GFR) – the rate of filtration in the kidneys

Glucagon – an important hormone in carbohydrate metabolism

Glucocorticoids – a class of corticosteroid so named because it increase blood sugar levels. Glucocorticoids are mainly used for their anti-inflammatory effect

Glutamate – an amino acid that acts as a neurotransmitter and is a key molecule in cellular metabolism, playing an important role in the body's disposal of excess or waste nitrogen

Gonadotropes – cells in the anterior pituitary gland that produce the gonadotropins known as luteinizing hormone and follicle-stimulating hormone

Gonadotropin-releasing hormone (GnRH) – stimulates the release of FSH and LH from the anterior pituitary gland

Gout – a disease caused by a congenital disorder of uric acid metabolism; metabolic arthritis

Graafian follicles – matured and grown ovarian follicles; these egg-containing tubes grown and develop between puberty, sexual maturation, and menopause

Gram stains – sequential procedures involving crystal violet and iodine solutions followed by alcohol that allow rapid identification of organisms as Gram-positive or Gram-negative types

Gram-negative – microorganisms that stain red or pink with Gram stain

Gram-positive – microorganisms that stain blue or purple with Gram stain

Grand mal – generalized seizure characterized by full-body tonic and clonic motor convulsions

Granule – a very small pill, usually gelatin- or sugar-coated, containing a drug to be given in a small dose

Graves' disease – an autoimmune disorder that involves overactivity of the thyroid gland (hyperthyroidism)

Growth hormone (GH) – secreted by the anterior pituitary gland in response to growth hormone-releasing hormone (GHRH)

Gynecomastia – enlargement of breast tissue in males

H

Half-life – the time it takes for the plasma concentration (e.g., of a drug) to be reduced by 50 percent

Hallucinations – false or distorted sensory experiences that appear to be real perceptions

Helicobacter pylori – a bacterial species that is associated with several gastroduodenal diseases

Hematoma – blood that has seeped from a blood vessel and collects in tissue, organs, or space

Hemodynamic – related to blood circulation or blood flow

Hemolysis – the destruction or dissolution of red blood cells, with release of hemoglobin

Hemostasis – a process that stops bleeding in a blood vessel

Heparin – a potent anticoagulant naturally obtained from the liver and lungs of domestic animals; in humans, it is usually found in basophils or mast cells

Hepatic portal circulation – the circulation of blood through the liver

Heterogeneous – consisting of a diverse range of different items

Hirsuitism – excessive hair growth on the face, abdomen, breasts, and back

Histamine – a chemical substance naturally found in all body tissues that protects the body from factors in the environment that produce allergic and inflammatory reactions

Histamine H$_2$-receptor antagonists – drugs that block the action of histamine on parietal cells in the stomach, decreasing acid production

Hormone – a chemical messenger that serves as a signal to target cells; are produced by nearly every organ system and type of tissue

Human immunodeficiency virus (HIV) – a retrovirus that infects helper T cells of the immune system, leading to AIDS

Hydroxocobalamin – is involved in the metabolism of protein, fats, and carbohydrates, aids in hemoglobin synthesis, is essential for normal functioning of all cells, and is important in energy metabolism; also known as vitamin B_{12}

Hyperactive – abnormally and easily excitable or exuberant

Hyperalimentation (total parenteral nutrition) – Also known as "TPN," this treatment is used to supply complete nutrition to patients when the enteral route cannot be used; all needed nutrients are injected into the body intravenously

Hypercalcemia – an excessive amount of calcium in the blood

Hyperemesis gravidarum – pernicious vomiting during pregnancy

Hyperkalemia – high blood level of potassium

Hyperlipidemia – an increase in triglycerides and cholesterol

Hypermetabolic – burning energy and nutrients at a higher rate than normal

Hyperpituitarism – a condition that results in the excess secretion of hormones that are secreted from the pituitary gland

Hypertension – an abnormal increase in arterial blood pressure

Hyperthyroidism – a condition of excessive amounts of thyroxine

Hypervitaminosis – an abnormal condition resulting from excessive intake of toxic amounts of one or more vitamins, especially over a long period

Hypnotics – drugs given to promote sleep

Hypoactive – abnormally inactive

Hypogonadism – a condition of little or no production of sex hormones, usually due to poor function or inactivity of either the testes or the ovaries

Hypokalemia – low blood level of potassium

Hypomagnesemia – an abnormally low level of magnesium in the blood

Hyponatremia – low blood level of sodium

Hypoprothrombinemic – the amount of prothrombin factor II in the circulating blood

Hypothalamus – the part of the brain that lies below the thalamus; it regulates body temperature, certain metabolic processes, and other autonomic activities

Hypothyroidism – a deficiency disease that causes cretinism (mental and physical retardation) in children

Hypotonic – having a lesser osmotic pressure than a reference solution

Hypovitaminosis – a condition related to the deficiency of one or more vitamins

I

Idiosyncratic reaction – experience of a unique, strange, or unpredicted reaction to a drug

Impotence – inability to achieve or maintain penile erection

Infection – the invasion of pathogenic microorganisms that produce tissue damage within the body

Infiltration anesthesia – anesthesia produced by injecting a local anesthetic drug into tissues

Insomnia – the inability to fall asleep or stay asleep

Insulin – a hormone secreted by the pancreas that regulates carbohydrate and fat metabolism, especially the conversion of glucose to glycogen

Insulin-dependent diabetes mellitus – a disorder caused by complete lack of insulin secretion by the pancreas

Intracranial – within the cranium (skull)

Intrinsic factor – a substance that is secreted by the gastric mucus membrane and is essential for the absorption of vitamin B_{12} in the intestines

Investigational new drug (IND) application – an application for human drug testing that is submitted to the FDA once enough data has been collected on a new drug

Iodine – an essential micronutrient of the thyroid hormone (thyroxine)

Iritis – inflammation of the iris

Iron (Fe) – A common metallic element essential for the formation of hemoglobin and myoglobin, as well as the transfer of oxygen to the body tissues

Iron deficiency anemia – anemia characterized by low serum iron, increased serum iron-binding capacity, decreased serum ferritin, and decreased marrow iron stores

K

Keratomalacia – a condition, usually in children with vitamin A deficiency, characterized by softening, ulceration, and perforation of the cornea

Kernicterus – yellow staining and degenerative lesions in basal ganglia associated with high levels of unconjugated bilirubin in infants; also known as bilirubin encephalopathy

L

Laceration – cut or break in the skin

Legend drug – a prescription drug

Leukotriene modifiers – a relatively new class of drugs designed to prevent asthma and allergic reactions

before they occur by either inhibiting leukotriene production, or preventing leukotrienes from binding to cellular receptors

Leukotrienes – substances that contribute to the inflammation associated with asthma

Liniment – a liquid preparation for external use, usually applied by friction to the skin

Lipid solubility – the ability to dissolve in a fatty medium

Lipophilic – able to dissolve much more easily in lipids than in water

Lipoprotein – a class of blood chemicals whose molecules are comprised of a lipid portion and a protein portion

Local anesthesia – provision of a pain-free state in a specific area of the body

Localized infection – involve a specific area of the body such as the skin or internal organs

Lozenge – a small, disk-shaped tablet composed of solidifying paste containing an astringent, an antiseptic, or an oil-based drug used for local treatment of the mouth or throat and is held in the mouth until dissolved; also known as a troche

Lubricant laxative – a substance, such as mineral oil, that works by increasing water retention in the stool to soften it

Lugol's solution – Lugol's iodine; a solution of iodine often used as an antiseptic, disinfectant, or starch indicator, to replenish iodine deficiency, to protect the thyroid from radioactive materials, and for emergency disinfection of drinking water

Luteinizing hormone (LH) – secreted by the anterior lobe of the pituitary gland that is necessary for proper reproductive function

M

Magnesium – an important ion for the function of many enzyme systems, and is the second most abundant action of the intracellular fluids in the body

Malaria – a severe generalized infection caused by the bite of an *anopheles* mosquito that is infected with a *Plasmodium* protozoon

Malignant – cellular growth that is severe and becomes progressively worse, often becoming life-threatening

Malignant hypertension – an uncontrollable, severe, and rapidly progressive form of hypertension with many complications

Malignant hyperthermia – a rare, genetic hypermetabolic condition that is characterized by severe overproduction of body heat with rigidity of skeletal muscles

Mania – a severe medical condition characterized by extremely elevated mood, energy, and unusual thought patterns; a characteristic of bipolar disorder

Mast cell stabilizers – substances that work to prevent allergy cells (called mast cells) from breaking open and releasing chemicals that help cause inflammation; they work slowly over time

Mast cells – large cells found in connective tissue that contain many biochemicals, including histamine; mast cells are involved in inflammation secondary to injuries and infections, and are sometimes implicated in allergic reactions

Mechanical digestion – the breakdown of large food particles into smaller pieces by physical means

Melatonin – an important hormone secreted from the pineal gland that is believed to induce sleep

Menadione – a water-soluble injectable form of the product of vitamin K_3

Metabolism – the conversion of a drug within the body; also known as biotransformation

Metastasize – to spread from one part of the body to another

Metered dose inhaler (MDI) – a hand-held pressurized device used to deliver medications for inhalations

Mineralocorticoids – steroid hormones that influence salt and water balance; they are released from the adrenal cortex

Minerals – inorganic substances occurring naturally in the earth's crust having characteristic chemical compositions

Miosis – contraction of the pupil of the eye

Mitotic inhibitors – drugs that block cell growth by stopping cell division

Mixture – a mutual incorporation of two or more substances, without chemical union, in which the physical characteristics of each of the components are retained

Monoamine oxidase inhibitor (MAOI) – a class of drugs effective for the treatment of depression

Mucolytic – destroying or dissolving the active agents that make up mucus

Mycoplasms – ultramicroscopic organisms that lack rigid cell walls and are considered to be the smallest free-living organisms

Mycoses – fungal diseases

Mydriasis – dilation of the pupil

Myocardial infarction (MI) – an area of dead cardiac muscle tissue, with or without hemorrhage

Myxedema – condition of thyroid insufficiency or resistance to thyroid hormone

N

Narcotics – drugs that produce a sedative or pain relieving affect

Narrow-spectrum antibiotics – antibiotics that are effective against only a few organisms

Necrosis – death of a group of cells or tissues

Negative feedback system – method by which regulation of hormones is achieved; released in response to concentration in the blood

Neonatal period – the time from birth to approximately 28 days of age

Neoplasm – a tumor; tissue that is composed of cells that grow in an abnormal way

Neuroleptic drugs – the major therapeutic modality for psychotic disorders; also known as antipsychotic drugs

Neurotransmitter – a biochemical that is formed in and released from a neuron in order to stimulate or inhibit the actions of another cell

Niacin – contains parts of two enzymes that regulate energy metabolism and is essential for a healthy skin, tongue, and digestive system; also known as vitamin B_3 or nicotinic acid

Nicotinic acid – contains parts of two enzymes that regulate energy metabolism and is essential for a healthy skin, tongue, and digestive system; also known as niacin or vitamin B_3

Nitrates – drugs used for the treatment of angina

Nitrosoureas – alkylating agents; they act by the process of alkylation to inhibit DNA repair

Nocturnal enuresis – nighttime bedwetting

Nonsteroidal anti-inflammatory drugs (NSAIDs) – drugs that have analgesic and antipyretic effects

Norepinephrine (noradrenaline) – released from the medulla of the adrenal glands, and is also a central nervous system and sympathetic nervous system neurotransmitter

Nystagmus – rhythmical oscillation of the eyeballs

O

Obsession – a recurrent, persistent thought, impulse, or mental image that is unwanted and distressing, and comes involuntarily to mind despite attempts to ignore or suppress it

Obsessive-compulsive disorder – anxiety characterized by recurrent, repetitive behaviors that interfere with normal activities or relationships

Ointment – a semisolid preparation usually containing medicinal substances and is intended for external application

Opioid – a natural or synthetic narcotic substance

Opioid agonists – drugs that can combine with receptors to initiate drug actions

Opioid antagonists – drugs that oppose or resist the action of others

Organogenesis – from implantation to about 60 days after, the time when major fetal organs form

Osteoarthritis (OA) – arthritis characterized by erosion of articular cartilage that mainly affects weight-bearing joints in older adults

Osteomalacia – a disease in which the bone softens and becomes brittle

Otitis media – an inflammation of the middle ear

Over-the-counter (OTC) – nonprescription drugs

Oxytocin (OT) – also acts as a neurotransmitter in the brain; in women, it is released during labor and lactation

P

Pain – an unpleasant sensation associated with actual or potential tissue damage

Palliation – treatment to relieve or reduce intensity of uncomfortable symptoms, but not to produce a cure

Panic attacks – of sudden onset, reaching peak intensity within ten minutes; symptoms may include trembling, shortness of breath, heart palpitations, chest pain (or chest tightness), sweating, nausea, dizziness (or slight vertigo), light-headedness, hyperventilation, paresthesias (tingling sensations), and sensations of choking or smothering

Panic disorder – anxiety characterized by intense feelings of immediate apprehension, fearfulness, and terror

Pantothenic acid – a member of the vitamin B complex widely distributed in plant and animal tissues and that may be an important element in human nutrition; also known as vitamin B_5

Parasympathomimetic – producing effects similar to those produced when a parasympathetic nerve is stimulated

Parathyroid hormone (PTH) – also called parathormone, is secreted by the parathyroid glands and increases the levels of calcium in the blood

Parkinson's disease – a neurological syndrome usually resulting from deficiency of dopamine because of degenerative, vascular, or inflammatory changes in the basal ganglia

Partial seizure – seizure originating in one area of the brain that may spread to other areas

Passive transport – the most common and important mode of traversal of drugs through membranes; diffusion

Patent ductus arteriosus – a condition in which the normal channel between the pulmonary artery and the aorta fails to close at birth

Pediatric period – the period from birth to approximately age 18

Pellagra – a disease caused by a deficiency of niacin and protein in the diet, characterized by skin eruptions, digestive and nervous system disturbances, and eventual mental deterioration

Peptic ulcer – a lesion located in either the stomach (gastric ulcer) or in the duodenum (small intestine)

Percutaneous transluminal coronary angioplasty (PTCA) – reduces obstruction by means of invasive procedures requiring cardiac catheterization; the catheter contains an inflatable balloon that flattens the obstruction

Periosteum – a thick, fibrous membrane covering the entire surface of a bone except its articular cartilage and where it attaches to tendons and ligaments

Pharma food – A system of receiving nourishment by breathing in nutritional microparticles

Pharmacodynamic interactions – differences in effects produced by a given plasma level of a drug

Pharmacodynamics – the study of the biochemical and physiological effects of drugs

Pharmacokinetic interactions – differences in the plasma levels of a drug achieved with a given dose of that drug

Pharmacokinetics – the study of the absorption, distribution, metabolism, and excretion of drugs

Pharmacology – the science concerned with drugs and their sources, appearance, chemistry, actions, and uses

Pheochromocytoma – a usually benign tumor of the adrenal medulla or the sympathetic nervous system in which the affected cells secrete increased amounts of epinephrine or norepinephrine

Phlebothrombosis – clotting in a vein without primary inflammation

Phosphorus – is essential for the metabolism of protein, calcium, and glucose, aids in building strong bones and teeth, and helps in the regulation of the body's acid-base balance

Pill – a small, globular mass of soluble material containing a medicinal substance to be swallowed

Placebo – an inert substance given to a patient instead of an active medicine

Plaster – a solid preparation that can be spread when heated and then becomes adhesive at the temperature of the body

Pneumonia – an inflammation or infection of the pulmonary parenchyma; caused by viruses, bacteria, mycoplasmas, and aspiration of foreign substances

Pneumonitis – inflammation of the lungs

Polypharmacy – the practice of prescribing multiple medicines to a single patient simultaneously

Porphyria – a group of enzyme disorders that cause skin problems (such as purple discolorations) and/or neurological complications

Post-traumatic stress disorder – anxiety characterized by a sense of helplessness and the re-experiencing of a traumatic event

Potassium – the major electrolyte in intracellular fluids, helping to regulate neuromuscular excitability and muscle contraction

Powder – a dry mass of minute separate particles of any substance

Preanesthetic medications – drugs given before the administration of anesthesia

Preeclampsia – the development of elevated blood pressure and protein in the urine after the twentieth week of pregnancy; it may also cause swelling of the face and hands

Primary hypertension – idiopathic (occurring spontaneously from an unknown cause); also known as essential hypertension

Pro-drug – inactive or partially active drug that is metabolically changed in the body to an active drug

Progesterone – secreted primarily by the ovarian cells in the corpus luteum at the time of ovulation during the female reproductive years

Prolactin (PRL) – a hormone that is primarily associated with lactation; it is secreted from the anterior pituitary gland

Prothrombin – a glycoprotein formed and stored in the parenchymal cells of the liver and present in the blood; a deficiency of prothrombin leads to impaired blood coagulation

Protozoa – single-celled parasitic organisms, many of which are motile (able to move spontaneously)

Pyridoxine – a water-soluble vitamin that is part of the B complex and acts as a co-enzyme essential for the synthesis and breakdown of amino acids; also known as vitamin B_6

R

Radiation therapy – cancer treatment method whereby drugs are used to treat cancer either before or after surgery

Reabsorption – the movement of water and selected substances from the tubules to the peritubular capillaries

Recombinant DNA technology – techniques wherein genes from one organism are spliced into the chromosomes of another organism; also known as genetic engineering

Red man syndrome – a rash on the upper body caused by vancomycin

Replication – the process of reproduction or copying of genetic material

Respiratory distress syndrome (RDS) – the result of the absence, deficiency, or alteration of the components of pulmonary surfactant

Respiratory syncytial virus (RSV) – the major cause of bronchiolitis and pneumonia in infants under one year of age; caused by a virus and exhibits mild cold-like symptoms

Retinol – a fat-soluble vitamin essential for skeletal growth, maintenance of normal mucosal epithelium, reproduction, and visual acuity; also known as vitamin A

Reye syndrome – an acquired encephalopathy of young children that follows an acute febrile illness; strongly associated with aspirin use

Rhabdomyolysis – a potentially fatal destruction of skeletal muscle, characterized by the presence of myoglobin in the urine; it is also associated with acute renal failure in heatstroke

Rheumatoid arthritis (RA) – a chronic and progressive condition that affects more women than men, focusing mainly on the joints of the hands and feet, and leading to deformity and disability

Riboflavin – one of the heat-stable components of the B complex, it is involved as a co-enzyme in the oxidative processes of carbohydrates, fats, and proteins; also known as vitamin B_2

Rickets – a deficiency disease resulting from a lack of vitamin D or calcium and from insufficient exposure to sunlight, characterized by defective bone growth and occurring mostly in children

Rickettsia – intercellular parasites that need to be in living cells to reproduce

S

Salicylates – salts or esters of salicylic acid

Saline laxatives – substances that create an osmotic effect to increase water content and stool volume

Schizophrenia – a mental illness characterized by distortion of reality, disorganized thought patterns, social withdrawal, hallucinations, and poor judgment

Sclerotic – hardening, toughening

Secondary hypertension – results from renal (e.g., nephrosclerosis) or endocrine (e.g., hyperaldosteronism) disease, or pheochromocytoma, a benign tumor of the adrenal medulla; in this type of hypertension, the underlying problem must be resolved

Sedative-hypnotics – drugs that when given in lower doses, produce a calming effect, and when given in higher doses, produce sleep

Seizure – abnormal discharge of brain neurons that causes alteration of behavior and/or motor activity

Selective serotonin reuptake inhibitor (SSRI) – a class of drugs used as antidepressants; they block resorption of serotonin in nerve cells in the brain

Septae – walls of the bronchioles

Septicemia – bacteremia associated with active disease, whether localized or systemic

Serotonin – a neurotransmitter that regulates appetite, sleep, arousal, mood, temperature, and hormone release

Serotonin syndrome – a rare condition resulting from intentional self-poisoning with serotonin, use of the drug therapeutically, or from inadvertent drug interactions characterized by progressively worsening symptoms such as: mental confusion, shivering or muscle twitching, sweating or fever, hallucinations, hypertension, tachycardia, headache, tremor, nausea, diarrhea, coma, and death; also known as serotonin toxicity

Sickle cell anemia – an inherited disorder characterized by the presence of abnormal hemoglobin; hemoglobin contains hemoglobin S (HbS)

Silent angina – a condition that occurs in the absence of angina pain

Social anxiety disorder – characterized by an intense, irrational fear of situations in which one might be scrutinized by others, or might do something that is embarrassing or humiliating; also known as social phobia

Social phobia – characterized by an intense, irrational fear of situations in which one might be scrutinized by others, or might do something that is embarrassing or humiliating; also known as social anxiety disorder

Sodium – one of the most important elements in the body; sodium ions are involved in acid-base balance, water balance, transmission of nerve impulses, and contraction of muscles

Solution – a liquid dosage form in which active ingredients are dissolved in a liquid vehicle

Somnolence – prolonged drowsiness that may last hours to days

Spasticity – a type of increase in muscle tone at rest, characterized by increase resistance of the muscles to stretching

Spermatogenesis – the process by which male gametes develop into mature spermatozoa

Spinal anesthesia – a type of regional anesthesia produced by injecting a local anesthetic drug into the subarachnoid space of the spinal cord

Spirits – alcoholic or hydroalcoholic solutions of volatile substances

Spores – bacteria in a resistant stage that can withstand an unfavorable environment

Sprain – injury to supporting ligaments of a joint

Statins – a class of drugs that inhibits the activity of an enzyme that forms cholesterol in the body; so named because all of their generic names end with "-statin" (e.g., lovastatin)

Status epilepticus – an emergency situation characterized by continual seizure activity with no interruptions (another term for seizure)

Steatorrhea – elimination of large amounts of fat in the stool

Steroids – numerous naturally occurring or synthetic fat-soluble organic compounds that include sterols, bile acids, adrenal hormones, sex hormones, digitalis compounds, and certain vitamin precursors

Stimulant laxatives – substances that stimulate bowel mobility and increase secretion of fluids in the bowel

Stool softeners – substances that decrease the consistency of stool by reducing surface tension

Strain – injury resulting from overstretching a muscle, results in tear of muscle or muscle and tendon

Stroke volume – the volume of blood pumped with each heartbeat

Substantia nigra – pigmented cells in the midbrain responsible for the production of dopamine

Sulfur – necessary to all body tissues and is found in all body cells

Superficial mycoses – involving a surface or a shallow depth of tissue

Suppository – a small, solid body shaped for ready introduction into one of the orifices of the body other than the oral cavity (e.g., rectum, urethra, or vagina), made of a substance, usually medicated, that is solid at ordinary temperature but melts at body temperature

Suspension – a liquid dosage form that contains solid drug particles floating in a liquid medium

Sustained release (SR) capsule – a capsule with a controlled release of the dosage over a special period of time

Sympatholytic – inhibiting or opposing adrenergic nerve function; sympatholytic agents are also known as adrenergic blocker agents

Sympatholytic drugs – a group of drugs that blocks or inhibits the effects of epinephrine or norepinephrine on the cells that normally react to them

Sympathomimetic – adrenergic, or producing an effect similar to that obtained by stimulation of the sympathetic nervous system

Synapse – a specialized junction at which a nerve cell communicates with a target cell

Syrup – a liquid preparation in a concentrated aqueous solution of a sugar used for medicinal purposes or to add flavor to a substance

Systemic infection – impacts the whole body rather than a specific area of the body

Systemic mycoses – relating to or affecting an entire body or an entire organism

Systolic blood pressure – the pressure measured at the moment the heart contracts

T

Tablet – a solid dosage form containing medicinal substances with or without suitable diluents

Target sites – the areas where a drug's greatest action takes place at the cellular level

Teratogenic – causing developmental malformations

Testosterone – stimulates the development of the male secondary sex characteristics, initiates the production of sperm, and enhances the functional capacity of the penis and accessory sex organs

Thiamine – a water-soluble, crystalline compound of the B complex, essential for normal metabolism and health of the cardiovascular and nervous systems; also known as vitamin B_1

Thrombin – enzyme occurring in blood during the clotting process

Thrombocytopenia – decrease in the number of platelets in circulating blood

Thrombogenic – substances causing blood clots

Thrombolytics – drugs designed to dissolve blood clots that have already formed within a blood vessel

Thrombophlebitis – venous inflammation with thrombus formation

Thromboplastin – substance to cause clotting

Thrombosis – the formation of a clot

Thrombus – a clot in the cardiovascular system formed during life from constituents of blood

Thyroid-stimulating hormone (TSH) – a substance secreted by the anterior lobe of the pituitary gland that controls the release of thyroid hormone and is necessary for the growth and function of the thyroid gland

Thyroxine (T4) – the major hormone secreted by the follicular cells of the thyroid gland

Tincture – an alcoholic solution prepared from vegetable materials or from chemical substances, used as a skin disinfectant

Tocopherol – a fat-soluble vitamin essential for normal reproduction, muscle development, resistance of erythrocytes to hemolysis, and various other biochemical functions; also known as vitamin E

Tolerance – reduced responsiveness of a drug because of adaptation to it

Tonic-clonic seizure – an alternate contraction (tonic phase) and relaxation (clonic phase) of muscles, a loss of consciousness, and abnormal behavior

Trade name – brand name given to a drug by its manufacturer (such drugs are marked with the symbol®). Trade names are also called *proprietary* or *brand* names

Tremor – repetitive, often regular, oscillatory movements caused by alternate, or synchronous, but irregular contraction of opposing muscle groups

Tricyclic antidepressant (TCA) – a class of antidepressants; they inhibit reabsorption of serotonin, norepinephrine, and dopamine in the brain

Troche – a small, disk-shaped tablet composed of solidifying paste containing an astringent, antiseptic, or oil-based drug used for local treatment of the mouth or throat and is held in the mouth until dissolved; also known as a lozenge

Tubular secretion – the active secretion of substances such as potassium from the peritubular capillaries into the tubules

U

Uveitis – inflammation of the uvea (the vascular middle layer of the eye, including the iris, ciliary body, and choroid)

V

Vasodilators – drugs used to relax or dilate vessels throughout the body

Vasospastic angina – decubitus angina; characterized by periodic attacks of cardiac pain that occur when a person is lying down

Venous stasis – injury to the veins causing loss of proper function of the vein and impairing the ability of blood flow to return to the heart

Viruses – intracellular parasites that take over the metabolic machinery of host cells and use it for their own survival and replication

Vitamin A – a fat-soluble vitamin essential for skeletal growth, maintenance of normal mucosal epithelium, reproduction, and visual acuity; also known as retinol

Vitamin B complex – a pharmaceutical term applied to drug products containing a mixture of the B vitamins, usually B_1 (thiamine), B_2 (riboflavin), B_3 (nicotinamide), and B_6 (pyridoxine)

Vitamin B_1 – a water-soluble, crystalline compound of the B complex, essential for normal metabolism and health of the cardiovascular and nervous systems; also known as thiamine

Vitamin B_{12} – is involved in the metabolism of protein, fats, and carbohydrates, aids in hemoglobin synthesis, is essential for normal functioning of all cells, and is important in energy metabolism; also known as cyanocobalamin

Vitamin B_2 – one of the heat-stable components of the B complex, it is involved as a co-enzyme in the oxidative processes of carbohydrates, fats, and proteins; also known as riboflavin

Vitamin B_3 – contains parts of two enzymes that regulate energy metabolism and is essential for a healthy skin, tongue, and digestive system; also known as niacin or nicotinic acid

Vitamin B_5 – a member of the vitamin B complex widely distributed in plant and animal tissues and that may be an important element in human nutrition; also known as pantothenic acid

Vitamin B_6 – a water-soluble vitamin that is part of the B complex and acts as a co-enzyme essential for the synthesis and breakdown of amino acids; also known as pyridoxine

Vitamin B_7 – a water-soluble B complex vitamin that aids in fatty acid production, and in the oxidation of fatty acids and carbohydrates; also known as biotin

Vitamin B_9 – essential for cell growth and the reproduction of red blood cells; also known as folic acid

Vitamin C – a water-soluble vitamin that is essential for the formation of collagen and fibroid tissue for teeth, bones, cartilage, connective tissue, and skin; also known as ascorbic acid

Vitamin D – a fat-soluble vitamin chemically related to steroids that is essential for the normal formation of bones and teeth and important for the absorption of calcium and phosphorus from the GI tract; also known as calciferol

Vitamin E – a fat-soluble vitamin essential for normal reproduction, muscle development, resistance of erythrocytes to hemolysis, and various other biochemical functions; also known as tocopherol

Vitamin K – essential for the synthesis of prothrombin in the liver

Vitamins – organic compounds essential in small quantities for physiologic and metabolic functioning of the body

Volatile liquids – liquids that evaporate upon exposure to the air

X

Xanthine derivatives – a substance that is effective for relief of bronchospasm in asthma, chronic bronchitis, and emphysema

Xerophthalmia – extreme dryness of the conjunctiva resulting from an eye disease or from a systemic deficiency of vitamin A

Z

Zinc (Zn) – A trace element that is essential for several body enzymes, growth, glucose tolerance, wound healing, and taste acuity

Zollinger-Ellison syndrome – peptic ulceration with gastric hypersecretion and tumor of the pancreatic islets

Index